The Bottom Line or
Public Health

The Bottom Line or Public Health

*Tactics Corporations Use to Influence
Health and Health Policy,
and
What We Can Do to Counter Them*

EDITED BY
WILLIAM H. WIIST

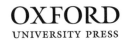

OXFORD
UNIVERSITY PRESS

2010

OXFORD
UNIVERSITY PRESS

Oxford University Press, Inc., publishes works that further
Oxford University's objective of excellence
in research, scholarship, and education.

Oxford New York
Auckland Cape Town Dar es Salaam Hong Kong Karachi
Kuala Lumpur Madrid Melbourne Mexico City Nairobi
New Delhi Shanghai Taipei Toronto

With offices in
Argentina Austria Brazil Chile Czech Republic France Greece
Guatemala Hungary Italy Japan Poland Portugal Singapore
South Korea Switzerland Thailand Turkey Ukraine Vietnam

Library of Congress Cataloging-in-Publication Data
CIP data on file
ISBN 978-0-19-537563-3

9 8 7 6 5 4 3 2 1
Printed in the United States of America
on acid-free paper

Alvin, Judy, Cynthia M. G.

Aiden and Addy.

May you live in a beautiful and sustainable world filled with peace, health, and happiness; free from tyranny and with democracy for all.

Preface

There are two things the reader needs to know about this book before proceeding further:

1. The book takes a point of view, a viewpoint that is critical of the institution known as the corporation, its practices, and the economic philosophy and legal rulings upon which the corporation is founded and by which it operates. The focus of the book is on the fundamental characteristics of the corporation, not the operations of specific corporations or industries that have an influence on health. That information is merely illustrative of the corporate institution. The book is not intended to provide a balanced perspective about corporations, including the benefits society may derive from corporations. The ideology and beliefs that underpin the corporation are already ubiquitous and promulgated by most news media (e.g., Wall Street Journal, CNBC), publishers, policy institutes, the educational system, particularly business schools, legislatures, and the courts. While harmful practices or products of a single company or an entire industry are sometimes criticized, the above institutions rarely critique the fundamental nature of the corporation or its operating principles. The conventional wisdom is that the corporation as it is currently structured and operates is necessary and always beneficial. Therefore, it is unnecessary for this book to present that viewpoint.

2. This book is intended for both academic and advocacy audiences. The chapters were written by both academics familiar with research about corporations and by staff of organizations who are working directly on issues related to the corporation.

Readers may think that my perspective as a university professor working for government is entirely theoretical without the benefit of firsthand experience that would give me a more favorable viewpoint about corporations. To the contrary, my personal experience with a publically traded, for-profit corporation and a private, for-profit corporation contributed to my academic interest in further studying the corporation as an institution.

For many years prior to completing my formal education, I worked at the minimum wage on an assembly line in a factory. This was the same factory at which my father worked for 30 years and that did not have a retirement plan, and where he was likely exposed to the substance that ended his life two years after retirement.

More recently, during my professional career, I was employed by a small privately held corporation that operated in an informal manner with considerable employee involvement in corporate decision making. Employees were well acquainted with each other and most were on a first name basis with the owner, the board, and other officials. When the corporation was purchased by a larger, publically traded corporation, the goals, operations, and management style quickly changed. One morning, not long after the new management took over, I dropped off my company laptop with the technicians for repairs. As usual, the technicians were pleasant and in a cheerful mood. They promised to have the laptop ready in 2 hours. When I returned at the designated time to retrieve the laptop, the technicians were not in their office. As I looked for my laptop, a stranger walked in and asked if he could help me. He informed me that the two technicians no longer worked there and that he was now in charge. Although many employees still worked closely with top corporate officials, those officials used the sudden, unexpected termination procedure many times over the coming years to terminate numerous employees working at all levels.

Because of my personal experience working on a factory assembly line and for the corporation described above, I understand, in a way that many academics do not, firsthand how the corporation operates.

Due to space limitations, the chapters in this book are not the "last word" on a topic nor do they provide a comprehensive review of the subject matter. The chapters serve as an introduction to the topics and as a stimulus for further scholarship and advocacy by others who might be willing to work on in this new frontier for public health, "the corporation." In making the arguments they make, the chapter authors courageously take positions contrary to conventional wisdom.

Often those who are experts in a field have vested interests in the status quo, particularly if they have ties to corporations from a consultancy, grants, and so forth that make their financial conflicts of interest so extensive that they are unwilling, or intellectually unable, to make the arguments that the authors in this book have made. Or, it may never have occurred to them to even consider examining the corporation in such a fundamental way as the chapter authors of this book have. The other individuals have simply accepted the conventional wisdom. The authors of chapters in this book are critical thinkers who do not accept the conventional wisdom. By definition they are radicals: they examine the root causes of the problem. Because of the nature of this book, the chapter authors have all provided a statement that they have no corporate conflicts of interests.

Chapter authors use both scholarly and journalistic sources: journals, books, popular press books, news media, magazines, Web sites and personal experience. Sources from outside traditional academic sources are also used, in part because, compared to a few scholars and advocacy organizations, relatively few academics critically examine the fundamental nature of the corporation as an institution, its source of power and influence, or the tactics the corporation uses. Few academics conduct research on the relationships between corporate or market variables and public health measures or publish such material in scholarly journals.

The thesis of the book is that because of the way the corporation, as an institution, was structured historically, mainly through court rulings, all corporations either use the same tactics to influence health policy or they have the same tactics available for their use. When I presented this thesis for the first time at the 2007 Annual Meeting of the American Public Health Association in Washington, D.C., I also laid out counter tactics that public health professionals and advocates can use. Based on this schema, the book is divided into three sections.

The first section of the book serves as an introduction to the topic. In Chapter 1, "The Corporation: An Overview of What It Is, Its Tactics and What Public Health Can Do" I provide an overview of the history of the corporation and the lessons that history holds for public health professionals, the prevailing economic model underlying the corporation, an enumeration of the six tactics the corporation uses, and provide examples of their use, and describe the key counter tactics public health professionals and advocates can use. In Chapter 2, "Corporations, Public Health and the Historical Landscape that Defines Our

Challenge" Shelley White provides a more thorough account of the historical events that created the corporation as we know it today. Public health professionals being focused on providing programs and services often do not appreciate the influence of distant historical events on their work. However, in order to understand how to rectify the influence of the corporation on health, an understanding of how the corporation came to have the rights is essential.

The chapters in the second section of the book "Corporate Tactics" highlight tactics that corporations have available to them and illustrate the use of those tactics by corporations operating in several major industrial sectors. This section begins with Chapter 3 "Limited Liability and the Public's Health," a reprinted journal article, in which Lainie Rutkow and Stephen Teret describe a key operational feature of the corporation that allows corporate stakeholders to avoid responsibility for the harmful effects on health or the environment that result from corporate operations, products or services, and present several tactics public health can use to address this characteristic of the corporation. In Chapter 4 "Public Relations and Advertising," Diane Farsetta describes some of the overt and covert public relations (PR) and advertising tactics corporations use to influence health and health policy. Corporations and their hired PR firms excel at subterfuge. They are so skilled at PR that most of the public never realizes that much of what they see in the electronic media or read in print about corporations, their products, about the economy, or about legislation, the government or regulations was created to deceptively appear as news and objective fact. Chapter 5, "Lobbying, the Revolving Door, and Campaign Contributions" taken from the Web site of the Center for Responsive Politics, presents information from the organization's databases about the current extent of lobbying, campaign financial contributions, and the revolving door. The increasing use of these tactics has given the corporation greater power than any other institutional influence and is primarily responsible for government's abdication of its responsibility to first protect and promote the common good of its human citizens.

The following chapters give industry case studies of corporate tactics to illustrate how specific industries utilize those tactics to corrupt science, foist harmful or unhealthful products on the public, manipulate government, deceive the public, force operational costs onto tax payers, and damage the environment, and to do these on a global scale.

In Chapter 6 "The Tobacco Industry," Ruth Malone describes the industry that opened up the eyes of public health professionals to how the corporation operates. Because of the access to tobacco corporation documents obtained through litigation, we have had an insider's viewpoint of the corporation. In Chapter 7 "The Pharmaceutical Industry, Disease Industry: A Prescription for

Illness and Death" David Egilman and Emily Ardolino introduce readers to the "poster child" for the corporation's magnitude of use of tactics, probably greater than any other health-related industry. In Chapter 8 "Motor Vehicle Industry," Leon Robertson recounts many events that he personally observed during his longtime work on motor vehicle safety, events that show the close ties between industry and government. In Chapter 9 "Alcohol Industry Interests, Global Trade Agreements and Their Impact on Public Health" Don Zeigler describes how the alcohol industry has taken advantage of the lack of health protections in international trade agreements to extend the promotion of their products around the world. In Chapter 10 "Food and Agriculture Industry," Judith Pojda describes the threats to health that have resulted from one of the greatest changes in the U.S. society: consolidated industrialization of our food sources, distribution and sales, a change that has become global.

Perhaps after the descriptions in the previous sections of the huge, powerful, and dominating force that the corporation is, accomplishing change may seem overwhelming or impossible. However, the authors of chapters in the last section "Tactics to Counter the Corporation" give us numerous, effective tactics we can use. And, they provide us with hope for the possibility of creating a different world, of an alternative way of conducting business that protects health, the environment, and democracy. In Chapter 11, "Using Charters to Redesign Corporations in the Public Interest" Charlie Cray focuses on some of the specific ways society might redesign the corporation so that health, the environment, and citizenship would have priority over profit. In Chapter 12, "A New Democracy in Action" Mari Margil presents a new form of democratic action that local communities can use to stop the corporation from overwhelming the rights of human citizens to protect their environment. Stephen Gardner and Katherine A. Campbell present cases in Chapter 13, "Legal Strategies: You Are What They Say You Are Eating" many from their personal experience litigating against corporations that illustrate how laws can be used to cause the corporation to stop unhealthful practices. In chapter 14, "Anti-corporate Social Movements: A Global Phenomenon" Tom Mertes shows how a worldwide movement has arisen in opposition to the corporation and the model by which it operates. The identification of some of the organizations involved in this movement gives concerned public health professionals and advocates comfort that they are not alone as they take up tactics to counter the corporation. They can join the networks, coalitions and organizations and contribute their skills as they learn about this new area.

In some parts of the world, the labor movement and workers have taken the lead in organizing to focus on redressing the influence of the corporation and in developing new ways of using the power of workers. In Chapter 15 "Labor

Movement Strategies to Address Corporate Globalization" Jane Lethbridge describes some of the activities of the international labor movement.

Nicholas Freudenberg, in Chapter 16 "Campaigns to Change Health-Damaging Corporate Practices," reviews some of the campaigns that public health advocates have organized against specific corporations and industries, and describes the strengths and weakness of this approach to addressing the influence of corporations on health.

In Chapter 17 "Public Health Infrastructure: Toward a Blueprint for Change," René Jahiel proposes how Schools of Public Health could restructure their curricula and research to better address the influence corporations have on health, and other changes that could make public health institutions able to better monitor and regulate industry.

In Chapter 18, a reprinted book chapter, "Indigenous Peoples' Movements," Raymundo D. Rovillos provides a survey of some of the activities indigenous people's organizations are engaged in to assert their rights that are threatened by corporations and the neoliberal economic model. In Chapter 19, a reprinted journal article, "The New Politics of Consumption: Promoting Sustainability in the American Market Place," Maurie Cohen and colleagues survey several consumer movement activities. In the final Chapter, 20, "Spiritual Activism and Liberation Spirituality: Pathways To Collective Liberation," a reprinted web article, Claudia Horwitz and Jesse Maceo Vega-Frey present a thought-provoking and inspirational message of the spiritual connections to the work of those engaged in the struggle to make the world a better place for us all.

Acknowledgments

My first and strongest expression of appreciation is to the authors of the original chapters in this book. None of them undertook the challenge of contributing to the book because of anticipated monetary reward or acclaim. I believe that they invested their time, knowledge, and writing skills because they believe that the corporation has a significant effect on the health of the public and democracy, and because they want public health professionals to become more engaged in working toward mitigating and preventing the effect that corporations have on health and democracy. Some of the authors wrote their chapter without the benefit of financial support from their employer. Those authors who submitted their chapter by the scheduled deadlines have my special thanks.

I appreciate the organizations, authors, and journal and book editors who were so generous in allowing me to include articles and chapters from their work in the book, and without fee. My thanks for those permissions go to Ted Hutchinson, Editor of the Journal of Law, Medicine and Ethics; Vicky Tauli-Corpuz coeditor of the book, "Reclaiming Balance," Maurie Cohen , Massie Ritch of the Center for Responsive Politics, and Claudia Horwitz, and Jesse Maceo Vega-Frey. I appreciate Universal Press Syndicate approving the inclusion of the Calvin and Hobbes cartoon, which so succinctly conveys much of the message of this book. My thanks to John Nace for his inspiring book "Gangs of America," and for his permission to freely use material from his book.

I was gratified by the favorable and supportive comments I received from many people around the world when I shared the ideas planned for this book. Many mentioned how much such a book was needed and that they looked forward to its publication, including using it in university courses. I especially appreciated the encouragement of John Stauber, author, founder, and until recently, Executive Director, of the Center for Media and Democracy and its SourceWatch, PR Watch, and Weekly Spin publications. My thanks to Russel Mokhiber for publishing his interview with me about the book in the Corporate Crime Reporter.

Many in the movement to reform the corporation, and the complicit governments, believe that reform requires global solidarity. While I found that spirit in most of the contacts I made while planning this book, I was disappointed that a few prominent individuals from U.S. organizations and universities who are well known for their work in corporate reform were nonresponsive. The new world that the corporate reform movement seeks requires that we all support one another in our efforts. I hope this book will contribute to solidarity in the United States and globally.

In 1995 or 1996, I was listening to the radio in my car and heard an interview on Pacifica Radio that former California Governor Jerry Brown was conducting with David Korten about David's then new book, "When Corporations Rule the World." I thank David for the initial inspiration that interview and his book gave me for my work, and for the vision of a positive future in his continuing work. The favorable reception from audiences to my articles, presentations, and courses about the influence of corporations on health and health policy has reinforced my belief in the importance of this topic to the field of public health, and it encouraged me to move forward on this book.

One of the first times I formally presented information about the influence of corporations and international monetary policy on health to students was in a doctoral student seminar at Walden University in July 2003. That experience showed me how much the conventional wisdom about corporations dominated the thinking of health students and reaffirmed my commitment to the importance of sharing an alternative viewpoint, albeit challenging.

I am grateful for the protection of academic freedom provided to me as a tenured professor at Northern Arizona University (NAU) that enables me to study, write, and speak about the corporation's influences on health.

My thanks to the Director of the School of Public Health at the University of Chile, Giorgio Solimano, and the Coordinator of International Affairs, Leonel Valdivia, for the opportunity in August 2008 to discuss corporate influences on health with the School's faculty. In January 2009, they, with the financial support of the Pan American Health Organization, enabled me to teach a course at the school that focused on corporate influences on health, and to which the receptivity of the Chilean students was gratifying. My thanks to Leslie Schulz, Executive Dean of the NAU College of Health and Human Services, and to Vice Provost for Global Education, Harvey Charles, for providing financial assistance for my travel to Chile in August 2008.

My thanks to René Jahiel, Director of École Libre des Hautes Études (ELDHE) for the opportunity in February 2007 to present my concept of corporate tactics and my proposals for public health curriculum and research to ELDHE's Industrial and Corporate Diseases Study Group.

The many favorable comments I receive in response to my August 2006 article about the corporation in the *American Journal of Public Health* and the numerous individuals who continue to cite the article have been gratifying. I was further inspired by the positive response I received to my presentation about corporate tactics at the November 2007 session of the Trade and Health Forum at the Annual Meeting of the American Public Health Association, particularly the strong vocal support from many audience members such as Randi Cameon. My work with the Trade & Health Forum leadership group, particularly the founder, Ellen Shaffer, has informed this book.

I owe special thanks to the editors at Oxford University Press. I am grateful to William Lamsback, former Executive Editor who accepted my proposal for this book, to Regan Hofmann, Editor, who was quick and informative in responding to my questions and in providing guidance through the editing and production process, to Rachel Mayer, the book's Production Editor at Oxford, and Aloysius Raj, Project Manager at Newgen Imaging Systems (P) Ltd., for their attention to the many details during production and copyediting. My special thanks to Mark Fowler for his gracious, collaborative review of the book, and to the numerous colleagues who reviewed the book.

Finally, my thanks to my wife, Cynthia M. G., who encouraged me from the first moment that I proposed the idea for this book and who supported my efforts through the challenges of writing, editing, and publication.

Contents

PART I

Introduction

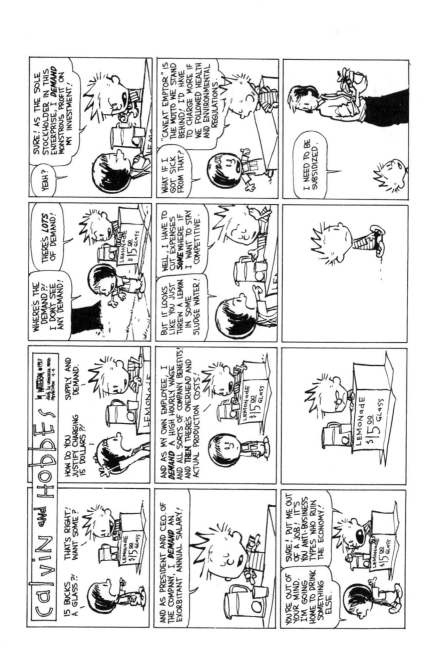

I

The Corporation: An Overview of What It Is, Its Tactics, and What Public Health Can Do

William H. Wiist

This chapter provides an overview of the concepts about how large, for-profit, publically traded corporations operate, particularly within the United States. It also serves as an introduction to the details provided in the chapters that follow. For those who are unfamiliar with this field of study and advocacy the chapter may also stand alone as an introduction to a new perspective about corporations.

The purpose of this chapter is to show that public health research and advocacy related to the influence of corporations on health should be focused on transforming the institution known as the corporation rather than focusing on a specific corporation, industry, product, service, or operation despite how egregious those may be. The chapter presents the view point of the book and is not intended to present balanced, opposing viewpoints. Opposing viewpoints, the conventional wisdom about corporations, are ubiquitous and available from many other sources. The chapter relies on sources of information from history, research reports, policy analysis, news reports, and opinion to present an advocacy viewpoint.

Introduction

A hallmark of the late 20th century was the facilitation of the globalization of commerce. The foundational force of that emphasis was, as it has been historically, the for-profit, transnational or multinational corporations. The terms multinational corporation (MNC) and transnational corporation (TNC) represent developmental stages and are somewhat overlapping. According to the United Nations' (UN's) MNCs own or control production or services outside the country in which they are based (Coleman, 2003). The term MNC may be used if the corporation is headquartered in one country but operating in several others and promoting loyalties among its shareholders, clients, and employees to itself rather than its country of origin. A TNC denationalizes by moving totally, including its capital, personnel, research, and development and is no longer tied to its nation of origin but is ready to settle wherever serves its own interests (Miyoshi, 1993).

For-profit corporations have extended their product design, production, marketing, and distribution operations around the globe. Developments in communications technology and transportation enable many industries of varied types, from manufacturers to financial institutions, to more easily conduct business globally. In addition, consolidation within industries such as communications media, energy, automobiles and agriculture have enabled the fewer remaining corporations to grow in size and revenue, while diversifying their holdings, thus increasing their influence and power. When corporations are large they have a disproportionate influence on policy.

For example, the global media market is dominated by seven corporations (Bennett, 2004) and chains own 80% of the newspapers in the United States (Cooper, 2007). The broadcast media frames public perception on issues and helps set the political agenda. Media consolidation undercuts culturally diverse programming and decreases the diversity of viewpoints, local programming and public interest programs, and results in politically biased reporting and programming (Cooper, 2007). Mainstream news media are biased in favor of center-right politics and they promulgate neoliberal policies and market strategies that support their business interests over their news function and overparticipatory democracy, including a tabloid focus on dysfunction in government (Bennet, 2004). And many business marketers obtain favorable news stories in exchange for buying advertisements (MS&L Worldwide, 2008). The mainstream media controlled by large corporations is a proponent of the conventional commercial viewpoint.

Another example of consolidation is agriculture. Agriculture has changed from family farming to consolidated industrial agriculture that is controlled from seed to supermarket by a few giant corporations earning increasingly huge profits. In 2005, 10 commercial seed corporations controlled 50% of the commercial seed market while five grain corporations controlled 75% of the world seed market in 2000. In 2002 the food sales of one grocery retailer was four times that of its nearest competitor, larger than the combined sales of the next four leading retailers. During one 7-year period of the 1990s the profits of one agriculture corporation grew from $110 million to $301 million (Barker, 2007).

It can reasonably be argued that corporations have become the most pervasive, the most dominant, and the most powerful organizational influence in the world. The top 200 corporations (the largest proportion being U.S. corporations) dominate sales, workforce, economic size, and influence (Anderson & Cavanagh, 2000). By 2000, the top 100 companies controlled 33% of the world's assets, but employed only 1% of the world's workforce (Lasn & Liacas, 2000). Almost every aspect of our lives is organized by, influenced by, or controlled by corporations. People earn their livelihood from corporations; we continuously use products and services of corporations; our access to health care and medicines are tied to corporations; we obtain our information from and communicate through corporate products and services; our political system and government is influenced by corporations; and we move about the world using corporate products and services. Corporations draw heavily from and affect the natural environment.

Concomitant with the growing influence and power of the corporation the public has grown less supportive of corporations and more skeptical of their contribution to society. A recent poll showed that 68% of people in the United States want corporations to have less influence versus 52% in 2001 (Meacham & Thomas, 2009). In 2007, only 38% of those surveyed said that they believe that corporations balance profits with public interest versus 43% in 1987 (Newsweek, 2009a). In 2000, between 72% and 82% said they believe that business has too much power over too many aspects of American life and 74–82% said that big corporations have too much influence over public policy, politicians, and policy makers in Washington (Anderson & Cavanagh, 2000).

Many products and services provided by corporations are useful (e.g., computers and word processing software) and may be without harm to health or the natural environment. So, what is "so bad" about the corporation? There are two concerns. First, in the absence of strong public spheres and the imperatives of a strong democracy, the corporation, lacking self-restraint, does not respect those human values that are not commoditized but that are central to a democratic civic culture (Giourx, 2002).

Second, the primary purpose of the corporation is to increase share-holder value. It has no other obligation to individuals, societies, or the planet. Competition in the marketplace drives corporations toward increasing prof-its which are often achieved through reduction in costs through cutting jobs, wages, or benefits or polluting the environment. Competition can lead to extremes in human behavior that can result in unethical, greedy, and risky managerial decisions to keep the corporation in business and competitive. Those managerial decisions are made within uncertain and conflicting pres-sures and within the corporate culture (Punch, 2000). Low standards can be-come the business norm. Decisions that may harm society or the environment are often made at a distance from the effected community and thus do not affect those who make the decision. Consumers of the corporation's products are often removed from the production site and are unaware of the produc-tion effects of their consumption. The corporation also concentrates wealth within a small proportion of individuals thus giving them inequitable amount of power over other citizens and a greater degree of independence from gov-ernmental oversight and control.

The increased power and influence of corporations and their surrogate organizations has raised increasing concern among some public health pro-fessionals about the effects of corporations' policies and practices on health, health policy, society, and democracy (Fort et al., 2004; Hart, 2004; Shaffer et al., 2005; Lee et al., 2009).

The Focus of Public Health

Most of the public health advocacy work related to health-damaging corpora-tions has been through campaigns against specific companies, industries, or products (Freudenberg et al., 2007) albeit with some emphasis on analysis of the corporation, policy, and the role of government and scientists (Freudenberg & Galea, 2007, ;Freudenberg & Galea, 2008; Huff, 2007; Spitzer, 2005). While focusing on the operations, products and policies of one single corporation or an industry, as a case study in how the corporation operates, can be instruc-tive (Jacques et al., 2003), targeting an egregious corporation or industry does not address the corporation as a foundational, societal institution that affects health.

Arguments have been made for the use of the ecological model in public health (Krieger, 2001), the examination of social determinants of health in public health and globalization (Raphael, 2006) and the applicability of the term colonialism in public health (Lang, 2001). Consistent with those concepts, a new perspective introduced to the public health field (Wiist, 2006), based on the work of corporate reformers such as Korten (1995) and the International Forum on Globalization (2002), is that the corporation is a distal, macro-level social structure that influences the health of the public, and that reform efforts need to be directed at the corporation as an institution rather than at individual corporations, industries, or products.

To address the corporation as a distal structural influence on health, public health professionals first need to better understand what a corporation is, its purpose, and the historical developments that gave corporations the rights they have and the significance of those rights.

The Purpose of the Corporation

The term "the corporation" is a generalized, broad term similar to "the government," "the church," "the schools," or "sports." Though run by human beings the corporation itself is inanimate and without human attributes. The corporation is a legal fiction; a piece of paper bearing official signatures and a government stamp. The corporation is a legal device that exists for the sole purpose of providing the greatest possible financial return to the owners or investors (usually small groups of owner-executives or institutional shareholders) by making a profit. Corporations are legally bound to that single purpose and it is the sole reason for the corporation's existence. If the sale of a product or services is insufficient to serve that purpose cost-cutting measures are introduced such as reduction of workforce, avoidance of taxation, and externalization of the costs of production.

Externalization of costs is a major corporate activity with a direct effect on human health and the natural environment. Externalization of costs refers a corporation's action to avoid bearing some cost of production or service by transferring those costs to society. In that way the cost does not detract from the company's bottom line (profit). While there are many examples of the externalization of costs, an easy example to visualize is a pipe extending from the back of a factory and carrying some liquid by-product of production into an adjacent river. The cost of the resulting pollution in the river is borne by those who swim or bathe in the river, use the water for irrigation or culinary purposes … society. Costs for cleaning up the pollution are borne by society through government rather than the corporation. Another example of externalization is when a corporation reduces or eliminates health insurance coverage for employees or increases employee's share of the premium. This results in the employee's medical care costs being externalized to the individual employee or to government when the employee seeks public services. Contemporary market demands, as well as technological developments and the regulatory climate has resulted in ever increasing pressures on corporations to demonstrate continued and increasingly larger profits and stock share price (Reich, 2007) and a reliance on cost-cutting measures such as externalization.

The corporation and the way it operates did not arise naturally or spontaneously and it is not an immutable entity. It was created and modified by humans. Corporations are a device to which legislatures and courts have given many rights, in some ways greater than those granted to human persons. Despite the human rights granted to the corporation it does not have human characteristics or attributes. A corporation cannot be "bad" or "good," "responsible" or "irresponsible" or "greedy," "evil" or "corrupt." A corporation cannot be demonized or vilified because it does not have a soul or a conscience. The corporation is better understood as a robot; a machine that does what it was designed and programmed to do.

Corporations that maximize profits are operating as we, society, have enabled them to operate. They are doing exactly what we require them to do, despite any harmful effects of their products or operations on humans or the environment. This is not to say that we should permit products or operations that are harmful but when we do so we are attacking symptoms, not the cause of the problem.

> "What corporations do well, what corporations are designed to be, is the problem."
>
> Richard Grossman

The real cause of the problem is the rights that we have given the corporation through court rulings and legislation (Table 1.1). The form we have given the corporation determines its function. It is important to understand why

TABLE 1.1. Some Rights of Corporations.

- Rights of personhood
- Right to sue and be sued
- Unlimited lifespan
- Shareholders subordinate to management
- Diversify and integrated; right to own stock
- Limited liability for shareholders
- Commercial and political speech
- Right to initiate and sign contracts

and how corporations came to hold those rights (Mayer, 1990), particularly the right of personhood and what that means (Gerencser, 2005), for society to effectively redress the corporation's influence on policy.

The History of the Corporation

In the United States we can trace the role and influence of corporations to the early European colonization of North American, and which may be the historical source of the bent of the United States toward corporate imperialistic hegemony (Korten, 2006). From their founding, the relatively young governments of the United States, Canada, New Zealand, and Australia were colonial settler states that imposed (in complicity with corporations), exploitation and destruction on the lives and lands of indigenous people, a colonialism that continues through TNCs with the facilitation of nation states (Choudry, 2001).

The framers of the Declaration of Independence, the Constitution, and the Bill of Rights were well aware of the tyranny of corporations and they set about to design a government that would not be subject to the overbearing rule of corporations. For the first 100 years after the Declaration of Independence corporations were deeply suspect and their operations and existence was tightly controlled (Lasn & Liacas, 2000). However, this wariness did not override the founding fathers principle interest in establishing a government that prioritized the protection of private property, including slaves, and private contracts of wealthy white men, the minority population of the country (Grossman, 1998; Kellman, 1999).

Before the colonizing of North American by Europeans the corporate entity formed in England had the purpose of pooling capital and spreading the corporate expenses across more than one individual and to provide the crown with income, in return for which the corporation was granted limited liability and monopolies. The East India Company, formed in 1600, became a dominant and more powerful world force than the British government itself in India, China, and North America until it was replaced in 1709 (Nace, 2003). In England during the 1690s numerous corporations were traded but by 1720 they were banned due to corruption and scandal, particularly related to the failure of one major company (Bakan, 2004).

In 1628, King Charles chartered the Massachusetts Bay Company to colonize the New World (Bleifuss, 1998) but by 1607 the London based Virginia Company had already founded the first permanent European settlement in North America, Jamestown, essentially a death camp for mistreated, English adults and children brought to the colony, most bonded and against their will, to supply the resources of North America to England and thereby provide corporate profit (Nace, 2003). Importation of slaves from the African continent followed in 1619.

From the inception of what would become the United States of America, North America was colonized for profitability. It was a source of raw materials, a source of agriculture products; all produced by cheap labor. It was a source of consumers for European products. The continent was an untapped resource for corporate harvesting. The European settlement of North America was an ever Westward expansion to acquire and sell those resources. While it is not the popularized version of history (i.e., that the European settlement of North America was for solely for religious freedom), the corporate quest for profit was integral to the founding of the United States. The quest meant that anyone or anything standing in the way had to be removed, including the indigenous people. Native Americans were removed from their homes, forced from one region to another, and were interned in camps, imprisoned, killed, and exterminated if expedient, on behalf of corporate commodification of the continent.

Similarly, corporations brought Africans to the North American continent as the ultimate cheap labor, slaves, to perform the work of industrial agriculture growing crops such as tobacco and cotton. The corporate purpose required removing Africans from their ancestral home, separating family members, imposing cruel punishments and squalid living conditions, and taking away their freedom. Later when the railroad corporations expanded, Chinese immigrants were similarly exploited for cheap labor for corporate profit. Along with women and children who labored in factories and on farms, non-Europeans and indigenous peoples were commodities, without rights, to keep corporate costs low.

Thus, North America became a corporate colony with all of the usual characteristics of colonialism: a dominant culture exploiting humans and nature; taking without sharing the benefits; forcing its products upon the colony, and imposing its will by violent force. To colonize can be equated with commodification, that is, to put a market buy and sell price on everything, including human life, nature, water, the oceans; anything that was previously considered free (Barber, 2007).

In 1776 Adam Smith, sometimes cited as a key proponent of the free market system, stated his belief that corporations concentrated and abused power, colluded with, captured, and corrupted governments and that those tactics led to oppression, imbalances of power, inefficiencies, destruction of local goods, and prohibited indigenous people's commerce and agriculture. He believed that large international corporations were the principal causes of those injustices and that they were intrinsic to the corporation because of the way the corporation was organized and the manner in which it operated.

He recognized that corporations only represent the public interest when their business interests overlap with broader societal interests (Muthu, 2008).

One can argue that today corporations do not operate much differently from their exploitative predecessors (Koenig-Archibugi, 2004). MNCs set up operations where the labor costs are the lowest, where the regulations to protect the environment are the weakest and where there are abundant mineral, forests, land, or other production resources to use until depleted. The corporation uses the legal rights it has, co-opting governments, including violent military intervention and using covert governmental agency operations, to force any country into allowing it to take that country's resources, acquire the services of its population for cheap labor, to operate with impunity, and to return little of its profits to that country.

Rebellion against the monopolies of the corporations in the American colony gained strength in the 1770s as the more affluent and influential leaders began to resist as well. The Boston tea party was an act of defiance against the efforts of the East India Company to force the distribution of its product on the colony. During the formation of the U.S. constitution great debate occurred over whether chartering of corporations would be at the federal or state level, a battle to avoid granting too much authority to the central government that might lead to creation of East India type of companies. Corporate charters were limited and chartering was left to the states (Nace, 2003).

The corporate charter is the privilege granted by the government to a group of investors to operate a company, originally granted only for the purpose of serving the public good. Early in the history of the United States charters were issued to carry out one specific purpose, such as to build a bridge, and over a limited time period, in a specific state. And, one corporation could not own another. In 1819 a U.S. Supreme Court ruling (*Dartmouth College v Woodward*), by overruling states' rights to revise corporate charters, began the erosion of governmental domination of corporations.

During the time of the Civil War the Union needed the advantage of the railroads to move goods and troops so that during the war and immediately afterward railroad companies became powerful and gained an expansion of the rights of corporations. Through an 1886 U.S. Supreme Court ruling on a railroad tax issue (*Santa Clara v Southern Pacific Railroad*), and several other cases during that period, corporations gained the right of natural personhood under the 14th amendment.

A key event in corporate history was the act of a court reporter, who served on a railroad board, whose unofficial notation of a prehearing comment made by a Justice, was incorporated into future court understandings of the rights of corporations. That particular Justice had been appointed to the court when Roscoe Conkling, a former U.S. senator, declined appointment. Conkling was apparently an unscrupulous and determined railroad employee who fabricated arguments (the "Conkling Deception") to deceptively convince the Supreme Court that the 14th amendment applied to corporations. Stephen Field, a Supreme Court Justice and circuit court judge, with close ties and sympathies with the railroads, argued in habeas corpus cases related to Chinese immigrants and railroad tax cases that the 14th amendment rights applied to corporations. Also, in the mid-1800s, the work of an influential Pennsylvania Railroad representative, Tom Scott, led to corporations gaining the right to own stock in another company. These rulings resulted in the form today's corporations take (Drutman & Cray, 2004; Korten, 1995; Nace, 2003).

> "... corporations have been enthroned ... an era of corruption in
> high places will follow ... until wealth is aggregated in a few hands
> ... and the Republic is destroyed"

> Abraham Lincoln

In 1916, Henry Ford decided to divert dividends from investors to customers by selling vehicles for a lower price. Investors sued and the judge ruled that company profits belong to the investors and that the primary purpose of a business is profit. This ruling established the principle of "best interests of the corporation" which is law in many countries (Bakan, 2004).

> "This is a government of the people, by the people, and for the
> people no longer. It is a government of corporations, by corporations,
> and for corporations."

> President Rutherford B. Hayes, 1876

In 1944, the UN Monetary and Financial Conference was held in July 1-44 Bretton Woods, NH. The meeting of 45 countries was led by the United States and the United Kingdom to plan post-war economic development and governance. The agreements reached there led to the founding of the International Bank for Reconstruction and Development, which became the World Bank (WB), the founding of the International Monetary Fund (IMF), and to the General Agreement on Tariffs and Trade (GATT) which in 1995 became the World Trade Organization (WTO).

The WTO was formed to ensure that international trade flowed smoothly, freely, fairly, and predictably. The WTO consists of 154 members, has a staff of 500 at its Geneva office, and controls more than 97% of world trade. Voting is based on a member country's share of trade. The WTO ensures adherence to rules and has a Dispute Settlement Understanding for dispute resolution (Peet, 2003).

The WTO dispute resolution process is confidential, no third parties can attend, transcripts or proceedings are not made public and only a nonconfidential summary report is released. A dispute resolution arises when a corporation or industry decides that it is at a competitive disadvantage in global trade because of the regulations, such as an environmental law or tariff, of a particular country. On behalf of that industry the government files a complaint with the WTO dispute resolution body. The WTO selects the small hearing panel restricted to WTO staff and their designated specialists. The process is conducted in secret. Civil society cannot be a part of the process and only a summary report of the decision is made public. The panel's decision carries the weight of law and is enforced, including with trade penalties and fines (Peet, 2003). (Note: "civil society" refers here to nonstate actors such as Nongovernmental Organizations (NGOs), citizen groups, Indigenous Peoples, or individuals not affiliated with or representing corporate interests.)

The rulings of the WTO and trade agreements supersede national and state laws and allow corporations to file suit against nations or states on the basis of claims for loss of profits and for potential loss of profits, such as was made in a mining company's threat against El Salvador under the Central American Free Trade Agreement (Mychalejko, 2008).

"The first truth is that the liberty of a democracy is not safe if
the people tolerate the growth of private power to a point where it
becomes stronger than their democratic state itself. That, in essence,
is fascism - ownership of government by an individual, by a group, or
by any other controlling power. Among us today a concentration of
private power without equal in history is growing."

Franklin Delano Roosevelt

In a 1978 case, the *First National Bank of Boston v Bellotti*, the Supreme Court affirmed the right of corporations to contribute cash to influence elections as a right of protected speech.

The economic model, or theory, by which particular governments have operated during different periods of time determine the constraints on the corporation. The underlying form of the capitalistic economic model driving corporate globalization in the past 30–40 years is known as "neoliberalism" in the South, and in the North, "neoconservative," "market fundamentalism, and "Washington Consensus" (the Washington, D.C. political and financial institutions, and *Wall Street*).

The neoliberal model was promulgated around the world by University of Chicago economists, particularly Milton Friedman, and their students. The underlying premises of the model are that tax incentives for the rich leads to entrepreneurship and creates jobs and provides incentives for the poor to work, and that public sector services can be run more efficiently by the private sector. According to the model, wealth creation is the highest priority and that is best accomplished by removing government obstacles (Balaam & Veseth, 2008), for example, through deregulation.

Neoliberalism emphasizes increased production, efficiency, free flow of currency and capital, free trade, open markets, market deregulation, privatization of government enterprises, minimal government intervention, reduction in the size and influence of government, a positive sum outcome for actors, and individual empowerment (Balaam & Veseth, 2008).

The Washington consensus principles emphasize fiscal discipline, re-direction of funding from public spending subsidies, trade liberalization of imports, tax reform (broadening the tax base, with targeted tax reductions for the wealthiest), competitive exchange rates, market determined interest rates, liberalization of direct foreign investment by corporations, privatization of public enterprises, deregulation, and the protection of property rights (Peet, 2003). Proponents of the neoliberal model do not accept that the common good such as education, environmental protections or health care may not be best served by for-profit methods. They resist the perspective that government can and should do things for citizens that individuals cannot do for themselves (e.g., health care).

A key to implementation of the neoliberal or Washington Consensus principles is the stringent and invariability of the application of those principles. The neoliberal model fueled "globalization," the worldwide economic integration and movement of goods, services, and capital accompanied by homogenization of economic, political, and social order (and culture) that has been largely driven by MNCs with the complicity of governments, and from which the economic benefits have not been equitably distributed (Guttal, 2007; Irogbe, 2005). Contemporary globalization is similar to corporate globalization of the 1550s and 1600s.

The neoliberal model was asserted in the policies of former U.S. President Reagan and former British Prime Minister Thatcher both of whom took steps to deregulate and privatize by weakening unions, reducing the size of government, cutting social programs, and selling off publically owned enterprises (Krieger, 1987). Former U.S. President George W. Bush implemented extensive privatization, including that of the Iraq war where most U.S. and Iraqi civilian, security, industry, and many military operations were conducted by private corporations (Klein, 2007).

Deregulation has also been supported by the policies of several Democratic presidents over the past 40 years. Under President Clinton's administration the 1933 Glass–Steagal Act that separated commercial banks from investment banking and which limited high-risk activity was replaced by the 1999 Financial Services Modernization Act, or Gramm–Leach-Bliley Act (Weissman & Donahue, 2009).

The change in banking law in the 1990s was promoted by Clinton administration officials who had formerly been heads of financial corporations that then benefited from the new law. The financial industry had lobbied for deregulation, spending over $5 billion during 1998–2008 on lobbying and campaign contributions for politicians in key positions with oversight of the industry (Weissman & Donahue, 2009). This change in law, along with lax regulation by government agencies, led to the 2008–2009 failure of many financial institutions due to their risky ventures, including mortgage derivatives, that resulted in a worldwide economic crisis. This required billions in government funds to "bail out" those same financial corporations that had pushed for deregulation to conduct those high-risk ventures.

Several former Clinton administration officials and others with direct and close ties to the finance industry have been appointed by President Obama to positions in which they oversee the industry and institutions with which they had been affiliated, institutions that had lobbied against financial industry regulatory reforms that President Obama himself proposed as a Senator (Ridgeway, 2008; Thomas & Hirsh, 2008). The support of both major parties for deregulation and privatization shows the pervasive influence of the neoliberal economic model and its proponents.

The increase in the influence and power of the corporation has flowed from the increasing adoption of the neoliberal model. One analysis comparing national government Gross Domestic Product (GDP) with corporate sales showed that 51 of the 100 world's largest economic entities are now corporations (Anderson & Cavanagh, 2000). In 2008, Chief Executive Officers (CEOs) of the S&P 500 corporations in the United States averaged $10.5 million compensation; 344 times the pay of the average American worker, and which through tax write offs and accounting mechanisms, the Officers compensation was subsidized by U.S. taxpayers (Anderson et al., 2008).

The implementation of the neoliberal model also led to disparities in the distribution of wealth between countries and within countries (Dembele, 2005; Irogbe, 2005) and has been devastating to numerous countries and their citizens (Klein, 2007) including an increase in mortality in postcommunist countries associated with privatization (Stuckler et al., 2009).

Under the neoliberal model the share of the national income obtained by the wealthiest 1% of the U.S. population grew from 14.6% in 2003 to 17.4% in 2005 (Gross, 2008), due in part to changes in the tax laws that favor the wealthy. In 2006 the 400 highest-income individuals reported $105 billion in income but paid approximately a 17% federal income tax rate whereas in 1955 they would have paid more than 50% of their income in taxes (Collins & Pizzigati, 2009).

This emphasis on market solutions to all problems, without government interference (except to benefit corporations), has fostered a new feudalism and colonialism controlled by TNCs. The definition of liberty and freedom has changed, consumption is idolized, everything is a commodity, decisions are made by private interests, and there is greater disparity between economic elites and the remainder of the population (Duvall, 2003). Under this model a corporation must be able to attract capital for its operations, keep its focus on short-term rapid growth, investment, expansion, and profit, with all of these consider above all other society priorities, including social good and the natural environment.

Lessons from History

While the above is an incomplete accounting of the history of the corporation, the importance of the historical events described is that those events created the corporate entity of today and gave the corporation its purpose and the rights to operate as it does.

The right of free speech that was given to the corporate entity via misuse of the 14th amendment enables corporations to advertise products that are harmful to health. The extension of the First Amendment to corporations enables them to make political contributions. The extension of Fifth Amendment rights to corporations enables them to keep inspectors and protesters off of corporation land. The Bellotti court ruling undermined the ability of governments to exert sovereign control over corporations (Drutman & Cray, 2004).

The state chartering process enables a company to move to another location if the health or environmental or other regulations or policies of the chartering state becomes less accommodating to them. By allowing a corporation to own other companies, a corporation that produces harmful products can ally itself with a more wholesome image and operations through ownership of a company that produces a healthful or less harmful product. This consolidation of ownership also makes the corporation so large and powerful that it is difficult for advocates and government regulators to obtain information, gain access to, or influence the corporation. It also increases the corporation's available finances that give them an increased ability to access legislators and elected officials and to promote a public image favorable to its own interests, even when contrary to the evidence.

The court ruling that set forth the principle that the returns of profits to investors is the sole purpose of corporations means that corporate social responsibility (CSR), "green" operations or any other corporate activity proposed as a social benefit or a social good, are all subservient to profit. A company cannot engage in those activities if the activity does not contribute to profit or if it decreases profits.

Another instructive lesson from the history of the corporation is that the courts are not impartial arbiters in cases involving corporations. The personal biases of judges that favor corporations can lead to court rulings that do not protect public health. The seats on the benches of courts are filled by human beings who have their own history and experience, usually a privileged history, and a history frequently entwined with corporate influence. Their experiences with corporations can color their perspective and favorably incline them toward corporations or business in general; they may have had direct experience with a corporation involved in a specific case; they may be personally acquainted with the corporate officers; and if in an elected judicial position, they may have received campaign financing from that corporation. A similar argument can be made about legislators.

Court rulings are often made, and legislation passed, at the behest of corporate interests asserted by specific individuals who cajole, pressure, and deceive in an attempt to gain advantage for the corporation. Today, much of that effort is carried out by public relations (PR) and lobbying firms at the behest of corporations and industries. The lobbyist or PR firm employees or owners are often former government officials who still have contacts in government and who know the procedures and process of government that they can use to accomplish the goals of their corporate clients.

The WTO is of particular relevance to contemporary public health. Trade agreements have successfully challenged or obstructed (as potential barriers to trade) measures that protect health and the environment; assure the safety and affordability of vital human services, including health care, water, education, and energy; limit exposure to harm from tobacco and alcohol; provide access to affordable prescription drugs; safeguard occupational safety and health; and limit unwarranted or unsafe use of infant formula. The WTO, particularly its dispute process, is undemocratic and lacks transparency. And, WTO rulings supersede national sovereignty, thus, in effect, allowing corporations to establish international law.

The neoliberal economic model upon which the corporation operates does not directly include the health of the public as a priority. Improved health can only be a hoped for, possible side-effect, or an assumed benefit of the wealth "trickledown" effect. Public health professionals are mistaken when they believe, and act upon the belief that corporations, counter to their purpose, can be made socially responsible and promote and protect health.

The global economic crisis of 2008 reemphasizes three history lessons that are important for public health professionals. First, the crisis showed again how the corporation has been given the right to take just about any action necessary to achieve increasing, short-term profits regardless of externalized costs to society. Second, government regulation of corporations is necessary to protect the health of the public, including regulation of the distal, macrolevel, social determinants of health such as corporate financial institutions. The third lesson is that public health professionals must work toward fair and equitable governmental policy and regulation to ensure that politicians and government officials of all political parties eliminate the conflict of interest in their ties to corporations.

Perhaps the most important lesson that public health professionals can learn from the history of the corporation is that the corporation was created by human governments, and is grounded in legality, located in a geographic space governed by elected representatives of the citizens. The corporation is subject to laws and therefore to the will of the people, the human citizens of that government. We, as human citizens of a democracy can change, dissolve, or recreate the corporation into whatever form we believe will best serve humanity and the planet.

The rights granted to corporations provide the power and influence that they wield and that enable them to use the tactics they apply to wield that power. One of the arguments proposed in this chapter and in this book is that it is these rights of the corporate entity that public health professionals and health advocates must join with others in reforming, or eliminating, to protect, promote, and ensure the health of the public. President Abraham Lincoln believed that the role of government is to do for people what they cannot as individuals alone do for themselves (Weisberg, 2009). Public health professionals and advocates must help restore governments' role as the regulator of the corporation.

Because all corporations have the same rights under those given to the corporate entity all corporations either use or have the right to use the same tactics to influence policy. Public health professionals and advocates need to be able to identify and to understand how and when the tactics are used so that they can take appropriate measures to counter the corporation.

Tactics of the Corporation

The tactics that corporations use to influence health policy and practices can be categorized into a model with five, somewhat overlapping, categories (Figure 1.1) (Wiist, 2007). The tactics may be used singularly or in combination. The examples of tactics in each category below are incomplete and meant to be illustrative and they may not be the most egregious examples.

Political Tactics

The numerous and varied political tactics available to corporations often overwhelm or undermine the democratic rights of real people (Sklair, 2002). The larger a corporation's revenue and the greater the regulatory pressures the greater will be the corporations' political activity (Hansen et al., 2004).

Lobbying

Corporate lobbying of Congress has grown to become a huge industry with thousands of lobbyist and millions of dollars spent by corporations for lobbyist. The number of registered lobbyist in Washington, D.C. increased from 3,400 to 32,890 between 1975 and 2005 and the amount of money spent on lobbying increased from about $200 million to over $2 billion between 1983 and

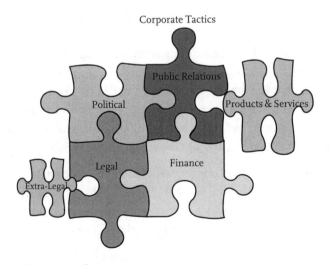

FIGURE 1.1. Categories of corporate tactics.

2005, with most of the increase being in the interest of corporations and not citizen groups (Reich, 2007). In 2008, the pharmaceutical and health product industry spent the largest amount on lobbying of any industry, over $230 million, (Open Secrets, nd). Lobbying continues to grow on specific topics such as climate change, for which the number of lobbyist increased 300% in the past 5 years, with 770 organizations spending $90 million in 2008; industry lobbyist outnumbered others 8 to 1 (Center for Public Integrity, 2009).

> "It is necessary that laws should be passed to prohibit the use of corporate funds directly or indirectly for political purposes; it is still more necessary that such laws should be thoroughly enforced."
>
> Theodore Roosevelt

Corporations lobby to gain an advantage over competitors or to prevent being disadvantaged, to increase government protections, and to increase government subsidies. One industry tried to pressure the U.S. government to stop funding the World Health Organization (WHO) because the corporations did not like the WHO nutrition guidelines related to their product (Boseley, 2003). Farm subsidies are more than $20 billion per year, of which two-thirds of farmers receive none (Barker, 2007).

One corporate CEO, highly praised in the business world for his fiscal management, lobbied Congress to try to avoid requirements that the corporation pay to clean up the polychlorinated biphenyls (PCBs) the corporation had dumped into a river (Multinational Monitor, 2001).

While federal legislation has been passed that places some limitations on campaign contributions and lobbying, there are still a variety of types of corporate campaign contributions to political activity (Baue, 2004). The suggestion is not that there is "buying of votes" or necessarily quid pro quo exchange of dollars for votes, but that because of their financial contributions corporations and their representatives gain access to legislators to present their position, opportunities that the average citizen does not have. Legislators often view corporate representatives as experts on the legislation under discussion and rely on that expertise to form their own position on the issue. Corporations can also be involved in drafting and/or reviewing legislative bills.

> "The real government of our country is economic, dominated by large corporations that charter the state to do their bidding. Fostering a secure environment in which corporations and their investors can flourish is the paramount objective of both [political] parties."
>
> Dan Hamburg, former Member, U.S. Congress

Corporations make political campaign contributions to candidates, particularly incumbents. Corporate Political Action Committee (PAC) contributions have been shown to influence legislators toward positions less favorable to labor (Moore et al., 1995). Corporations might collect campaign donations from their employees or colleagues and bundle them into one large donation. Many corporations also make large (including $1 million) "soft money" contributions to the political parties for their conventions (Corporate Accountability International, nd).

Corporations have made gifts to politicians and provided travel for them as well as invitations to speak at business meetings. Corporations have also provided so-called education sessions, sometimes at luxury resorts, to provide legislators and judges (Kendall & Sorkin, 2000) with the corporate or an industry's viewpoint on a particular topic. Some judges with corporate financial ties have made rulings favorable to the corporation with which they have such ties (Community Rights Counsel, 2007). Appointment of judges was used to promote one U.S. Presidents' project to use the Takings Clause of the Fifth Amendment to decrease regulation of corporations and business (Constitutional Accountability Center, nd).

Corporations have influenced the placement of industry officials on government oversight panels, advisory boards, and committees. Corporations use their contacts in government administration to influence the appointment of industry officials to high-level administrative positions in governmental regulatory agencies, review committees, or committees that have authority over their own industry. This enables them to control or delay the implementation of regulations affecting their industry and unduly influence the content of government reports that is critical of their industry. In fact the first regulatory agency in the United States, the Interstate Commerce Commission, established in 1887, was largely a creation of the large railroad corporations, established to protect the railroads from populist activism and from rate competition (Allison, 2006; Morris, 1998). Industrial agriculture views the US Department of Agriculture as its own agency and through its lobbying and the appointment of industry officials to the agency the industry often wields veto power over nutrition guidelines and policy (Mattera, 2004; Nestle, 2002). The National Highway Traffic Safety Administration knew about the proneness of sport utility vehicles to rollover that caused an increased number of deaths but did not take action and it delayed implementation of shoulder restraint seatbelts and airbags due to Presidential administration antiregulatory approaches and resistance of automobile manufacturers, including concealing data that showed vehicles to be unsafe (Kelley, 1992).

Some critics believe that federal regulatory agencies continue to lack accountability to citizens and are predominantly established and operate to serve corporate interests. Corporate and industry representatives dominate the advisory committees to the US Trade Representatives (Shaffer & Brenner, 2004). Ten members of a Food and Drug Administration (FDA) advisory committee that voted that a drug's benefits outweighed the risks had received consulting or research funds from the corporation that produced the drug (Rubin, 2005).

The cycle of corporate representative's employment in and then back out of government to work in a corporation or lobbying firm is termed "the revolving door" and threatens democracy in a variety of ways (Revolving Door Working Group, 2005). Their increased knowledge of the regulatory or legislative processes and their network of contacts in government enables them to manipulate and influence the governmental processes to favor the corporate interests in ways that are closed to the average citizen. The revolving door includes congressional representatives, senators, or their staff (Salant, 2007) and administration officials (PR Watch, 2009).

It is also in the interest of corporations to work toward limiting the size of government. When corporate officials and employees join the conservative chorus of calls to "reduce big government," "get government off our backs," "cut the government bureaucracy," and "reduce government spending" they, in reality, want a smaller government workforce so that the regulatory agencies will not have enough funds, inspectors, and auditors to monitor their activity and to enforce laws that affect the corporations.

> "Indeed, it is doubtful if free government can long exist in a country where such enormous amounts of money are ... accumulated in the vaults of corporations, to be used at discretion in controlling the property and business of the country against the interest of the public and that of the people, for the personal gain and aggrandizement of a few individuals."
>
> *Richardson v. Buhl*, Nebraska Supreme Court

Finance Tactics

Corporations use a variety of financial tactics to influence policy but perhaps the most direct is to decrease its costs by avoiding taxation. U.S. corporations pay lower taxes, as a percent of GDP (1.9%), than do other Organization for Economic Cooperation Countries (3.2%) (McIntyre, 2007). The U.S. Federal law requires that corporations pay income tax at a rate of 35% of profits but a study of 275 Fortune 500 corporations showed that in 2002 and 2003, the average rate was less than half that. From 2001 to 2003, pretax corporate profits grew by 26% while corporate federal income tax payments decreased by 21%. Between 2001 and 2003, 82 of the corporations paid no federal income taxes during at least 1 year but earned $102 billion in pretax profits (McIntyre & Nguyen, 2004). Out of the 275 corporations, 252 fully disclosed their state and local taxes and had paid 2.3% of their profits in state income taxes. During at least 1 year during the 2001 to 2003 period, 71 of the corporations had paid no state taxes. In 2003, 35 paid no state income taxes, and 46 paid zero or less federal income tax while reporting earnings of $42.6 billion in pretax profits. During that period the 252 corporations avoided $41.7 billion in state corporate income taxes. If those corporations had reported all of their profits to the Internal Revenue Service (IRS) and had been taxed at the 35% tax rate, they would have paid $370 billion in income taxes over the 3 years. Instead they paid a 3-year effective tax rate of 18.4% (McIntyre & Nguyen, 2005). During the U.S. financial crisis of 2008–2009, at least 13 corporations that received billions in federal bail out funds owed $220 million in back federal taxes (Associated Press, 2009).

In the 1950s, corporate taxes paid for a fifth of the U.S. Federal expenditures, 25% in the 1960s, 11% in the 1990s, and 6% in 2002 and 2003 (McIntyer & Nguyen, 2005). That continuing decrease in corporate income tax support to help meet societal needs placed a greater proportion of the burden on individuals. Since corporations pay less tax, individual citizens through their income taxes and through their contributions to churches and community charities must disproportionately bare the burden of supporting the common needs of society such as public health services, public libraries, education, and parks. Lower corporate tax contribution also reduces funds available to government agencies to monitor and regulate industry.

Corporate Influence on Universities

Universities have traditionally held the societal role of objectively discovering and transmitting knowledge, and engaging in discourse to foster democracy, freedom, equality, and a reduction in human suffering. Universities have served as the conscience of society, the guardian of civic freedoms (Giourx, 2002). Because of that role any influence of corporations on universities can be particularly pernicious.

The university has moved in management, culture, campus, and purpose toward a business operations model closely allied with corporations (Steck, 2003) and become privatized (CUPE Research, 2006), including a bureaucratization and corporatization of university administration, and a weakening of faculty governance (Aronowitz, 2000; Washburn, 2005). This has resulted from a variety of economic and cultural influences, many stemming from the direct influence of the corporation and from the manufactured but pervasive societal mythology that "government should operate like a business" (Beckett, 2000).

State legislatures, state boards of education, and university regents who control the curriculum and funding for state universities sometimes bring to those positions the corporate business perspectives and a lack of understanding of the university mission. That perspective sometimes includes the viewpoint that the private sector operates more efficiently and that, in reality, the private sector could do a better job running everything, including educational systems. University administrators also serve on corporate boards and are sometimes hired to bring the corporate perspective to their university positions (Washburn, 2005).

Legislators pass bills that favor tax reductions and reductions in the number and or size of government programs and cut so-called "entitlement" programs to reduce "big" government, including universities. Not accepting the viewpoint that information and education are part of "the commons" to which everyone has a free and equal right of access, they believe that knowledge is proprietary and force the for-profit model on the public sphere.

The corporatized approach to managing universities is viewed by some university faculty as detrimental to the mission of the university (Giroux, 2002). Critics believe that corporatization has moved the curriculum toward job training at the expense of teaching students to be citizens of democracy who should be able to, for example, critique the ethics of corporate leaders and analyze corporate culture and operations. In the corporate view social goals and concerns of education interfere with preparation in job skills. Corporatized management of the university also emphasizes part-time contractual instructors without faculty rights, reduces funding for liberal arts, hiring of business administrators who emphasize cost cutting, including the emphasis of profitable intellectual products over research and education for the public good such as public health (Giroux, 2002).

Corporations, corporate foundations, its officers, or former corporate officers make large financial gifts to support universities, sometimes focusing on business schools, and can thereby influence the philosophy, research agendas, courses offered, and facilities available for education and sports. The shortage of government funding for universities has caused them to allow corporations to purchase product advertising on campus, and naming rights for buildings and programs and concessions (Shaker, 2008).

Spending cuts to federal funding for research grants has led universities to turn to corporations to fund research. Through such grants corporations control the research agenda thus giving researchers less flexibility to pursue research that may not have an immediate commercial benefit. Corporations also support universities by forming joint or affiliated corporations with universities as well as licensing discoveries from faculty research thus providing both the university and faculty member royalty income. A key means to the corporate co-optation of the university was the Bayh–Dole Act of 1980, and subsequent Presidential policy, which enabled the privatization of public knowledge through university licensing to corporations (Washburn, 2005). This led to the increased influence of university patenting and licensing offices.

Two-thirds of medical school departments and their heads receive research equipment or funds from corporations and have personal consulting or board relationships with industry (Mangan, 2007). A survey found that in 2007 10 U.S. universities, hospitals, and research institutes earned more than $50 million in commercial licensing of their patents to corporations and 27 earned more than $10 million. Among 200 institutions surveyed 555 new start-up companies were formed to transfer the institutions' technological discoveries to market (Masterson, 2009).

One university formed a partnership with a petroleum corporation to fund an institute from which the corporation would benefit from university-conducted confidential research and would have rights to license the research results (Blumenstyk, 2007). Another university made a deal to establish a chair in sustainable development that was funded by a corporation that produces pesticides alleged to be harmful to animals and banned in several countries (Ranii, 2008; Vollmer, 2008). Some corporations prohibit university scientists from conducting research on their products, even if the scientists are favorable toward them (Pollack, 2009).

Corporations also use innovations developed with government-funded university research programs to develop products and services for the commercial market place and thereby avoid the costs of conducting that research themselves (Mintzberg, 2006). Reliance upon universities for basic research is another way corporations externalize their costs. Government does not recover those research costs through corporate taxes because corporate taxes have decreased.

Contributions to universities from corporations can lead to conflict of interest where there is a lack of clear demarcation between the independent university and faculty role from the role of entrepreneur and beneficiary (Corporations and Health, 2008; Krimsky, 2003). These financial ties can minimize the traditional faculty and university role as independent, objective observers, and social critics.

Studies have shown that research results are biased in favor of a particular product when the researcher received funding from the corporation that produces the product (Baird, 2003; Corporations and Health, 2008). A software corporation paid for a university study that showed that the antitrust case against it damaged state pension funds and corporation paid for newspaper ads signed by academics (Reich, 2007). Nutrition research funded by the food and drink industry had more favorable conclusions toward the financial interests of the funding industry (Lesser et al., 2007). Researchers are sometimes not aware of their biases and may deny a conflict of interest. It seems unlikely that institutions would have more self-insight into its own conflicts of interest.

"The rise of entrepreneurship in universities has resulted in an unprecedented rise in conflicts of interest, specifically in areas sensitive to public concern."

Sheldon Krimsky

When universities stand to lose so much money from corporations it seems unlikely that they would jeopardize that relationship by criticizing the corporation.

Business Associations and Corporate Foundations

Corporations either set up or participate in business and global trade groups that influence legislation, business strategy and tactics, and global trade policy, or they work together informally to influence policy (Bero, 2003). Examples include the influential Chamber of Commerce, and the WTO, neither of which are accountable to citizens. Thus decisions that have global effects on a wide range of societal concerns including human rights, the natural environment, and health services are transferred from the public sphere to private sector.

Some corporations set up foundations that make grants to not-for-profit health, educational or nongovernmental organizations (NGOs). By doing so the foundation sets the agenda and co-opts the NGO (Roelofs, 2003). Foundations do not usually provide funds for radical causes or those organizations that focus on root causes of problems or those organizations that seek to bring about fundamental structural changes in society (Roelofs, 2007).

Foundations may not use the leverage they have through their large stock holdings in corporations to influence health policy. For example, some of the largest foundations in the world, which hold billions of dollars of stock in corporations, will not use their power, through those stock holdings, to influence policy of those companies whose practices sometimes work in opposition to the foundation's programs (Piller, 2007). Some critics also claim that foundations that focus on public health actually serve the purpose of introducing corporate products into the less-developed countries (e.g., patented vaccines and drugs) as opposed to using less-commercialized approaches to disease prevention. Some accuse foundations of dominating public health policy (McNeil, 2008) and that foundations working in poor and less industrialized countries serve as vanguards for corporate hegemony in a role similar to that played by missionaries in the destruction of culture during the earlier periods of colonization (Korten, 2006).

A trend among corporations is to partner with NGOs and thus enable the NGOs to grow their staffs and program budgets, and to purportedly have greater influence on the policies and practices of corporations than through confrontation tactics (Schulte, 2007). Those NGOs can become more corporate-like in their hierarchy, bureaucracy, and operations, and become dependent on the corporation and less willing to criticize them for fear of losing funding.

> "The primary purposes of social policy are to narrow the inequalities generated in the marketplace and to reduce the impact on personal security and life changes of adverse events such as sickness, disability, and unemployment"
>
> Paul Starn

Corporations, such as tobacco companies, use philanthropic contributions and PR strategically to gain political influence (Tesler & Malone, 2008). The tobacco corporations conducted detailed research about the charitable causes with which elected officials identified and then strategically planned their corporate charitable contributions and publicity campaigns to leverage them to achieve their legislative objectives.

Corporations also make donations to NGOs such as youth sports (Maher et al., 2006), civil rights organizations, and other nonprofits and academic institutions (Jacobson, 2005). This funding can influence the agendas of the organizations and the messages that they convey, particularly those positions contrary to the donor's products or operations. It also creates a dependency that makes it difficult for the NGO to break away for fear of a losing its ability to provide services to its low-income, underserved populations for which there are insufficient government funds or programs to meet needs (due in part to low-corporate taxes).

Subsidies to Corporations

Corporations are also the beneficiaries of extensive governmental subsidies and tax breaks (Barlett & Steele, 1998). For example, U.S farms, mainly industrial agriculture, receive $20 billion per year in governmental subsidies (Barker, 2007) through tariff protection, export subsidies, price supports, production limiting subsidies, and policies that allow commodity dumping onto other countries.

Corporations set up competitions between states and local governments to obtain subsidies such as economic development incentives and tax breaks for locating a factory or other facility in a specific locale, at a large loss of tax revenue to government (LeRoy, 2005). They also receive direct public financing for corporate facilities such as sports stadiums. In return for all of these governmental subsidies and tax benefits corporations return fewer taxes to support to societal needs.

One critical issue that arises from society's reliance on corporate funding is that the priorities are determined by the corporation, or the foundation, by small groups of individuals, foundation officers, and board members, who are privileged members of society, well-educated, and affluent elite who may have little understanding of the problems and conditions faced by the poor and underserved communities. And, foundation officers and board members were not elected by citizens to make the determination about society priorities. They are not required to represent the best interests of society nor are they accountable to society. They can fund narrow interests without public justification and their decisions are made without transparency. In addition, many philanthropic donors obtained their wealth as a benefit of the inequitable distribution of the benefits of neoliberal corporate globalization.

In contrast, hypothetically, governmentally funded programs are determined by a democratic, transparent and accountable process and are prioritized to serve the best interests of society overall. Rescuing victims through philanthropy cannot substitute for democratically determined policies and publically funded program priorities that promote and protect the public's health. The fact that such programs are called "entitlement" programs for "special interest" groups such as the elderly, poor, women, or ethnic minorities shows the extent to which neoliberal perspective has permeated society, including philanthropy.

PR and Advertising Tactics

Public relations has become a huge industry whose aim, at least in part, is to abolish independent journalism and maintain for itself the appearance of independent media so as to have credibility (Miller, 2006). From its inception PR was founded on the principle of manipulation and the intention of controlling the public's thinking (Miller, 2008). PR efforts are a means of influencing opinion or perception to create good will or favorable impression or viewpoint for the company or industry, and which doesn't usually involve payment for promotional material for the corporation's product or service as is the case with advertising. PR purpose is broader than directly promoting sales of the corporate product or services. Its purpose is to shape perceptions about the corporation, its mission, goals, or operations. Some large PR firms, with high-level political connections and government ties, have represented industry on health issues (SourceWatch, nd). There are numerous avenues or methods of PR that corporations use (Babor, 2009; Bohme et al., 2005; Patel et al., 2005).

Spokespersons

Corporations directly or through their hired PR firms often use paid health professionals as expert spokespersons to represent their interests (Saul, 2008). Those experts may be professors, health-care practitioners, researchers, or "think tank" employees. Those spokespersons may represent the corporation or industry in advertisements, trial testimony, testimony before congress, or as content experts to the news media. The paid expert usually only presents information favorable to the corporation and its product and does not discuss negative or side effects of the product although portrayed as an independent, objective analyst. Usually the financial relationship between the corporation and the expert is not disclosed. In both respects the audience does not have the necessary information upon which to evaluate the information conveyed by the expert spokesperson. For example, a prominent mental health scientist, and former federal agency administrator, who moderated a science program on National Public Radio received corporate funding that was not disclosed to listeners (Folkenflik, 2008).

Corporations also sponsor education programs for health professionals, sometimes at resort locations, or as part of the meetings of professional organizations, over dinners, all of which may be promoted as continuing education opportunities. Information about the corporation's products, such as a medication, is presented but usually without presenting studies with contrary results, information about side effects or about alternative equally or more effective drugs. These events often serve as the major source of information about the product that health-care providers use in deciding whether to prescribe the product for their patients (Angell, 2005; Kassirer, 2005).

Funding Health Professions Organizations

Corporations fund professional organizations by making direct monetary donations or grants, by purchasing booth space at conventions, furnishing tote bags, or advertizing in the organization's publications. They also may sponsor continuing education seminars held in conjunction with the professional conference for which they prepare the curriculum, select and hire the speakers, and provide the educational materials, often without disclosing their role in the educational program (Angell, 2005; Kassirer, 2005).

Corporate sponsorships are not limited to physician, nutrition, or dental professional groups but also includes the American Public Health Association (APHA), albeit under APHA's conflict of interest policy. For example, some of the largest pharmaceutical corporations have purchased booth space at APHA annual meetings and had their name on the convention tote bag. Corporations also advertise in journals including the *American Journal of Public Health* and in the APHA annual meeting conference program, including one by a corporation that has been boycotted by public health professionals and advocates for many years (Baby Milk Action, nd).

Corporate sponsorships, advertisements, and the presence of the corporations at professional meetings lends legitimacy and credibility to the corporation. It can result in the professional organization being reluctant to criticize the corporation or its products for fear of jeopardizing revenue from the corporation.

Corporate "News"

Another way that corporations use their PR firms is by having the PR firm produce materials intended to resemble news. Historically, corporations have prepared and submitted written press or news releases to particularly newspapers, television, and radio stations. The media then either directly used those in public service announcements or news stories, with some editing or their reporters used them as research material for pieces they wrote. In more recent times, as electronic media have become more dominant the PR firms produce and distribute video news releases about the corporation (Peabody, 2008), particularly when a negative report about their product is made public. The video news releases are especially useful to local television stations that have limited budgets for investigative reporting who may use the video news releases unedited just as the PR firm produced them. They may be used by networks too with little investigation. One particularly deceptive technique used with video news releases is to record someone who appears to be a reporter standing in a TV studio with lots of TV monitors behind her or him. The "reporter" makes her or his "report" as an actual news reporter might. The "reporter" gives information about the corporation or its product that is favorable to the corporation and doesn't present the opposing facts nor disclose that the story was produced by or own behalf of the corporation under discussion.

The PR tools are sometimes used to divert attention from a public issue to a message favorable to the corporation or to portray the corporation's product or the company as having human characteristics and emotions, or the advertising material is emotionally laden to gain audience sympathy or identification with the corporation. For example, in 2008 at least two oil companies ran television (see web site: Chevron, 2001–2009) and magazine (BP, in 2008–2009 Newsweek) advertizing campaigns with messages about their creativity, the dedication of their employees (e.g., "we tap the greatest source of energy in the world, human energy") and their creativity, the company's concern for the future of the world (e.g., "we live on this planet too"), their investment in alternative fuels and their espousal of conservation. The ads use pleasant visuals and emotionally soothing music. These messages are in stark contrast to the realities that only a small percentage of the BP corporation's business was in alternative fuels (McKibben, 2006), and that the BP corporation was fined by the U.S. Justice Department for oil spills, refinery explosion leaks, and fraud (CorpWatch, 2007). One automobile manufacturer, known for a hybrid vehicle, promoted itself as environmentally responsible while participating with other manufactures in a suit to overturn a state law to reduce greenhouse gas from vehicles (Fugere, 2005).

The Corporate Junk Science Argument

Another PR technique used by corporations is to portray public health scientists whose research has shown the corporation's product to be harmful as "junk science" (Michaels, 2008). The corporation or industry groups may set up and fund "research" organizations or think tanks to produce biased or falsified materials to use in their PR campaigns to oppose public health findings that the corporations believe are contrary to their interests. A recent example includes the corporate-sponsored PR campaigns against the concept that global warming has occurred and that it has resulted from human activity, particularly use of fossil fuels (Mooney, 2005).

Corporate Spinning and Framing

Corporate PR efforts also includes manipulation of the actual content of public Web messages and "spinning" events into messages that reflect more positively on themselves. Corporations changed information about themselves on Wikipedia, making allegations against their detractors and altering and deleting messages to make the messages more favorable to themselves (PR Watch, 2007; SourceWatch, 2007). Corporations sometimes spin health risk messages related to their services into a positive health message (Wingert, 2008).

Corporate PR conceptual framing is pervasive and is used to promote the corporate agenda (Rowell, 1998). This framing creates a biased perspective in the minds of decision-makers and the public and helps set an agenda favorable to corporate interests. The use of phrases and terms such as "Free trade" "Social responsibility" "We don't want big government controlling our lives or meddling in our private affairs" "Business is good for everyone" "The market forces will take care of it," "Tax cuts for the wealthy are good for everyone/ middle class because they create investment," "Personal responsibility" (i.e., workers exposed to hazards should wear protective gear), "Corporate tax incentives will create jobs in the community," "tort reform" are purveyed in most forms of communication media, in stories about the economy, the environment, government programs, or taxes. Such messages have been conveyed generally unchecked and unopposed by the main stream media and in educational settings over many years. This has contributed to shaping public opinion related to specific issues and has helped create an uncritical, pro-business, anti-"big" government perspective among much of the public. A common corporate mantra when threatened with monitoring, regulation, or taxation is "if that bill is passed it will cost jobs" or "we will have to pass the cost on to the consumer." Corporations also perpetuate the concept that there is no option to their model for conducting global trade, or that there is no alternative way of conducting business.

The Oxymoron of CSR

One of the most significant corporate PR campaigns of recent times is the introduction of the concept of CSR and good corporate citizenship. These concepts have been promoted in magazines, scholarly journals, at conferences, by business schools, and by the news media. Referring to the corporation as being socially responsible or a good citizen is an oxymoron. These terms refer to concepts that are mythical and impossible because corporations (a) cannot deliver both short-term financial returns and long-term social benefits, (b) consumers will not drive ethics, (c) the corporate competitive race takes precedence over ethics, and (d) corporations will not compete to have the best ethical practices (Doane, 2005).

One corporate approach that supposedly demonstrates CSR is industry voluntary codes of conduct with standards that purportedly govern their processes, their performance, and their compliance with those standards (Hemphill, 2006; Koenig-Archibugi, 2004; Seidman, 2003). Corporations use the codes to protect their reputations but the codes have little public accountability, they can be difficult to enforce in ways other than through negative publicity, and they divert attention away from enforceable standards and compliance with laws. Monitoring of voluntary codes by third-party NGOs in partnerships with TNCs has been shown to be of limited effectiveness (Wells, 2007).

Corporate Front Groups

Corporations and business alliances set up or fund industry front groups that pose as consumer groups or think tanks and use names that seem innocuous or supportive of public health, free choice, and so on (The Center for Media & Democracy, nd). However, the fronts represent the industry or corporations' perspective, and often do not disclose that affiliation and funding. One study found 40 front organizations or affiliates that received more than $8 million dollars between 2000 and 2003 from one of the largest oil companies to try to undermine scientific findings on global climate change, including using celebrities to convey their message (Mooney, 2005). Readers may also remember the example of the television advertisement funded by industry in which an elderly couple convey opposition to President Clinton's health-care reform proposals, or the similar ads sponsored by industry against the Medicare drug bill.

A particularly blatant example was in a 2006 when two propositions about smoking were before the citizens of Arizona. The numbers of the propositions were one digit apart and one had a name that sounded like it was favorable to health when in actuality it would have liberalized nonsmoking laws. It was supported by tobacco interests. The other proposition restricted smoking and was sponsored by public health organizations. Defeat of the confusing, tobacco-funded proposition required extraordinary efforts to defeat, at high costs to public health advocates.

Advertising

Corporate advertising through sales representatives and direct-to-consumer advertisement influences health and health care. Direct advertisement of drugs to consumers through TV, magazines, and internet has been effective in increasing sales, particularly of a few specific types of medications and with influence on physician prescribing patterns. However, they offer little patient education benefit or public health benefit (Lyles, 2002). In Europe where there are restrictions on direct advertisement of pharmaceuticals to consumers, the corporations use alternatives tactics such as internet chat groups and drug or disease information web sites to market their products (Consumers International, 2006).

In the U.S. pharmaceutical sales representatives who provide samples to physicians for distribution to patients, provide office supplies and patient education materials to physicians and verbally serve as the physician's source of information about medications. Such methods influence the prescription patterns of physicians. The company keeps detailed records about physician's prescribing patterns and targets their marketing accordingly (Kassirer, 2005). The pharmaceutical corporations have expended large amounts of money on direct-to-consumer advertising of prescription medications via TV, web sites, and magazines (with mixed results) (Law et al., 2008).

A major concern with corporate PR and advertising is that they do not convey the risks or side effects of the corporation's products or that there are alternatives that may be as or more effective. They present only the most favorable viewpoint about the corporation or product to the public and are made to appear to be objective reporting.

Product and Service Tactics

Many public health professionals have been involved in campaigns in which they have taken action to confront corporations about their unsafe or unhealthful products, services, policies, or operations. In doing so they may have been faced with corporations that respond and adapt by changing their product or operations to avoid the criticism or regulation, or changed the production process, availability, or price, or apply patent laws to refine their target market segmentation and reposition themselves competitively.

Product Modification

One pharmaceutical corporation took its low cost, widely used HIV medication off the market after it released a new, more expensive medication (Carreyrou, 2007). This left many who were dependent upon the medication without treatment that they could afford.

Corporations also change the product slightly so that they can continue to have patent protection on essentially the same product and thus prevent others from producing the product (Mintzberg, 2006). This is easily accomplished by a pharmaceutical company that can slightly alter molecules of the chemicals in the drug so that they can extend the patent and prevent generic production. There is little innovation or improvement in pharmaceuticals and more money is spent on marketing than on research and development (Love, 2005).

Corporate Physical Location

Corporations may move their operations to geographic areas where costs are lowest based on labor costs and/or environmental regulations. The clothing products of some transnational clothing corporations that have large market shares and high profits are produced in low-income developing countries where workers, mostly women, are hired on short-term, temporary contracts, paid less than a living wage for working long hours in unsafe or unsanitary working conditions, and where worker efforts to organize may be repressed with layoffs, intimidation, and violence (Hearson, 2009; Connor , 2002).

Product Targeting at Vulnerable Populations

Corporations sometimes modify their products to increase revenue by almost imperceptively reducing the product's size (Dickler, 2008). Some corporations modify their products to better target vulnerable consumers. One athletic shoe company designed a running shoe specifically for Native Americans ostensibly to help address Native health issues such as diabetes (Benally, 2007). The alcohol beverage industry markets large container beer in minority neighborhoods (Jones-Webb et al., 2008) and they developed sweet tasting alcoholic beverages that appealed to the youth market (Center for Science in the Public Interest, 2002).

The food industry directly targeted children with unhealthful food products through advertizing (Nestle & Jacobson, 2000) and beverage and snack sales through contracts with schools for vending machine placement (Nestle, 2000). Some hospitals encourage new mothers to breast feed but then distribute infant formula and advertizing materials, provided by the corporation that makes the formula, to mothers when they leave the hospital after delivery (Shelton, 2008).

Tobacco corporations produce different types of products to market to youth, women, and African Americans (National Cancer Institute, 2008; Primack et al., 2007). Tobacco corporations located in developed countries use trade agreements to challenge tobacco control laws of low-income, developing countries as barriers to trade and thus make tobacco more accessible and increase its use in those countries (Shaffer et al., 2005). The food industry tailors packaging, appearance and ingredients, menus, tie-ins to children's show characters, and advertizing to better reach the children's market, and partners with African-American and Latino organizations to better target their products and messages to those populations (Institute of Medicine, 2006).

Corporations are able to target the design and marketing of their products because they conduct research to develop psychological profiles of consumers, and compile data bases that are shared, or sold, to most effectively target their product to consumers (CNBC, 2008).

Manipulation of Scientific Research and Information

As shown from the Tobacco Settlement documents (Bero, 2003) corporations will manipulate the research process about the effects of their products; control research studies; determine who the investigators are, who authors the manuscripts and conceal and falsify research (Egilman & Bohme, 2005); use paid medical writers to write articles for professional journals and then attach academic researchers names as authors (Tanner, 2008), all to prevent information about the harmful effects of their products from being known, or to promote incorrect information.

The FDA financed a study of antidepressants for pregnant women, published by authors, most of whom were paid consultants for the corporations that manufactured antidepressants (Reich, 2007). A manuscript reviewer for a prestigious U.S. medical journal who had received consulting and speaking fees from a pharmaceutical corporation sent, without authorization and contrary to customary ethics, a copy of a manuscript critical of one of the corporation's products to the corporation itself (Raloff, 2008).

Corporations fail to acknowledge the harmfulness of their products or operations. One automobile manufacturer did a cost-benefit analysis of the cost of human "burn deaths" and tried to keep that information secret (Public Citizen, nd). The lead industry continued to promote the use of lead water pipes and lead-based paint despite the known harmful effects, and it conducted campaigns to keep the information about the harmful effects from the public and to prevent regulation (Rabin, 2008). Pharmaceutical companies have been found to use similar tactics (Freudenberg & Galea, 2008). Twenty-one years after the Bhopal chemical release that killed and injured thousands of people, the corporation has not released the complete information about what happened and allegedly refused to respond to the public's charges that it has failed to give a full accounting or make full restitution (Hawken, 2007).

Corporations sometimes specifically establish and operate or fund research and policy institutes to produce papers or research to promote the false information, cause confusion, and misunderstandings about the harmful effects of their products, as a way to lend scientific credibility to their viewpoints, to control the manner in which research is conducted and the results released, or to withhold results (Baird, 2003; Mintzberg, 2006).

Corporations purchase other companies that make and sell more benign products and services to enhance their image or to help offset risk and costs. The parent corporation is protected from the liabilities of the subsidiary company and can be spun off with tax benefits. Tobacco corporations have owned many food corporations (Nestle, 2002). Corporations also change their name when the previous name has become associated with a negative aspect of the corporation's performance or a product (Newsweek, 2009b).

Legal Tactics

There are a wide variety of tactics within the judicial system that the corporation can use that influence health and health policy. Only a few are described here.

Liability

One of the key protections for the corporation is the limited liability of shareholders and officers. Since the corporation is a fictional person the shareholders, managers, or owners of the corporation are not held personally liable if, for example, they make decisions in their corporate role that result in corporate negligence for a harmful product (Rutkow & Teret, 2007). This can lead to human decisions on behalf of the corporation that are a business risk or are risky to human health or the environment without the decision maker being held responsible.

Corporate interests frequently call for tort law reform (Citizen Works, nd; Public Citizen, 2002) to, in part, purportedly to protect corporations from "sleazy lawyers and greedy consumers." In tort cases a harmed individual seeks redress against a corporation for its wrongful act that caused the individual to be injured. Tort reform refers to the idea that there is a need to limit the number of such injury claims pursued by personal injury lawyers and to limit the amount of money that could be awarded to the victim and attorneys (News Batch, 2006). Tort cases include injuries related to medical malpractice, automobiles, drugs, devices, and other products. Tort reform would enable corporations to externalize more of the costs of the harm caused by their products or operations.

Tort reform advocates fail to point out that there are more corporate law suits against other corporations than there are individual law suits against corporations. Corporate-related litigation is typically against their competitors relative to patents or copyrights, predatory practices, contracts, or liability. They also fail to point out that little money is awarded in punitive damages, insurance savings from reduced corporate liability are small, and the addition to insurance liability costs are a small fraction of the cost of the product (Citizen Works, nd). Corporations also expend large sums of money to influence judges who often make rulings in the corporation's favor (Kendall & Rylander, 2004). It has become common for corporations to require consumers, patients, or employees to agree to binding arbitration and to give up their right to file a lawsuit if they should have a dispute with the corporation (Perwin, 2005).

Punitive damage awards to individuals against corporations are necessary to deter corporations such as automobile manufacturers from ignoring safety complaints about their products (Public Citizen, 2001). Law suits provide a way to hold erring corporations accountable. Class action suits enable consumers, who usually do not have the financial resources that are available to a corporation, to sue the corporation.

Corporate legal action is often against government agencies in opposition to regulatory findings, enforcement, or development of safety regulations (Monforton, 2006). During the 1990s corporations appealed, in court, 80% of the Environmental Protection Agency's and 96% of the Occupational Safety and Health Administration's regulatory decisions (Shank, 1995). And, corporations often fail to comply with governmental regulation without governmental agencies filing suit against the corporation, or they reveal safety or health data only when pressured to by lawsuits.

When issues go through the judicial system corporations are frequently able to withhold information about the harmfulness of their product or operations, including use of confidentiality clauses that plaintiffs have to agree to when the corporation settles the case (Halperin, 1997), including consumer or patient law suits. The corporation agrees to give the consumer or patient a specified amount of money without acknowledging whether the consumer's complaint is valid. In turn the consumer must agree not to reveal the terms of the settlement and to keep all information confidential and undisclosed. Corporate legal strategy is to reach, at the most, this level of resolution to the case: settlement.

The corporate goal in lawsuits brought by consumers or the government is that the case never be heard on the facts or merits of the case. If the case should get to court information about their operations and products would be brought out during trial and become available to others, thus making the corporation vulnerable to additional legal action or regulation. The tactic also delays the legal process as long as it is possible to deplete the resources of the consumer and to delay presentation of the facts through pretrial depositions and evidence. Because of the confidential settlement of consumer lawsuits the harmful effects or mechanisms of many corporate products or operations are unproven or unknown.

Corporations Take On Their Opponents

Corporations have also taken legal action against, spied on, and tried to intimidate their individual critics. An automobile manufacturing corporation spied on an attorney because of his criticism of one of their cars and because of his efforts to improve automobile safety (Nelson, 2007). The beef industry sued a television and movie star about comments she made about her dietary preferences based on a disease found in cows (Public Broadcasting System, 1998). The tobacco industry tried many different ways to try to silence and stop the tobacco policy research of a public health scientist (Landman & Glantz, 2009).

Avoiding Taxes

Corporations avoid paying taxes through legal offshore tax havens (Komisar, 2005). In 2007, 7,937 U.S. entities controlled Caymans bank accounts; 732 companies on the U.S. stock exchange are incorporated in the Caymans (Vaughn, 2008). A corporation can reincorporate in an offshore tax haven without moving any of their operations. A U.S. Senator estimated that tax shelters and hidden offshore accounts cost the U.S. government nearly $100 billion a year in lost tax revenue (Delevingne, 2009).

Corporate Trials and Junk Science

Corporations have misused the uncertainties inherent in the scientific method to claim that research that shows their product or service to be faulty is unproven and to cast dispersions on the credentials of the public health scientist.

The corporate "junk science" view point was embedded in the U.S. justice system by the Supreme Court ruling in the Daubert case which allows either party in the case to challenge the expert testimony of the opposition, and that the admissibility of expert testimony is to be determined by the trial judge (Michaels, 2008). Therefore, scientific evidence supporting claims that citizens might bring against a corporation will likely be challenged by the corporation on the grounds that it is "junk science." The Daubert decision was reinforced by subsequent Supreme Court rulings that the scientific validity of individual research studies would be determined by the trial judge and that the validity of expert testimony that relies on judgment gained from experience, such as clinical expertise, can be challenged and then decided by the trial judge. Judges often lack sufficient background in the scientific method, the interpretation of research results, the concept of scientific uncertainty, and how conclusions are drawn based on the overall weight of the scientific evidence. Since most juries or judges don't understand the scientific method, they can fall prey to corporate false junk science claims.

Corporate Dominance of International Organizations

Corporations also benefit from dispute resolution or development of health and trade agreements through organizations whose development and operation was shaped by corporate interests. Those processes may not be transparent or accountable to elected government, and civil society is excluded from participation or outnumbered in participation by corporations. Corporate dominance is often the case even when the organizing body is supposed to be internationally inclusive of countries, such as the WHO's Codex Alimentarius committees (Sklair, 2002) or the WTO (as in the dispute resolution described above).

Under the investor's rights chapter of North American Free Trade Agreements (NAFTA) corporations can and have sued governments (federal, state, and local) for alleged violations of the act, including for loss of future potential profits because of health and environmental laws and regulations (Shaffer et al., 2005).

Free Passes from the U.S. Department of Justice

Within the U.S. justice system there are two procedures that enable corporations to escape prosecution for their wrong doing. The first type is called "Deferred Prosecution." In this situation the U.S. Department of Justice brings a criminal charge against a company and if the company agrees not to violate the law for 2 years, the company won't be prosecuted. The second type is called a "Non Prosecution Agreement." In this case the U.S. Justice Department fines the company but doesn't file criminal charges. The Department doesn't prosecute the company and company does not plead guilty but pays a fine (Spivack & Ramans, 2008). The corporation may not pay court imposed fines for years.

Using the Constitution

Courts have ruled that the First Amendment gives the corporation the right of free speech and thereby allowing the corporation to make political campaign contributions, lobby, advertize, and the right to refuse to speak. The Fourth Amendment against unreasonable searches and seizures has been used by the corporation to refuse or delay government inspection of its property thereby giving time to destroy evidence of unhealthful or illegal practices and challenge information obtained under search warrant. In 1978, the Supreme Court ruled that the federal Occupational Safety and Health Administration had to obtain a search warrant to enter a corporation's property to investigate worker health and safety complaints (Kellman, 1999). Under the Fifth Amendment, that in part prohibits taking of property for public use without compensation, has been used by the corporation to challenge governments actions to protect the environment and for the corporation to claim compensation for property value and loss of potential profits (Edwards & Valencia, nd).

Perhaps the most egregious corporate misappropriation of rights under a Constitutional Amendment is the use of Fourteenth Amendment. The 14th amendment to the U.S. constitution was passed post-civil war, in 1868, to ensure that all citizens/people received due process of law and had equal protection of the law, specifically to ensure provision of these rights by States to freed slaves. However, because of the deceit-instigated and corporate-influenced Supreme Court ruling of 1886 sighted above, corporations received the right of personhood. Within about the first half-century of its adoption the 14th amendment was used by corporations 11 times more than for the protection of former slaves (Lee, 1936). During the first 50 years less than one-half of 1% of the amendment-related cases before the Supreme Court were for the protection of former slaves or their descendents while 50% were for protection of corporate rights (Women's International League for Peace & Freedom, 1999). Between 1886, when the amendment was ratified, and 1896 the Supreme Court heard 150 cases involving the Fourteenth Amendment of which 15 involved blacks and 135 involved business entities (Hammerstrom, nd).

Unregulated Activity

The corporation uses whatever means is available, or that it can create, to achieve its purpose. If the means is not regulated those who represent corporate interests will go to great lengths to avoid regulation of those means whether there is consensus about their value and benefit. For example, corporations have used derivatives, a financial instrument that allows buyers of debt that have collateral, to sell the instrument back to the original holder, to falsely inflate the worth of company. Derivates played a key role in the financial collapse of several corporations in the U.S. in 2008–2009. Some officials of those corporations that were deeply involved in the financial collapse, with heavy reliance on derivatives, were former high-level federal government officials who, during their revolving door government service, opposed regulation of derivatives (Thomas & Hirsh, 2008).

Premption

A right granted to the federal government in the commerce clause of the United States. Constitution is the regulation of commerce between states. Decisions of the Supreme Court, beginning in 1898, limited the ability of individual states to regulate corporations. Using the commerce clause, the Supreme Court struck down 83 state laws between 1910 and 1919 but only 13 since 1990 (Connors, nd). These decisions expanded the power of the corporation by in effect prohibiting states from establishing laws to protect human health or the environment that corporations perceive to be an infringement on their conduct of business. The Supreme Court rulings went a long way toward convincing state legislators to cease their attempts to regulate corporations. However, more recently the Supreme Court denied that preemption applied in all cases in its ruling related to a suit against drug manufacturers of drugs approved by the FDA (Wolbert, 2007). Some state courts have ruled that local nonsmoking ordinances are not preempted by state law (O'Connor et al., 2008). However, in 2008 the U.S. Supreme Court supported the FDA's regulatory position that preemption of states applies to devices that the FDA had approved before going to market (Jacobstein, 2008). Concerns have arisen about whether federal nutrition laws preempt local laws that require nutrition labeling (Rutkow et al., 2008).

Corporations try to get the court jurisdiction in legal proceedings changed to obtain the most favorable hearing and to cause delay in the case. After its case was heard in the United States, a large oil corporation wanted its pollution dumping case to be heard outside the United States in another country because it claimed the country's courts were competent, fair, and impartial. However, after receiving a large fine for the cleanup costs from that country's court, the corporation claimed the country's courts were corrupt, illegal, and biased (Taillant, 2008). A chemical company used this tactic multiple times to fight agriculture worker's suit claiming sterility from the company's pesticide, that was banned in the United States but exported for use on bananas outside the United States (Bohme, 2008).

Extralegal Tactics

The term "extra-legal" is used here to refer to corporate activities outside the usual moral or ethical conventions of civil society or actions by corporations or their surrogates that are illegal. Corporate intimidation, harassment, and spying on their opponents fall within the definition of "extra-legal." Bribing of individuals or governments, fraud, and physical violence against their opponents are usually illegal.

Corporate Infiltration of Opposition Groups

A baby food corporation's representative infiltrated an opposition group and spied on the group to monitor their planned campaign activities against the corporation (Swiss ATTAC, 2008). A private security firm was hired by a fast food restaurant to have employee pose as a student and infiltrate and spy on a student organization that was working to get fast food restaurants to improve the working conditions and wages of farm workers (Corporate Crime Reporter, 2008). Tobacco corporations have also conducted covert monitoring of antitobacco groups (Bero, 2003). One individual who became a long-time, prominent, national activist in the gun control movement worked for the firearms association (Ridgeway et al., 2008).

Corporate Illegal Activity

At times corporations act illegally, usually when they are not likely to get caught or when the cost of getting caught is less than the profit benefit of acting illegally.

Illegal corporate activities cost the United States billions of dollars each year and thousands of lives, much of the activity is not identified or prosecuted, and is much more costly to society than the well-publicized violent street crime (Mokhiber, nd). Some of the top 100 corporate activities identified and prosecuted in recent decades include fraud, antitrust violations, food and drug violations, obstruction of justice, environmental violations, violations of campaign finance laws, illegal exports, bribery, tax evasion, public corruption, worker death, illegal boycott, and obstruction of justice. These crimes were committed by pharmaceutical, oil, agriculture, metals, cruise lines, banks, technology, health-care insurance, automobile, and airline corporations (Mokhiber, nd).

A mining corporation paid large amounts of money into the personal bank accounts of Indonesian officials to bride them to allow the company's waste disposal into the river (Riech, 2007). An agriculture chemical corporation was fined by the U.S. Securities and Exchange Commission for bribing foreign government officials to remove the requirement for environmental assessment of their genetically modified cotton (Patel et al., 2005). A large bank was required by a U.S. court to pay $780 million in fines, penalties, interest, and restitution as a result of knowingly assisting U.S. customers to set up accounts to hide income and avoid taxes (Barrett, 2009).

Corporations, particularly petrochemical, petroleum, automobile and electrical industries, sometimes illegally dispose of waste products, including having hired organized crime syndicates to do the dumping for them. (Simon, 2000). Corporations or their agents have used intimidation, harassment, spying, bribes, and physical violence against their opponents, including labor groups, individuals and organizations, particularly in subcontract firms located outside the United States (Klein, 2002, 2002b). Workers in contract factories have experienced union busting and efforts to prevent workers from organizing for labor rights and for healthful and safe working conditions. In factory zones in developing countries where goods are produced for prominent US. companies and the U.S. markets, there are documented situations of cheating workers out of their wages, confiscating passports, breaking labor laws, gathering illegal donations from workers, not allowing pickets or demonstrations, requiring overtime, employing short-term workers without contracts, using fire/rehire contracts to prevent the workers from gaining permanent employee status, all in servitude that amounts to slave labor (Greenhouse & Barbaro, 2006; Wehrfritz et al., 2008). Agriculture workers in the U.S. are being held as slaves and forced to work (Patel, 2009).

In 2007, a large international fruit corporation agreed to pay a $25 million fine by the U.S. Justice Department for paying a terrorist paramilitary group from 1997 to 2004 (Evans, 2007). Another corporation paid a government's military to use force against environmental protestors and offered to bribe trial witnesses to testify against environmental activists (Simon, 2000).

> "Corporate criminals are the only criminal class in the United States
> that have the power to define the laws under which they live."
>
> *Corporate Crime Reporter*

Some tobacco corporations participate in or support smuggling of their products. Duties not paid on the products imported into other countries, and United States sales taxes that are not paid open up areas to the product that are otherwise closed or restricted (Collin, et al., 2004; Guevara & Willison, 2008;). In 2007 the loss of sales tax on smuggled cigarette sales cost the State of New York $1 billion (Guevara & Willson, 2008).

An understanding of the tactics that the corporation uses leads to the identification of tactics and strategies that public health professionals and advocates can use to counter the influence and power of the corporation.

Counter Tactics

The field of public health needs to refocus our research and programs, reframe our way of thinking about and acting toward corporations, disconnect our programs, research and professional preparation from the corporation, and join in efforts to redesign the corporation.

Refocus

We need to refocus our programs, research and professional preparation education away from the medical model that focuses on individual risk factor reduction and to a focus on the social determinants of disease, including the corporation. And, rather than focusing our research and advocacy campaigns on a specific harmful product (e.g., tobacco) or on specific companies (e.g., Nestle, WalMart, etc.) we need to focus on the legal entity defined as the corporation.

The schools of public health and related academic programs need to add courses and redesign courses in the curriculum of public health professional education programs to focus on the corporate entity and on how to address the tactics used by the corporation (Wiist, 2006). Illustrative examples of the health-damaging operations and products of corporations could be integrated across the curriculum, including in the required core courses of biostatistics, epidemiology, administration and policy, environmental health, and the social and behavioral sciences. Public health students need to understand the corporate entity and its tactics, economics, how to deconstruct the corporation's activities and messages, know about the influence of court decisions on corporate operations and policies, understand how to conduct corporate-related policy analysis and development, and be able to plan and conduct advocacy activities to address the corporation.

The field of public health needs to conduct ecological research in which the variables of interest reflect activities and outcomes of the corporation and how they may influence traditional public health status measures (Wiist, 2006). For example, research could be conducted on the relationship between corporate activity such as profits, per share costs, CEO and worker compensation, and public health measures such as years of potential life lost, morbidity, infant mortality, disability, or quality of life (Wiist, 2006).

Reframe

Public health needs to adopt the characterization of corporations as an institution that does not have human characteristics, emotions, or behaviors and understand that the purpose of a corporation is singular: to make a profit and provide the largest possible return to investors.

Public health professionals must accept that corporations do not have a social mission or goal and that corporations only undertake such activities so long as they contribute to profit. The corporation is not a moral being. Some corporations benefited from supporting Nazi Germany, including operating concentration camps, such as a predecessor conglomerate corporate of Bayer (Coalition Against Bayer Dangers Germany, 2003). Corporate officials may be "nice" ethical people with their family and friends, but when acting in their corporate roles they cannot, by law, be "socially responsible" if doing so conflicts with their duty to ensure that the corporation makes a profit. Conveying the message that companies can be more "socially responsible" distracts from the work of getting laws passed and regulations implemented that will address the underlying corporate causes of disease. Singling out a single highly profitable company for its unhealthful practices or products misses the point. Such a corporation is operating the way the corporate system we established requires.

"Corporate 'social responsibility' is as meaningful as cotton candy."

Robert Reich

The precautionary principle is of particular relevance as a rationale for addressing the corporations' influence on policy. The precautionary principle proposes, among other elements, that we determine whether something is harmful before we introduce it into society, and that the burden of proof for lack of harm rests on those who would introduce the substance (Kriebel & Tickner, 2001). If there is a risk the item should be banned even if the evidence about its harmfulness is uncertain. Corporations have long fought public health policy and regulations based on this fundamental public health principle (Rosner & Markowitz, 2002) because of the view that precaution and prevention interfere with innovation, economic development, and progress.

Disconnect

The public health field must be willing to disconnect from its reliance on funding from corporate sponsorship, and find other ways of sustaining its activities. We need to disconnect from corporate advertisements in publications, sponsorship of conferences, funding of research, training grants, and fellowships. Even a consistent acknowledgement of corporate sponsorship does not prevent conflicts of interest such as the inability to objectively recognize or acknowledge bias, the prioritization of the corporate agenda, or a reluctance to focus on a corporate caused health problem. Money can cloud judgment. It can induce us to overlook evidence, avoid criticism of the corporation, or avoid actions that oppose the corporation. "He who pays the piper names the tune" and the tune, or goals, of the corporate entity and public health are different, and, in fact, are often in opposition.

Redesign

Redesigning or restructuring the corporation as an institution is the most fundamental way to address the global influence of corporations. Redesign addresses the root, underlying cause of the problem and will go further to improve health, the natural environment, and democracy than any other counter strategy or tactic.

> "Inspiration … resides rather in humanity's willingness to restore, redress, reform, rebuild, recover, reimagine and reconsider."
>
> Paul Hawken

There is a large and growing movement of organizations worldwide that advocates for such a fundamental change in the design or structure of the corporation (Marx et al., 2007; Mayer, 2007; White & Kelly, 2007). The recommendations of that movement include the following, among others:

1. Ban all corporate political activity of any type, including political campaign funding and lobbying. This would necessitate eliminating the free speech right of the corporation and removing its designation as a citizen. This is probably the single most important proposed action. It would free up legislators and the administration to reprioritize their representation to the interests of human citizens rather than corporations.

2. Conduct periodic charter reviews for renewal or revocation of corporate charters. Include worker health, environmental protection, sustainability standards, and contributions to the social good as criteria that must be met for charter renewal, perhaps through a constitutional Social Responsibility Amendment (Learner, nd). (Note: few proposed amendments have ever passed.) Corporations not meeting the criteria could be dissolved or banned from operating in that country or state; that is, revoke the corporation's charter (Linzey, 1996). A clause could be included in corporate charters mandating that profit will not take precedence over social and environmental effects. Corporate charters could be made self-revoking if the corporation externalizes costs.

3. Allow citizens to make presentations about corporations' actions directly to grand juries at the state level, thereby passing some corporate bias in the judicial system.

4. Remove the corporate right of personhood (Women's International League for Peace and Freedom, nd), and therefore citizenship, perhaps through a constitutional amendment (Chelsea Green, 2008). Alternatively, use the right of personhood to prosecute the crimes of corporations as would be done with a human citizen's crimes (Gerencser, 2005).

5. Eliminate or reduce limited liability for shareholders and officers. Hold parent corporations directly liable for the activities of all of its subsidiaries (Gregor & Ellis, 2008).

6. Remove corporations' right to sue, to challenge legitimately enacted laws and regulations in court.

7. Strengthen government regulatory agencies so they can effectively carryout monitoring, inspections, independent research, and enforcement of laws and regulations related to all corporations.

8. Strengthen and enforce antitrust laws for contemporary circumstances such as the many and complex linkages between institutions, such as board membership, corporate subsidiaries, and financial transactions. For example, transactions between the banking, mortgage and hedge-fund corporations that enabled the 2008–2009 economic crises.

9. Eliminate government subsidies to corporations through tax laws including for such items as research and development, price supports, and marketing. Include in corporate charters a clause that the corporation cannot receive government assistance or subsidies.

10. Prohibit appointments of individuals with corporate or industry ties to positions in governmental regulatory bodies and review panels that have oversight authority over industries in which they have recently worked.

11. Strengthen restrictions on (e.g., extend the time before they can become lobbyist) or completely prohibit government officials from lobbying after leaving government service.

12. Make any voluntary codes agreed to by corporations transparent and enforceable, and with frequent independent, external audits for which the results are made public.

13. Give shareholders a direct voice in such corporate governance matters such as determining executive compensation, and corporate policies and practices, such as in human rights and health care (Interfaith Center on Corporate Responsibility, nd).

14. Enforce corporate adherence to the UN "Norms on Responsibilities of Transnational Corporations and Other Business Enterprises with Regards to Human Rights," (United Nations, 2003) and the UN Global Compact: "Advancing Corporate Citizenship" adopted in 2000 (United Nations, nd).

15. Renegotiate or abrogate bilateral and multilateral trade agreements in which corporate interests trump public health, worker rights, the environment, or democratic sovereignty.

16. Reform the WTO by increasing civil society participation, democratic decision making, transparency, and accountability to civil society and government. Implement reforms specific to various industries, such as agriculture (Barker, 2007) and health (Blouin, 2007).

17. Establish an alternative organization to WTO that serves a similar purpose but which is subject to and operated by civil society, perhaps through the UN, with transparency, accountability, and that ensures that health, human rights, nature, and democracy have precedence over commerce. It should be free of the current corporate influence on the UN (Lewit, 2000).

18. Pass and enforce laws that would allow workers their right to organize into unions without interference of the corporation.

19. Disentangle universities from corporate influence through such means as modifying the Bayh–Dole Act, establishing strong conflict of interest regulations, and providing additional independent research funding (Washburn, 2005).

In addition to proposals for direct reform of the corporation, there are a number of suggestions for alternatives to the corporate way of conducting business (International Forum on Globalization, 2002; Marx et al., 2007; White & Kelly, 2007), that include the following, among others:

1. Work with corporations to get them to operate in more benign ways. Corporations can produce, ship, and market their products in ways that are profitable but with less detrimental effect on the natural environment and human health. One of the largest MNCs is purportedly taking steps to reduce its carbon footprint and save money by packaging and transporting products in ways that use less petroleum (Karabell, 2008).

2. Build and support local businesses and show preference to independent enterprises (e.g., local communications media and local food growers). Local groups or individuals buy out absentee owners so that the new management can understand and be more responsive to the local community and economy, customers, and natural environment.

3. Create alternative local, national, and global operating systems in energy, transportation, agriculture and food, manufacturing systems, and news media.

4. Educate future corporate leaders about saving money and increasing profits with sustainable products and operations that protect workers and the environment, through, for example, "Green" MBA curricula (Locke, 2007).

5. Develop and use new measures of economic health. Commonly used measures such as GDP, Gross National Product (GNP), or Consumer Price Index (CPI) do not consider quality of health, the environment, health care, quality of life, and so on.

6. Establish and charter institutional forms such as community development corporations, trusts, and cooperatives to serve the public interest. Eliminate the IMF and WB and set up alternative organizations that are democratically accountable to all governments.

7. Institute a small percent tax on all international speculative financial transactions ("Tobin Tax") to encourage the financial and monetary industry to make productive, long-term investment and provide additional funding for society's needs (Engler, 2008).

Both of the two types of proposals above (redesigning the corporation and alternative business practices) are undergirded by the principles of relocalization and subsidiarity; that is, local economies, local production, local labor;

with power and decisions devolved to the lowest governmental, local community, or regional level appropriate to the goal and with the competence to deal with the issue (International Forum on Globalization, 2000). Those who might be the most directly affected by or gain from a change would make the decisions on such matters as the location of corporate facilities, CEO compensation, any worker layoffs, or the disposal of production waste.

There are additional, specific actions that public health professionals can take in several areas related to the influence of the corporation, including the following:

1. Work toward strengthening the public health infrastructure, such as laboratories, so that national and local public health agencies can conduct independent research on corporate products, provide surveillance, and monitor the health and environmental effects of corporate products and operations. This would enable policy makers to use independent data as the basis of health standards, for regulatory purposes and for setting health policy rather than using corporate produced data such as the FDA relies on.

2. Public health professionals can join in the work of groups such as the APHA's Trade & Health Forum whose members' focus on researching the relationship between trade policies and practices and public health measures, and engaging in advocacy activities. A priority of members is to get public health representation on the Advisory Committees of the U.S. Trade Representative which has been largely absent (Shaffer & Brenner, 2004). Also, join in working to hold the U.S government and corporations to the provisions of the WTO 1994 Trade Related Aspects of Intellectual Property (TRIPS), the Doha Declaration, and the U.S. 2002 Trade Promotion Authority (TPA) Act so that access to medicines and the public's health are given priority.

3. Use direct actions such as boycotts, litigation, media campaigns, and protests. However, the financial costs of campaigns are high, they take a lot of energy and resources to sustain, the public and the news media lose interest; campaigns scatter energy, time, and recourses across many different issues, and chances are great that the message will not be heard above or have influence greater than the voice of corporate interests (Corporations and Health Watch, nd). Also, in the post-9/11 climate, campaigns may have civil rights repercussions such as government violations of individual privacy and may lead to accusations that participating individuals violate national security.

The Global Movement

To accomplish any of the above public health must build and strengthen alliances with the global network, or movement, that is working for social justice, economic equality, worker's rights, indigenous peoples' rights, and environment sustainability. What is different about the organizations in the network compared to earlier social movements is that in this movement all of the organizations have the same perspective and the same targets, they make the connection between local issues and global issues, and the movement is global. Joanna Macy called this world-wide movement a "great turning" (Macy, 2000). Others have called it the Global Justice Movement (Reitan, 2007) or the "movement of movements," that includes 1–2 million organizations (Hawken, 2007).

The organizations recognize that there is a connection between the hegemonic neoliberal model and the corporation and the resulting inequities, lack of democracy, and harmful health and environmental effects. They are working toward reform, developing alternatives, and rebuilding state control over corporations (Badawi, 2004; Green & Griffith, 2002). These organizations have diverse but connected interests including social entrepreneurship, human rights, slow food, health care, education, sustainable development, indigenous rights, biopiracy, ecology, alternatives to global capitalism, poverty reduction, and so on.

Some of the organizations, such as Via Campesina, a large rural-based network of small- and medium-size farmers, agriculture workers, and fishers, the People's Global Action, a network against capitalism that arose from the Zapatistas in Mexico, and international meetings such as the World Social Forum have become large and world wide (Fisher & Ponniah, 2003; Reitan, 2007). Among the organizations working toward social and economic justice there are many organizations that specifically focus on reforming and redesigning the corporation (see Appendix).

> "Tyranny cuts off the singer's head. But the voice from the bottom
> of the well returns to the secret springs of the earth and rises out of
> nowhere through the mouths of the people."

> Pablo Neruda

Underlying this global movement is an adoption of a similar perspective of causation that links local concerns with global issues, and a common critique of the corporation by different nations, classes, religions, and ethnic groups (Hawken, 2007; Lowy & Betto, 2003; McNally, 2006; Reitan, 2007; Starr, 2000, 2005). There are two foci to the movement: the common target, and the process of change. The target of the movement is the neoliberal economic model of corporate globalization fostered by the WTO, IMF, and WB.

The movement views globalization as corporate expansion across borders that threatens national sovereignty; an ideology that promotes itself as beneficient and unstoppable. It is not a specific corporation or a specific industry that is responsible for these problems but it is the logic of the corporation itself that is the root problem and that needs to be addressed. The corporate, neoliberal model is a recolonization of and structural violence against the South and the nonelites of the North that creates inequalities by class (Navarro, 2007). Business rights are not legitimate if they infringe on human rights or damage the natural environment. The Corporation is antidemocratic; suppressing free speech and freedom of information and reducing citizens to consumers. Corporate globalization has created large inequalities in the distribution of wealth, the corporation is extractive and has destroyed the environment, depleted resources and commoditized human labor, information, and nature, including essential water and human genes. Public good cannot and should not be determined by the corporation.

These organizations use a wide range of tactics and approaches to critique neoliberal economic globalization and the corporation. The tactics emphasize direct confrontation and civil disobedience rather than lobbying, including independent media groups, cultural jamming, street actions, occupying vacant buildings and land, frivolity, fake presentations at business conferences and press conferences, violence against property, and suicide (Starr, 2000, 2005; The Yes Men, 2004). The rallying cries of these organizations reflect their tactics: "Ya Basta" ("no more") and "Our world is not for sale."

The second focus of the movement is nothing less than a remaking of the governance of the world. The movement is doing this through direct participatory democracy in which discussion and socio-economic decisions and related priorities are made by the population itself, the people, not through representatives, and not through hierarchical practices. Power is collective and communal through local sovereignty that will protect the local political economy. Processes are decentralized and without pressures to conform and are temporary. They use informal affirmation, group development, rotating individual roles, and give attention to group process. Competition and dispute are replaced with cooperation, sharing, fraternity, and solidarity, including recognizing the rights of nature (Community Environmental Legal Defense Fund, 2008). All forms of racial, gender, and economic exploitation are resisted, with some attention give to reparations for slavery and colonialism.

There is a consciousness about reducing consumerism and for decommodification, and an emphasis on the type of development that will not compromise future generations to meet present needs. Quality of life is emphasized over the corporate globalization's quantitative measures such as GDP and stock prices. The movement accepts responsibility to produce alternatives to corporate globalization, neoliberalism, and imperialism, and recognizes that criticism alone is insufficient.

One aspect of the movement is termed "globalization from the below" (Brecher et al., 2000) because the goal is to remake the world by the people, without dominance, without central authority, and to recover the authority of the state to regulate corporations. This international populist movement is based on the belief that networks and global alliances between human and indigenous rights groups, labor, and environmental groups and others can make corporations and governments accountable to people instead of dictation by the elites (Hawken, 2007; Lowy & Betto, 2003; McNally, 2006; Reitan, 2007; Starr, 2000, 2005). Some of these beliefs and goals were formalized in The Earth Charter (Earth Charter Initiative, 2000).

Indigenous Peoples' Leadership

Indigenous Peoples have taken a lead in the movement against neoliberal corporate globalization, as a continuation of historical colonialism, and its agents the WTO, IMF, and WB. Indigenous Peoples, along with women and children, have often suffered the most directly from corporate globalization (Mander & Tauli-Corpuz, 2006). However, the rationale for Indigenous Peoples' resistance to corporate globalization, if it is indeed that (Yashar, 2007), is preceded by an imperative to remember ceremony, return to homeland, and the liberation from the myths of colonialism from an earlier era and from continuing imperialism (Alfred & Corntassel, 2005).

Corporations have sought patents on Indigenous Peoples' seeds and medicinal plants that they have cultivated for centuries (Mushita & Thompson, 2007). Corporations search their blood and DNA for additional patentable technologies (Tsosie, 2007). When corporations log forests or build dams that flood the countryside, or mine for minerals or drill for oil, Indigenous Peoples often lose their usual source of livelihood, their homes, ceremonies, communities, language, and sacred places. When they are thus driven from their ancestral land they often migrate to the fringes of urban areas where they live in poverty and unhealthful conditions.

Indigenous Peoples are fighting for their rights, for their sovereignty, to retain their traditional ways, develop in their own way, and to retain or recover their land. Their work has resulted in numerous institutional gains, including resolutions, declarations, policies, constitutional provisions and national commissions and councils in several countries and regions. The UN has a

"Declaration on the Rights of Indigenous Peoples," a Permanent Forum on Indigenous Issues, and a Special Rapporteur on the Situation of Human Rights and Fundamental Freedoms of Indigenous Peoples (Mander & Tauli-Corpuz, 2006). International groups of Indigenous Peoples recently adopted the "Declaration of the International Conference on Extractive Industries and Indigenous Peoples" (Manila Declaration, 2009).

> "Only some kind of psychospiritual conviction, training, and insight goes deep enough to support the necessary radical social shift."
>
> Ken Jones

Ethics and Spirituality

Finally, but fundamentally, if we are to regain human citizen control over the corporation we must emphasize the ethical, or spiritual, aspects of life. The tactics for doing so are both practical and philosophical.

First we need to teach children, serve as exemplars of, and promote societal values in which the acquisition of material goods, consumerism, materialism, growth in production and consumption, and the measurement of personal success by financial wealth are not viewed as the highest values of human life.

From 2003 to 2008 consumer spending in the United States accounted for 70% of the GDP, or $1 trillion more than in 1980. There are over 1.4 billion credit cards; and household debt in 2008 was 139% of personal disposable income, compared to 103% in 2000 (Samuelson, 2008). We must foster the understanding that the pursuit of material wealth may not be conducive to our own health (DeAngelis, 2004), nor to the well-being of the planet (Mayell, 2004). Even "green" consumption uses up our limited and dwindling resources.

A corporatized, commercialized environment infantilizes teens and adults and serves only the need of the market place for economic growth. To satisfy this reliance the neoliberal marketplace requires consumption and it substitutes these false and manufactured needs for real needs (Barber, 2007).

We must work to change the accepted conventional "wisdom" that public policies should be judged by whether they improve the efficiency of the economy regardless of their effect on health, the environment, inequality, peace, fairness, accountability, and so on. We must encourage, teach, and act from altruism, with regard for the entire community rather than only for our individual self.

Second, we need to reassert our citizen role over our consumer role. Only citizens have sovereignty, not consumers (Barber, 2007) and our consumer role has usurped our role as citizens (Riech, 2007). For example, as information consumers we use a corporate Web Search Engine that, as citizens of a democratic country we allow to help totalitarian governments suppress democracy (Bray, 2006).

We need to teach, foster, and develop new democratic structures, process, and practices based on direct citizen participation; processes that are economically and culturally inclusive, with real influence, real involvement, and meaningful participation of those affected by decisions. We need to develop democratic processes that will protect the health and well-being of us all ... one of the fundamental purpose of democracy, and a fundamental purpose of government.

"Democracy isn't the work of the market; it is the work of real hands"

Naomi Klein

There is a growing recognition among people from various religions (Carmichal & Barnes-Davies, 2007; Rifkin, 2003), evangelicals (Wallis, 2006) (e.g., Sojourners Magazine), Catholics (e.g., Center of Concern), Buddhists (Daniels, 2005; Loy, 2003), Judaism (e.g., Tikkun Magazine), and interfaith groups such as the Network of Spiritual Progressives, and people of varied moral beliefs (Benatar, 2005), that a long-term regard for all of humanity and for the planet must be the primary purpose and goal of society, not short-term corporate profits, economic growth, and consumption (Mander, 2007; Simmer-Brown, 2002).

What is needed is the refined awakening of spiritual consciousness about taking care of the Earth, the possibilities for democratic self-governance, and a recognition that the diversity of all life is of the same sacred origin. That awakening will enable us to overcome imperialism and create a new, higher order human community (Hawken, 2007; Korten, 2006).

Some people may believe that the changes suggested here are impossible to achieve. It is true that they will take reprioritizing, determination and persistence, wise effort, and strong alliances. But impossible? No! We can take courage in several other recent human achievements. Apartheid in South Africa was overthrown. Slavery, once common (and still practiced in places) is now illegal in most of the world. In the United States "Jim Crow" racial discrimination was defeated. Child labor, once common in industrialized Europe, was outlawed. The Berlin Wall came down and democracy replaced many repressive governments. U.S. women obtained the legal right to vote. Women in many countries have become the leader of their country. And recently, an African American was elected President of the United States.

Humans create social institutions. If those institutions are not working in a beneficial way we can change them. We cannot wait for others or wait for future generations to begin the necessary work. We cannot wait for or rely only on a powerful and magnetic leader to emerge who has the vision and will to "save" the world. It is up to us; now, to begin the work. "We are the ones we've been waiting for" as the late Lisa Sullivan said (Wallis, 2006). A character in a Broadway show and Hollywood movie asked the question that concisely summarizes the long-term motivation that we must hold onto: "If you don't have a dream, how can you have a dream come true?" We must hold onto our dream that generations to come will have health, happiness and freedom, equality, and be able to enjoy life on a healthy and beautiful planet. We humans are the citizens and it is we who can create the changes that guarantee that world.

REFERENCES

Alfred T, Corntassel J. *Being Indigenous: Resurgences Against Contemporary Colonialism.* Oxford, UK: 'The Politics of Identity,' Government and Opposition Ltd; 2005.

Allison J, Allison T, Hutchinson S, Rawland M, Rasmussen V, Crosby, R. Challenge Corporate Power/Assert People's Rights: A Campaign of the International League for Peace and Freedom, U.S. Section. Session I, Reading 3, 1–7. Available at: http://www.wilpf.org/docs/ccp/corp/2006-I-CompleteSession.pdf. Revised edition published 2006. Accessed September 18, 2009.

Anderson S, Cavanagh J, Collins C, Pizzigati S, Lapham M. *Executive Excess 2008: How Average Taxpayers Subsidize Runaway Pay: 15th Annual CEO Compensation Survey.* Institute for Policy Studies and United for a Fair Economy; 2008. Available at: www.ips-dc.org.

Anderson S, Cavanagh J. *Of the World's 100 Largest Economic Entities, 51 Are Now Corporations and 49 Are Countries.* Washington, D.C. Institute for Policy Studies. Available at: http://www.corporations.org/system/top100.html. Published 2000. Accessed September 15, 2009.

Anderson S, Cavanagh J. *Top 200: The Rise of Corporate Global Power.* Washington, D.C. Institute for Policy Studies; 2000.

Angel M. *The Truth about the Drug Companies: How They Deceive Us and What To Do about It.* New York: Random House; 2005.

Aronowitz S. *The Knowledge Factory: Dismantling the Corporate University and Creating True Higher Learning.* Boston: Beacon Press; 2000.

Associated Press. *13 Firms Receiving Bailouts Owe Back Taxes.* Available at: http://www.msnbc.msn.com/id/29773472/. Published March 19, 2009. Accessed September 16, 2009.

Baby Milk Action Nestle Boycott. Available at: http://www.babymilkaction.org/pages/boycott.html. Accessed September 15, 2009.

Badawi AA. The social dimension of globalization and health. *Perspectives on Global Development and Technology* 2004;3(1–2):73–90.

Baird P. Getting it right: industry sponsorship and medical research. *CMAJ.* 2003;168(10):1267–1269.

Bakan J. *The Corporation: The Pathological Pursuit of Profit and Power.* New York: Free Press; 2004.

Balaam DN, Veseth M. *Introduction to International Political Economy.* Upper Saddle River, New Jersey: Pearson; 2008.

Barber BR. *Consumed: How Markets Corrupt Children, Infantilize Adults, and Swallow Citizens Whole.* New York: W.W. Norton & Company; 2007.

Barbor TF. Alcohol research and the alcoholic beverage industry: issues, concerns and conflicts of interest. *Addiction* 2009;104(Suppl. 1):34–47.

Barker D. *The Rise and Predictable Fall of Globalized Industrial Agriculture.* San Francisco, CA: The International Forum on Globalization; 2007.

Barlett DL, Steele JB. Corporate welfare. *Time Magazine* November 9, 1998.

Barrett D. *USB to Pay $780M, Open Secret Swiss Bank Records.* Available at: http://abcnews.go.com/business/wirestory?id=6908025. Published February 18, 2009. Accessed September 19, 2009.

Baue W. *Corporations Fight to Keep Political Contributions in the Closet. Sustainability Investment News.* Available at: http://www.socialfunds.com/news/article.cgi/1586.html. Published December 9, 2004. Accessed September 15, 2009.

Beckett J. The "Government Should Run Like a Business" Mantra. *The American Review of Public Administration* 2000;30:185–204.

Benally K. Nike opportunism: Turning Native plight into profit? *Navajo Hopi Observer* October 11, 2007; A5.

Benatar SR. Moral imagination: the missing component in global health. *PLoS Med.* 2005;2(12):1207–1210.

Bennet WL. Global media and politics: transnational communication regimes and civic cultures. *Annual Rev Polit Sci.* 2004;7:125–148.

Bero L. Implications of the tobacco industry documents for public health and policy. *Annu Rev Public Health.* 2003;24:267–288.

Bleifuss J. Know thine enemy: a brief history of corporations. In These Times. Women's International League for Peace & Freedom. Available at: http://www.wilpf.org/docs/ccp/corp/2006-II-CompleteSession.pdf. Published February 8, 1998. Accessed September 15, 2009.

Blouin C. Trade policy and health: from conflicting interests to policy coherence. *Bull World Health Organ.* 2007;85:169–173.

Bohme SR. Cross-border hazard and cross-border justice: the case of DBCP. Presented at the *136th Annual Meeting and Expo of the American Public Health Association,* San Diego, CA; October 27, 2008.

Bohme SR, Zorabedian J, Egliman DS. Maximizing profit and endangering health: corporate strategies to avoid litigation and regulation. *Int J Occup Environ Health.* 2005;11:338–348.

Boseley S. *Sugar Industry Threatens to Scupper WHO*. Guardian.co.uk. Available at: http://www.guardian.co.uk/society/2003/apr/21/usnews.food. Published April 21, 2003.

Blumenstyk G. BP gets good terms in U. of California deal. *Chronicle of Higher Education*. November 23, 2007;A21.

Bray H. Google China censorship fuels calls for US boycott: Some American users also urging investors to sell service's stock. The Boston Globe. Available at: http://www.boston.com/news/world/asia/articles/2006/01/28/google_china_censorship_fuels_calls_for_us_boycott/. Published January 26, 2006. Accessed September 15, 2009.

Brecher J, Costello T, Smith B. Globalization from below. *The Nation. Women's International League for Peace & Freedom*. Available at: http://www.wilpf.org/cvd. Published December 4, 2000.

Carreyrou J. Inside Abbott's tactics to protect AIDS drug. Pittsburgh Post-Gazette. Available at: http://www.post-gazette.com/pg/07003/750966-28.stm. Published January 3, 2007.

Cassandra Carmichael C, Barnes-Davies R. Environment, faith, and corporate influence. *Justice Rising: Grassroots Solutions to Corporate Domination*, 2007;2(4):12.

Center for Media and Democracy. *Front Groups*. Available at: http://www.sourcewatch.org/index.php?title=Front_groups. Published September 8, 2007. Accessed September 15, 2009.

Center for Science in the Public Interest. *Kids in the Crosshairs of Big Booze*. Available at: http://www.cspinet.org/new/200207161.html. Published July 16, 2002. Accessed September 15, 2009.

Chelsea Green Publishing. Why We Need the 28th Amendment to the Constitution: Separation of Corporation and State (VIDEO). Available at: http://www.alternet.org/water/106645/why_we_need_the_28th_amendment_to_the_constitution%3A_separation_of_corporation_and_state_%28video%29/. Posted November 11, 2008.

Chevron. *Human Energy*. Available at: http://www.chevron.com/stories/. Published 2001–2009. Accessed September 15, 2009.

Choudry A. *Bringing It All Back Home: Anti-globalisation Activism Cannot Ignore Colonial Realities*. Available at: http://www.converge.org.nz/pma/indbring.htm. Published August 2, 2001.

Citizen Works. Democracy: Tort Reform. Available at: http://www.citizenworks.org/issues/democracy/demo-issuepapers-tort_ref.php. Accessed September 15, 2009.

CNBC. Big brother, big business. March 30, 2008.

Coalition Against Bayer Dangers Germany. Materials about Bayer's past: Letter to the Editor of "The Jewish Chronicle." Available at: http://www.cbgnetwork.org/365.html. Published September 2003. Accessed September 15, 2009.

Coleman D. The United Nations and Transnational Corporations: from an inter-nation to a "Beyond-state" Model of Engagement. *Global Society*. 2003;17(4):339–357.

Collin J, LeGresley E, MacKenzie R, Lawrence S, Lee K. Complicity in contraband: British American Tobacco and cigarette smuggling in Asia. *Tobacco Control.* 2004;13(Suppl II):ii104–ii111.

Collins C, Pizzigati S. Obama is right to take on the very rich. Christian Science Monitor. Available at: http://www.csmonitor.com/2009/0224/p09s02-coop. html. Published February 24, 2009. Accessed September 15, 2009.

Community Environmental Legal Defense Fund. Ecuador approves new constitution: Voters approve rights of nature. Available at: http://www.celdf.org/Default. aspx?tabid=548. Published September 28, 2008.

Community Rights Counsel. News Release: Exxon, Punitive Damages, and Judicial Junkets. Available at: http://www.communityrights.org/Newsroom/ crcNewsReleases/Exxon%20Release%203_21_07.asp. Published 2007. Accessed September 15, 2009.

Connors T. We are not machines: despite some small steps forward, poverty and fear still dominate the lives of Nike and Adidas workers in Indonesia. Oxfam. Available at: http://www.cleanclothes.org/documents/we_are_not_machines. pdf. Published 2002. Accessed September 15, 2009.

Constitutional Accountability Center. The Takings Project: Using Federal courts to attack community and environmental protection. Available at: http://www.theusconstitution.org/upload/filelists/166_chapter1.pdf. Accessed September 15, 2009.

Consumers International. Branding the Cure: A consumer perspective on corporate social responsibility, drug promotion and the pharmaceutical industry in Europe. London, UK. Available at: www.consumersinternational.org/pharma. Published 2006.

Cooper MN, ed. *The Case Against Media Consolidation: Evidence on Concentration, Localism and Diversity.* Donald McGannon Center for Communications Research, Fordham University; 2007:458.

Corporate Accountability International. INFACT 2000 People's Annual Report: Challenging corporate influence in the 2000 U.S. elections.

Corporations and Health. Corporations and Campus Research: How private industry dollars influence scientific discovery and threaten public health. Available at: http://corporationsandhealth.org/campus_research.php. Accessed April 9, 2008. Published 2008.

Corporations and Health Watch. What are the limitations of campaign-building as a strategy to modify health damaging corporate practices? Available at: http:// www.corporationsandhealth.org/faq.php#faq6. Accessed September 15, 2009.

Corporate Crime Reporter. Burger King spies on activists. *Corporate Crime Reporter.* May 12, 2008;22(19):5.

CorpWatch. US: BP fined $373m by US government. Available at: http://www. corpwatch.org/article.php?id=14774. Published October 26, 2007.

CUPE Research. Privatization & U: Changing the face of our universities. Available at: http://cupe.ca/updir/the_changing_face_of_our_public_universities.pdf. Published October 13, 2006.

Daniels PL. Economic systems and the Buddhist world view: the 21st century nexus. *J Socio Econ.* 2005;34:245–268.

DeAngelis T. Consumerism and its discontents. APA online. *Monitor on Psychology.* 2004;35(6):51. Available at: http://www.apa.org/monitor/jun04/discontents.html. Accessed September 15, 2009.

Delevingne L. Trouble in tax paradise: Offshore havens may have to take the welcome mat if world leaders have their way. Available at http://money.cnn.com/2001/04/01/new/international/tax_havens.fortune/index.htm?section=money_pf_taxes. Published April 1, 2009. Accessed September 19, 2009.

Dembele DM. The International Monetary Fund and World Bank in Africa: a "disastrous" record. *Int J Health Serv.* 2005;35(2):389–398.

Dickler J. The incredible shrinking cereal box. Available at: http://money.cnn.com/2008/09/09/pf/food_downsizing/index.htm. Published September 10, 2008. Accessed September 15, 2009.

Doane D. The myth of CSR. Stanford Social Innovation Review. Available at: http://www.ssireview.org/articles/entry/the_myth_of_csr/. Published Fall, 2005. Accessed September 15, 2009.

Drutman L, Cray C. *The People's Business: Controlling Corporations and Restoring Democracy.* San Francisco: Berrett-Koehler, Inc.; 2004.

Duvall T. The new feudalism: globalization, the market, and the great chain of consumption. *New Polit Sci.* 2003;25(1):81–97.

Earth Charter Initiative. The Earth Charter. Available at: http://www.earthcharterinaction.org/invent/images/uploads/echarter_english.pdf. Published June 29, 2000. Accessed September 15, 2009.

Edwards J, Valencia A. Corporate Personhood and the "Right" to Harm the Environment. Women's International League for Peace & Freedom. Available at: http://www.wilpf.org/docs/ccp/corp/ACP/corp_harm_environment.pdf. Accessed September 15, 2009.

Egilman DS, Bohme SR. Over a barrel: corporate corruption of science and its effects on workers and the environment. *Int J Occup Environ Health.* 2005;11(4):331–337.

Engler M. There is an alternative to corporate rule. Available at: http://www.alternet.org/workplace/96806/there_is_an_alternative_to_corporate_rule/. Published September 1, 2008. Accessed September 15, 2009.

Evans M. Para-politics goes bananas. *The Nation.* April 4, 2007.

Fisher WF, Ponniah T, eds. *Another World Is Possible: Popular Alternatives to Globalization at the World Social Forum.* New York: Zed Books; 2003.

Folkenflik D. Controversy follows science host's industry ties. National Public Radio. Available at: http://www.npr.org/templates/story/story.php?storyId=97488556. Published November 25, 2008. Accessed September 15, 2009.

Fort M, Mercer MA, Gish O. *Sickness and Wealth: The Corporate Assault on Global Health.* Cambridge, MA: South End Press; 2004.

Freudenberg N, Bradley SP, Serrano M. Public health campaigns to change industry practices that damage health: an analysis of 12 case studies.

Health Educ Behav Online First, published on December 12, 2007 as doi:10.1177/1090198107301330.

Freudenberg N, Galea S. Corporate practices. In: Galea S, ed. *Macrosocial Determinants of Health* (pp. 71–104). New York: Springer; 2007.

Freudenberg N, Galea S. The impact of corporate practices on health: implications for health policy. *J Public Health Policy.* 2008;29:86–104.

Fugere D. Toyota's green commitment: fact or fiction? *Friends of the Earth Newsmagazine.* 2005;35(4):4–7.

Gerencser S. The Corporate person and democratic politics. *Polit Res Q.* 2005;58:625–635.

Giroux HS. The corporate war against higher education. *Workplace.* October 2002;5(1). Available at: http://louisville.edu/journal/workplace/issue5p1/giroux.html. Accessed September 15, 2009.

Greenhouse S, Barbaro M. An ugly side of free trade: sweatshops in Jordan. *New York Times.* May 3, 2006;C1, C7.

Green D, Griffith M. Globalization and its discontents. *Int Aff.* 2002;78(1):49–68.

Gregor F, Ellis H. Fair law: legal proposals to improve corporate cccountability for environmental and human rights abuses. European Coalition for Corporate Justice. Available at: http://www.corporatejustice.org/IMG/pdf/ECCJ_FairLaw.pdf. Published 2008. Accessed September 15, 2009.

Gross D. To the rich, from America. *Newsweek.* January 28, 2008;17.

Grossman R. Part I: Can corporations be accountable. *Rachel's Environment & Health Weekly* #609. Women's International League for Peace & Freedom. Available at: http://www.wilpf.org/docs/ccp/corp/2006-II-CompleteSession.pdf. Published July 30, 1998. Accessed September 15, 2009.

Guevara MW, Willison K. Big tobacco's New York black market: How America's top cigarette firms fueled a billion-dollar trade. Center for Public Integrity. Available at: http://www.publicintegrity.org/investigations/tobacco/articles/entry/1084/. Published December 19, 2008. Accessed September 18, 2009.

Guttal S. Globalisation. *Dev Pract.* 2007;17(4–5):523–531.

Halperin D. Discovery abuse: how defendants in products liability lawsuits hide and destroy evidence. Public Citizen Congress Watch. Available at: http://www.citizen.org/congress/civjus/archive/tort/tortlaw/articles.cfm?ID=918. Published 1997. Accessed September 15, 2009.

Hammerstrom D. The Hijacking of the Fourteenth Amendment Women's International League for Peace & Freedom. Available at: http://www.wilpf.org/docs/ccp/hijacking_of_14.pdf.

Hansen WL, Mitchell NJ, Drope JM. Collective action, pluralism, and the legitimacy tariff: corporate activity or inactivity in politics. *Polit Res Q.* 2004;57:421–429.

Hart JT. Health care or health trade? A historical moment of choice. *Int J Health Serv.* 2004;34(2):245–254.

Hawken P. *Blessed Unrest: How the Largest Movement in the World Came into Being and Why No One Saw It Coming.* New York: Penguin; 2007.

Hearson M. Cashing in: giant retailers, purchasing practices, and working conditions in the garment industry. Clean Clothes Campaign. Available at: http://www.

cleanclothes.org/bb-news/1270-ccc-cashing-in-research-report-launched. Published 2009. Accessed September 15, 2009.

Hemphill TA. Physicians and the pharmaceutical industry: a reappraisal of marketing codes of conduct. *Business and Society Review.* 2006;111(3):323–336.

Huff J. Industry influence on occupational and environmental public health. *Int J Occup Environ Health.* 2007;13:107–117.

Institute of Medicine. Brief Summary: Institute of Medicine Regional Symposium: Progress in Preventing Childhood Obesity: Focus on Industry. December 1, 2005. The National Academy of Sciences: National Academies Press. Available at: http://books.nap.edu/openbook.php?record_id=11614&page=R1. Accessed September 15, 2009.

Interfaith Center on Corporate Responsibility. About ICCR. Available at: http://www.iccr.org/about/. Accessed September 15, 2009.

International Forum on Globalization. *Alternatives to Economic Globalization: A Better World Is Possible.* San Francisco: Berrett-Koehler Publishers, Inc.; 2002.

Irogbe K. Globalization and the development of the underdevelopment of the third world. *Journal of Third World Studies.* 2005;XXII(1):41–68.

Jacobson MF. Lifting the veil of secrecy from industry funding of nonprofit health organizations. *Int J Occup Environ Health.* 2005;11:349–355.

Jacobstein JM. Federal regulatory pre-emption of state tort claims against the manufacturers of medical devices and pharmaceutical drugs. *J Law Med Ethics.* 2008;36(3):594–597.

Jacques P, Thomas R, Foster D, McCann J, Tunno M. Wal-mart or world-mart? A teaching case study. *Rev Radic Polit Econ.* 2003;35:513–533.

Jones-Webb R, McKee P, Wall M, Pham L, Erickson D, Wagenarr A. Alcohol and malt liquor availability and promotion and homicide in inner cities. *Subst Use Misuse.* 2008;43:159–177.

Karabell Z. Green really means business. *Newsweek.* September 22, 2008:E6.

Kassirer J. *On the Take: How Medicine's Complicity with Big Business Can Endanger Your Health.* New York: Oxford University Press; 2005.

Kelley B. How the auto industry sets read blocks to safety: remember the Susuki Samari. *Business and Society Review.* 1992;83:50–53.

Kellman P. Labor must challenge corporate rule. By What Authority. Available at: http://www.wilpf.org/docs/ccp/corp/2006-VI-CompleteSession.pdf. Published Spring 1999. Accessed September 18, 2009.

Kendall D, Rylander J. Tainted justice: how private judicial trips undermine public trust in the federal judiciary. Community Rights Counsel. Available at: http://www.theusconstitution.org/upload/filelists/163_Chap4.pdf. Published 2004. Accessed September 15, 2009.

Kendall D, Sorkin E. Nothing for free. How Private Judicial Seminars are Undermining Environmental Protections and Breaking the Public's Trust. Community Rights Counsel. Available at: http://www.theusconstitution.org/upload/filelists/152_Chapter2.pdf. Published 2000. Accessed September 15, 2009.

Klein N. *Fences and Windows.* New York: Picador; 2002.

Klein N. *No Logo.* New York: Picador; 2002b.

Klein N. *The Shock Doctrine: The Rise of Disaster Capitalism*. New York: Picador; 2007.

Koenig-Archibugi M. Transnational corporations and public accountability. *Government and Opposition, Ltd.* 2004;39(2):234–259.

Komisar L. Profit laundering and tax evasion: the dirty little secret of financial globalization. *Dissent.* 2005;Spring:48–54.

Korten DC. *When Corporations Rule the World*. San Francisco: Berrett-Koehler Publishers, Inc.; 1995.

Korten DC. *The Great Turning: From Empire to Earth Community*. San Francisco: Berrett-Koehler Publishers; 2006.

Kriebel D, Tickner J. Reenergizing public health through precaution. *Am J Public Health.* 2001;91(9): 1351–1355.

Krieger J. Social policy in the age of Reagan and Thatcher. *Socialist Register.* 1987;23:177–198. Available at: http://socialistregister.com/index.php/srv/article/view/5545/2443.

Krieger N. Theories for social epidemiology in the 21st century: an ecosocial perspective. *Int J Epidemiol.* 2001;30:668–677.

Krimsky S. *Science in the Private Interest: Has the Lure of Profits Corrupted Biomedical Research?* Lanham, JD: Rowman & Littlefield Publishers, Inc.; 2003.

Landman A, Glanz S. Tobacco industry efforts to undermine policy-relevant research. *Am J Public Health.* 2009;99(1):45–58.

Lang T. Public health and colonialism: a new or old problem? *J Epidemiol Community Health.* 2001;55:162–163.

Lasn K, Liacas T. 1600–1886: the birth of the corporate "I": the birth. Adbusters. Women's International League for Peace & Freedom. Available at: http://www.wilpf.org/docs/ccp/corp/2006-III-CompleteSession.pdf. Published August/September 2000. Accessed September 15, 2009.

Law MR, Majumdar SR, Soumerai SB. Effect of illicit direct to consumer advertising on use of etanercept, mometasone, and tegaserod in Canada: controlled longitudinal study. *BMJ.* 2008;337(a1055):1–7.

Learner, M. (nd). The Social Responsibility Amendment. Network of Spiritual Progressives Available at: http://www.spiritualprogressives.org/article.php/socialjustice. Accessed September 15, 2009.

Lee ET. Should not the 14th Amendment to the Constitution of the United States be amended? An Address to the Gary, Indiana, Bar Association. Women's International League for Peace & Freedom. Available at: http://www.wilpf.org/docs/ccp/corp/2006-III-CompleteSession.pdf. Published November 20, 1936. Accessed September 15, 2009.

Lee K, Sridhar D, Patel M. Bridging the divide: global governance of trade and health. *Lancet.* 2009;373:416–422.

LeRoy G. The great American jobs scam. CorpWatch. Available at: http://www.corpwatch.org/article.php?id=12540. Published August 10, 2005. Accessed September 15, 2009.

Lesser LI, Ebbeling CB, Goozner M, Wypij D, Ludwig DS. Relationship between funding source and conclusion among nutrition-related scientific articles. *PLoS Med.* 2007;4(1):e5. doi:10.1371/journal.pmed.0040005.

Lewit D. Who runs the U.N.?: a half century of corporate influence. The Alliance for Democracy. Available at: http://www.thealliancefordemocracy.org/html/eng/1629-AA.shtml. Published 2000. Accessed September 15, 2009.

Linzey T. A citizen's guide to corporate charter revocation under state law. The Community Environmental Legal Defense Fund. Available at: http://www.celdf.org/DocumentCenter/tabid/101/Default.aspx. Published 1996. Accessed September 15, 2009.

Locke M. Green MBAs: new programs teach balancing profit and the plane. *Arizona Daily Sun.* September 30, 2007; D1, D5.

Love J. Pharmaceutical research and development and the patent system. *Int J Health Serv.* 2005;35(2):257–263.

Lowy M, Betto F. Values of a new civilization. In: Fisher WF, Ponniah T, eds. *Another World Is Possible: Popular Alternatives to Globalization at the World Social Forum.* New York: Zed Books; 2003.

Loy D. *The Great Awakening: A Buddhist Social Theory.* Boston, MA: Wisdom Publications; 2003.

Lyles A. Direct marketing of pharmaceuticals to consumer. *Annu Rev Public Health.* 2002;23:73–91.

Macy J. The great turning. *Yes! Magazine.* 2000;Spring. Available at: http://www.yesmagazine.org/pdf/Macy_Great_Turning.pdf. Accessed September 15, 2009.

Maher A, Wilson N, Signal L, Thomson G. Patterns of sports sponsorship by gambling, alcohol and food companies: an Internet survey. *BMC Public Health.* 2006;6(95):1–9.

Mander J, ed. Manifesto on global economic transitions. *The International Forum on Globalization.* The Institute for Policy Studies, & the Global Project on Economic Transitions; 2007.

Mander J, Tauli-Corpuz *Paradigm Wars: Indigenous Peoples' Resistance to Globalization.* San Francisco: Sierra Club Books; 2006.

Mangan K. Medical schools see many ties to industry. *Chronicle of Higher Education.* October 26, 2007;LIV(9):A31.

Manila Declaration. *Declaration of the International Conference on Extractive Industries and Indigenous Peoples.* Legend Villas, Metro Manila, Philippines; March 23–25, 2009.

Marx M, Margil M, Cavanagh J, et al. Strategic Corporate Initiative: Toward a Global Citizens' Movement to Bring Corporations Back Under Control. Corporate Ethics International. Available at: http://corpethics.org/downloads/SCI_Report_September_2007.pdf. Published 2007. Accessed September 15, 2009.

Masterson A. Research and inventions earn big bucks for American Universities. *Chronicle of Higher Education.* February 6, 2009;A16.

Mattera P. USDA Inc.: how agribusiness has hijacked regulatory policy at the U.S. Department of Agriculture. Available at: http://www.agribusinessaccountability.org/clearinghouse/viewDoc.php?id=204. Published 2004. Accessed September 15, 2009.

Mayell H. As consumerism spreads, earth suffers, study says. National Geographic. Com/News. January 12, 2004.

Mayer C. Personalizing the impersonal: corporations and the bill of rights. *Hastings Law J.* 1990;41 Hastings 577:1–82.

Mayer C. The corporation and the constitution. Taming the giant corporation: a national conference on corporate accountability. Available at: http://video.google.com/videoplay?docid=9200589775601266335#. Published 2007. Accessed September 15, 2009.

McIntyre B. United States Remains One of the Least Taxed Industrial Countries. Citizens for Tax Justice. Available at: http://www.ctj.org/pdf/oecd07.pdf. Published April 26, 2007. Accessed September 15, 2009.

McIntyre RS, Coo Nguyen TD. State Corporate Income Taxes 2001–2003. Citizens for Tax Justice and the Institute on Taxation and Economic Policy; February 2005.

McIntyre RS, Coo Nguyen TD. Corporate Income Taxes in the Bush Years. Citizens for Tax Justice and the Institute on Taxation and Economic Policy; September 2004.

McKibben B. Hype vs. hope: Is corporate do-goodery for real? Mother Jones. Available at:http://www.motherjones.com/news/feature/2006/11/hype_vs_hope.html. Published November/December 2006. Accessed September 15, 2009.

McNally D. *Another World Is Possible: Globalization & Anti-capitalism.* Winnipeg, Manitoba: Arbeiter Ring Publishing; 2006.

McNeil DG. Gates Foundation's Influence Criticized. *New York Times.* February 16, 2008.

Meacham J, Thomas E. We are all socialists now. *Newsweek.* February 16, 2009.

Michaels D. *Doubt Is Their Product: How Industry's Assault on Science Threatens Your Health.* New York: Oxford University Press; 2008.

Miller D. Democracy and Corporate Spin's part in its downfall. Republished from SpinWatch. Available at: http://www.guerrillanews.com/headlines/9180/Democracy_and_Corporate_Spin_s_part_in_its_downfall. Published May 19, 2006. Accessed September 15, 2009.

Miller D. The corporate takeover of reason and science. SpinWatch: Monitoring PR and Spin. Available at: http://www.spinwatch.org/-articles-by-category-mainmenu-8/41-corporate-spin/5130-the-corporate-takeover-of-reason-and-science. Published August 8, 2008. Accessed September 15, 2009.

Mintzberg H. Patent nonsense: evidence tells of an industry out of social control. *CMAJ.* 2006;175(4):1–7.

Miyoshi M. A borderless world? From colonialism to transnationalism and the decline of the nation-state. *Crit Inq.* 1993;19:726–751.

Mokhiber R. Top 100 Corporate Criminals of the Decade: 1990s. Corporate Crime Reporter. Available at: http://www.corporatepredators.org/top100.html. Accessed September 15, 2009.

Monforton C. Weight of the evidence or wait for the evidence? Protecting underground miners from diesel particulate matter. *Am J Public Health.* 2006;96:271–276.

Mooney C. As the world burns: some like it hot. Mother Jones. Available at: http://www.motherjones.com/environment/2005/05/some-it-hot. Published May/June 2005. Accessed September 15, 2009.

Moore WJ, Chachere DR, Curtis TD, Gordon D. The Political Influence of Unions and Corporations on COPE Votes in the U.S. Senate, 1979–1988. *J Labor Res.* 1995;XVI(2):203–221.

Morris JA. Sheep in wolf's clothing. By what authority, 1(1). Program on Corporations, Law and Democracy. Available at: http://www.poclad.org/bwa/fall98.htm. Published 1998. Accessed September 15, 2009.

MS&L Worldwide. 19% of senior marketers-or one in five- say their organizations have bought advertising in return for a news story. Available at: 200http://www.mslworldwide.com/in-the-news/press-releases/19-of-senior-marketers-or-one-in-five-say-their-organizations-have-bought-advertising-in-return-for-a-news-story. Published July 30, 2008. Accessed September 15, 2009.

Multinational Monitor. Editorial: You don't know Jack. Available at: http://www.multinationalmonitor.org/mm2001/01july-august/julyaug01editorial.html. Published July/August 2001. Accessed September 15, 2009.

Mushita A, Thompson CB. *Biopiracy of Biodiversity: Global Exchange as Enclosure.* Trenton, NJ: African World Press, Inc.; 2007.

Muthu S. Adam Smith's critique of international trading companies: theorizing "globalization" in the age of enlightment. *Political Theory.* 2008;36(2):185–212.

Mychalejko Canadian company threatens El Salvador with free trade lawsuit over mining project. Upside Down World. Available at: http://upsidedownworld.org/main/content/view/1637/1/. Published December 19, 2008. Accessed September 15, 2009.

Nace T. *Gangs of America: The Rise of Corporate Power and the Disabling of Democracy.* San Francisco: Berrett-Koehler; 2003.

National Cancer Institute The role of the media in promoting and reducing tobacco use. NCI Tobacco Control Monograph Series # 19. U.S. Department of Health and Human Services; 2008.

Navarro V. Neoliberalism as a class ideology; or, the political causes of the growth of inequalities. *Int J Health Serv.* 2007;37(1):47–62.

Nelson M. Somewhere to go. *The Chronicle of Higher Education.* January 26, 2007;B16.

Nestle M. Soft drink "Pouring Rights": marketing empty calories to children. *Public Health Rep.* 2000;115(4):308–319.

Nestle M. *Food Politics: How the Food Industry Influences Nutrition and Health.* Berkely, CA: University of California Press; 2002.

Nestle M, Jacobson MF. Halting the obesity epidemic: a public health policy approach. *Public Health Rep.* 2000;115(1):12–24.

News Batch. Tort reform. Available at: http://www.newsbatch.com/tort.htm. Published 2006. Accessed September 15, 2009.

Newsweek (a)(January 26, 2009). The Demographics: Swing to the Left. p 49

Newsweek (b). Sorry, don't know anyone by that name. March 2, 2009:9.

O'Connor JC, MacNeil A, Chriqui JF, Tynan M, Bates H, Eidson SKS. Preemption of local smoke-free air ordinances: the implications of judicial opinions for meeting national health objectives. *J Law Med Ethics*. 2008;36(2):403–412.

Open Secrets (nd). Lobbying: Top Industries 2008. Available at: http://www. opensecrets.org/lobby/top.php?showYear=2008&indexType=i. Accessed September 16, 2009.

Patel R. Apartheid in America. Corporation Watch <corporation-watch@countercorp. org>. March 12, 2009.

Patel R, Torres RJ, Rosset P. Genetic engineering in agriculture and corporate engineering in public debate: risk, public relations, and public debate over genetically modified crops. *Int J Occup Environ Health*. 2005;11:428–436.

Peabody J. When the flock ignores the shepherd - corralling the undisclosed use of video news releases. *Federal Communications Law Journal*. 2008;60(3):577–596.

Peet R. *Unholy Trinity: The IMF, World Bank and WTO*. New York: Zed Books; 2003.

Perwin A. Mandatory binding arbitration: civil injustice by corporate America. White Paper No. 13. Center for Justice and Democracy; August 2005.

Piller C, Sanders E, Dixon R. Dark cloud over good works of Gates Foundation. *Los Angeles Times*, January 7, 2007. Available at: http://www.latimes.com/news/ nationworld/nation/la-na-gatesx07jan07,0,6827615.story?page=1. Accessed September 16, 2009.

Pollack A. crop scientists say biotechnology seed companies are thwarting research. *New York Times*, February 20, 2009. Available at: http://www.nytimes. com/2009/02/20/business/20crop.html?_r=1&pagewanted=print. Accessed September 16, 2009.

Primack BA, Bost JE, Land SR, Fine MJ. Volume of tobacco advertising in African American markets: systematic review and meta- analysis. *Public Health Rep*. 2007;122(5):607–615.

Public Broadcasting System. What's your beef? News Hour with Jim Lehrer transcript. Available at: http://www.pbs.org/newshour/bb/law/jan-june98/ fooddef_1-20.html. Published January 20, 1998. Accessed September 16, 2009.

Public Citizen. How our civil justice system protects consumers. Available at: http:// www.citizen.org/congress/civjus/articles.cfm?ID=7545. Published April 29, 2002. Accessed September 16, 2009.

Public Citizen. Limiting punitive damages: what will deter bad corporate conduct now? Available at: http://www.citizen.org/congress/civjus/archive/tort/ tortlaw/articles.cfm?ID=835. Published March 25, 2001. Accessed September 16, 2009.

Public Citizen. Profits over lives—long-hidden documents reveal GM cost-benefit analyses led to severe burn injuries; disregard for safety spurred large verdict. Available at: http://www.citizen.org/congress/civjus/archive/tort/tortlaw/articles. cfm?ID=570. Accessed September 16, 2009.

Punch M. Suite violence: why managers murder and corporations kill. *Crime Law Soc Change*. 2000;33:243–280.

PR Watch. Wikis prove tricky for PR firms. *PR Week*, August 31, 2007. Available at: http://www.prwatch.org/node/6413. Accessed September 16, 2009.

PR Watch. Connaughton's New Job: Greenwashing Constellation. Available at: http://www.prwatch.org/node/8236. Published February 23, 2009. Accessed September 16, 2009.

Rabin R. The lead industry and lead water pipes: "a modest campaign." *Am J Public Health.* 2008;98:1584–1592.

Raloff J. Diabetes drug and conflicts of interest. *Science News.* February 9, 2008;173:92.

Ranii D. Group urges NCSU to end deal with Bayer News Observer. Available at: http://www.newsobserver.com/news/story/1384337.html. Published January 29, 2009. Accessed September 16, 2009.

Raphael D. Social determinants of health: present status, unanswered questions and future directions. *Int J Health Serv.* 2006;36(4):651–677.

Reich RB. *Supercapitalism: The Transformation of Business, Democracy, and Everyday Life.* New York: Knopf; 2007.

Reitan R. *Global Activism.* New York: Routledge; 2007.

Revolving Door Working Group. A matter of trust: how the revolving door undermines public confidence in government—and what to do about it. Available at: www.revolvingdoor.info. Published October 2005.

Ridgeway J. It's the deregulation, stupid. Mother Jones. Available at: http://www.motherjones.com/politics/2008/03/its-deregulation-stupid. Published March 28, 2008. Accessed September 16, 2009.

Ridgeway J, Schulman D, CornD. There's something about Mary: unmasking a gun lobby mole. Mother Jones. Available at: http:// http://www.motherjones.com/politics/2008/07/theres-something-about-mary-unmasking-gun-lobby-mole. Published July 30, 2008. Accessed September 16, 2009.

Rifkin I. *Spiritual Perspectives on Globalization: Making Sense of Economic and Cultural Upheaval.* Woodstock, VT: Skylight Paths Publishing; 2003.

Roelofs J. The mask of pluralism. Available at: http://www.icdc.com/~paulwolf/oss/maskofpluralism.htm. Published 2003. Accessed September 16, 2009.

Roelofs J. Foundations and collaboration. *Crit Sociol.* 2007;33:479–504.

Rosner D, & Markowitz G. Industry challenges to the principle of prevention in public health: the precautionary principle. *Public Health Reports.* 2002;117:501–512.

Rowell A. *The Dangers of Co-optation with Corporations.* Spinwatch: Monitoring PR and Spin; 1998. Available at: http://www.spinwatch.org/-articles-by-category-mainmenu-8/41-corporate-spin/17-the-dangers-of-co-optation-with-corporations. Accessed September 16, 2009.

Rutkow L, Teret SP. Limited liability and the public's health. *J Law Med Ethics.* 2007;35(4):599–608.

Rutkow L, Vernick JS, James, G, Hodge, Jr, JG, Teret SP. Preemption and the obesity epidemic: state and local menu labeling laws and the nutrition labeling and education act. *J Law Med Ethics.* 2008;36(4):772–789.

Rubin R. "Too cozy" with drugmakers? *USA Today,* March 3, 2005.

Salant J.D. Pfizer, Halliburton Grab Democrats as Hearings Loom. Bloomberg.com. Available at: http://www.bloomberg.com/apps/news?pid=20601070&sid=a8fyOQYvbFQ8. Published January 31, 2007. Accessed September 16, 2009.

Samuelson RJ. The great shopping spree. *R.I.P. Newsweek.* April 28, 2008;49.

Saul S. US: Pfizer to end Lipitor ads by Jarvik. *The New York Times,* February 26, 2008. Available at: http://www.corpwatch.org/article.php?id=14948. Accessed September 16, 2009.

Schulte B. Teaming up with the enemy. *U.S. News & World Report,* November 19, 2007;54–56.

Seidman GW. Monitoring multinationals: lessons from the anti-apartheid era politics society. *Politics & Society.* 2003;31:381–406.

Shaffer E, Brenner J. Advice and no dissent: public health and the rigged U.S. trade advisory system. *Multinational Monitor.* 2004;25(11):1–8.

Shaffer ES, Brenner JE, Houston TP. International trade agreements: a threat to tobacco control policy. *Tob Control.* 2005;14:19–25.

Shaffer ER, Waitzkin H, Brenner J, Jasso-Aguilar R. Global trade and public health. *Am J Public Health.* 2005;95:23–34.

Shaker E. Corporate Initiatives on Campus: A 2008 Snapshot. Canadian Center for Policy Alternatives. Available at: www.policyalternatives.ca. Published 2008.

Shank JW. The case for regulation-some—republican anti-business regulation stance. *Washington Monthly,* March 1995.

Shelton DL. Hospitals send formula home with baby while encouraging mother to breast-feed. *Chicago Tribune,* September 2, 2008. Available at: http://archives. chicagotribune.com/2008/sep/02/health/chi-formula-samples_tuessep02. Accessed September 16, 2009.

Simon DR. Corporate environmental crimes and social inequality: new directions for environmental justice research. *Am Behav Sci.* 2000;43:633–645.

Simmer-Brown J. Remedying globalization and consumerism: joining the inner and outer journeys in "Perfect Balance." *Buddhist-Christian Studies.* 2002;22:31–46.

Sklair L. The transnational capitalist class and global politics: deconstructing the corporate-state connection. *International Political Science Review.* 2002;23:159–174.

Spitzer S. A systemic approach to occupational and environmental health. *Int J Occup Environ Health.* 2005;11:444–455.

Spivack P., Raman S. Regulating the 'New Regulators': current trends in deferred prosecution agreements. *Am Criminal Law Review.* 2008;45(2):150–193.

SourceWatch SourceWatch Project on Tracking Attempts to Spin Wikipedia. Available at: http://www.sourcewatch.org/index.php?title=SourceWatch:Project:Track ing_attempts_to_spin_Wikipedia. Published September 8, 2007. Accessed September 16, 2009.

SourceWatch. Burson-Marsteller. SourceWatch Encyclopedia. Available at: http:// www.sourcewatch.org/index.php?title=Burson_Marsteller. Accessed September 16, 2009.

Starr A. *Naming the Enemy: Anti-corporate Movements Confront Globalization.* New York: Zed Books; 2000.

Starr A. *Global Revolt: A Guide to the Movements Against Globalization.* New York: Zed Books; 2005.

Steck H. Corporatization of the university: seeking conceptual clarity. *Ann Am Acad Pol Soc Sci.* 2003;585:66–83.

Stuckler D, King L, McKee M. Mass privatization and the post-communist mortality crisis: a cross-national analysis. *Lancet.* 2009;373(9661):399–407.

Swiss ATTAC. Nestlé/Attac/Securitas: legal complaint against X. Available at: http://www.suisse.attac.org/druckformat.php3?id_article=1822. Published June 13, 2008. Accessed September 16, 2009.

Taillant JD. Chevron lobbyist reveals imperialist corporate attitude. Center for Human Rights and Environment. escr-corp-accountability@yahoogroups.com. August 29, 2008.

Tanner L. Ghostwriters for medical research criticized, reforms urged. Available at: http://www.newsvine.com/_news/2008/04/15/1432771-ghostwriters-for-medical-research-criticized-reforms-urged?threadId=251414. Published April 15, 2008. Accessed September 16, 2009.

Tesler LE, Malone RE. Corporate philanthropy, lobbying, and public health policy. *Amer J Public Health.* 2008;98(12):2123–2133.

The Center for Media and Democracy. Source Watch: Front Groups. Available at: http://www.sourcewatch.org/index.php?title=Front_groups.

The Center for Public Integrity. Latest Center analysis reveals explosive growth in the climate change lobby: Washington now boasts more than four climate lobbyists for every member of congress. Available at: http://www.publicintegrity.org/news/entry/1187/. Published February 25, 2009.

The Yes Men [DVD]. Los Angeles, CA: United Artists. Available at: http://theyesmen.org/. Published 2004.

Thomas E, Hirsh M. Rubin's detail deficit. *Newsweek,* December 8, 2008;45.

Tsosie R. Cultural challenges to biotechnology: Native American genetic resources and the concept of cultural harm. *J Law Med Ethics.* 2007;35(3):396–411.

United Nations Sub-Commission on the Promotion and Protection of Human Rights Resolution. Norms on the responsibilities of transnational corporations and other business enterprises with regard to human rights. U.N. Doc. E/CN.4/Sub.2/2003/L.11 at 52. Available at: http://www.unhchr.ch/huridocda/huridoca.nsf/(Symbol)/E.CN.4.Sub.2.2003.12.Rev.2.En?Opendocument. Published 2003. Accessed September 16, 2009.

United Nations. The principles of the global compact. Available at: http://www.unglobalcompact.org/docs/news_events/8.1/after_the_signature.pdf. Accessed September 16, 2009.

Vaughn M. Senate probes increase in offshore accounts. *Wall St J.* July 24, 2008. Available at: http://online.wsj.com/article/SB121686880772780155.html?mod=djemITP. Accessed September 16, 2009.

Vollmer S. Italy is latest to ban sale of Bayer pesticide. *News and Observer,* September 19, 2008. Available at: http://www.newsobserver.com/business/nc/story/1224224.html. Accessed September 16, 2009.

Wallis J. *God's Politics: Why the Right Gets It Wrong and the Left Doesn't Get It.* New York: HarperCollins Publishers; 2006.

Washburn J. *University, Inc.: The Corporate Corruption of American Higher Education.* New York: Basic Books; 2005.

Wehrfritz G, Kinetz E, Kent J. Bottom of the barrel: millions of Asian workers producing good sold here are trapped in servitude. *Newsweek,* March 24, 2008; 41, 43.

Weisberg J. Obam's big-picture problem. *Newsweek,* February 2, 2009; 37.

Weissman R, Donahue J. Wall Street's best investment: ten deregulatory steps to financial meltdown. *Multinational Monitor.* January/February, 2009;30(1). Available at: http://www.multinationalmonitor.org/mm2009/012009/ weissman.html. Accessed September 16, 2009.

Wells D. Too weak for the job: corporate codes of conduct, non-governmental organizations and the regulation of international labour standards. *Global Social Policy.* 2007;7:51–73.

White A, Kelly M, eds. Summit on the future of the corporation: paper series on corporate design. Corporation 20/20 & Society for Organizational Learning. Available at: http://www.corporation2020.org/pdfs/SummitPaperSeries.pdf. Published 2007. Accessed Septmber 16, 2009.

Wiist WH. Public health and the anticorporate movement: rationale and recommendations. *Am J Public Health.* 2006;96:1370–1375.

Wiist WH. Corporate strategies to influence trade & health policies. Oral presentation at the *Annual Meeting of the American Public Health Association,* November 7, 2007; Washington, D.C.

Wingert P. Teens, tans and truth. *Newsweek,* May 19, 2008, 42.

Wolbert CJ. Tort Law: Desiano and the Second Circuit's Repudiation of de jure Tort Reform. *J Law Med Ethics.* 2007;35(3):500–502.

Women's International League for Peace & Freedom. WILPF's Campaign to Challenge Corporate Power and Assert the People's Rights, October, 1999. Session I, Reading 3, 1–7. Available at: http://www.wilpf.org/docs/ccp/ corp/2006-I-CompleteSession.pdf. Accessed September 16, 2009.

Women's International League for Peace and Freedom. Declaration to abolish corporate personhood. Available at: http://wilpf.org/docs/ccp/corp/ACP/ declaration.pdf. Accessed September 16, 2009.

Yashar DJ. Resistance and identity politics in an age of globalization. *Ann Am Acad Pol Soc Sci.* 2007;610:160–181.

2

Corporations, Public Health, and the Historical Landscape that Defines Our Challenge

Shelley K. White

> Corporations have emerged as the dominant governance
> institutions on the planet, with the largest among them
> reaching into virtually every country of the world and exceed-
> ing most governments in size and power. Increasingly, it is
> the corporate interest rather than the human interest that
> defines the policy agendas of states and international bodies.
> (Korten, 2001:60)

When was it that public health began taking a backseat to corporate
profits? How is it that we have reached a point today where
the rulings of our global courts permit corporations to dump
toxins into our environment and punish governments that try to
intervene? Since when have such indicators as infant mortality been
subordinated to indicators such as trademark protection? Today's
corporations have at their disposal a deep bag of powerful strategies
for avoiding losses and obligations and for maximizing their returns,
often at great cost to public health and human protections. But
where did this unprecedented level of power come from? How did
corporations gain the legal, political, and social capital they have
today to maneuver so powerfully in our global society?

The powers and privileges corporations enjoy today were
certainly not a mainstay throughout history. In fact, although
corporate dominance has historical precedence, anticorporate

movements and the wane of corporations have also characterized major historical periods in America's history. Our nation's very founding and early days centered on limiting the excesses of corporations. When we examine the history of corporations, we can conceive of the negotiation between private and public interests—between corporations and our governance structures—as a pendulum swinging. When it swings one way, corporations are largely unregulated and left to their own devices in the free market. When it swings the other way, the public pushes back on the private, and corporations and markets are more carefully regulated.

The dominance corporations hold today was arrived at incrementally, and sometimes explosively, over time, but at each step of the way, corporations have faced some level of negotiation with our governments and courts, as well as with public citizens and academics. During every historical period, and with each movement of this metaphoric pendulum of corporate rights, citizens have played a critically important role. The powers that corporations acquire never expand unquestioned, and the counterstrategies we have available to us today are built in part from a powerful history of citizen movements that have defended human rights and public health in the face of corporate infringements. Likewise, academics (particularly those from economics and business) have held an important place in shaping this debate, in guiding conventional wisdoms, and even in shaping the very government policies that ultimately determine the appropriate extent of regulation of markets and corporate entities.

In examining the history that this chapter presents, it becomes quite clear that public health professionals, in their roles as citizens, academics, and practitioners, have a critical role to play in this debate, and in shaping this next era of corporate rights and human welfare. Although the rights of corporations today largely interfere with our capacity to protect and promote public health, the long history of corporate development ensures us that change is possible. Indeed, the contemporary state of corporate privilege is already beginning to crack. The recent environment of economic recession, epidemic sub-prime mortgage foreclosures, and government bailouts have created a public dialogue about the integrity of the unfettered free markets that have guided us through this most recent pendulum swing (Berenson, 2008; National Public Radio, 2008; Theil, 2008). It has also created an historical opening for reinfusing public health principles into the regulation of corporate practices, and thus requires the concerted efforts of the public health profession to guide us through this next historical chapter. First, however, it is important to explore the history of how we arrived to this point.

Early Corporations Spur Colonial American Resistances

The earliest corporate entities emerged during the 16th and 17th centuries under the British and Dutch crowns. Evolving from earlier partnership-style guilds, merchant and trading companies, these new entities initiated some of the most important features of modern corporations—joint-stock pooled capital, limited liability and corporate immortality. Prior to this, businesses had been limited as to how much capital they could raise, as they were both funded and managed by small partnerships of individuals. Even early trading companies were limited to raising funds from individual voyage to voyage, which curbed the lifespan of these companies and left investors liable for short-term losses (Bakan, 2005; Hartmann, 2002; Nace, 2003).

Joint-stock companies were formed as larger-scale commerce and overseas exploration developed in the late 1500s. Trading companies began to experiment with pooled capital, allowing investors to share risk with others and invest in companies over a period of time or over many voyages. The British East India Company (BEIC), chartered in 1600 to explore trade and colonize in foreign lands, was the first to fully develop joint-stock shareholder mechanisms (Drutman & Cray, 2004). It moved from raising funds per voyage, to raising funds for limited time periods, to ultimately issuing permanent stock in 1613 (Nace, 2003). This mechanism of pooling capital was a critical development for corporations as it separated owner from manager and expanded the possible scope of funds companies could raise through the sale of tradable public shares.

Moreover, the corporation came to exist as a single entity, rather than an association of partners, and gained a legally separate identity from its owners. This is significant because it allowed for corporate immortality: corporations could now outlive their owners and could potentially exist forever. It also opened the door for limited liability whereby owners' financial liability could be limited, for example, to the sum of their investment. Thus, owners could be free from responsibility for debts assumed by their companies, as the business was now legally separate from its owner (Bakan, 2005; Nace, 2003).

The British East India Company is an important historical example of corporate power. Beyond the economic power it consolidated, the company also quickly gained global geopolitical standing. Through the corporate charter and broad rights it gained from the British crown, it formed an army larger than any other standing army in the world and fought local and European forces to gain control over India and its surrounding islands. It effectively governed India, setting up laws and courts, taxes and broad military forces, for nearly a century beginning in the 1750s. It also dominated the opium trade in China and managed a slave trade out of Madagascar (Osborne, 2007).

At home, the BEIC became so politically entrenched that a third of Parliament's members held its stock, 10% of the British government's revenues derived from a tax on its tea, and the King depended upon loans from the company (Nace, 2003). Companies like the BEIC played a key role in the expansion of the British Empire and its colonies, and set up corporate practices of exploiting labor and extracting wealth globally to create returns at home. In exchange for such benefits, the crown granted such corporations special privileges and monopoly rights, and bribes and corruption were not uncommon (Osborne, 2007). This transfer of wealth from colony to empire was an important foreshadowing of today's corporate transfer of wealth from global south to global north countries that often benefits America's elite. Similarly, the tendency toward exploitative labor practices that would have raised public health concerns then is still with us today.

The BEIC also dominated America during its reign, establishing the first colony of Jamestown in 1606 via its affiliate, the Virginia Company. The company thrived through its use of conscripted labor, capturing and transporting thousands of Britain's dispossessed to work as forced laborers in the colony, 80% of whom died during their 7-year tenure (Nace, 2003). By 1770, the BEIC controlled nearly all trade into and out of America, but was almost bankrupt from its rapid global expansion. An important threat to the company's viability was competition from small colonial businesses importing tea and other provisions either independently or in cooperation with BEIC's Dutch competitors. With its strong favor already established in Parliament, the BEIC pressured Britain to pass laws expanding its monopoly, including the 1773 Tea Act that tipped off the Boston Tea Party (Hartmann, 2002).

As a precursor to what we know as corporate welfare today, the Tea Act lifted tariffs on the BEIC's tea so it could dump its excess product into the colonies, increase its profitability, and drive smaller competitors out of business, to ensure its long-term monopoly over the global tea trade. Small businessmen and entrepreneurs, both British and American, organized protests and resistances against this early multinational corporate maneuver and the government complicity behind it. In the most consequential response, Boston Tea Party protestors dumped over 90,000 pounds—today's equivalent of one million dollar's worth—of BEIC's tea into Boston Harbor. This resulted in Britain closing Boston Harbor for more than a year and a half, and eventually led to the famed battles of Lexington and Concord (Hartmann, 2002). The American Revolution itself, then, was instigated by a popular anticorporate movement. Following the Revolution, America's founding leaders expressed deep suspicions about corporations and were determined to protect the new nation from their associated corruption (Drutman & Cray, 2004; Meyers, 2000).

America's Founders Envision Citizen Protections

In the years following the American Revolution, as the federal government was newly organizing and drafting the constitution, very few corporations existed. Corporations were not seen as a necessity in American society by most, and were seen as a potential threat by many. At the Constitutional Convention of 1787, James Madison (with Benjamin Franklin's support) proposed authorizing federal control over corporations, but the states resisted this concentration of power as reminiscent of the conditions that created the BEIC. Instead, the constitution ultimately omitted all reference to corporations, leaving the granting of corporate charters to individual states. It was judged that keeping corporate matters as local as possible would restrict the potential power and corruption of corporations, and that their exclusion from the constitution would in fact serve as a protection from their gaining broad political influence (Drutman & Cray, 2004; Nace, 2003).

As the constitution was drafted and then circulated to the states for ratification, Thomas Jefferson was also drafting a Bill of Rights that he unsuccessfully tried to include in the original constitution. Among the natural rights he included was a freedom from corporate monopolies. He wrote to Madison concerning the deficiencies of the newly written constitution in 1787: "I will now tell you what I do not like... First, the omission of a Bill of Rights, providing clearly, and without the aid of sophism, for freedom of religion, freedom of the press, protection against standing armies, *restriction of monopolies*, the eternal and unremitting force of the habeas corpus laws, and trials by jury..." (as quoted by Hartmann, 2002:70; emphasis added) Jefferson envisioned a system of strong self-governance that at the same time protected people from three potentially threatening institutions: governments, organized religion, and commercial monopolies. In particular, he was concerned about the consolidation of power and wealth that could infringe on the natural freedoms of individuals (Hartmann, 2002).

While Jefferson's Bill of Rights was ultimately ushered through Congress by Madison in 1791 and became part of the Constitution, the freedom from monopolies he so strongly believed in was removed from the final list of rights. The more pro-corporate Federalist Party was successful in resisting its inclusion (Hartmann, 2002). Still, the initial stance toward corporations in the new nation was one of restriction and accountability, and states were empowered to carefully control the activities of corporations (Meyers, 2000).

During this period of history, economic thought was greatly influenced by the writings of Adam Smith. Smith, often considered the father of economic liberalism, wrote in his 1776 *Wealth of Nations* how unimpeded, free markets naturally reach equilibrium and efficiency as if guided by an invisible hand. His theory became central to arguments against government interventions in market affairs or corporate regulation, and is often still called on today (Kennedy, 2005). However, free market champions seldom choose to recall that Adam Smith himself was suspicious of joint-stock companies as they separated owner and manager and had the potential to corrupt workers (Drutman & Cray, 2004; Werhane, 1991). Smith also believed that markets function best in conditions of relative equality and perfect information, and wrote extensively about issues of morality (Chomsky, 2002; Stiglitz, 2002). In fact, Smith's writings on morality contributed significantly to Jefferson's thinking as he advocated for the separation of church and state at the Constitutional Convention (McLean, 2007).

The Civil War Creates an Opening for Corporate Maneuvering

Early corporate charters issued by the states were quite limited, both in scope of privileges and activities, and in length of time, allowing for frequent and active review of corporate undertakings. Charter restrictions limited each corporation to a single purpose; restricted land and real estate holdings; prevented corporations from owning other corporations; required stockholder involvement in the business as well as liability for corporate actions; prevented political contributions; and even limited expansion and profitability, sometimes setting product prices within monopoly industries (Adams & Grossman, 2001; Hartmann, 2002; Meyers, 2000; Nace, 2003). State governments also explicitly required corporations to serve the public's interest, and charters were revoked if this function was not fulfilled. For example, the Virginia Supreme Court opined that charters would not be granted if the business' "object is merely private or selfish; if it is detrimental to, or not promotive of, the public good" (Nace, 2003:61).

By 1800, there were only 334 corporations nationwide, and many corporations of the early 19th century served to create public infrastructure, such as roads, railways, banks, bridges and canals (Drutman & Cray, 2004). While corporate shareholder structures persisted, the corporate features of immortality and limited liability enjoyed to date were eliminated through much of the 19th century. Imposing quite the opposite approach as Britain, many states used a "double liability" standard, whereby stakeholders were liable for two times the sum of their investment—a standard included in the bank charters of seven states through the 1870s (Nace, 2003). Thus, this early period of American history was one in which the pendulum had swung largely in favor of government oversight and intervention.

Railroad companies soon became a central player in this history, however, and would quickly work to turn the tide in favor of corporations. By 1840, within 10 years of launching the first railway, seven states had been connected. As tracks were laid across America, and economic activity came to depend upon this network, these businesses also laid the legislative tracks to becoming the most powerful corporations in American history to date. The Civil War helped to greatly consolidate this power. President Lincoln—himself a former lawyer for the Illinois Central Railroad Company—passed the Pacific Railroad Bill in 1862, authorizing government loans and land concessions to expand railways as a military necessity (Hartmann, 2002). The government even named a lobbyist of the Pennsylvania Railroad Company, Tom Scott, as the Assistant Secretary of War.

Scott's ability to coordinate the complex railway system to efficiently move troops and equipment was seen as key to the North's success, which secured Scott's political influence after the war. When he returned to his railroad company, he took with him the trust of state and national government officials and became intimately involved in the selection of candidates and appointees for both parties during the next 20 years. Indeed, he has even been credited by some with having determined the outcome of the contested 1876 Presidential election between Rutherford Hayes and Samuel Tilden. Scott also used his vast influence during these years to create a new corporate creature, the holding company (which purchases stocks to own at least part, if not all, of other companies) that allowed him to consolidate power over railways across the entire southern region (Nace, 2003).

Toward the end of the Civil War, President Lincoln came to recognize, with great fear, the implications of having empowered the corporation. In 1864, he wrote to a friend, "As a result of the war, corporations have been enthroned and an era of corruption in high places will follow, and the money power of the country will endeavor to prolong its reign by working upon the prejudices of the people until all wealth is aggregated in a few hands and the Republic is destroyed. I feel at this moment more anxiety than ever before, even in the midst of war. God grant that my suspicions may prove groundless" (as quoted in Hartmann, 2002:88).

Ironically, one of Lincoln's great accomplishments—the passing of amendments to abolish slavery—would become a vehicle for further corporate empowerment.

Corporate Personhood Ushers in the Gilded Age

Since it was passed into legislation in 1868, the 14th Amendment, which granted freed slaves due process, became a legal basis upon which corporate lawyers argued for corporate personhood. That is, they reasoned that the law should view corporations as *natural persons* that should enjoy the same rights as all people. After two decades of persistent failed attempts to establish their sovereignty, the corporations were finally successful in the 1886 *Santa Clara County v. Southern Pacific Railroad* Supreme Court case. While the case revolved around the company's refusal to pay state taxes on a technicality, its lawyers used the case to argue for corporate personhood under the 14th Amendment (Meyers, 2000).

Prior to his official ruling in this case, Chief Justice Waite made a statement before the court that corporations are persons under section one of the 14th Amendment. Because this statement was not an official opinion of the court, no discussion or dissenting opinions were offered, nor was any explanation as to why this was so. Yet, the statement became law, even though corporations had lost every Supreme Court case in which they argued for 14th Amendment rights in the decade prior (Hartmann, 2002; Meyers, 2000).

As soon as the door had been opened to amendment rights, corporate lawyers took hold. During the 50 years following the Santa Clara case, 50% of cases applying the 14th Amendment did so for corporations, while less than one-half of one percent did so for African Americans (Mayer, 1990). Between 1908 and 1914, the Supreme Court struck down a large and wide-ranging variety of public health and public safety regulations on the basis of corporate personhood, including minimum wage, child labor, and worker's compensation laws. Over the years, corporations also invoked Bill of Rights protections, successfully claiming 5th Amendment rights to extend their property protections, 1st Amendment rights to free speech so they could lobby and make political campaign contributions, and 4th Amendment rights to privacy so they could avoid health and environmental inspections, among other things (Mayer, 1990). In 1986, for example, corporations claimed the right to refuse surprise inspections by the Environmental Protection Agency (EPA) and the Occupational Health and Safety Administration (OSHA), severely limiting the public health and safety function of these organizations (Drutman & Cray, 2004; Mayer, 1990).

While efforts were certainly put forth to contain the corporation over time, such as the Sherman and Clayton Antitrust Acts (passed in 1890 and 1914 respectively), corporate-friendly courts and legislatures through the years did little to enforce their provisions (Hartmann, 2002). Also acting to support the corporations, the courts were quick to issue injunctions to prevent worker strikes: Between 1877 and 1930, over 1800 such injunctions were issued (Nace, 2003). Over a period of just a few decades, therefore, corporations vastly expanded their domain, and the corporate charter system that had contained their privileges and ensured the public good was destroyed. This came to be known as the Robber Baron era; corporations, and the individuals running them, were amassing huge fortunes and had at their disposal the legal escape routes and mechanisms to ensure their continued success. During this era, the pendulum shifted strongly in favor of corporate sovereignty.

Corporations also gained influence over state legislatures, and thus began a domestic race to the bottom in which states competed against one another to attract corporations by slackening restrictions. New Jersey was the first to dismantle corporate regulations, and as such quickly became a safe-haven state for corporations. In 1896, New Jersey passed the General Revision Act, which allowed for massive mergers and acquisitions, perpetual charters, and incorporation for any lawful purpose (Derber, 2000). By 1900, 95% of all American corporations with at least $25 million in assets based themselves in New Jersey to escape the regulations of their home states (Nace, 2003). In 1901, John D. Rockefeller and J.P. Morgan combined 112 corporate directorates under one massive corporation in New Jersey, whose $22 billion worth of assets was double the assessed value of all property in 13 southern U.S. states (Korten, 2001).

Significant about this period is not just the incredible consolidation of wealth and power made possible through the transformation of the corporate entity, but also the dramatic shift in the court's—and to some extent, the public's—mindset about corporations. Corporations came to be seen not as vehicles for furthering the public good, but as naturally private entities whose rightful purpose was profit-seeking, and whose responsibility was to its shareholders alone. As sociologist Charles Derber explains, "by 1900, the corporation had the blessing of the Court as a new citizen of the Republic... This turned the old notion of public control over the corporation into a violation of the same set of constitutional privileges enjoyed by the public itself" (Derber, 2000:130).

The Great Depression Revives Anticorporate Sentiment

Beginning in the late 1920s, after a period of incredible reign, the powers of corporations were challenged anew. As the Great Depression shook America, citizen outrage and blame centered on corporate leaders and the politicians and judges who had facilitated their great wealth and leverage. Franklin D. Roosevelt (FDR) successfully ran for President on a populist platform that challenged corporations, stating in 1932, "[I]f the process of concentration goes on at the same rate, at the end of another century we shall have all American industry controlled by a dozen corporations, and run by perhaps a hundred men. Put plainly, we are steering a steady course toward economic oligarchy, if we are not there already" (Nace, 2003:156).

Franklin D. Roosevelt carried out an agenda of regulatory reform through the beginning of WWII, putting in place social safety nets for workers and empowering the government to intervene more in markets. The New Deal of 1934 included provisions to regulate corporate power, and through his long presidency FDR pressured the Supreme Court and appointed new justices to prevent further expansion of corporate rights. As a result, between 1922 and 1970, only one Supreme Court case expanded such rights (Hartmann, 2002; Nace, 2003).

Over this period of American history, then, the excesses of corporate privilege were brought into better check in favor of citizen rights. Over three decades, beginning in the mid-1940s, America experienced a "great leveling" in which the wealth gap of the Gilded Age was squeezed to create greater equality and expand the middle class (Rasmus, 2007). Between 1929 and 1944, the number of American millionaires declined from 20,000 to 13,000, and the proportional wealth of the top 0.5% of households fell from 32.4% to 19.3% between 1929 and 1949 (Korten, 2001). Several important public health and environmental initiatives were also created during this era, continuing through Richard Nixon's presidency ending in 1974, including Medicare, Medicaid, Social Security, the EPA, and OSHA.

With the changing tides of public sentiment, corporations also initiated new practices in an attempt to shore up their image, including corporate social responsibility (CSR) programs. The first writings on CSR appeared in the 1950s, and proliferated during the 1960s, centering on the obligations of business to take action in line with broad social values beyond profit-seeking. However, in the late 1960s and 1970s, the literature began to strongly emphasize that CSR must be voluntary and not coerced, and also began to more transparently advance the instrumental (profit-returning) value of CSR (Carroll, 1999). Ultimately, writings on CSR even went so far as to conflate wealth creation and social welfare, suggesting that the business pursuit of profit itself should naturally lead to social improvements (Windsor, 2001).

While CSR may have boosted corporate images at a much needed point in history, its emphasis on voluntary participation successfully prevented its meaningful formalization into a broad code of conduct that might have set the basement standard for business ethics. During the late 1970s, the International Labor Organization (ILO), the Organization for Co-operation and Development (OECD), and the United Nations Center on Transnational Corporations (UNCTC) each attempted to create mandatory international codes of conduct for corporations. However, the former two ultimately complied with the call of businesses to create suggestive codes without penalties for noncompliance, and the latter never achieved consensus to adopt its recommended accountability structures. Without a universal standard, CSR's application was ultimately quite limited in the face of shareholder obligations that compel business executives to privilege profit above all else (Kolk, Van Tulder, & Welters, 1999).

Nonetheless, during the early New Deal era, the pendulum did swing in favor of government interventionism. The theories of British economist John Maynard Keynes were quite influential in American domestic and international policy. Keynesian economics did not view markets as perfectly self-righting, and thus advocated government involvement in stimulating economic demand by lowering taxes and interest rates and increasing expenditures (Stiglitz, 2002). Keynes himself was present to debate such interventionist approaches as the Allied nations came together to design a post–WWII global economic system.

In July 1944, representatives of the 44 Allied nations met in Bretton Woods, New Hampshire, for the United Nations Monetary and Financial Conference. In an attempt to prevent future economic depressions (and their associated political strife), the delegates formed three global economic institutions. The World Bank was charged with funding post–war reconstruction. The General Agreement on Tariffs and Trade (GATT), which would later become the World Trade Organization (WTO), aimed to decrease tariffs and thereby facilitate trade between nations. The International Monetary Fund (IMF) would create and monitor a fixed global exchange system (the gold standard) and make short-term loans to stabilize countries. As economist Joseph Stiglitz points out, "In its original conception, then, the IMF was based on a recognition that markets often did not work well... [It] was founded on the belief that there was a need for *collective action at the global level* for economic stability." (Stiglitz, 2002:12, emphasis original)

However, while the spirit of Bretton Woods was collective, the United States still emerged as the central player in these institutions, a position that would later, almost inevitably, lead to the global expansion of American corporations. Even as of the 1960s, the benefits of America's dominance in the post–war era were paying off. American multinational corporations (MNCs) had quietly risen to dominate the world market, and U.S. foreign direct investment (FDI) represented a full half of total worldwide FDI (Miyoshi, 1993).

Neoliberalism and Reaganism Spark Corporate Resurgence

Between the Great Depression and the 1970s, America's businesses were not enjoying the freedoms they had enjoyed during the Gilded Age. The government had enacted legislation to protect workers and prevent market excesses, and public sentiment toward business was low. As late as 1977, only 15% of Americans believed that business fairly balanced profit-seeking and public interest (Nace, 2003), and consumer leaders like Ralph Nader were leading a charge against business practices that were deceptive and harmful to the public's health (Nader, 1976). Meanwhile, new social and environmental restrictions, especially at the federal level, were cutting into profits (Mayer, 1990). Many in the business world sensed that it was time to organize.

The early 1970s were just that: an era of businesses coming together to organize and create long-term planning to protect free enterprise. Lewis Powell, Jr., an accomplished corporate lawyer who shortly became a Nixon-appointed Supreme Court justice, drafted a confidential memo that became an important organizing tool. Titled "Attack on American Free Enterprise System," this 1971 document called for inter-sector business cooperation to launch counterstrategies against government and even social science (recognizing how it shaped public opinion) (Nace, 2003). The memo became a call to action and, among other things, sparked a new era of corporate political organizing. The Business Roundtable was formed to organize the nation's top CEOs, alongside new legal councils, business publications, public relations organizations, and foundations. The Heritage Foundation, a conservative think tank and advocate of extreme free market economics, was founded in 1973, representing one of many newly created corporate-friendly think tanks (Nace, 2003).

Such new cooperation paid off. As of 1975, when the legal uses of Political Action Committees (PACs) were expanded, corporations aligned to take hold of this traditional union tool and soon dominated soft money political contributions (Clawson, Neustadtl, & Weller, 1998; Drafan, 2003). Since soft money contributions are not explicitly allocated to affect elections, they are unregulated and unlimited, and translate into vast political influence. The number of registered lobbyists soared from 3,400 in 1975 to 32,890 in 2005. Over 500 American companies had opened offices in D.C. by the 1990s, employing over 60,000 lobbyists, including lawyers involved in lobbying (Reich, 2007). By the 2008 presidential campaign, businesses were outspending labor organizations 29 to 1 in campaign contributions (Center for Responsive Politics, 2008).

Along with the concentrated efforts of businesses descending on Washington, winds were shifting in economic theory during this period as well. Beginning in the early 1970s with the oil crisis brought on by production cutbacks of the Organization of the Petroleum Exporting Countries (OPEC), and continuing into the early 1980s with the debt crisis of World Bank and IMF borrower countries, confidence in Keynsian economics waned. Economist Milton Friedman and his University of Chicago colleagues were arguing for a new approach to deal with these woes, pushing for the privatization of industries (including public good industries such as education and healthcare) and the removal of government oversight. Unfettered free markets became viewed as the most efficient mechanisms for delivering all goods and services (Friedman, 1962). These theories ushered in the era of neoliberalism (a resurgence of Adam Smith's invisible-hand liberalism without Smith's moral concerns about equity), and a renewed belief in market supremacy and deregulation.

President Reagan was deeply influenced by University of Chicago economists—he asked Milton Friedman to serve on the President's Economic Policy Advisory Board, and later honored him with the Presidential Medal of Freedom (Friedman, 2005)—and the Reagan Administration was characterized by neoliberal, corporate-friendly policies. Reagan facilitated a new era of mergers and acquisitions, new corporate tax laws, and a strategic dismantling of unions that quickly expanded the size and influence of corporations (Miyoshi, 1993). The pendulum had swung again, and dramatically so in favor of corporations.

One of Reagan's first acts as president was to override the striking air traffic controller's union, Professional Air Traffic Controllers Organization (PATCO), and force workers back to work. He successfully rallied public opinion against unions and contributed to their slow decline, from a high of 34% of the national workforce in 1954 to only 15% in 2000 (Derber, 2000). This weakening of unions eliminated one very important counter-balance to corporate power in America.

Reagan also set in motion corporate expansion by slackening antitrust laws meant to prevent monopolies (Sackrey, Schneider, & Knoedler, 2002). Such mergers allowed giant corporations to achieve monopolies, or at least oligarchies, over entire industries. As such, by 2005, just four businesses controlled 60% of the nation's grain market, four controlled 70% of the meatpacker market, and ten controlled 60% of the retail grocery market (Brock, 2005). In perhaps an even more frightening consolidation, corporations gained increasing control over our mass media, and thereby acquired control over the very filter of our most widely used and publicly available sources of information. While in 1983, 50 conglomerates controlled America's newspapers, magazines, radios, televisions, books, and movies, by 2004, mergers left only 5 corporations largely in charge of our news and information sources (Bagdikian, 2004).

Reagan also assisted corporations with a dramatic tax reform. He cut taxes for the wealthy from 70% to 30%, and cut the corporate tax rate as much as 12% for some industries (Hartmann, 2007; Mandel, 2004). With this, the "great leveling" that the New Deal had set in motion 70 years prior was inverted. Between 1977 and 1987, the ratio of income between the top 1% of wealthy families and the bottom 10% increased from 65 to 1 all the way to 115 to 1. Furthermore, during the 1980s, while the bottom 10% lost 15% of their real annual income, the top 1% increased theirs by 50% (George, 1999). Business profits boomed, and CEO salaries soared. In 1980, CEOs made on average 35 times more than their company workers and by 2000, this ratio peaked at 525 times (Rasmus, 2007; United for a Fair Economy, 2008).

Corporations also benefited greatly in the global arena. In 1971, the gold standard crashed, eliminating it as the international fixed exchange system established at Bretton Woods. The IMF's purpose was shaken, and the institution shifted its focus to global development and lending. Thus, the IMF and World Bank largely converged in purpose and policy approaches beginning in the 1980s, and were heavily influenced by the United States, the largest shareholder government in both institutions. They initiated Structural Adjustment Programs (SAPs) for lending that were infused with neoliberal logic touting privatization and deregulation (Stein, 2004; Stiglitz, 2002).

SAPs required recipient nations to privatize public entities, deregulate national markets, and open up their economies to foreign investment. As such, entry for foreign MNCs and investors was made easier, and governments of developing countries were disempowered to regulate corporate activities even within their own borders. The international race to the bottom took off. Corporations enjoyed huge profits and many times these profits resulted from their capacity to externalize costs (or shift them to the public domain) by skirting public health and environmental protections (Chan, 2003). These trends were reinforced and formalized with the creation of the WTO and multinational trade agreements.

International Free Trade Agreements Open the Door Further

The era of neoliberalism began with Reagan, and has been supported by each subsequent administration. The Clinton Administration oversaw the creation of modern expansive free trade agreements (FTAs) and formed the World Trade Organization (WTO). The development of such free trade initiatives fortified corporate and trade dominance globally, and often at the expense of government sovereignty, environmental protection, and public health and welfare.

The North American Free Trade Agreement (NAFTA), for instance, although technically a trade agreement between the United States, Canada, and Mexico, extends far beyond the scope of trade agreements seen prior. Passed in 1994, NAFTA not only eliminates tariffs and quotas (the traditional realm of trade agreements), but also limits food safety measures, upholds patents that increase medication prices, and prevents governments from limiting toxic waste dumping, amongst other provisions—each of which has raised clear public health concerns (Public Citizen). Ultimately, NAFTA privileges the rights of investors above social welfare and environmental concerns to ensure that barriers to trade are minimized. Its private, non-transparent tribunal, for example, ruled against the Mexican municipality of Guadalacazar in 2000 for preventing the U.S. Metalclad Corporation from creating a toxic waste landfill in an ecologically protected zone. Furthermore, it ruled that Mexico must pay Metalclad over $16 million dollars in compensation (Wallach & Woodall, 2004).

The Metalclad case illuminates some important features of NAFTA and the agreements it has inspired since. Under NAFTA's Article 1110, corporations can sue governments for expropriation (which is interpreted as much broader than the traditional meaning of taking over of land) and can expect compensation for losses of anticipated profits (Stone, 2003). Also, NAFTA's national treatment principle ensures that foreign corporations can expect the same treatment as domestic corporations so that governments cannot privilege local labor or materials and cannot expect local investment or returns from the dealings of foreign corporations (Wallach & Woodall, 2004).

The principles of NAFTA are meant to promote harmonization; that is, they intend to make the trade and industry laws of its signatory countries the same so that MNCs and investors can move more easily from place to place. NAFTA laid the groundwork, though, to create an even broader playing ground for MNCs. One year after NAFTA was in place, the even more expansive WTO was created at the Uruguay Round of the GATT, becoming the world's most powerful global trade institution. GATT was included as one of 18 agreements summarized in the WTO's 800-pages of rules. Its new agreements grossly expanded patent rights, pushed to commodify public goods like water, healthcare, and education, (under GATS, the General Agreement on Trade in Services) and undermined environmental, product, and food safety standards. They also required countries to liberalize finance and investment industries by slackening regulations (Wallach & Woodall, 2004).

The creation of the WTO represented the historic peak of formal corporate rule at the global level. WTO rules are set up to protect the interests of business. That social welfare, public health, and environmental protections are not included in the WTO's agreements is unsurprising when one notes that the United States had 500 corporations acting as official government advisors during the WTO drafting process. Issue per issue, the Clinton Administration favored corporate experts over citizen experts, business proponents over public health proponents. For example, a former lobbyist for a corporate producer of genetically modified foods was chosen to consult on WTO rules regarding this issue over a Consumer Union-nominated scientist (Hartmann, 2002).

Despite popular pushback, the WTO has balked at suggestions to include labor standards in its agreements, and/or to collaborate with the ILO to ensure basic human rights protections for workers worldwide. Furthermore, in all but two of its cases dealing with social and environmental challenges through 2004, the WTO's non-transparent judicial system viewed protective regulations as barriers to trade (Wallach & Woodall, 2004). Thus, the international race to the bottom that was facilitated by IMF and World Bank SAPs was formalized and expedited under the WTO. With the access to the global market that the WTO created, corporations can easily move into and out of countries in search of the most favorable conditions, meaning conditions where costs such as wages and healthcare are minimized, and public health and environmental oversight can be negotiated. Corporations can also dismiss government concerns about ethics in purchasing, as the WTO now prevents governments from banning products based on "noncommercial values." As such, governments cannot, for instance, ban products made by child labor, or corporations whose production is connected with genocide (Global Exchange, 2002).

Neither the WTO nor NAFTA have strong records of promoting conditions for good public health, and the broad prosperity that each promised has been unfulfilled. For example, while Mexico's manufacturing exports increased under NAFTA, growth in manufacturing sector employment has been dismal as assembled parts from the United States replaced the need for many workers. Furthermore, 1.3 million farmers lost their livelihoods when the United States used NAFTA's provisions to flood Mexico's markets with corn priced at 30% below production cost (Audley et al., 2004). This created greater public health needs as fewer families had the capacity to sustain themselves. However, even while the need for coordinated public health services may increase, governments are being compelled to turn over health and public sector services to the private sector under GATS, thus weakening their capacity to ensure affordable healthcare access—a dismal picture indeed (American Public Health Association, 2001).

Corporations have certainly emerged as winners in this era of neoliberalism, today representing 51 of the top 100 economies worldwide (including national economies). However, people and governments have struggled

(Anderson, Cavanagh, & the Institute for Policy Studies, 2000). Nonetheless, the push for additional FTAs has continued. While the United States attempt to create the Free Trade Agreement of the Americas (FTAA)—to include all of Latin America—ultimately failed in 2005, the expansive Central American Free Trade Agreement (CAFTA) was ratified the same year. Even today, the U.S. Trade Representative's office that drives these FTAs is guided by 42 big business representatives on its advisory committees and only three public health representatives (the latter whom were added only after years of organizing for representation) (Center for Policy Analysis on Trade and Health).

A Way Forward: Mobilizing for Public Health

Free trade initiatives have created unprecedented global corporate privileges in the contemporary era, but they have also prompted powerful counter movements. The 1999 Seattle protest, where more than fifty thousand "teamsters and turtles" descended on the WTO ministerial, represented a powerful and visible pushback on corporate supremacy. It also spurred a decade of more or less continual protest at the global meetings of the financial elite, successfully blocking key expansions of the WTO (Derber, 2002). At the 2003 WTO ministerial in Cancún, Mexico, 70 developing countries successfully blocked WTO agreements that would have sustained unfair agricultural subsidies (Mutume, 2003). This built upon another success in 2001 when the WTO was pressured by global resistances to create the Doha Declaration. The declaration conceded expanded access to life-saving generic HIV/AIDS medications by allowing exceptions to WTO drug patent rules in cases of public health emergencies (World Health Organization).

The popular pushback on the WTO, and particularly the Doha Declaration that reflected the values of protecting and promoting the public's health, opened the door for public health principles to take precedence over corporate protections. However, persistence must follow as implementation of the Doha Declaration is still unresolved, and generic HIV/AIDS medications remain unavailable to millions in high-burden countries (Stop AIDS Campaign, 2006). Such initial victories should represent the first of many in a concerted effort to protect our public's health in an age where corporations have become more powerful even than the governments and institutions concerned with promoting our public's health and social welfare.

Public health professionals have a critical role to play in shaping and countering the corporate practices that undermine human health, safety, and welfare. The rights that corporations have acquired both domestically and globally threaten our very capacity to meet the obligations of our profession—to protect and promote the public's health. With the confluence of IMF, World Bank, and WTO regulations, governments worldwide have been pressured to privatize healthcare delivery systems, water and sanitation, and even entitlement programs meant to ensure basic survival and welfare. Meanwhile, corporations have won lawsuits and new trade protections that allow them to dump toxins in our environment, prevent generic drug production, and dismantle food and product safety protections. At home and abroad, while corporate CEOs salaries have soared, worker's wages and protections have been steadily undermined.

A concentrated effort of public health professionals could help to bring about a new pendulum swing in favor of our public, a goal that is clearly aligned with the aims of our profession to address structural disease causation (Wiist, 2006). This kind of swing is possible, given our current climate of economic recession and renewed public critique of corporate dominance, and the thriving contemporary surge in critical countercampaigns. Such campaigns include those focused on our global economic institutions, such as the anti-WTO and debt-relief campaigns, but also include such broad campaigns as the Fair Trade, anti-sweatshop, local, alternative development and green trade and consumption movements. There are many potential areas for collaboration between the public health profession and these numerous social movements, which offer rich opportunities for advancing the public's health and welfare. The coordinated response of the public health profession is critical, however, to ensure that public health considerations are at the forefront of future regulations of, and responses to, corporations.

REFERENCES

Adams F, Grossman R. Taking care of business. In: Ritz D, ed. *Defying Corporations, Defying Democracy: A Book of History and Strategy.* New York: Apex Press; 2001.

American Public Health Association. *Threats to Global Health and Equity: The General Agreement on Trade in Services (GATS), and the Free Trade Area of the Americas (FTAA).* Available at: http://www.apha.org/advocacy/policy/policysearch/default.htm?id=260. Published 2001. Accessed October 8, 2008.

Anderson S, Cavanagh J, The Institute for Policy Studies. *Top 200: The Rise of Corporate Global Power.* Available at: http://www.ips-dc.org/downloads/Top_200.pdf. Published 2000. Accessed October 10, 2008.

Audley JJ, Papademetriou DG, Polaski S, Vaughan S. *NAFTA's Promise and Reality: Lessons from Mexico for the Hemisphere.* Carnegie Endowment for International Peace. Available at: http://www.carnegieendowment.org/files/nafta1.pdf. Published 2004. Accessed September 26, 2008.

Bagdikian BH. *The New Media Monopoly*. Boston: Beacon Press; 2004.

Bakan J. *The Corporation: The Pathological Pursuit of Profit and Power*. New York: Free Press; 2005.

Berenson A. Power Plays: How Free Should a Free Market Be? *The New York Times*. October 4, 2008. Available at: http://www.nytimes.com/2008/10/05/weekinreview/05berenson.html?_r=1&scp=3&sq=free%20market&st=cse. Accessed December 6, 2008.

Brock J. Merger mania and its discontents: the price of corporate consolidation. *Multinational Monitor*. July/August, 2005;26:7, 8. Available at: http://multinationalmonitor.org/mm2005/072005/brock.html. Accessed October 16, 2008.

Carroll AB. Corporate social responsibility: evolution of a definitional construct. *Business Society*. 1999;38:268–295.

Center for Policy Analysis on Trade and Health. CPATH Responds to NY Times: Health Key to Trade and Prosperity. Available at: http://www.cpath.org/id4.html. Accessed December 6, 2008.

Center for Responsive Politics. *2008 Overview: Business-Labor-Ideology Split in PAC & Individual Donations to Candidates and Parties*. Available at: http://www.opensecrets.org/overview/blio.php. Published 2008. Accessed December 1, 2008.

Chan A. A "race to the bottom": globalization and China's labor standards. *China Perspectives*. 2003;46:41–49. Available at: http://rspas.anu.edu.au/~anita/pdf/AChancp461.pdf. Accessed February 10, 2008.

Chomsky N. *Understanding Power: The Indispensible Chomsky*. New York: New Press; 2002.

Clawson D, Neustadtl A, Weller M. *Dollars and Votes: How Business Campaign Contributions Subvert Democracy*. Philadelphia: Temple University Press; 1998.

Derber C. *Corporation Nation: How Corporations Are Taking Over Our Lives and What We Can Do About It*, 2nd ed. New York: St. Martin's Press; 2000.

Derber C. *People Before Profit: The New Globalization in the Age of Terror, Big Money, and Economic Crisis*, 1st ed. New York: St. Martin's Press; 2002.

Drafan G. *The Elite Consensus: When Corporations Yield the Constitution*. New York: The Apex Press; 2003.

Drutman L, Cray C. *The People's Business: Controlling Corporations and Restoring Democracy*. San Francisco: Berrett-Koehler Publishers, Inc.; 2004.

Friedman M. *Capitalism and Freedom*. Chicago: University of Chicago Press; 1962.

Friedman M. Autobiography. *Nobel Foundation*. Available at: http://nobelprize.org/nobel_prizes/economics/laureates/1976/friedman-autobio.html. Published 2005. Accessed September 26, 2008.

George S. A short history of neoliberalism: twenty years of elite economics and emerging opportunities for structural change. *Conference on Economic Sovereignty in a Globalizing World*, 1999. Available at: http://www.zmag.org/CrisesCurEvts/Globalism/george.htm. Accessed August 1, 2007.

Global Exchange. *Top Reasons to Oppose the WTO.* Available at: http://www.globalexchange.org/campaigns/wto/OpposeWTO.html. Published 2002. Accessed October 8, 2008.

Hartmann T. *Unequal Protection: The Rise of Corporate Dominance and the Theft of Human Rights.* Emmaus, PA; New York: Rodale; St. Martin's Press [Distributor]; 2002.

Hartmann T. *Roll Back the Reagan Tax Cuts.* Available at: http://www.thomhartmann.com/index.php?option=com_content&task=view&id=1&Itemid=38. Published August 6, 2007. Accessed September 26, 2008.

Kennedy G. *Adam Smith's Lost Legacy.* New York: Palgrave MacMillan; 2005.

Kolk A, Van Tulder R, Welters C. International codes of conduct and corporate social responsibility: can transnational corporations regulate themselves? *Transnational Corporations.* April 1999;8(1):143–181.

Korten DC. *When Corporations Rule the World,* 2nd ed. San Francisco; Bloomfield, CT: Berrett-Koehler Publishers; Kumarian Press; 2001.

Mandel MJ. *Reagan's Economic Legacy: his Policies Helped Spur the 1980s Boom and were Integral to the High-tech Revolution. But the Poor Paid a Price.* Available at: http://www.businessweek.com/magazine/content/04_25/b3888032_mz011.htm. Published 2004. Accessed October 8, 2008.

Mayer CJ. Personalizing the impersonal: corporations and the bill of rights. *Hastings Law J.* 1990;41:577–667.

McLean I. Adam Smith at the Constitutional Convention. *Presented at the 2007 Annual Meeting of the American Political Science Association,* 2007. Available at: http://www.nuffield.ox.ac.uk/Politics/papers/2007/AdamSmi.pdf. Accessed October 5, 2008.

Meyers W. *The Santa Clara Blues: Corporate Personhood versus Democracy. III Publishing.* Available at: http://www.mcn.org/e/iii/afd/santaclara.html. Published 2000. Accessed September 3, 2008.

Miyoshi M. Summer. A borderless world? From colonialism to transnationalism and the decline of the nation-state. *Crit Inq.* 1993;19:726–751.

Mutume G. Hope seen in the ashes of Cancún: WTO trade talks collapse, as Africa and allies stand firm. *United Nations Economic and Social Development,* 2003. Available at: http://www.un.org/ecosocdev/geninfo/afrec/vol17no3/173wto.htm. Accessed October 8, 2008.

Nace T. *Gangs of America: The Rise of Corporate Power and the Disabling of Democracy.* San Francisco: Berrett-Koehler Publishers, Inc.; 2003.

Nader R. *Taming the Giant Corporation.* New York: W.W. Norton & Company, Inc.; 1976.

National Public Radio; Talk of the Nation. *Bailout Pits Free-Market Against Gov't Regulation.* Available at: http://www.npr.org/templates/story/story.php?storyId=95215972. Published September 30, 2008. Accessed December 2, 2008.

Osborne E. *The Rise of the Anti-Corporate Movement: Corporations and the People Who Hate Them*. Westport, CT: Praeger Publishers; 2007.

Public Citizen. The Ten Year Track Record of the North American Free Trade Agreement: The Mexican Economy, Agriculture and Environment. Available at: http://www.citizen.org/documents/NAFTA_10_mexico.pdf. Acccessed September 26, 2008.

Rasmus J. The Trillion Dollar Income Shift, Part 1. *Z Magazine* 2007. Available at: http://zmagsite.zmag.org/Feb2007/rasmuspro207.html. Accessed August 1, 2007.

Reich RB. *Supercapitalism*. New York: Alfred A. Knopf; 2007.

Sackrey C, Schneider GE, Knoedler JT. *Introduction to Political Economy*, 3rd ed. Cambridge, MA: Dollars and Sense, Economic Affairs Bureau; 2002.

Stein H. The World Bank and the IMF in Africa: Strategy and Routine in the Generation of a Failed Agenda [online]. Available at: http://www.macua.org/Howard_Stein.pdf. Published 2004. Accessed August 5, 2007.

Stiglitz J. *Globalization and Its Discontents*. New York: W.W. Norton & Compnay, Inc.; 2002.

Stone M. Summer. NAFTA Article 1110: Environmental friend or foe? *Georgetown International Environmental Law Review* 2003. Available at: http://findarticles.com/p/articles/mi_qa3970/is_200307/ai_n9295426. Accessed September 26, 2008.

Stop AIDS Campaign. On the 5th Anniversary of the Doha Declaration the world's poor have little to cheer but broken promises. Available at: http://64.233.169.104/search?q=cache:3XkJqkzi40YJ:www.stopaidscampaign.org.uk/downloads/press%2520releases/DohaRelease06.doc+doha+medication+access&hl=en&ct=clnk&cd=1&gl=us. Published 2006. Accessed October 8, 2008.

Theil S. Adam Smith's Return. *Newsweek*, December 8, 2008. Available at: http://www.newsweek.com/id/171314. Accessed December 6, 2008.

United for a Fair Economy. CEO Pay Charts 1990–2005. Available at: http://faireconomy.org/news/ceo_pay_charts. Accessed October 8, 2008.

World Health Organization. The Doha Declaration on the TRIPS Agreement and Public Health. Available at: http://www.who.int/medicines/areas/policy/doha_declaration/en/index.html. Accessed October 8, 2008.

Wallach L, Woodall P. *Whose Trade Organization?: A Comprehensive Guide to the WTO*. New York: The New Press; 2004.

Windsor D. The future of corporate social responsibility. *The International Journal of Organizational Analysis*. 2001;9(3):225–256.

Werhane P. *Adam Smith and His Legacy for Modern Capitalism*. New York: Oxford University Press; 1991.

Wiist WH. Public health and the anticorporate movement: rationale and recommendations. *Am J Public Health*. 2006;96(8):1370–1375.

PART II

Corporate Tactics

3

Limited Liability and the Public's Health

Lainie Rutkow and Stephen P. Teret

Corporations, through their products and behaviors, exert a strong effect on the well-being of populations. Public health practitioners and academics have long recognized the harms associated with some corporations' products. For example, firearms are associated with approximately 30,000 deaths in the United States each year[1] and over 200,000 deaths globally.[2] Motor vehicles are associated with about 40,000 deaths in the United States each year[3] and over 1.2 million deaths globally.[4] Tobacco products kill about 438,000 people each year in the United States[5] and about 4.9 million people worldwide.[6] In addition to producing unsafe or harmful products, some corporations behave in ways that negatively impact the public's health, such as marketing alcohol to youth[7] and other vulnerable populations.[8] Given these observations, one can conclude that it is possible to quantify the public health impact of individual industries, such as firearms, motor vehicles, tobacco, and alcohol.[9] Health professionals can then target these individual industries to prevent or lessen the harms they cause.

Though focusing on individual industries can have a significant public health impact, this type of single issue research and advocacy does not consider what might be a more general facilitator of widespread morbidity and mortality. Most industries, including those previously listed, are composed of corporations, which are legal fictions[10] designed to provide limited exposure to liability, through

This article reprinted by permission from *Journal of Law, Medicine & Ethics.* 2007;35(4), 599–608.

a variety of mechanisms, for their investors and directors. Thus, corporate structure and function allow—and even encourage—corporations to act in ways that harm the public's health.[11]

To fully appreciate the ramifications of this statement, one must first understand the corporate form, which, while varying slightly among countries, maintains certain essential elements. By law, corporations are obligated to act in their own best interests, which usually means maximizing profits.[12] The responsibility of a corporation is to its shareholders, to enhance their wealth. Often, attempts to maximize profits run counter to protecting the public's health.[13] In addition, corporate shareholders benefit from limited liability. Limited liability, a concept that originated several centuries ago,[14] allows individuals to be held responsible only for the money they have invested in a company.[15] A principle separate from limited liability holds that, because the corporation itself (as a "person" under the law) is liable for its actions, its directors and managers generally will not be held personally responsible for any wrongdoing in which the corporation has engaged.[16] This means that, even if a court determines that a corporation is liable for a tort, such as negligently manufacturing a product that has caused harm, the individuals who own the corporation and who made the decisions regarding the product will not be held personally responsible. When actions are taken under the auspices of a corporate entity, the individuals responsible, in either financial or administrative capacities, will not face personal liability for the negative results of those actions. To illustrate this point, this article provides examples of corporate products or practices that have caused harm in the United States and elsewhere, and considers the role that limited liability played in these cases.

Given this explanation of corporate function and limited liability, it is useful for health professionals to consider what steps can be taken to reduce corporations' negative impact on public health. This article concludes by considering strategies that may modify or eliminate some of the aspects of limited liability. By becoming knowledgeable about these alternatives, health professionals can strengthen their efforts to prevent injuries and other health-related harms caused by corporate entities. Because criminal liability for corporations involves a different set of considerations and raises unique issues,[17] this article focuses only on civil liability for corporations.

Corporate Function

The concept of a corporation, with slight variations, has existed for several centuries.[18] Some of the earliest companies, such as those chartered by the British to explore the Americas and the East Indies, were formed as a means to accumulate capital.[19] Because exploration was dangerous with many attendant risks, a single person could not afford to finance an entire voyage. This led to two innovations, both of which have remained fundamental aspects of modern corporations. First, the company made discrete portions, or shares, of itself available to investors. These shares were offered and traded through some type of public market[20] which served as a precursor to modern markets like the New York Stock Exchange. Investors were motivated to buy these shares because, if the voyage was successful, the company's worth, and the worth of their shares, would increase. However, investors also had to worry about the debts they would incur if the voyage was not a success and the company lost its ships and cargo. These concerns ultimately led to the idea of limited liability for investors.[21]

Company owners reasoned, correctly, that investors would not offer financial support to risky ventures unless they were protected. As it evolved, limited liability came to mean that if the company encountered financial difficulties and incurred debt, individual investors would only be liable for the amount of their personal investment in the company.[22] Therefore, beyond their own investment in the company, they would bear no responsibility for the company's debts. These two innovations—freely transferable shares and limited liability—remain hallmarks of today's corporations.

Modern corporations are creations of the state. As such, they enjoy a unique status: although they are owned and operated by actual people, corporations retain a separate legal identity as fictional persons.[23] This concept of a separate legal identity is crucial to understanding the relationship between corporations and their owners and managers. Although a corporation's actions are determined by the real people who manage it, those people are insulated from being held responsible for their actions by the existence of the fictional corporate "person."

The people who run a corporation, including its directors and managers, are legally obliged to act in the corporation's best interest.[24] Academics and commentators,[25] as well as courts,[26] have confirmed that this charge generally means that a corporation's managers should seek to maximize the corporation's profits, and, in turn, enhance its shareholders' wealth. Corporate managers are legally prevented from taking action, on a corporation's behalf, to improve the environment or create a safer product, unless this action is ultimately designed to increase the corporation's profits either directly or indirectly.[27] While corporate mangers can pursue public health and/or humanitarian goals with their own money as private citizens, they cannot do so in their role as corporate managers without demonstrating that such pursuits directly or indirectly enhance the financial status of the corporation.

In recent decades, the rise of the corporate social responsibility (CSR) movement has presented a challenge to this mandate. CSR questions whether corporate directors and managers also have obligations to society as a whole rather than just to their shareholders.[28] CSR initiatives range from promoting the use of environmentally friendly paper products[29] to participating in programs designed to increase access to pharmaceuticals in developing nations.[30] Though these initiatives are, of course, welcome examples of corporations making constructive social contributions, one must understand where CSR fits within a corporate entity's existence. Because corporations are ultimately expected to maximize profits, corporations must engage in CSR with this goal in mind.[31] For this reason, some corporations have engaged in campaigns to publicize their CSR initiatives, relying on the theory that consumers will want to give their business to a socially responsible company.[32] To this end, CSR has become a specialty of public relations firms.[33] However, in terms of its legal rights and responsibilities, a corporation, as a legal entity, must carefully consider what, if any, CSR initiatives it will pursue.

Corporate Structure

To officially exist as a legal entity, a corporation must be registered with a state or national government,[34] depending on the laws of the country in which it is based. Once it has been registered and recognized by the government, the corporation is subject to laws and regulations that determine the extent of its rights as a fictional person. These rights generally include, inter alia, the ability to sue and be sued as well as the power to initiate and sign contracts for goods and services.[35] These rights make it easy to confuse a corporate entity with an actual person, but it is important to remember that a corporation's existence, and any accompanying rights, is entirely dependent on the government's creation and recognition of its status as a fictional person. For example, while a corporation can, according to its charter, exist in perpetuity,[36] the state can also revoke its charter and end its existence.

Today's largest corporations are publicly owned. Their shares, also known as stock, are traded on public markets, like the New York, Tokyo, or London Stock Exchanges, and their investors enjoy limited liability. Publicly owned corporations can, in theory, amass the capital of unlimited numbers of people.[37] In recent years, this has allowed them to expand their operations into countries throughout the world, leading to the development of multinational corporations.[38]

Though a public corporation is owned by its shareholders, it is governed by a board of directors whom the shareholders elect.[39] The board then chooses managers, such as a chief executive officer, who run the corporation's day-to-day operations.[40] In this model, the corporation is owned by one group of people and managed by a different group of people. Because this article is primarily concerned with the public health impact of limited liability, the ensuing discussion will focus on large, publicly owned corporations and their subsidiaries. However, it is useful to note that modern corporations can also be privately owned. These corporations, known as close corporations, have no publicly traded shares.[41] Instead, they are usually owned and managed by a small group of people.

In addition to the rights mentioned above, corporations can own stock in other corporations.[42] Sometimes this will mean that a corporation owns stock in another corporation as an investment, the same way that an individual investor might own a corporation's stock. In other instances, one corporation will own the majority or all of a second corporation's stock. In this case, the owner corporation is known as the parent, and the owned corporation is known as the subsidiary. There are several reasons why one corporation might choose to completely own a second corporation, but the one most relevant to this article involves the exposure to risk. Because the parent corporation, as the investor, has only limited liability toward the subsidiary corporation, the subsidiary corporation can engage in high-risk business ventures with limited risk to the parent.[43] This means that if a subsidiary company owns a ship that causes a major oil spill along a country's coastline, the parent corporation would have limited liability for any debt that the subsidiary incurs. The parent corporation would only be liable for the amount of money that it had already invested in the subsidiary. In fact, the ability of one corporation to create and own a subsidiary corporation is an inducement for corporations to engage in risky behavior through the subsidiary while protecting the assets of the parent.

The Behavioral Implications of Limited Liability

Since commerce has existed, participants in business activities have looked for ways to limit their responsibilities and minimize their losses.[44] From a purely financial perspective, this makes sense: individuals want to maximize their wealth, not their debt. Therefore, it is no surprise that limited liability has become a fundamental principle for corporate entities.[45] Today, as a quid pro quo, investors will provide capital for a corporation as long as their financial obligations based on the actions of the corporation cannot exceed the amount of their investment.[46]

One then wonders, if a corporation's investors and its managers bear only a limited responsibility for potentially dangerous products and behaviors of the corporation, is there anyone else who shoulders the remainder of this burden? The answer rests in the concept of an externality, which is defined as "the effect of a transaction … on a third party who has not consented to or played any role in the carrying out of that transaction."[47] An externality can be positive or negative. For example, a positive externality results from vaccinations. When a company produces a vaccine, the vaccine must then be administered to individuals to confer immunity. And, if a certain percentage of a population receives the vaccine, then non-vaccinated individuals will benefit from herd immunity.[48] According to the tenets of herd immunity, a measure, such as a vaccination, can dramatically lessen the number of people who are susceptible to a given disease. This decrease of susceptible persons protects the entire "herd," since non-vaccinated persons are then much less likely to come into contact with a person who can expose them to the disease.[49] The non-vaccinated persons benefit from a positive externality: they did not participate in the vaccine transaction, yet they also receive protection from the disease.

While corporate activity can lead to this type of positive externality, it is necessary to recognize the host of negative externalities that accompany corporate behavior. A common example of a negative externality involves pollution. When, through the manufacturing process, a company produces large amounts of toxin-filled smoke and other particulate matter, the air becomes polluted.[50] This pollution will impact the quality of the air inhaled by persons who have nothing to do with the company or the products it manufactures. Moreover, the company may not be held responsible for the costs these individuals incur, such as medical bills for breathing-related conditions. In this example, the costs of the company's pollution are borne by individuals rather than the company and are thus externalized.

Limited liability promotes externalization of costs. For example, since corporate managers know that their investors cannot be held personally responsible for the air pollution generated by their corporation, they have little incentive to lessen their pollution-causing activities.[51] The corporate managers know that other parts of society will absorb these costs. The managers can therefore focus on ways to increase their investors' profits while continuing to impose certain negative outcomes, such as pollution, on society.

The incentives that accompany limited liability dramatically influence the ways in which corporations, and the individuals who run them, act. Economists, whose expertise involves individual and market responses to incentives, have frequently considered the effects of limited liability on behavior. Some economists have suggested that limited liability fosters innovation.[52] Because corporate managers know they can take risks without jeopardizing their investors' assets, they are more likely to take on projects that offer a small chance of producing large financial gains. For instance, corporate managers can pour resources into the research and development of drugs that may never prove effective. But, if the company creates a single drug that is extremely effective, its sales could spectacularly increase profits.

On the other hand, economists have noted that limited liability can also lead to negative consequences on a global scale. When corporate managers take risks, the results do not always lead to innovation.[53] In fact, the incentive to take risks frequently leads to colossal public health disasters, as discussed later in this article. For example, corporate managers may choose to develop products using a relatively unexplored, but potentially risky, chemical compound. They may reason that, while risky, developing even one extremely popular new product will increase their profits. Because of limited liability, these managers know that their investors' personal assets are safe, even if the corporation produces and sells a seemingly innovative product that actually causes significant public health harm. When injured persons sue the corporation, only the corporation's own assets will be available to compensate victims.

In addition to increasing the potential for injury, limited liability can lead managers to devote resources to hazardous activities, such as pesticide or other toxic chemical production. Since the managers know that, through limited liability, their investors' personal assets are protected, they can pursue extremely high-risk ventures,[54] such as constructing chemical production plants with sub-standard safety and precautionary systems. The company's managers pursue these ventures because they know that despite the risk, a successful plant can lead to increased company profits. However, if one of these plants experiences a catastrophic incident, such as a massive dispersal of toxic chemicals into the environment, the company's investors will not be financially harmed beyond their investment. Therefore, the company's managers have great incentive to pursue high-risk, but potentially highly profitable, ventures.

Given these observations, some economists have considered what would happen under a system of unlimited liability for corporate investors.[55] Unlimited liability would mean that investors could be held personally responsible for the corporation's actions, which would allow creditors to have access to the investors' personal assets. This would greatly change the incentives that currently drive corporate managers. Before assuming any liability, investors would want to know about the activities in which the corporation was engaged, and the attendant risks. In addition, some of the costs that are currently externalized by corporations would become apparent in the price of the corporation's stock: "If shareholders faced full liability for potential tort losses, share prices would incorporate available information about the full extent of these possible losses."[56] The price of individual shares would rise and fall to reflect the risk engendered by the corporation's products and behaviors. But, of course, unlimited liability presents significant drawbacks. Unlimited liability could make it difficult for corporations to quickly amass large amounts of capital. It could also discourage the kind of risk-taking that can lead to positive innovations that improve health on a global scale.

Limited liability can also impact the behavior of governments. In their willingness to take risks to enhance the likelihood of profits, corporate managers seek out states, regions, or countries that will allow them to take such risks while bearing the smallest amount of responsibility for any adverse consequences that result from the engagement. This means that corporations are always looking for places that, either through laws or regulations, offer the most business-friendly environment.

In the United States, this so-called "race to the bottom" has occurred during the last 150 years as states have sought to entice corporations and the purported economic stimulation that their presence can bring.[57] Delaware is known for its business-friendly laws, particularly in terms of how managers and directors are treated; this reputation has led about 90 percent of large corporations in the United States to incorporate there.[58] Other states often offer incentives, including corporate tax breaks, to encourage corporations to relocate.[59]

With the rise of multinational companies, governments around the world have attempted to make their countries more attractive to corporations.[60] For some, this has meant relaxing regulations that protect workers and/or the environment. These actions have led multinational corporations to further encourage the race to the bottom, as they look for international venues that offer the most business-friendly environment. This strategy is particularly useful for corporate subsidiaries that are wholly owned by a parent company.[61] As explained earlier, this financial arrangement allows the subsidiary to engage in extremely high-risk business ventures while largely protecting the parent corporation from liability for the results of those activities. As part of this strategy, a parent corporation may undercapitalize its subsidiary corporation. This means that the subsidiary corporation's assets will be less than those necessary to cover its potential debts.[62] As a result, the subsidiary will have even greater incentive to pursue high-risk ventures: because of limited liability, it can only be held responsible for its own assets. If the subsidiary's risky activities lead to the accumulation of debt, then limited liability holds that the assets of the parent corporation are safe. The parent corporation will only be held responsible for its investment in the subsidiary.

The Public Health Ramifications of Limited Liability

To better illustrate the issues associated with limited liability and public health, this article now draws on two examples intended to showcase the health impact of limited liability. As the examples illustrate, limited liability has the potential to greatly influence behavior by removing the threat of personal responsibility for actions taken under the auspices of a corporate entity.

Germany's Law on Pharmacies

For the last few years, large corporate pharmacies have challenged several provisions of Germany's Law on Pharmacies. This law, which derives from practices that began during the Middle Ages, insists that only a pharmacist can own and operate a pharmacy "on [his or her] own responsibility."[63] For centuries, this has meant that German pharmacists are held personally liable for their professional mistakes, including dispensing and other errors.[64] The law goes on to state that, with the exception of certain legal forms, "[s]everal persons can not operate a pharmacy together … ,"[65] which effectively prohibits large corporate pharmacies from entering the German market.

Recently, the managers of DocMorris, a large Dutch pharmacy corporation, have sought to set up franchises in Germany. DocMorris has argued that this expansion will provide a public service, by offering drug prices much lower than those of small privately owned pharmacies.[66] However, DocMorris's ambitions also contravene Germany's Law on Pharmacies and would dramatically shift the country's assignment of liability. While German pharmacists are currently held personally responsible for their mistakes, the introduction of corporate pharmacy ownership would come with the accompanying limited liability that corporations enjoy.[67]

German pharmacists have suggested that this will introduce a two-tiered system, both in terms of prices and safety, among Germany's pharmacies.[68] Because they are personally responsible for their mistakes, prices set by German pharmacists must reflect the debts they may incur, much like in the unlimited liability scheme discussed earlier in this article. Although there are other aspects of this situation, including a potential conflict between Germany's law and the law of the European Union regarding the freedom to establish a business,[69] Germany's pharmacists have focused on the potential ramifications of a shift in liability. Pharmacists and their lobbying groups have suggested that personal liability allows for more attentiveness and fewer mistakes, which ultimately leads to better health outcomes for customers.[70] This intuitively makes sense: currently, if a pharmacist makes a dispensing error and is then sued by a customer who subsequently becomes ill, then the pharmacist must personally compensate the victim. Therefore, pharmacists have great incentive to make as few mistakes as possible.

If Germany's law is altered, however, and limited liability for corporate-owned pharmacies is introduced, one might expect to find an increase in pharmacist errors and negative health outcomes, since the pharmacists responsible for dispensing drugs will be able to hide behind the veil of corporate limited liability. In other words, if Germany's law is changed, then pharmacists at corporate-owned pharmacies would not take on personal responsibility for their actions. Also, according to the tenets of limited liability, the corporation's investors would not take on any additional responsibility. To compensate injured persons, the corporation would rely on its own resources, which may or may not be sufficient to cover its debts. The European Court of Justice will likely rule on this situation later this year.

Dow Corning and Silicone Breast Implants

In 1943, Corning Glass Works (now Corning, Incorporated) and The Dow Chemical Company formed Dow Corning. Dow Corning is a wholly owned subsidiary, with ownership shared by Corning and Dow Chemical.[71] Dow Corning was created "specifically to explore the potential of silicones."[72] In the 1940s, silicone was a relatively unknown, but potentially highly profitable, product. By forming a wholly owned subsidiary, Dow Chemical and Corning could enter the risky silicone market without compromising the financial well-being of either parent corporation.[73] The limited liability associated with Dow Corning, their subsidiary, would protect the parent companies from losing any money beyond their initial financial investments in the new company.

Within two decades, Dow Corning had developed several silicone-based products, including breast implants composed of silicone gel encased by a silicone wrapper. Plastic surgeons began implanting the devices in 1962, although Dow Corning scientists had not thoroughly assessed the safety of the implants through human studies.[74] In time, it became apparent that some implants would rupture, allowing their silicone gel to ooze out. Usually the gel would remain in the vicinity of the implant, but sometimes it would travel throughout a woman's body. This led to a series of lawsuits by women who believed that their ruptured implants were linked to autoimmune diseases such as rheumatoid arthritis and/or breast cancer.[75] During the first of these trials, Dow Corning documents emerged and offered confirmation that the company was both aware of the potential for its implants to leak and had conducted no studies to research the long-term safety of the implants for women.[76]

By 1992, thousands of women who had received Dow Corning's silicone implants had sued the company as individuals or joined a class action lawsuit against the company. Eventually, although the science linking silicone breast implants to certain diseases and conditions was controversial,[77] Dow Corning and other implant manufacturers agreed to a multi-billion dollar settlement. However, as more women came forward, the settlement could not hold, and Dow Corning declared bankruptcy in 1995[78] because it did not have the assets to make its settlement payments. Nine years later, Dow Corning emerged from bankruptcy, and, since 2004, has been processing claims related to its silicone implants.[79]

Dow Corning's fate can partially be explained by undercapitalization. Because its parent companies knew that it was developing high-risk products, they had incentive to deliberately undercapitalize Dow Corning.[80] Thus, if Dow Corning created a product, such as breast implants, which led to lawsuits and a multi-billion dollar settlement, Dow Corning could then only be held responsible for its own assets. Due to Dow Corning's limited liability, the assets of Dow Chemical and Corning, its parent companies, were untouchable.[81] As a result, Dow Corning's undercapitalization allowed it to declare bankruptcy, leading to nine years of reorganization, because it did not have the assets to fund a multi-billion dollar settlement.

Addressing Limited Liability as a Public Health Threat

Several possibilities exist or have been suggested for minimizing the potential for damage to the public's health presented by limited liability. Perhaps the most direct and aggressive possibility is to eliminate the existence of limited liability altogether, as mentioned earlier, by the rewriting of corporate law. Although some scholars have argued that unlimited shareholder liability is a viable policy option,[82] this possibility is immensely unlikely to occur. It is politically infeasible because all states and nations would then have to eliminate limited liability; if even just one state continued to offer it, all corporations would choose to be chartered there. Business, which is a potent political force, would understandably oppose any effort to abolish limited liability. Also, limited liability probably confers significant social benefits, such as an inducement to invest in speculative products like new drugs or safety devices, and that inducement should not be lost. Short of the abolition of limited liability, however, is an established legal strategy that might reduce the negative public health effects of limited liability.

Piercing the Corporate Veil

Piercing the corporate veil is a legal maneuver designed to hold personally responsible an individual wrongdoer who is improperly hiding behind a corporate curtain. (When speaking of an individual in this sense, it may be an actual person, or a parent corporation that owns a subsidiary corporation.) The individual's "improper" invocation of corporate limited liability can be evidenced by several factors, such as an underfinanced corporation, sole ownership of the corporate stock, or failure to follow the legally prescribed governance process of a corporation. In such cases, the corporation is alleged to be a sham, or merely the "alter ego" of the individual, and the legal theory is that under such circumstances, the individual loses the corporate benefit of limited liability.

Litigation that attempts to pierce the corporate veil is the most prevalent type of lawsuit against corporations in the United States,[83] and these cases have built what scholars deem to be an awkward body of law. The cases use terms such as alias, alter ego, corporate double, nominal entity, puppet, and shell to describe the particular corporation whose practices are being examined.[84] Thus, the very language of piercing law is contentious. In an early piercing case, the esteemed Judge Benjamin Cardozo, sitting on the New York Court of Appeals, struggled to define the circumstances under which a parent corporation will be held liable for the wrongs of its subsidiary corporation, by means of piercing a corporate veil. Cardozo, in 1916, wrote the following:

> The whole problem of the relation between parent and subsidiary corporations is one that is still enveloped in the mists of metaphor. Metaphors in law are to be narrowly watched, for starting as devices to liberate thought, they end often by enslaving it. We say at times that the corporate entity will be ignored when the parent corporation operates a business through a subsidiary which is characterized as an "alias" or a "dummy." All this is well enough if the picturesqueness of the epithets does not lead us to forget that the essential term to be defined is the act of operation. Dominion may be so complete, interference so obtrusive, that by the general rules of agency the parent will be a principal and the subsidiary an agent. Where control is less than this, we are remitted to the tests of honesty and justice.[85]

The difficulties of clearly defining the circumstances under which a corporate veil will be pierced have persisted into modern times, resulting in a less than fully predictable state of the law. In some cases, courts have been willing to find individuals and parent corporations personally liable, beyond the limits of their investments, for the wrongs of a corporation. Robert Thompson, in a creative study of the epidemiology of veil-piercing cases, looked at about 1,600 reported legal cases through 1985 in which there was an attempt to pierce a corporate veil. In about 40 percent of the cases, courts did pierce the veil.[86]

However, in a prominent U.S. Supreme Court case decided in 1998, the limits of a parent corporation's responsibility for a subsidiary corporation were more strictly defined. In United States v. Bestfoods,[87] the Court examined the responsibility of a parent corporation under the Comprehensive Environmental Response, Compensation and Liability Act (CERCLA, or the Superfund Act). Bestfoods had acquired a subsidiary corporation that operated a polluting chemical manufacturing facility that required cleanup. The question for the Supreme Court was whether Bestfoods was responsible for the cleanup costs. The Court found that the "respect for corporate distinctions" between a parent and a subsidiary corporation is a "bedrock principle" of corporate law that is not disrupted by CERCLA.[88] While the Court recognized that piercing a corporate veil was also a traditional part of the law, its ruling stipulated that piercing would take place in a Bestfoods type of situation only if the corporate form was misused to accomplish wrongful purposes, such as fraud.

Some scholars have advocated for a change in the law that would clarify situations under which a shareholder could be held personally responsible for the wrongs of a corporation, i.e., clarity in veil piercing. Nina Mendelson has argued, for example, that shareholders, who control the actions of a corporation by the size of their investment, should be held fully responsible for the torts of the corporation. This, she argues, would motivate such shareholders to internalize the costs of the corporation's risky ventures, rather than having innocent parties, such as individuals injured by a corporation's product, bear the brunt of externalized costs.[89]

Piercing the corporate veil is not restricted to United States jurisprudence. Limited liability is a hallmark of corporate law in many countries, and therefore, attempts to go beyond the limits of liability, such as through veil piercing, have found fertile soil in places other than the United States. A recent law review article[90] reports that in 1994, China adopted its Company Law which recognizes limited liability forms of business, but which initially failed to provide for veil piercing. However, the article points out that an amendment to the law, effective in 2006, now recognizes corporate veil piercing.

Other Strategies for Addressing Corporate Behavior

Piercing the corporate veil is the strategy that most directly relates to corporations' limited liability as a public health problem. Other aspects of how corporations are organized and how they function can also present difficulties for protecting the public's health. For example, and as described earlier in this article, the statutory mandate for a corporation to maximize its profits and its return to its shareholders can lead to corporate conduct that poses risks to others. This problem is not addressed directly by attempts to pierce the corporate veil. Therefore, others have suggested that a revision to the standard language in corporate charters could materially minimize the problem. Presently, most states create or charter corporations with very general language such as, "This corporation may engage in or transact any or all lawful activities or business permitted under the laws of the United States, the state of [name], or any other state, county, territory, or nation."

Robert Hinkley, a corporate lawyer who previously represented major corporations, has suggested that, with 28 additional words in the corporate charter, the conduct of corporations could be materially changed. Those words are: "... but not at the expense of the environment, human rights, public health and safety, dignity of employees, and the welfare of the communities in which the company operates."[91]

Additional strategies, some of which are part of the corporate social responsibility movement, address the issues of changing the norms for corporate conduct and minimizing the risk of corporate criminal activity.

Conclusion

These observations reinforce the need for health professionals to understand the impact that limited liability has on public health. This knowledge is important for several reasons. For one, it serves to reorient health professionals' attention to corporations as causative agents of illness and injury. Also, it allows health professionals to understand how limited liability allows corporations to externalize risk. Given this knowledge, it would be useful if health professionals developed ways to quantify the significant detriment that limited liability poses for public health. Even without this quantified knowledge, there are ways that limited liability can be addressed. As this article explained, health professionals should be aware and supportive of measures such as legislative and common law changes that would make it less likely for corporations to engage in risky behavior that negatively impacts public health.

REFERENCES

1. Centers for Disease Control and Prevention, U.S. Department of Health and Human Services, "Webbased Injury Statistics Query and Reporting System (WISQARS)," Available at <http://www. cdc.gov/ncipc/wisqars/> (last visited August 22, 2007).

2. W. Cukier and V. W. Sidel, The Global Gun Epidemic (Westport, CT: Greenwood Publishing, 2006).

3. National Highway Traffic Safety Administration, U.S. Department of Transportation, Traffic Safety Facts 2005, at 2.

4. Pan American Health Organization, "Deaths from motor vehicle traffic accidents in selected countries of the Americas, 1985–2001," Epidemiological Bulletin 25, no. 1 (2004): 2-5.

5. Centers for Disease Control and Prevention, U.S. Department of Health and Human Services, "Tobacco-Related Mortality," Available at <http://www.cdc.gov/ tobacco/data_statistics/Factsheets/ tobacco_related_mortality.htm> (last visited August 21, 2007).

6. World Health Organization, "An International Treaty for Tobacco Control," Available at <http://www.who.int/features/2003/08/ en/> (last visited August 21, 2007).

7. D. H. Jernigan, Global Status Report: Alcohol and Young People, World Health Organization, Geneva, 2001, at 10-13.

8. S. P. Teret and A. P. Michaelis, "Litigating for Native American health: the liability of alcoholic beverage makers and distributors," Journal of Public Health Policy 26, no. 2 (2005): 246-59.

9. See Corporations and Health Watch, "Corporate Practices," Available at <http:// www.corporationsandhealth.org> (last visited August 22, 2007).

10. By the term "legal fictions," we mean that corporations are a creation of the law, and exist only because the law has authorized their existence.

11. W. H. Wiist, "Public health and the anticorporate movement: rationale and recommendations," American Journal of Public Health 96, no. 8 (2006): 1370-75.

12. J. Bakan, The Corporation: The Pathological Pursuit of Profit and Power (New York: Free Press, 2004): at 37.

13. S. L. Hills, ed., Corporate Violence: Injury and Death for Profit (Totowa, NJ: Rowman & Littlefield, 1987): at 190-91.

14. R. W. Hillman, "Limited liability in historical perspective," Washington and Lee Law Review 54 (Spring 1997): 615-27.

15. T. E. Rutledge, "Limited liability (or not): reflections on the holy grail," South Dakota Law Review 51, no. 3 (2006): 417–49, at 419-21.

16. K. B. Davis, Jr., "Once more, the business judgment rule," Wisconsin Law Review 2000, no. 3 (2000): 573-95.

17. See, e.g., N. Frank, "Murder in the workplace," In Hills, ed., supra note 13, at 103-07.

18. J. Micklethwait and A. Wooldridge, *The Company: A Short History of a Revolutionary Idea* (New York: Modern Library, 2003).

19. Id., at 17-21.

20. Id.

21. See Bakan, supra note 12, at 11-13.

22. Id.

23. Id., at 158.

24. Id., at 37.

25. S. M. Bainbridge, "The Case for Limited Shareholder Voting Rights," *UCLA Law Review* 53 (February 2006): 601-36, at 625; M. Friedman, "The Social Responsibility of Business Is to Increase Its Profits," *New York Times Magazine,* September 13, 1970.

26. E.g., Dodge v. Ford Motor Co., 204 Mich. 459, 507 (1919) ("A business corporation is organized and carried on primarily for the profit of the stockholders. The powers of the directors are to be employed for that end. The discretion of the directors is to be exercised in the choice of means to attain that end, and does not extend to a change in the end itself...").

27. See Bakan, supra note 12, at 37, 50.

28. C. A. Harwell Wells, "The Cycles of Corporate Social Responsibility: An Historical Retrospective for the Twenty-First Century," *University of Kansas Law Review* 51, no. 1 (2002): 77-140.

29. See, e.g., Starbucks Corporation, *Corporate Social Responsibility Fiscal 2006 Annual Report* (Seattle: Starbucks Coffee Company, 2007): at 57.

30. See, e.g., Pfizer, *A Prescription for Access* (New York: Pfizer, 2004).

31. See D. C. Korten, *When Corporations Rule the World* (Bloomfield, CT: Kumarian Press, 2001): at 202-4.

32. See, e.g., Starbucks Corporation, supra note 29, at 10.

33. See, e.g., Ogilvy Public Relations Worldwide, "Expertise: Corporate Social Responsibility," available at <http://www.ogilvypr.com/expertise/corporate-social-responsibility.cfm> (last visited August 21, 2007).

34. M. Ventoruzzo, "'Cost-Based' and 'Rules-Based' Regulatory Competition: Markets for Corporate Charters in the U.S. and in the E.U.," *NYU Journal of Law & Business* 3 (Fall 2006): 91-153.

35. M. A. Eisenberg, *Corporations and Other Business Organizations* (New York: Foundation Press, 2000): at 100.

36. Id.

37. See Bakan, supra note 12, at 8.

38. P. I. Blumberg, "Limited Liability and Corporate Groups," *Journal of Corporation Law* 11, no. 4 (1986): 573-631.

39. See Eisenberg, supra note 35, at 203.

40. Id.

41. D. K. Moll, "Minority Oppression & the Limited Liability Company: Learning (or Not) from Close Corporation History," *Wake Forest Law Review* 40, no. 3 (2005): 883-976, at 888.

42. See Blumberg, supra note 38.

43. Id., at 575.

44. See Hillman, supra note 14.

45. F. H. Easterbrook and D. R. Fischel, "Limited Liability and the Corporation," *University of Chicago Law Review* 52, no. 1 (1985): 89-117.

46. See Eisenberg, supra note 35, at 219.

47. See Bakan, supra note 12, at 61.

48. G. L. Armstrong et al., "The Economics of Routine Childhood Hepatitis A Immunization in the United States: The Impact of Herd Immunity," *Pediatrics* 119, no. 1 (2007): e22-e29.

49. L. Gordis, Epidemiology (Philadelphia: W. B. Saunders Company, 2000): at 19-20.

50. D. C. Christiani and M. A. Woodin, "Urban and Transboundary Air Pollution," in M. McCally, ed., *Life Support: The Environment and Human Health* (Cambridge: The MIT Press, 2002): 15-37.

51. See Eisenberg, supra note 35, at 233.

52. See Blumberg, supra note 38, at 616.

53. H. Hansmann and R. Kraakman, "Toward Unlimited Shareholder Liability for Corporate Torts," *Yale Law Journal* 100, no. 7 (1991): 1879-1934, at 1894.

54. Id., at 1882-83.

55. Id.; see Blumberg, supra note 38.

56. See Hansmann and Kraakman, supra note 53, at 1907.

57. See Bakan, supra note 12, at 22.

58. See Micklethwait and Wooldridge, supra note 18, at 141.

59. C. Derber, *Corporation Nation* (New York: St. Martin's Griffin, 1998): at 168.

60. Id., at 43-48.

61. See Blumberg, supra note 38, at 575-77.

62. L. M. Lopucki, "The Death of Liability," *Yale Law Journal* 106, no. 1 (1996): 1-92, at 20-23.

63. See German Law on Pharmacies, § 7, quoted in C. Lafontaine, *National Law on Pharmacies and its Non-Application by a Member State's Public Authorities* (Saarbrucken, Germany: Law Web Saarbrucken, 2006): at 304, available at <http://www. jura.uni-saarland.de/projekte/Bibliothek/text.php?id=432> (last visited August 21, 2007).

64. E. Harris, "Germany Attempts to Update Pharmacy Laws," *Morning Edition*, National Public Radio Programs, November 14, 2006.

65. See German Law on Pharmacies, § 8, quoted in Lafontaine, supra note 63, at 304.

66. A. Cullen and S. Bauer, "Drug Chain Rattles Markets in Germany," *International Herald Tribune*, April 17, 2007.

67. See Harris, supra note 64.

68. Id.

69. M. Thompson, "Government Urges ECJ to Retain German Ban on Foreign Ownership of Pharmacies," *Global Insight*, August 20, 2007.

70. W. Boston, "Pills + Politics," *Time*, September 24, 2006; see Harris, supra note 64.

71. See "Dow Corning at a Glance," Dow Corning Web site, available at <http://www. dowcorning.com/content/about/> (last visited May 25, 2007).

72. Id.

73. See Blumberg, supra note 38, at 575-77.

74. D. E. Bernstein, "The Breast Implant Fiasco," *California Law Review* 87, no. 2 (1999): 457-510, at 462.

75. B. J. Feder, "Dow Corning in Bankruptcy Over Lawsuits," *New York Times*, May 16, 1995.

76. See Bernstein, supra note 74, at 464.

77. See, e.g., N. R. Rose and M. Potter, "The Silicone Controversy: Towards a Resolution," *Immunology Today* 16, no. 10 (1995): 459-60.

78. See Feder, supra note 75.

79. "Dow Corning Emerges from Bankruptcy," New York Times, June 2, 2004.

80. See, e.g., *Radaszewski v. Telecom Corp.*, 981 F.2d 305, 311 (8th Cir. 1992) ("The doctrine of limited liability is intended precisely to protect a parent corporation whose subsidiary goes broke.")

81. See Blumberg, supra note 38, at 575-77.

82. See Hansmann and Kraakman, supra note 53, at 1880.

83. R. B. Thompson, "Piercing the Veil: Is the Common Law the Problem?" *Connecticut Law Review* 37 (Spring 2005): 619-34, at 619.

84. C. S. Krendl and J. R. Krendl, "Piercing the Corporate Veil: Focusing the Inquiry," *Denver Law Journal* 55, no. 1 (1978): 1-60.

85. *Berkey v. Third Avenue Railroad Co.*, 244 N.Y. 84 (1926).

86. R. B. Thompson, "Piercing the Corporate Veil: An Empirical Study," *Cornell Law Review* 76 (July 1991): 1036-74.

87. 524 U.S. 51 (1998).

88. Id., at 56.

89. N. A. Mendelson, "A Control-Based Approach to Shareholder Liability for Corporate Torts," *Columbia Law Review* 102, no. 5 (2002): 1203-1303.

90. B. C. Reed, "Clearing Away the Mist: Suggestions for Developing a Principled Veil Piercing Doctrine in China," *Vanderbilt Journal of Transnational Law* 39, no. 5 (2006): 1643-75.

91. A. Cooper, "Twenty-Eight Words That Could Change the World," *The Sun*, September 2004, available at <http://www. thesunmagazine.org/345_Hinkley. pdf> (last visited August 21, 2007).

4

Public Relations and Advertising

Diane Farsetta

It was toward the end of a 3-day conference organized by the nuclear power industry. A thin man in a dark suit ascended the stage at one end of a large conference room. The words "Energizing a Low-Carbon Future" loomed behind him, in large type. Stylized graphics of a watery surface, a child's silhouette and a floating globe appeared over his other shoulder.

"First, I want to talk a little bit about what my company does," began Craig T. Smith, an executive with one of Washington DC's best-known polling firms. He then gave an unusually frank description of corporate communications.

"Penn, Schoen and Berland is a company that does market research to develop strategies on positioning ideas, individuals, organizations in the public policy marketplace," Smith continued. "Many of you may have heard of our firm because of the political work we do—Bill Clinton, Tony Blair, [Silvio] Berlusconi, Michael Bloomberg. ... But actually 80 percent of the work we do is for corporations, [to] help position them in the public policy marketplace. Not their products, but their image, their ideas and what they're trying to do."

As the audience of reactor operators, owners and other nuclear proponents listened intently, Smith assessed attempts to "shape the image of nuclear power," as of mid-2008. While nuclear power had recently been repositioned as a low-carbon energy source and part of the solution to global warming, he said, "You still have a challenge of what to do with used fuel." One way to allay public concerns about the radio-active waste is to promise a technological fix: reprocessing it into material that can again be used to fuel reactors. But call it recycling, not reprocessing, Smith suggested. "Recycling is a message that resonates with people. ... It resonates with audiences that don't necessarily support, or are somewhat agnostic, with nuclear power" (Smith, 2008).

Smith is a pollster by trade, with a background in politics (Penn, Schoen web site, undated). His work lies at the intersection of public relations (PR) and marketing. The interrelated nature of polling, PR, and advertising practices is further illustrated by the fact that Mark Penn, the cofounder and president of Smith's polling firm, also heads the major PR firm Burson-Marsteller (Burson-Marsteller web site, undated).

Indeed, the body seen as the incubator for the modern PR industry closely studied and borrowed from the advertising industry. The U.S. government established the Committee on Public Information in 1917, to "sell" World War I to a reluctant public. One history of the war effort called the Committee "perhaps the most effective job of large-scale war propaganda which the world had ever witnessed" (Stauber & Rampton, 1995). Its chair later described the Committee as "the world's greatest adventure in advertising" (Creel, 1920).

Edward Bernays and Walter Lippmann—two of the most influential early PR practitioners—assisted the Committee on Public Information. The experi-ence left them convinced that democracies require extensive PR operations. However, their view of communications and governance severely minimizes the role of public debate and participation.

"The conscious and intelligent manipulation of the organized habits and opinions of the masses is an important element in democratic society," wrote Bernays. "No serious sociologist any longer believes that the voice of the people expresses any divine or specially wise and lofty idea. ... Fortunately, the sin-cere and gifted politician is able, by the instrument of propaganda, to mold and form the will of the people" (Bernays, 1928).

Lippmann, who coined the phrase "the manufacture of consent," called the idea of enlightened self-government a "democratic fallacy." While the manipu-lation of public opinion "was supposed to have died out with the appearance of democracy ... it has not," he wrote. "It has, in fact, improved enormously in technic [technique]. ... The practice of democracy has turned a corner. ... Persuasion has become a self-conscious art and a regular organ of popular government" (Lippmann, 1922).

Today's PR professionals are usually not so blunt. Acutely aware of their profession's poor public image, they point to PR ethics codes that stress trans-parency and public engagement (Public Relations Society of America, 2000).

However, nothing is done to enforce these codes and, far too often, PR tactics are used to confuse issues and manipulate public debates.

Perhaps the most common misleading PR approach is the third party technique. Simply described, it involves putting the PR client's words into someone else's mouth. It's effective because a seemingly independent testimonial on behalf of a product or company has much more credibility than the same message relayed by someone directly and openly affiliated with that company.

A member of Nuclear Energy Women, a now-defunct group established by the nuclear industry in 1975, experienced this phenomenon firsthand. She worked "in the public relations department of a utility company," and when she spoke as a representative of the utility, "her 'credibility was next to zero'," as she described it; "audiences were hostile and media coverage was inadequate and critical. However, when she spoke as a representative of Nuclear Energy Women, she usually received sympathetic press coverage and her audiences were more open to her pro-nuclear arguments" (Useem & Zald, 1997).

Nuclear Energy Women is an example of a front group, an organization that presents itself as independent, but unwaveringly supports the interests of the company or industry association that founded it and is often its sole source of funding. Other applications of the third party technique include paying "experts"—sometimes people with dubious or irrelevant credentials— who publicly promote the company or product; skewing online conversations by paying bloggers, posting comments or launching fake blogs that hide or misrepresent the identity of the author(s); and ghostwriting favorable opinion columns or academic papers, which are then published as the work of individuals unaffiliated with the company or product. Overwhelmingly, the ties between the endorser and the company or product being endorsed are not disclosed. While doing so would honor professional and ethical standards, it would undermine the PR impact of the third party technique.

For example, the Washington, DC-based PR firm LawMedia Group (LMG) has been linked to several ghostwritten op/ed columns. In July 2008, an LMG-written column was published under the name of the president of the Southern Christian Leadership Conference (SCLC), without his approval. The SCLC protested publicly, because two of its corporate funders were mentioned disapprovingly in the column. The op/ed column criticized a bill that would lower credit card fees. Presumably it was part of LMG's work for the Electronic Payments Coalition, a group of credit card and financial companies that opposed the bill (Birnbaum, 2008). However, LMG knew that presenting a civil rights group like the SCLC as the public face of opposition to the bill would be much more persuasive than having credit card companies speak out against it themselves.

A step beyond the covert recruitment of supporters is the insertion of corporate-funded PR segments into news programming. In television, these segments are called video news releases (VNRs); in radio, they're audio news releases (ANRs). VNRs and ANRs are not like print press releases, which are most commonly used to encourage reporters to include mention of the company's activities or perspective in independently generated reports. Instead, ANRs and VNRs are broadcast segments that PR professionals script, record, edit, distribute, and promote to resource-strapped newsrooms.

VNRs and ANRs effectively replace reporters with publicists, substituting PR and marketing messages for news. Worse, a series of studies on television stations' use of VNRs found that stations failed to disclose VNR footage to viewers 98% of the time. In addition, nearly 85% of VNR-derived news segments contained no independently gathered video. The sole source for visuals and information in these segments were the VNR and accompanying PR materials (Farsetta & Price, 2006a, 2006b, 2007).

Health-related VNRs and ANRs are especially popular. Station producers see health segments as "news you can use," and PR professionals can easily work in mentions of any of a wide range of products. In 2004, the head of a major VNR firm remarked, "Our medical stories are consistently generating more than 100 placements per project per year" (Simon, 2004).

VNRs and ANRs pose problems more serious than the commercialization of health news. Sometimes, they contain inaccurate, misleading, or even blatantly false information. For example, in February 2006, an anchor on New York City's WCBS-2 introduced a health story by claiming that a recent study showed that "popular supplements ... deliver a one–two punch to ease the pain" of arthritis. The segment featured glowing testimony about the over-the-counter supplements, glucosamine, and chondroitin sulfate. The story was derived entirely from a VNR funded by a company that makes glucosamine/chondroitin pills.

WCBS-2, the third most watched local newscast in the United States, didn't tell its viewers that the segment was a VNR. The station also didn't fact-check the claims made in the VNR. That allowed the supplement company's distortion of the study to air, unchallenged by the facts. Contrary to the VNR's claims, the study, which was published in the *New England Journal of Medicine*, actually concluded that "glucosamine and chondroitin sulfate alone or in combination did not reduce pain effectively" (Farsetta & Price, 2006a).

Using news programming to plug products is one example of the increasing convergence of marketing and PR. Historically, the distinction between PR and advertising was clear. If the favorable product or company mention was paid for, it was advertising, which was distinct from news or entertainment content. If the favorable mention wasn't paid for, but obtained through reporter cultivation, it was PR. Traditionally, PR shapes news content by creating events or relaying persuasive materials. Reporters and editors then act as journalistic "gatekeepers," deciding whether the subject of the PR pitch merits news coverage.

Recently, marketing communications or "marcom" practices have further blurred the distinction between PR and advertising. One marcom approach is the "paid placement" or "secured" VNR. While most VNRs are provided to stations for free, to air or not as they see fit, the airtime for secured VNRs is purchased, as it is for ads. The benefits of this approach include "the ability to target specific demographics and to conduct a post-buy analysis of audience delivery," in addition to ensuring that the VNR is aired (Mandese, 2005).

Sometimes, marcom approaches blur the distinction between news and promotional content. The broadcast PR firm Medialink Worldwide offers clients what it calls "branded journalism": the close association of a product or company with a newscast (Mandese, 2005). Another firm, ARAnet, provides sponsored articles to "more than 65 of the nation's top 100 newspapers," according to an August 2008 account. ARAnet's president describes the articles as "high-quality consumer content" that "just happen to be underwritten by our clients." The articles are often flagged as sponsored content online, but not when they appear in print (Reinan, 2008).

In 2000, the Ackerman McQueen advertising agency launched "Branded News," a practice that creates and runs video-rich online "news" sites. The firm's clients include the National Rifle Association and the American Clean Skies Foundation, a front group run and funded by the natural gas company Chesapeake Energy (Hughes, 2008). Branded News says its goal is "narrowcasting": providing in-depth news on a particular issue to a relatively small but influential audience. When mainstream news doesn't adequately cover an issue, "why shouldn't brand leaders fill this void?" asks the firm's web site (Branded News web site, undated).

Tech Central Station, a news and opinion web site launched by a lobbying firm in 2000, used a similar approach. Its columns invariably reflected the interests of the lobbying firm's clients. Not only did Tech Central Station columns appear on its web site, they were "cited hundreds of times in the mainstream media and reprinted on op/ed pages across the country," according to a 2003 article that dubbed the practice "journo-lobbying" (Confessore, 2003). In 2006, the lobbying firm, DCI Group, sold Tech Central Station to the site's editor (O'Dwyer's, 2006). A statement on the site, now named TCS Daily, says its "previous sponsorship agreements have expired," but does not explain how the site is currently funded (TCS Daily web site, undated).

The net effect of these and many other communications tactics is to privilege the corporate viewpoint, since corporations can best afford to purchase PR, advertising, polling, and lobbying services. As a result, independent voices are marginalized, and news coverage of issues damaging or irrelevant to corporate agendas dwindles.

As the article on Tech Central Station warned, "The new game is to dominate the entire intellectual environment in which officials make policy decisions, which means funding everything from think tanks to issue ads to phony grassroots pressure groups." While the media is "the institution that most affects the intellectual atmosphere," it "has proven the hardest ... to influence—until now" (Confessore, 2003).

Burnishing Public Images

"If you choose to drink bottled water, please choose to make a difference," implores the print advertisement. The text appears under a blue-tinted picture of actor Matt Damon squatting next to three African children, tracing something in the sand near their feet. A small picture of Ethos brand bottled water—the product being promoted—appears in the lower right corner. To the left is the logo for the organization H2o Africa. The group's logo is larger than the Ethos label on the water bottle (Zmuda, 2008).

The emphasis on charity is no mistake. Ethos, which is owned by the Starbucks coffee chain but packaged, distributed, and marketed by Pepsi-Cola, made its national debut in early 2008, as bottled water sales continued to slowdown. To differentiate itself in a crowded market, Ethos partnered with H2o Africa, an organization cofounded by Damon that works to bring clean drinking water to African communities. For each bottle of Ethos water sold, five cents are given to the Ethos Water Fund of the Starbucks Foundation. The Ethos ad proclaims, "Every bottle makes a difference" (Pepsi-Cola, 2008).

Ethos' ad campaign glosses over numerous ironies and contradictions. Perhaps foremost is that the vast majority of those who buy bottled water—especially a brand like Ethos, which was advertised in Vanity Fair, GQ, Sports Illustrated, and Time, among other magazines (Zmuda, 2008)—has easy access to clean tap water. In addition, both Starbucks and Pepsi declined an earlier opportunity to partner with a bottled water company that gives all of its proceeds to charity (Hein, 2008). That's not to mention the energy and environmental concerns inherent to bottling large volumes of water, then transporting and eventually disposing of the plastic bottles.

Still, a company's charitable or socially responsible practices can make for potent PR. Positive media coverage can help boost sales, recruit, and retain staff, and increase share value. Having a good public image also makes it easier for companies to persuade community members and policy makers to support their business plans and policy agendas.

The only drawback to this approach—called "cause-related marketing" by advertisers and "corporate social responsibility" (CSR) by PR professionals—is that it leaves the company open to charges of hypocrisy. If enough people perceive the company's do-gooder claims as misleading, false, or totally self-serving, the campaign could actually damage the company's public image.

The oil industry has had a particularly difficult time with CSR campaigns, even though oil companies persist in attempts to promote their environmental and other social initiatives. When BP launched a $200 million PR and marketing campaign to rebrand itself as "Beyond Petroleum" in 2000, charges of "greenwashing"—making disingenuous "green" claims, in an attempt to whitewash a poor environmental record—came from all sides. A *New York Times* review of the "Beyond Petroleum" campaign protested, "BP remains an oil company, deriving the vast majority of its profits from the black stuff that— from drilling rig to oil tanker to refinery to gas station—scars the earth, pollutes the air and eventually warms the planet" (Frey, 2002).

Some firms have concluded that the best way for companies to win or regain the public's confidence is for them to partner with nongovernmental organizations (NGOs). "Amplify relationships with centrist NGOs," recommended the head of the major PR firm Edelman, during a February 2001 presentation. "Make sure they are part of the solution, that they have a stake in the outcome." NGOs—at least, established centrist groups, not "radical" ones— are key allies, he argued, because they are more widely trusted than business or government. Plus, they can have a "halo effect" on associated companies (Richard Edelman, 2001). "We recognized before anyone that NGOs, such as Greenpeace and Amnesty International, were influencing corporate social responsibility by highlighting environmental and labor practices," Edelman's web site counseled clients. "Open your channels of communication so when an issue becomes a problem stakeholders are more predisposed to listen" (Edelman web site, 2004).

Partnering with NGOs is a newer variation on a standard corporate PR tactic: donating to charitable groups. Whether the donations are monetary or in-kind, made by the company directly or via a corporate foundation, they help foster goodwill and create a record of positive community engagement. Often, companies limit their donations to groups relevant to their products or services, affiliated with their employees, or active in communities near their facilities.

Focusing corporate largesse in this manner maximizes the PR impact on three key audiences: potential customers, employees and their families, and people living near the company.

Many pharmaceutical companies follow this approach, sometimes giving millions of dollars to patient groups, organizations that advocate for people with certain medical conditions. Donating to patient groups not only allows a drug maker to cultivate potential customers, but may also provide it with "third party" advocates willing to support the company's policy agenda and defend it in the court of public opinion.

For example, in mid-January 2008, a study was published questioning the effectiveness of the cholesterol drug Vytorin. The following day, the American Heart Association released a statement that said the study "was not large enough or long enough to determine whether" Vytorin "is more or less effective than" a cheaper, more established treatment, "in reducing heart attacks or deaths" (American Heart Association, 2008).

"What the association did not note in its statement," reported the *New York Times*, "was that the group receives nearly $2 million a year from Merck/ Schering-Plough Pharmaceuticals, the joint venture that markets Vytorin." The American Heart Association said its statement was not motivated by the industry funding, and was simply meant to clear up confusion among patients (Saul, 2008). However, the association failed to criticize Merck and Schering-Plough for delaying the study's publication for nearly 2 years. Medical doctors and members of Congress harshly criticized the delay, which also led to legal action against the drug companies (Thomaselli, 2008).

Related pharmaceutical industry practices include sponsoring medical conferences, organizing continuing education courses—as the ad firm Interpublic does for its pharmaceutical clients (Petersen, 2008)—and otherwise cultivating doctors, the powerful "gatekeepers" who stand in between drug companies and the consumers of their products. "Pharmaceutical companies spend billions of dollars annually to ensure that physicians most susceptible to marketing prescribe the most expensive, most promoted drugs to the most people possible," concluded an academic paper. "Physicians are susceptible to corporate influence because they are overworked, overwhelmed with information and paperwork, and feel underappreciated" (Fugh-Berman & Ahari, 2007).

More traditional cause-related marketing campaigns have been used to boost revenue and deepen consumer loyalty since at least the 1980s. American Express pioneered the use of charitable donations as marketing with its Statue of Liberty campaign. During the last quarter of 1983, American Express pledged one cent for every credit card transaction and one dollar for every new credit card issued, toward efforts to restore the Statue of Liberty. The campaign netted the credit card company massive amounts of positive media coverage and a 28% increase in business (Stole, 2006).

The same approach is widely used today. "Breast cancer in particular has been an increasingly popular cause for marketers to align with," noted *Advertising Age*. During October, National Breast Cancer Awareness Month, companies specially market products ranging from cars to cosmetics, pledging a share of the proceeds to breast cancer research. Campbell Soup "doubled sales of its top varieties to its biggest grocery customer" in October 2006, by adding a pink ribbon—a sign of breast cancer awareness—to its labels and donating 3.5 cents per can sold to a breast cancer advocacy group (Thompson, 2006).

The proliferation of breast cancer-related marketing ploys led the grass-roots group Breast Cancer Action to launch its "Think Before You Pink" project in 2002. The project encourages people to question breast cancer-related marketing. It also targets what the group calls "pinkwashers": "companies that purport to care about breast cancer by promoting a pink ribbon campaign, but manufacture products that are linked to the disease," such as yogurt containing recombinant bovine growth hormone (Breast Cancer Action web site, undated).

The (RED) campaign, launched in 2006 by rock star Bono and Bobby Shriver to raise funds for Africa, is perhaps the highest profile cause-related marketing effort today. Companies pay for the ability to market (RED) products, like Apple's (RED) iPod and Gap's (RED) clothing line, and donate some percentage of (RED) product sales to the Global Fund to Fight AIDS, Tuberculosis, and Malaria. In return, the companies benefit from the (RED) campaign's marketing, including celebrity endorsements, as well as the "halo effect."

In its first year, the (RED) campaign raised $25 million for AIDS medications in Africa. Supporters called it "found money," pointing out that participating companies would not have otherwise supported the Global Fund. Critics advocated for direct donations to charities instead. "Join us in rejecting the ti(red) notion that shopping is a reasonable response to human suffering," urges the web site buylesscrap.org (Buy (Less) Crap web site, undated). Other (RED) critics asked whether the campaign's marketing budget exceeded its charitable donations—a question the campaign could not answer, because neither it nor its participating companies were willing to make the financial details public (Arnoldy, 2007).

Organizations that benefit from cause-related marketing campaigns or corporate partnerships argue that it's a win-win situation. Yes, their name and cause are used to sell products, but at least some of that money is then used to do good. However, as the PR firm Edelman has admitted, "cooperation with business [may] lead to subversion of NGO credibility" (Richard Edelman, 2001). Moreover, as communications professor Inger Stole has pointed out, such partnerships are "driven by the need to increase a businesses' return on its investment. ... Non-profits that do not fit a corporate profile or appeal to the customer group that businesses want to reach are ignored, even if they do vital work, while groups that provide good marketing vehicles receive a disproportionate amount of interest" (Stole, 2006).

Responding to Criticism or Threats

"CIW is an attack organization lining the leaders [sic] pockets by attacking restaurant companies," wrote a commenter on the video-sharing web site YouTube, referring to the Coalition of Immokalee Workers, a farmworker advocacy group. "They make up issues and collect money from dupes that believe their story. To [sic] bad the people protesting don't have a clue regarding the facts. A bunch of fools!" (Bennett Williams, 2008b).

At the time, the Coalition of Immokalee Workers (CIW) was pressuring Burger King to pay a penny more per pound for its tomatoes. McDonald's and Taco Bell had already agreed to the same modest raise for tomato pickers, who work long hours in Florida's produce fields for such low pay that the extra penny would nearly double their wages (Grech, 2008).

In early 2008, 2 years into its Burger King campaign, CIW sought to increase pressure on the fast food company through protests and a possible boycott. That's when the anti-CIW comments started appearing online, and reporters received similar accusations via email. At the same time, shadowy individuals contacted CIW and its allies, offering help. A CIW-affiliated student group allowed one of these people to join its planning meetings. She claimed to be a student but, they soon realized, actually owned a security and espionage firm (Bennett Williams, 2008a).

Burger King was responsible for all these activities. The fast food company claimed that it hired the spy firm "to protect its employees and assets from potential harm," even though CIW uses nonviolent protest tactics (Schlosser, 2008). Two executives, including one who started working for Burger King as a consultant from the PR firm Edelman (Silversmith, undated), were behind the online smears against CIW. The resulting uproar forced Burger King to fire the two executives, sever ties with the spy firm, and finally agree to pay the tomato pickers more (Bennett Williams, 2008c).

Burger King's actions might seem extreme, but they're not unusual. Companies gain a significant PR advantage, when they obtain even a little advance information about their critics' plans. For example, the National Rifle Association used a longtime corporate spy, Mary Lou Sapone (also known as Mary McFate), to infiltrate gun control groups. In early 2008, she pushed U.S. groups to take part in a United Nations meeting on gun control, putting herself in a position "to learn what the anti-gun forces were planning ... including the delegates they intended to lobby, and the arguments they would highlight" (Ridgeway, Schulman, & Corn, 2008). From 1995 to 2001, the Maryland-based security firm Beckett Brown International "produced intelligence reports for public relations firms and major corporations involved in environmental controversies," sometimes based on information gleaned from dumpsters outside environmental groups' offices (Ridgeway, 2008). While Beckett Brown no longer exists, its former executives now work for at least three other security firms (Farsetta, 2008).

Another way corporations counter critics is to initiate frivolous but damaging legal actions against them. These are called SLAPP suits, for "strategic lawsuits against public participation." As the First Amendment Project explains, "While most SLAPPs lose in court, they 'succeed' in the public arena. This is because defending a SLAPP, even when the legal defense is strong, requires a substantial investment of money, time, and resources. The resulting effect is a 'chill' on public participation in, and open debate on, important public issues" (First Amendment Project web site, undated).

These aggressive tactics belong to a subset of PR referred to as crisis management or crisis communications. Eric Dezenhall, a crisis management expert who's been called "the pit bull of public relations" (Javers, 2006), believes that companies that admit to wrongdoing or make changes in response to activist campaigns lose on both the business and public opinion fronts. "In their marketplace battles, environmental radicals, consumer activists and trial lawyers are the darlings of the press," Dezenhall once explained. "But my clients have learned how to hit back, strike the attackers first and sometimes even position themselves as the victims in the media melodrama" (Dezenhall, 2002).

Not all crisis management is so confrontational. Johnson & Johnson's response to the 1982 Tylenol capsule poisoning deaths is widely deemed the "gold standard" in crisis communications. After seven people in the Chicago area died from ingesting poisoned capsules, the company was lauded for its quick response and willingness to share information with the press and public.

In 2007, *Fortune* magazine measured corporate responses to recent scandals against the Tylenol yardstick. JetBlue earned high marks for its actions, after thousands of airline customers were stranded during a snowstorm.

JetBlue's CEO "appeared on Letterman, recorded a YouTube video addressed to JetBlue customers, and issued a passenger bill of rights," the magazine noted approvingly (Yang, 2007).

Yet, as the PR trade publication *O'Dwyer's* reported, the Johnson & Johnson/Tylenol "gold standard" is a "fairy tale." Johnson & Johnson's CEO at the time never held a press conference and didn't even call a staff meeting until the week following the Chicago deaths. The company also "tried to localize the problem," limiting its initial recall to "two batches that were circulated in the Chicago area." It didn't launch a wider recall until "after another attempted poisoning using Tylenols took place on the following Tuesday," in California. Most seriously, Johnson & Johnson didn't change the design of the Tylenol capsules, which made them vulnerable to tampering, until another Tylenol poisoning occurred, 4 years later (*O'Dwyer's*, 2007).

Issue management is a related subset of PR that seeks to avoid crisis situations, to deal with their lingering aftereffects or to manage problems that don't rise to the crisis level. At the heart of issue management is the identification of company weaknesses and external threats. Issue management often involves repositioning the company or its challenges in the public's mind. Common tactics include emphasizing the company's charitable contributions or CSR programs; highlighting the personal stories of its employees, to "humanize" the company; and building coalitions or recruiting "third party" advocates who have credibility on issues that are challenging to the company.

For example, when CIW first asked McDonald's to pay tomato pickers more, the fast food company responded by joining the "socially accountable farm employer" program. However, the program had no credibility in labor rights circles and was eventually linked to CBR Public Relations, one of McDonald's PR firms, which specializes in "activist response management" (Lydersen, 2005).

When Purdue Pharma faced legal challenges over its misleading marketing of the addictive painkiller OxyContin, the pharmaceutical company hired a well-connected third party advocate, Rudolph Giuliani. The former New York City mayor and his consulting firm, Giuliani Partners, had credibility with the audiences most critical of Purdue. "Among Mr. Giuliani's missions was the job of convincing public officials that they could trust Purdue because they could trust him," reported the *New York Times*. Giuliani served as a liaison between Purdue and the U.S. Drug Enforcement Administration, and helped keep at least one lawmaker, former Pennsylvania Representative Curt Weldon, from publicly criticizing Purdue (Meier & Lipton, 2007).

The pharmaceutical industry's response to the debate over the cost of prescription drugs is one example of issue management through repositioning. The industry claims that drugs are expensive because drug companies invest heavily in research and development (R&D), in order to offer new, life-saving treatments. This claim is specious on multiple levels. First, it ignores drug companies' reliance on publicly funded research. "Of the nation's twenty-one most important drugs introduced between 1965 and 1992, fifteen were developed using knowledge from federal-funded research," as reporter and author Melody Petersen has noted (Petersen, 2008). The industry's claim also contradicts drug companies' actual financial practices. An independent academic study found that "pharmaceutical companies spend almost twice as much on promotion as they do on R&D" (Gagnon & Lexchin, 2008).

Advertising is often used in crisis response or issue management campaigns to directly communicate the company's side of the story to the general public. While ads have less credibility than testimonials from seemingly independent sources, they can be used to reinforce the PR campaign's messages. Ads designed as communications from company leaders or affiliated experts can also be used to portray the company as penitent, concerned, or simply wanting to clear up misunderstandings.

For example, Pfizer ran ads in several major newspapers in May 2008, as part of a wider campaign to respond to concerns about the safety of its antismoking drug, Chantix. The ads were framed as a message from Pfizer's medical director, explaining Chantix's "risk-benefit balance." Shortly afterwards, Pfizer hosted "round-table discussions on Chantix for members of the media" (Mundy & Johnson, 2008). The campaign was based on the premise that Pfizer merely needed to explain the facts, not change or recall its drug. The company resumed its direct-to-consumer television ads for Chantix 4 months later, after adding additional warnings about side effects (Herper, 2008).

In 2004, after its drug Vioxx was finally recalled, due to its causing strokes and other heart problems, Merck ran a series of full-page ads in prominent newspapers, including the *New York Times, Wall Street Journal,* and *Financial Times.* The ads called Merck's actions on Vioxx "consistent with putting the interests of patients first" and claimed the company demonstrated "faithful adherence to the best principles of scientific discipline and transparency." The ads echoed statements made by Merck executives, to reporters and before Congress. The main message was that Merck had acted, as soon as problems with Vioxx became apparent. Internal company documents would soon prove otherwise, but PR professionals faulted Merck's response on only one point—it lacked "third party" advocates (Agovino, 2004).

Impacting Public Policy

"It is now more crucial than ever that we have a debate which is properly informed by the science," explained Bob Ward. "The next IPCC [Intergovernmental Panel on Climate Change] report should give people the final push that they need to take action and we can't have people trying to undermine it" (Adam, 2006).

Ward, the Royal Society's senior manager of policy communication, was explaining his September 2006 letter to ExxonMobil. The letter—the first one that Britain's leading scientific body had ever sent a company, asking it to change its practices—urged ExxonMobil to stop distorting the science around global warming. It expressed the Royal Society's "disappointment at the inaccurate and misleading view of the science of climate change" presented in ExxonMobil documents. It also urged ExxonMobil to stop funding think tanks and other groups that have "misrepresented the science of climate change by outright denial of the evidence" (Ward, 2006).

ExxonMobil has become infamous for its efforts to stall action on global warming. From 1998 to 2006, the oil giant gave an estimated $23 million to dozens of think tanks and organizations that question whether climate change exists and whether human activities contribute to global warming. Many of the groups also lobby against policies designed to address climate change (Greenpeace, 2007). In addition, ExxonMobil's lobbying firm, DCI Group, and DCI's Tech Central Station web site have tried to call climate change into question, using newspaper columns, VNRs, and online videos (Farsetta & Price, 2006b).

ExxonMobil's funding helped create and legitimize an "echo chamber" of authoritative-seeming climate change skeptics. Instead of promoting the company or its products, ExxonMobil's cadre of "third party" supporters helped stall policies that the oil giant was concerned would hurt its bottom line. Years passed before ExxonMobil was pressured to account publicly for its role in distorting public and policy maker discussions. After the Royal Society's critical letter, the company pledged to stop funding climate change skeptics, but continued to do so. A year later, in mid-2008, ExxonMobil once again promised to cut funding to the groups (Center for Science in the Public Interest, 2008).

ExxonMobil's actions are just the most visible part of an industry-wide campaign. In a 1998 memo, the American Petroleum Institute—an association representing the U.S. oil and natural gas industry—recommended reframing the climate change issue, by challenging the science. "The advocates of global warming have been successful on the basis of skillfully misrepresenting the science and the extent of agreement on the science, while industry and its partners ceded the science and fought on the economic issues," the memo stated. "If we can show that science does not support the Kyoto treaty," the first international agreement to reduce greenhouse gas emissions, "this puts the United States in a stronger moral position and frees its negotiators from the need to make concessions as a defense against perceived selfish economic concerns" (American Petroleum Institute, 1998).

In challenging the science behind climate change, the oil industry was taking a page out of the tobacco industry's playbook. For decades after the link between smoking and health problems had been established, the tobacco industry funded scientists and studies that claimed otherwise. In a "Smoking and Health Proposal" from 1969, a Brown & Williamson employee explained, "Doubt is our product. … With the general public the consensus is that cigarettes are in some way harmful to health. If we are successful in establishing a controversy at the public level, then there is an opportunity to put across the real facts" (Brown & Williamson, 1969).

Indeed, PR efforts are most effective at influencing policy when aimed not at particular bills, but at framing the issues, shaping the ideas and even changing the words used to describe policies. That's one reason why corporations readily fund antiregulatory, "free market" think tanks and pressure groups like Americans for Tax Reform, the Competitive Enterprise Institute and Frontiers of Freedom.

Promoting a pro-business worldview through a network of corporate-funded organizations is nothing new. In a 1971 memo to the U.S. Chamber of Commerce, written before he joined the Supreme Court, Lewis Powell suggested that the Chamber lead an organized response to consumer and left-wing activism. Powell warned that "the ultimate issue may be survival—survival of what we call the free enterprise system." He suggested funding pro-business programs on college campuses, demanding equal time from the media, and strategically arguing cases before the judiciary. In a section that foreshadows the current role of "free market" think tanks, Powell wrote, "It is especially important for the Chamber's 'faculty of scholars' to publish. One of the keys to the success of the liberal and leftist faculty members has been their passion for 'publication' and 'lecturing.' A similar passion must exist among the Chamber's scholars" (Powell, 1971).

Wide-ranging efforts are necessary to fundamentally shift the intellectual and political environment in which policies are developed. However, corporations are frequently confronted with a smaller scale, more immediate challenge: how to limit or avoid independent oversight. Such challenges commonly arise after incidents that highlight a company's or industry's negative impact on public health, the environment, worker safety, or other aspects of civic life. A particularly effective corporate PR response to such challenges is to develop and promote voluntary codes of conduct.

Voluntary codes give the appearance of taking responsibility and responding to a problem. However, these corporate-designed and -implemented codes tend to be very limited in scope, with minimal public reporting and weak or nonexistent enforcement mechanisms. In short, such codes serve a PR purpose. They give the company something with which to respond to criticism, but rarely result in any significant change in corporate policies or practices.

For example, concerns about increasing rates of childhood obesity led major food, drink, and restaurant companies to sign the "Children's Food and Beverage Advertising Initiative" in November 2006. Participating companies promised that their ads directed toward children younger than 12 would be kept distinct from entertainment content, and would market food in the context of a balanced meal. The entity overseeing the agreement, the Children's Advertising Review Unit (CARU), was created by the advertising industry and has been widely criticized as ineffective (Shin, 2006).

Ten companies, including General Mills, Kraft, McDonald's, and Coca-Cola, additionally pledged to CARU that they would promote healthy food and lifestyle choices in half their overall advertising to children under 12. The companies also agreed to limit the use of cartoon characters in ads, and to stop advertising in elementary schools. "But the truth," observed *Advertising Age*, "is that at least five of the marketers who signed on ... already operate well within the guidelines," while the others "have been treading carefully in their ad efforts, fearing the ever-lurking threat of litigation or legislation." At the announcement of the supposedly "groundbreaking" initiative, "no details were provided to frustrated journalists seeking examples of what real changes the new effort might create" (Thompson & Teinowitz, 2006).

More recently, the industry group Pharmaceutical Research and Manufacturers of America (PhRMA) announced a voluntary ban on pens, mugs, and other common small gifts to medical doctors. PhRMA's "Code on Interactions with Health Care Professionals" was announced in July 2008, after a few states passed legislation requiring drug companies to disclose payments to doctors, and support for a similar measure was growing in Congress.

In contrast to the bills, which require disclosure of all gifts or payments over a certain dollar amount, PhRMA's code "provides no definite limits on the millions of dollars spent on speaking and consulting arrangements that drug makers have forged with tens of thousands of doctors," noted the *New York Times*. "Nor does it ban routine provision of office breakfasts and lunches, or the occasional invitation to educational dinners at fancy restaurants." In addition, any drug company that assures PhRMA in writing that it has relevant "policies and procedures in place" is automatically considered to be in full compliance with the gift ban (Harris, 2008).

Adapting to a Changing Media Landscape

Few media outlets take it upon themselves to fact-check or otherwise vet advertising content. Instead, most rely on the famed news/advertising "wall" to insulate reporters from advertiser pressures, and to keep ad space open to a wide variety of messages. However, the media watchdog group FAIR annually details instances where advertisers have influenced news content. Its 2008 report listed a newspaper business column sponsored by a bank and a television health segment sponsored by a hospital, among many other examples (Jackson & Hart, 2008).

Public relations is inherently different. It relies on reporters to relay PR messages to news audiences. Ideally, reporters would reject PR that's misleading or manipulative, always disclose the relevant connections of "third party" advocates, and balance promotional material with independent information and views. Yet, problematic PR is frequently incorporated without challenge into news content. Why?

One reason is the consolidation of media ownership. "In 1983, the men and women who headed the fifty mass media corporations that dominated American audiences could have fit comfortably in a modest hotel ballroom. ... By 2003, five men controlled all these media," wrote media scholar Ben Bagdikian. The five major companies—Time Warner, Walt Disney, News Corporation, Viacom, and Bertelsmann—own media properties ranging from radio and television stations to newspapers and book publishers to motion picture studios. Each of the Big Five enjoys "more communications power than was exercised by any despot or dictatorship in history," according to Bagdikian (2004).

As fewer companies gained control of more media outlets, owners increasingly judged news operations by their ability to turn profits. To maximize profits, newsroom budgets were often slashed. The trend was most apparent in television, where many stations expanded news programming as newsroom staff levels stayed the same or even decreased. "Stations did fewer reporter packages and less original reporting and enterprise" or investigative pieces, "relying more on second-hand material," concluded the Project for Excellence in Journalism's 2007 report (Project for Excellence in Journalism, 2007).

Media consolidation also leads to a "reduced emphasis on local issues," as ownership shifts from local families to national conglomerates. One study found a general decrease "in the quality and quantity of [news] coverage, with local stories suffering most." Ownership impacts have been documented on news and editorial coverage of partisan, electoral, financial, and media policy issues. For example, during the debate over a 1996 bill that allowed television stations free use of additional digital spectrum, every newspaper "whose own-ers got little TV revenue editorialized against the spectrum 'giveaway,' whereas every one with high TV revenues editorialized in favor of giving broadcasters free use of spectrum" (Cooper, 2006).

Currently, print media—especially daily newspapers—are witnessing their economic model implode. Subscriptions are down, as is classified adver-tising, which once brought in "more than 40 percent of a newspaper's revenues and more than half of its profits" (Farhi, 2008). As a result, many newspapers have cut staff, made formatting changes or, in a few cases, have transitioned to publishing online (*Capital Times*, 2008).

What's bad for journalism is good for PR and advertising firms. Fewer reporters are trying to generate the same or more news content. That means overextended journalists, who may be more receptive to PR pitches or, in the case of broadcast outlets, wholly PR-generated VNR or ANR "reports." In October 2008, ABC News Now producer Jessica Guff informed one PR exec-utive that PR firms should send newsrooms "fully formed four minute seg-ments, with visuals, spokespeople and news hook all conceived." She added, "Don't just send me a pitch letter or a book which requires me to put together the piece," because "we are short staffed" (Richard Edelman, 2008).

News operations expected to turn larger profits may also stop costly inves-tigative reporting and begin seeking nontraditional sources of income. "With TV stations facing pressure on advertising revenue ... U.S. product placement, media and branded entertainment agencies say they are increasingly being pitched by local stations to integrate their clients' products into news program-ming in exchange for buying commercial time or paying integration fees," according to a 2006 article (Schiller, 2006).

The rise of the Internet has destabilized mainstream media's economic models and fragmented news audiences. At the same time, it's allowed many more groups and individuals to publish their own news, commentary, and media criticism. Even traditionalists acknowledge that vital reporting can be and is being done online. In 2008, Talking Points Memo became the first Internet-only news organization to win the prestigious George Polk Award (The George Polk Awards, 2008).

Yet, independent news sites face resource limitations more serious than those of traditional newsrooms, and lack the training and vetting resources of more established news operations. In addition, television—perhaps the medium most compromised by marketers and PR professionals—remains the most popular news source in the United States.

Worse, PR firms are honing their pitches to web publishers and perfecting such deceptive techniques as "branded" news sites, fake blogs, and marketer-sponsored "community" web sites. In late 2008, the broadcast PR firm DS Simon Productions extolled the online potential for sponsored video content. It conducted a survey of more than 200 "influential" web sites and found that 65% already use video, and nearly 80% expect to increase their video content over the next year. "We need to understand the content needs of these Web Influencers if we hope to communicate successfully in the online world," explained the firm's president (O'Malley, 2008).

In December 2008, pharmaceutical and medical device companies' use of online videos was challenged. The consumer group Prescription Project filed a formal complaint with the U.S. Food and Drug Administration, pointing out that the companies' online videos often lacked the required health risk information. One of the companies named in the complaint, Medtronic, responded by removing a video that its PR firm had produced from the popular web site YouTube (Snowbeck, 2008). Abbott Laboratories, which was also named in the complaint, promised it would add risk information to videos it posted on YouTube (Japsen, 2008).

Overall, current trends suggest that PR will become more influential—at least, until new economic models for news operations are developed. That makes developing the skills to evaluate news content, in part by understanding how the PR and ad industries work, more important than ever.

REFERENCES

Adam D. Royal society tells exxon: stop funding climate change denial. *The Guardian* September 20, 2006.

Agovino T. Merck steps up public relations campaign after recall. *Associated Press* November 22, 2004.

American Heart Association. Statement from the American Heart Association on ENHANCE study results. Available at: http://www.americanheart.org/presenter. jhtml?identifier=3053094. Accessed January 15, 2008.

American Petroleum Institute. Global climate science communications action plan (draft). Available at: http://www.environmentaldefense.org/documents/3860_ GlobalClimateSciencePlanMemo.pdf. Accessed April 3, 1998.

Arnoldy B. Buy a red T-shirt to fight AIDS. But does it help? *Christ Sci Monitor* March 12, 2007.

Bagdikian BH. *The New Media Monopoly*. Boston: Beacon Press; 2004, pp. 3, 27.

Bennett Williams A. Tomato pickers feeling spied on: aide says infiltrators have been at meetings. *The News Press* (Fort Myers, Florida), April 13, 2008.

Bennett Williams A. Burger King VP puts self on grill: daughter says dad wrote anti-coalition postings. *The News Press* (Fort Myers, Florida), April 28, 2008.

Bennett Williams A. Tomato pickers celebrate deal with Burger King: after three years, immokalee workers receive increase. *The News Press* (Fort Myers, Florida), May 24, 2008.

Bernays E. *Propaganda*. New York: H. Liveright, 1928. Republished by Ig Publishing; 2005, pp. 37, 109.

Birnbaum JH. The Man Behind the Byline Isn't Behind the Article. So, Who Is? *Washington Post*, July 29, 2008.

Branded News web site. *Our Company*. Available at: http://www.brandednews.com/. Accessed September 2008.

Breast Cancer Action's Think Before You Pink web site. *Focus on Pinkwashers*. Available at: http://www.thinkbeforeyoupink.org/Pages/FocusOnPinkwashers. html. Accessed October 2008.

Brown, W. *Smoking and Health Proposal*. Available at: http://legacy.library.ucsf.edu/ tid/rgy93f00. Published 1969.

Burson-Marsteller web site. *Mark J. Penn, Worldwide President & CEO*. Available at: http://www.burson-marsteller.com/About_Us/Global_Leadership/ Lists/GlobalLeadership/DispForm.aspx?ID=1&nodeName=Global%20 Leadership&SubTitle=Mark%20J.%20Penn. Accessed September 2008.

Buy (Less) Crap web site. Available at: http://buylesscrap.org. Accessed December 2008.

Capital Times Changes: Focuses on Web, Two Weekly Editions. *The Capital Times* (Madison, Wisconsin), February 7, 2008.

Center for Science in the Public Interest. Exxon announces cutoff for warming skeptics—again. *Integrity in Science Watch* Available at: http://www.cspinet.org/ integrity/watch/200806021.html. Accessed June 2, 2008.

Confessore N. Meet the press: how James Glassman reinvented journalism—as lobbying. *Washington Monthly*, December 2003.

Cooper M. *Media Ownership and Viewpoint*. Comments of Consumers Union, Consumer Federation of America and Free Press to the Federal Communications Commission. Available at: http://www.stopbigmedia.com/ filing/part_2.pdf. Accessed October 23, 2006.

Creel G. *How We Advertised America*. New York: Harper & Brothers; 1920, p. 4.

Dezenhall E. How arafat wags the dog. *Jewish World Review*, June 18, 2002.

Edelman web site. Edelman: our approach—the relationship imperative. Archived page of the Edelman firm's web site at http://web.archive.org/ web/20040821000431/http://www.edelman.com/about_us/relationship_ imperative/index.asp. Accessed August 2004.

Edelman R. Presentation to the Conference Board on Global Corporate Citizenship. *The Relationship Among NGOs, Government, Media and Corporate Sector: Proprietary Research by Strategy One and Edelman PR Worldwide*. Available at: http://www.sourcewatch.org/images/f/ff/EdelmanNGOPresentation_-_2-28-01. pdf. Accessed February 2001.

Edelman R. *Networks Fight Back.* Edelman blog 6 A.M. Available at: http://www.edelman.com/speak_up/blog/archives/2008/10/networks_fight.html. Accessed October 10, 2008.

Farhi P. Don't blame the journalism: the economic and technological forces behind the collapse of newspapers. *American Journalism Review* October/November 2008.

Farsetta D, Price D. *Fake TV News: Widespread and Undisclosed.* Center for Media and Democracy. Available at: http://www.prwatch.org/fakenews/execsummary. Accessed April 6, 2006a.

Farsetta D, Price D. *Still Not the News: Stations Overwhelmingly Fail to Disclose VNRs.* Center for Media and Democracy. Available at: http://www.prwatch.org/fakenews2/execsummary. Accessed November 14, 2006b.

Farsetta D, *Know Fake News.* Center for Media and Democracy. Available at: http://www.prwatch.org/fakenews3/summary. Accessed October 11, 2007.

Farsetta D. A bad week for corporate spies. *PR Watch*, April 14, 2008.

The First Amendment Project. *Guarding Against the Chill: A Survival Guide for SLAPP Victims.* Available at: http://www.thefirstamendment.org/antislappresourcecenter.html. Accessed October 2008.

Frey D. How green is BP? *New York Times*, December 8, 2002.

Fugh-Berman A, Ahari S. Following the script: how drug reps make friends and influence doctors. *PLoS Med* 2007;4(4). Available at: http://dx.doi.org/10.1371/journal.pmed.0040150. Accessed April 24, 2007.

Gagnon M-A, Lexchin J. The cost of pushing pills: a new estimate of pharmaceutical promotion expenditures in the United States. *PLoS Med* 2008:5(1). Available at: http://dx.doi.org/10.1371/journal.pmed.0050001. Accessed January 3, 2008.

The George Polk Awards. *Long Island University Announces 2007 George Polk Awards in 14 Categories.* Available at: http://www.brooklyn.liu.edu/polk/glance07.html. Accessed February 19, 2008.

Grech D. A cent too far for Burger King: Burger King's two-year battle with Florida tomato pickers over a penny-per-pound raise is coming to a head with the news that BK has begun planning to buy tomatoes elsewhere. *Marketplace*, January 16, 2008.

Greenpeace USA. *ExxonMobil's Continued Funding of Global Warming Denial Industry.* Available at: http://www.greenpeace.org/usa/assets/binaries/exxon-secrets-analysis-of-fun. Accessed May 2007.

Harris G. Drug industry to announce revised code on marketing. *New York Times*, July 10, 2008.

Hein K. Beverage bigs battle bottle backlash. *Brandweek*, February 17, 2008.

Herper M. Can chantix make a comeback? *Forbes*, September 12, 2008.

Hughes S. CleanSkies.TV enjoys backing of top natural gas executive. *Dow Jones Newswires*, August 8, 2008.

Jackson J, Hart P. Fear & favor 2007: how power still shapes the news. *FAIR's Extra!* Available at: http://www.fair.org/index.php?page=3323. Accessed March/April 2008.

Japsen B. Abbott to add safety information in YouTube ads after group complains. *Chicago Tribune*, December 3, 2008.

Javers E. 'The Pit Bull of Public Relations': Eric Dezenhall serves clients such as exxonmobil by going after their foes. *BusinessWeek*, April 17, 2006.

Lippmann W. *Public Opinion*. New York: Macmillan; 1922. Republished by Simon & Schuster; 1997, pp. 196, 158.

Lydersen K. McDonald's vs. the Tomato Pickers. *The NewStandard* via AlterNet, December 20, 2005.

Mandese J. The art of manufactured news. *Broadcasting & Cable*, March 28, 2005.

McCullagh D. "Wanted: Writers for D.C. Tech Lobby Group, Secrecy Mandatory," CNET News, August 14, 2008.

Meier B, Lipton E. Under attack, drug maker turned to Giuliani for help. *New York Times*, December 28, 2007.

Mundy A, Johnson A. Pfizer seeks to Counter Chantix concerns. *Wall St J*. May 29, 2008.

Penn, Schoen & Berland Associates web site. Bios: Craig T. Smith. Available at: http://www.psbresearch.com/who_bios_CraigSmith.htm. Accessed September 2008.

See, for example, the Public Relations Society of America's member code of ethics, revised in 2000. Available at: http://www.prsa.org/aboutUs/ethics/preamble_en.html. The preamble to the Code admits, "Emphasis on enforcement of the Code has been eliminated."

DCI Sells TCS. *Jack O'Dwyer's Newsletter*, November 1, 2006.

Fortune Lauds Tylenol PR. *O'Dwyer's PR Daily*, May 22, 2007.

O'Malley G. Video use will continue to rise, per web influencers. *MediaPost*, October 20, 2008.

Oil lobbyist's 'news' denies inconvenient truths. In: Farsetta D, Price D, eds. *Still Not the News: Stations Overwhelmingly Fail to Disclose VNRs*. Center for Media and Democracy. Available at: http://www.prwatch.org/fakenews2/vnr40. Accessed November 14, 2006.

Pepsi-Cola press release. Ethos water and H2o Africa Join Forces to help alleviate the world water crisis. Pepsi-Cola North America, March 6, 2008.

Petersen M. *Our Daily Meds: How Pharmaceutical Companies Transformed Themselves into Slick Marketing Machines and Hooked the Nation on Prescription Drugs*. New York: Sarah Crichton Books; 2008, pp. 68, 130.

Powell LF, Jr. "Confidential Memorandum: Attack of American Free Enterprise System," to Mr. Eugene B. Sydnor, Jr., Chairman, Education Committee, U.S. Chamber of Commerce. Available at: http://www.mediatransparency.org/story.php?storyID=22. Accessed August 23, 1971.

Prescription-strength spin at WCBS-2. In: Farsetta D, Price D, eds. *Fake TV News: Widespread and Undisclosed*. Center for Media and Democracy. Available at: http://www.prwatch.org/fakenews/vnr30. Accessed April 6, 2006.

Project for Excellence in Journalism. Local TV: News Investment. In: *The State of the News Media 2007: An Annual Report on American Journalism*. Available at: http://www.stateofthenewsmedia.org/2007/narrative_localtv_newsinvestment.asp?cat=5&media=7. Accessed March 12, 2007.

Reinan J. Advertising that doesn't look like advertising. *MinnPost.com*, August 18, 2008.

Ridgeway J, with Corn D, Wedekind J, Schulman D, Baumann N. Cops and former secret service agents Ran Black ops on green groups. *Mother Jones*, April 11, 2008.

Ridgeway J, Schulman D, Corn D. There's something about Mary: unmasking a gun lobby mole. *Mother Jones*, July 30, 2008.

Saul S. Heart group backs drug made by Ally. *New York Times*, January 24, 2008.

Schiller G. Newscasts adopt product placements: crossing the line. *Hollywood Reporter*, March 17, 2006.

Schlosser E. Burger with a side of spies. *New York Times*, May 7, 2008.

Shin A Ads aimed at children get tighter security: firms to promote more healthful diet choices. *Washington Post*, November 15, 2006.

Silversmith K. LinkedIn profile. Available at: http://www.linkedin.com/in/kevasilversmith. Accessed October 2008.

Simon A, quoted in "D S Simon Productions Releases Survey of TV News Stations," D S Simon Productions press release. Available at: http://www.dssimon.com/releasehealthsurvey.html. 2004. Accessed September 15, 2009)

Smith CT, presentation on "Nuclear Energy and the Public: A New Understanding," given at the Nuclear Energy Assembly at The Fairmont in Chicago, Illinois, on May 7, 2008. Also see Diane Farsetta, "When Recycling Isn't: Lessons from a Nuclear Industry Conference," *PR Watch*. Available at: http://www.prwatch.org/node/7316. Accessed May 9, 2008.

Snowbeck C. Medtronic pulls video from YouTube after complaint. *St. Paul Pioneer Press* (Minnesota), December 3, 2008.

Stauber J, Rampton S. *Toxic Sludge Is Good for You! Lies, Damn Lies and the Public Relations Industry.* Maine: Common Courage Press; 1995, pp. 21–24.

Stole I. 'Cause-Related Marketing': why social change and corporate profits don't mix. *PR Watch*, July 14, 2006.

TCS Daily web site. About TCS Daily. Available at: http://www.tcsdaily.com/about.aspx. Accessed October 2008.

Thomaselli R. Merck, schering wage PR battle after Vytorin Backlash: newspaper ads look to comfort consumers worried about drug's effectiveness. *Advertising Age*, January 22, 2008.

Thompson S. Breast cancer awareness strategy increases sales of Campbell's soup: pink-labeled cans a hit with Kroger customers. *Advertising Age*, October 3, 2006.

Thompson S, Teinowitz I. Big food's big deal not such a big concession—analysis: move makes sense, but most of titans were already onboard. *Advertising Age*, November 20, 2006.

Useem B, Zald MN. From pressure group to social movement: efforts to promote use of nuclear power. In: Zald MN, McCarthy JD, eds. *Social Movements in an Organizational Society: Collected Essays* (p. 283). Edison, NJ: Transaction Publishers; 1997.

Ward B, Senior Manager of Policy Communication for the Royal Society, Letter to
    Nick Thomas, Director of Corporate Affairs for Esso UK Limited. Available
    at: http://image.guardian.co.uk/sys-files/Guardian/documents/2006/09/19/
    LettertoNick.pdf. Accessed September 4, 2006.
Yang JL. Getting a handle on a scandal: Johnson & Johnson's response to the 1982
    tylenol poisonings remains the gold standard in crisis control. *Fortune*, May 22,
    2007.
Zmuda N. Pepsi partners with starbucks water brand: also teams with Matt Damon's
    Group to push charitable message behind ethos. *Advertising Age*, March 10,
    2008.

5

Lobbying, the Revolving Door, and Campaign Contributions:

The Center for Responsive Politics

William H. Wiist

Editor's Note

The amount of money spent and the number of lobbyist have increased during the past 10 years (see Figures 5.1 and 5.2) and the lobbying industry is a big business (see Tables 5.1, 5.2, 5.3, and 5.4). The corporation uses lobbying of government officials to obtain legislation and regulation favorable to the bottom line, for competitive advantage, subsidies, lower taxes, and less regulation, or to shape law and regulation (Table 5.8 shows examples of the number of lobbyist trying to influence specific Congressional bills). While political scientists do not all agree as to the effectiveness of lobbying, the increasing amount of money that corporations and their industry organizations have been spending on lobbying suggests that corporate officials perceive that lobbying is beneficial. Through corporate and industry organizations' lobbying the corporation gains access to policy makers that human citizen groups do not have. The information that a corporate lobbyist or official shares with the government official carries weight as expert information even though the information may be biased, or incomplete, or erroneous. Similar to lobbying, political campaign contributions also gain the large donor access to officer seekers and

The information in this chapter provided courtesy of the Center for Responsive Politics (www.Opensecrets.org)

Total Lobbying Spending	
1998	$1.43 Billion
1999	$1.43 Billion
2000	$1.53 Billion
2001	$1.62 Billion
2002	$1.80 Billion
2003	$2.03 Billion
2004	$2.17 Billion
2005	$2.41 Billion
2006	$2.60 Billion
2007	$2.84 Billion
2008	$3.24 Billion

FIGURE 5.1. The Total Amount of Money Spent on Lobbying the U.S. Federal Government 1998–2008.

Number of Lobbyists	
1998	10,693
1999	13,332
2000	12,754
2001	12,075
2002	12,351
2003	13,166
2004	13,407
2005	14,443
2006	14,876
2007	15,398
2008	15,138

FIGURE 5.2. The Total Number of Lobbyist Registered to Lobby the U.S. Federal Government 1998–2008.

elected officials that human citizen groups or individual humans do not have. Large campaign contributions are made by a wide variety of business sectors and industries and go to both major political parties (see Tables 5.6 and 5.7). In addition to campaign contributions, legislators take trips sponsored by organizations intent on influencing the position of the legislator. These tactics of the corporation create an imbalance in the democratic process in favor of commercial interests often to the detriment of public health. The corporation also leverages the Revolving Door (see Table 5.5) to its advantage, sometimes as a result of lobbying and political campaign contributions. When corporate officials, because of their knowledge of their industry, are appointed to government positions, they sometimes have direct responsibility for regulating the

TABLE 5.1. Lobbying Expenditures by Specific Organizations to Lobby the U.S. Federal Government All Years 1998–2008.

Lobbying Client	Total
U.S. Chamber of Commerce	$461,529,680
American Medical Assn	$200,002,500
General Electric	$182,468,000
American Hospital Assn	$163,621,485
AARP	$154,692,064
Pharmaceutical Research and Manufacturers of America	$147,253,400
Northrop Grumman	$127,385,253
Edison Electric Institute	$123,495,999
Business Roundtable	$120,620,000
National Assn of Realtors	$118,360,380
Blue Cross/Blue Shield	$111,193,172
Exxon Mobil	$111,036,942
Lockheed Martin	$105,910,681
Boeing Company	$103,748,310
General Motors	$99,831,483
Freddie Mac	$96,164,048
Southern Company	$94,710,694
Verizon Communications	$87,796,908
Ford Motor Company	$82,569,808
Microsoft Corporation	$82,115,000

TABLE 5.2. Lobbying Expenditures by Specific Lobbying Firm to Lobby the U.S. Federal Government All Years 1998–2008*.

Lobbying Firm	Total
Patton Boggs LLP	$312,212,000
Cassidy & Associates	$282,725,000
Akin, Gump et al.	$253,575,000
Van Scoyoc Associates	$204,053,000
Williams & Jensen	$149,654,000
Hogan & Hartson	$136,593,907
Ernst & Young	$132,777,536
Barbour, Griffith & Rogers	$114,430,000
PMA Group	$113,715,132
Quinn, Gillespie & Associates	$113,253,500
Greenberg Traurig LLP	$109,228,249
Holland & Knight	$97,779,544
PriceWaterhouseCoopers	$93,324,084
Verner, Liipfert et al.	$88,595,000
Alcalde & Fay	$86,300,660
Carmen Group	$84,700,000
Dutko Worldwide	$83,251,766
Clark & Weinstock	$79,195,000
Timmons & Co	$75,818,000
Washington Group	$74,957,000

*Each quarterly filing is treated as a separate report, and each may mention multiple firms

TABLE 5.3. Total Lobbying Expenditures to Lobby the U.S. Federal Government, by Industry Sector All Years 1998–2008.

Sector	Total
Finance, insurance, and real estate	$3,441,172,596
Health	$3,275,568,883
Misc business	$3,158,766,843
Communications/electronics	$2,843,615,210
Energy and Natural Resources	$2,365,262,733
Transportation	$1,817,478,201
Other	$1,765,931,084
Ideological/Single-Issue	$1,166,294,075
Agribusiness	$1,063,930,905
Defense	$989,941,961
Construction	$378,378,842
Labor	$354,016,328
Lawyers & Lobbyists	$275,173,377

TABLE 5.4. Total Lobbying Expenditure to Lobby the U.S. Federal Government by Industry Types All Years 1998–2008*.

Industry	Total
Pharmaceuticals/Health Products	$1,550,614,839
Insurance	$1,173,504,366
Electric Utilities	$1,076,638,452
Computers/Internet	$871,470,290
Business Associations	$825,565,261
Education	$749,587,621
Oil & Gas	$742,273,214
Real Estate	$726,644,338
Hospitals/Nursing Homes	$686,054,332
Misc Manufacturing & Distributing	$684,569,851
Health Professionals	$634,600,215
Civil Servants/Public Officials	$603,397,018
TV/Movies/Music	$597,866,332
Securities & Investment	$595,978,224
Air Transport	$559,509,867
Automotive	$545,959,294
Misc Issues	$524,857,671
Telecom Services & Equipment	$523,907,551
Telephone Utilities	$466,697,468
Defense Aerospace	$435,217,553

*Each quarterly filing is treated as a separate report, and each may mention multiple industries.

TABLE 5.5. U.S. Government Agencies That Have Employed the Greatest Number of Former Lobbyists—or Sent the Greatest Number of Former Employees to Lobbying Firms and Interest Groups.

Agency	Number of Revolving Door People Profiled
White House Office	455
US House of Representatives	303
Federal Communications Commission	127
Dept of Commerce	116
Dept of State	114
Dept of Defense	113
Dept of Treasury	112
Office of the Attorney General	110
Obama-Biden Transition Project	107
Environmental Protection Agency	102
Office of Management & Budget	100
Office of U.S. Trade Representative	98
Dept of Army	91
Federal Trade Commission	90
Dept of Energy	86
U.S. Attorney's Office	86
U.S. Senate	82
Dept of Health & Human Services	81
Securities & Exchange Commission	81
Dept of Transportation	72

industry they left, or are able to have an effect indirectly through their influence with other agencies, or through their access to decision makers. When government officials leave their posts, they carry specialized knowledge about regulations, the regulatory and legislative process with them. In addition, they also carry their networks of contacts with decision makers in the administration and legislature. In the private sector, lobbying role on behalf of the corporation has advantages of knowledge and access that the average person does not have. Thus, the Revolving Door creates an imbalance in democracy in favor of the corporation over the public's health. The information provided below is from The Center for Responsive Politics, an organization that continuously monitors, in great detail, lobbying, campaign contributions, the Revolving Door, government official's investments and income, and other information. The following includes only a sampling of information in the databases the center maintains that can be used to analyze corporate tactics from a variety of perspectives. The information provided below just begins to show the extent and scope of

TABLE 5.6. Political Campaign Contributions to Democratic and Republican Candidates by Business Sector in 2008.*

Sector*	Total	To Dems	To Rep
Agribusiness	$9,406,329	$3,750,254	$5,627,030
Communications/Electronics	$45,794,358	$35,673,670	$9,967,504
Construction	$20,389,766	$9,096,459	$11,243,916
Defense	$2,926,610	$1,684,346	$1,227,274
Energy & Natural Resources	$11,078,167	$4,256,622	$6,809,790
Finance, Insurance & Real Estate	$130,557,659	$69,823,872	$60,605,254
Health	$41,162,622	$27,243,954	$13,819,417
Lawyers & Lobbyists	$95,877,472	$74,566,938	$21,241,646
Transportation	$7,808,633	$2,839,475	$4,949,535
Misc Business	$81,856,314	$51,736,624	$29,917,612
Labor	$1,123,927	$1,079,982	$42,595
Ideological/Single-Issue	$38,560,985	$25,012,973	$13,489,761
Other	$168,238,513	$110,153,793	$57,502,864

*All the numbers are for the 2008 election cycle and based on Federal Election Commission data released electronically on Monday, March 2, 2009.

TABLE 5.7. The Top Political Campaign Contributions to Candidates by Industry in 2008.*

Industry	Total
Retired	$108,614,867
Lawyers/Law Firms	$91,192,535
Securities & Investment	$45,460,655
Real Estate	$39,056,205
Homemakers/Nonincome earners	$36,849,690
Education	$31,846,780
Misc Business	$28,273,213
Health Professionals	$26,519,514
Business Services	$24,575,292
Misc Finance	$19,205,402
Democratic/Liberal	$16,356,768
TV/Movies/Music	$15,525,053
Computers/Internet	$15,384,720
Civil Servants/Public Officials	$14,976,708
Republican/Conservative	$10,988,066
Hedge Funds	$10,012,816
Printing & Publishing	$9,999,853
Commercial Banks	$9,854,751
Insurance	$9,119,104
General Contractors	$6,811,260

Methodology: The totals on this chart is calculated from PAC contributions and contributions from individuals giving more than $200, as reported to the Federal Election Commission. Individual contributions are generally categorized based on the donor's occupation/employer, although individuals may be classified instead as ideological donors if they've given more than $200 to an ideological PAC.
*All the numbers are for the 2008 election cycle and based on Federal Election Commission data released electronically on Monday, March 2, 2009.

TABLE 5.8. The Number of Lobbyist Who Filed and Reported Lobbying on Specific Issue Bills Before the U.S. Congress in 2008.

Bill Number	Congress	Bill Title	No. of Clients
H.R.2638	110	Making appropriations for the Department of Homeland Security for the fiscal year ending September 30, 2008, and for other purposes.	1,225
H.R.3043	110	Making appropriations for the Departments of Labor, Health and Human Services, and Education, and related agencies for the fiscal year ending September 30, 2008, and for other purposes.	978
S.1710	110	An original bill making appropriations for the Departments of Labor, Health and Human Services, and Education, and related agencies for the fiscal year ending September 30, 2008, and for other purposes.	910
H.R.2764	110	Making appropriations for the Department of State, foreign operations, and related programs for the fiscal year ending September 30, 2008, and for other purposes.	864
H.R.2419	110	To provide for the continuation of agricultural programs through fiscal year 2012, and for other purposes.	837
H.R.1424	110	A bill to provide authority for the Federal Government to purchase and insure certain types of troubled assets for the purposes of providing stability to and preventing disruption in the economy and financial system and protecting taxpayers, to amend the Internal Revenue Code of 1986 to provide incentives for energy production and conservation, to extend certain expiring provisions, to provide individual income tax relief, and for other purposes.	747
H.R.2641	110	Making appropriations for energy and water development and related agencies for the fiscal year ending September 30, 2008, and for other purposes.	727
H.R.3074	110	Making appropriations for the Departments of Transportation, and Housing and Urban Development, and related agencies for the fiscal year ending September 30, 2008, and for other purposes.	719

(Continued)

TABLE 5.8. Continued

Bill Number	Congress	Bill Title	No. of Clients
H.R.3222	110	Making appropriations for the Department of Defense for the fiscal year ending September 30, 2008, and for other purposes.	710
H.R.6	110	An Act to move the United States toward greater energy independence and security, to increase the production of clean renewable fuels, to protect consumers, to increase the efficiency of products, buildings, and vehicles, to promote research on and deploy greenhouse gas capture and storage options, and to improve the energy performance of the Federal Government, and for other purposes.	704

lobbying, political contributions, and the Revolving Door. The Center's web site can be used to conduct more detailed analyses. My thanks to the Center for granting permission to include this information from their web site.

Lobbying

Lobbying data that form the basis of this site are compiled using the quarterly lobbying disclosure reports filed with the Secretary of the Senate's Office of Public Records (SOPR) and posted to their web site.

Lobbying firms are required to provide a good-faith estimate rounded to the nearest $10,000 of all lobbying-related income for each quarterly filing period. If income does not exceed $5,000, it does not have to report a figure, and the center treats it as zero. (Lobbying firms sometimes double as law, accounting, or public relations firms—the income for nonlobbying activity is supposed to be excluded from the lobbying reports.) Organizations that hire lobbyists must provide good-faith estimates rounded to the nearest $10,000 of all lobbying-related expenditures in quarterly period that exceed $5,000. However, an organization that spends less than $5,000 in any quarter does not have to state its expenditures. In those cases, the center again treats the figure as zero.

There are three different filing methods. Two options are largely identical (one for for-profit groups, the other for nonprofit groups) and use a definition of lobbying provided by the Internal Revenue Code (IRC). The third follows the definition of lobbying contained in the Lobbying Disclosure Act of 1995 (LDA).

Filers using the IRC methods must report state and grassroots lobbying costs, which are not included in LDA reports. However, the list of covered public officials under the IRC is much narrower than the set covered by the LDA. Thus, lobbying expenditures may not be strictly comparable among organizations.

Where an organization "self-files" (reports spending by in-house lobbyists), the center generally uses that figure to represent their total lobbying expenditure for the period. Where an organization does not "self-file," the sum of its contracts with outside lobbying firms is used to represent their total lobbying expenditure for the period.

Annual lobbying expenditure and income totals on this site are calculated by adding quarterly totals. Whenever a lobbying report is amended, income/expense figures from the amendment are generally used instead of those from the original filing. Similarly, where a termination report is filed, generally figures from that report replace those of the original filing. Often, however, center staff determine that the income/expenditures on the amendment or termination report are inaccurate. In those instances, figures from the original filing are used.

Occasionally, income that an outside lobbying firm reports receiving from a client is greater than the client's reported lobbying expenditures. Many such discrepancies can be explained by the fact that the client and the outside firm use different filing methods. When both organizations use the same method, discrepancies are generally due to filer error. In cases that are not resolved in the previous reports and where the discrepancy exceeds the $10,000 that can be attributed to rounding, the client's expenditures—the smaller amount—rather than the lobbying firm's reported income are used. The only exception is when a client reports no lobbying expenditures, while the outside lobbying firm lists an actual payment. In such cases, the figure reported by the lobbying firm is used.

In cases where the data appear to contain errors, official Senate records are consulted and, when necessary, the center contacts SOPR or the lobbying organizations for clarification. The center standardizes variations in names of individuals and organizations to identify them clearly and more accurately represent their total lobbying expenditures.

In cases where both a parent and its subsidiary organizations lobby or hire lobbyists, the center attributes lobbying spending to the parent organization. Therefore, the lobbying totals reported by the center for a parent organization may not reflect its original filing with the Senate, but rather the combined expenditures of all related entities.

However, to calculate lobbying expenditures by sector and industry, each subsidiary is counted within its own sector and industry, not those of its parent. The center makes this distinction when it has the information necessary to distinguish some or all of the subsidiary's lobbying expenditures from either the subsidiary's own filing or from the receipts reported by outside lobbying firms. For example, tobacco giant Altria Group owns Kraft Foods. Although Altria Group's filing included lobbying for Kraft in its expenditures, the center isolated Kraft's payments to outside lobbyists and included them in "Food Processing and Sales."

When companies merge within any 2-year election cycle, their lobbying expenditures are combined and attributed to the new entity. This is done in order to correlate lobbying data to campaign contribution data for each particular organization and industry.

In addition to campaign contributions to elected officials and candidates, companies, labor unions, and other organizations spend billions of dollars each year to lobby Congress and federal agencies. Some special interests retain lobbying firms, many of them located along Washington's legendary K Street; others have lobbyists working in-house.

Lobbying Issues

Lobbying disclosure forms ask filers to disclose which "specific lobbying issues" they worked on during the period. "Specific" is up for interpretation, however, as some filers name bills by number and title while others provide vague descriptions that offer little information. Here we've counted up the number of filers that reported lobbying on a particular piece of legislation, to the extent that can be counted.

Revolving Door

Although the influence powerhouses that line Washington's K Street are just a few miles from the U.S. Capitol building, the most direct path between the two doesn't necessarily involve public transportation. Instead, it's through a door—a Revolving Door that shuffles former federal employees into jobs as lobbyists, consultants, and strategists just as the door pulls former hired guns into government careers. While members of the executive branch, Congress and senior congressional staffers spin in and out of the private and public sectors, so too does privilege, power, access, and, of course, money.

Whether they are a presidential appointee plucked from an elite position in corporate America to run a government commission or an outgoing member of Congress looking for a more lucrative job in the influence industry, OpenSecrets.org's Revolving Door database tracks anyone whose résumé includes positions of influence in both the private and public sectors. Government employees may have had the president's ear or may have simply been the doorkeeper of the congressional cloakrooms. Influence-peddlers merely have to be in a position to influence government policy on someone else's behalf, commonly as a "hired gun" at a K Street firm, an executive of a professional trade association, or as a vice president of government relations for a large company.

The Center for Responsive Politics's Revolving Door project intends to identify those people whose career trajectory has taken them from Capitol Hill, the White House and Cabinet office suites to K Street, and vice versa. The center's Revolving Door database is the most comprehensive source to date to help the public learn who's who in the Washington influence industry, and to uncover how these people's government connections afford them privileged access to those in power.

The purpose of this project is to reveal the relationships between those who represent special interests and those in government who regulate those interests. The intent is not to accuse people of benefiting from a conflict of interest; there is a whole set of statutes, regulations, and executive orders that define ethical boundaries for current and former government employees and appointees. This database provides no evidence that any of these boundaries have been crossed. Users are free to interpret the relationships identified by the center as they please, and are urged to consult additional sources to both confirm the information in this database and to find additional information. To interpret these relationships properly, be sure to examine the center's conceptualization and operational definition of the Revolving Door project.

Conceptualization

The concept of the Revolving Door is open to interpretation, so the center has chosen to draw the theoretical boundaries for the Revolving Door broadly, yet precisely. Generally, the Revolving Door database consists of any person with previous or current government experience who also has held, or currently holds, a professional position in the private sector where they can reasonably be expected to influence, or be seeking to influence, public policy decisions. Private sector employment certainly includes traditional lobbyists, but may also include people who lead organizations that are in a position to influence public and elite opinions, who advise clients on regulatory or political law, who counsel organizations on public affairs strategies, who publish opinions on public policy matters, or who otherwise serve in a capacity to contribute ideas to the public sphere that may ultimately affect policy decisions in Washington.

Clearly, the most observable employment that meets these qualifications is that of a registered lobbyist. Traditional lobbyists and policy advocates engage in "inside lobbying" when they communicate policy preferences to federal government policy makers on behalf of their clients. However, this commonsense understanding of lobbying, and the statutory definition of "lobbyist" under the Lobbying Disclosure Act, remains overly narrow to recognize every person employed in Washington's influence industry. The center's practical characterization of influence includes professionals engaged in all methods of influencing policy decisions, including traditional lobbying (personal contacts with policy makers), invited testimony at public hearings, grassroots lobbying, formal comment submissions to administrative rulemakings, amicus curiae filings in federal court, legal and strategic advice on political and policy matters and any other attempts of a person to manipulate (or help their clients manipulate) the outcome of a public policy debate. People with past government experience who use their expertise, professional networks, and policy background to engage in "outside lobbying"—or efforts to mobilize the public in an effort to influence policy makers—or to engage in political consulting are just as significant for the Revolving Door as are traditional lobbyists. These professionals indirectly influence public policy through grassroots lobbying campaigns, public relations operations, coalition-building, public discourse, and political strategy development, all with the ultimate goal of shaping public policy. Because traditional lobbying is only one of many ways to affect policy change, the center has chosen to give equal weight to these other means by which former government employees trade their access and expertise for a living.

Operational Definition

In practice, the center has defined several criteria to determine whether or not a person appropriately belongs in the Revolving Door database. Specifically, a person qualifies to be included in the Revolving Door if they have been, or are currently:

1. employed in the federal government, or;
2. appointed to a noncompensated federal government advisory board, independent commission, or congressional-, presidential-, or Cabinet-member-appointed entity, including blue ribbon commissions, task forces, working groups, and other boards.

And that person has been, or is also:

1. employed as a registered lobbyist according to the Lobbying Disclosure Act, or;

2. employed as a registered representative according to the Foreign Agents Registration Act, or;

3. employed as a treasurer, manager, or other official in an organization that has an associated political action committee registered with the Federal Election Commission under the Federal Elections Campaign Act, or qualifies with the Internal Revenue Service as an independent expenditure organization under section 527 of the Internal Revenue Code, or;

4. employed as or appointed as a noncompensated member of the board of directors, governors or trustees of an organization or institution that is (1) registered according to the Lobbying Disclosure or Foreign Agents Registration Act, (2) has an affiliated political action committee identified by the center, or (3) is an independent expenditure organization identified by the center under section 527 of the Internal Revenue Code, or;

5. employed as an executive, general counsel, public affairs, or consultant specializing in public affairs for an organization or institution that is (1) registered according to the Lobbying Disclosure or Foreign Agents Registration Act, (2) has an affiliated political action committee identified by the center, or (3) is an independent expenditure organization identified by the center under section 527 of the Internal Revenue Cod;

6. employed as a professional in a law, lobbying, or public relations firm that represents an organization or institution that is (1) registered according to the Lobbying Disclosure or Foreign Agents Registration Act, (2) has an affiliated political action committee identified by the center, or (3) is an independent expenditure organization identified by the center under section 527 of the Internal Revenue Code, or;

7. employed as a professional in a campaign strategy, public-opinion polling, or other firm engaged in political, government contracting, or policy consulting services, or;

8. employed as an executive, editor, producer, author, journalist, faculty member, fellow, scholar, or professional research position at a periodic publication, broadcast, cable, or satellite television or radio program, university or think tank that contributes credible ideas to public policy debates in published format.

For all of these criteria, the center's staff makes judgments based on verifiable facts, not on opinions about the relevance of individuals' employment histories. Likewise, there are many people who clearly meet these criteria, but the center has yet to identify or verify their employment histories. The Revolving Door database will be continually updated, refined, and expanded as information becomes available.

Data Sources

The information that forms the basis of this database is compiled from a combination of proprietary and publicly available sources. The primary source for the core data is a set of 7,745 people with details, biographical, or education entries in the comprehensive online directory of lobbyists published by Columbia Books, Inc., at www.lobbyists.info, as of September 29, 2006. For those people whose biographies were supplied by Columbia Books, the original text of their entries as of that date is included in their summary pages. In addition, the center's research staff uses internal resources and publicly available sources to continuously update this original core data set with new biographical information about people existing in the Revolving Door Database, and with information about new people who meet the criteria for inclusion.

At all times the center has done its best to choose whether a person qualifies for the Revolving Door based on imperfect information, such as informal job titles or incomplete descriptive narratives. If there are any errors or omissions for a person's summary, or if there are suggestions of any person who may be added to or excluded from the center's Revolving Door project, please contact our research staff at revdoor@crp.org.

Data Summaries, Searches, and Other Information

The Revolving Door database allows users to view the data conveniently through summaries and searches. Summary data ranks the top employers of people within the data set, organized by members of Congress, federal agencies, congressional committees, lobbying firms, and other organizations. Unless otherwise indicated, these summaries will include any person in the data set that is identified as ever having worked for a particular employer. Thus, these lists include both people who currently work for and people who formerly worked for a specific employer.

Similarly, the center lists people identified as having worked for a particular presidential administration, or for an elected official affiliated with either the Democrat or Republican parties. The data for political parties is determined by the party affiliation of the employer; the center has made no attempt to determine actual party registration or identification of any nonelected person in the database.

In addition, for those people in the Revolving Door database who are also registered to lobby under the Lobbying Disclosure Act, the center has calculated scale variables to measure the composition of their clientele and their policy specializations.

Industries Represented

The charts located under the "Industries Represented" tab approximate concentrations of industries represented by lobbyists and organizations registered with the Senate Office of Public Records according to the Lobbying Disclosure Act. The center identified five top industries for individual lobbyists and for their clients from semiannual lobbying disclosure reports. For individual lobbyists, the industry-representation is calculated by summing the amounts spent by all of a lobbyist's clients. These amounts are then aggregated according to the center's industry-coding system. For employers, industry-representation is calculated by summing the amounts earned from all of the firm's registered clients (or spent by an organization that represents itself). These amounts are then aggregated by industry.

Expertise and Interests

The charts located under the "Expertise & Interests" tab charts approximate lobbyists' policy expertise and the policy interests of their clients registered with the Senate Office of Public Records (SOPR) according to the Lobbying Disclosure Act. The center identified five top issue areas for individual lobbyists and for their clients from semiannual lobbying disclosure reports. For individual lobbyists, policy expertise is calculated by counting the number of semiannual reports that mention an issue for each of their clients. These totals are then aggregated according to the center's industry-coding system. For registered clients, policy interests are calculated by counting the number of semiannual reports that mention an issue for all of their clients. These totals are then aggregated by industry.

Top Agencies

Former employees of federal agencies can often find good (and lucrative) jobs as lobbyists, capitalizing on the connections that they forged while in public service. An Environmental Protection Agency administrator may go on to lobby his former colleagues on environmental issues, and a White House staffer can tap her West Wing connections when she starts a new job on K Street. The White House is traditionally the executive branch's largest supplier of fresh lobbyists; the office of the president employs a large team of staffers of varying seniority. But public servants switching to careers as lobbyists (and back again) come from agencies as varied as the Department of Defense, NASA, and the Smithsonian Institution. Agency employees strolling through the Revolving Door include those as powerful—and well connected—as secretaries of state and as far from Washington as Peace Corps volunteers.

6

The Tobacco Industry

Ruth E. Malone

Introduction

In November 2008, in a cavernous convention hall in Durban, South Africa, diplomatic representatives from more than 130 countries gathered to negotiate guidelines for implementing the Framework Convention on Tobacco Control (FCTC), the world's first global public health treaty. The delegates, mostly high-level diplomatic, trade, or health officials in their countries, spent a week negotiating language aimed at helping governments stem an epidemic of tobacco-caused disease that will, if unchecked, claim 1 billion lives in this century (World Health Organization, 2008a). They recommended that countries raise awareness about tobacco industry interference with tobacco control policies; limit interactions with the industry and ensure transparency in those that must occur; reject partnerships and voluntary agreements with the industry; and recognize that activities described as "socially responsible" by the tobacco industry constitute another form of tobacco marketing and should be denormalized and regulated. On the meeting's last day, the body of delegates—working by consensus, not majority rule—declared as a guiding principle that *"there is a fundamental and irreconcilable conflict between the tobacco industry's interests and*

Ruth Malone owns one share apiece of Altria/Philip Morris USA, PM International, and Reynolds American tobacco company stock for research and advocacy purposes.

155

public health interests" (Conference of the Parties to the WHO Framework Convention on Tobacco Control, 2009).

Why would so many nations band together to issue such an unprecedented statement, explicitly naming an entire industry the inherent enemy of public health? First, the deadliness of the tobacco industry's products means that *everything* tobacco companies do to achieve their business success harms health. However, we also know more about tobacco corporations than about any other corporate entities, due to an unusual set of circumstances that resulted in the release of millions of pages of internal company documents, many of which were once considered "confidential" and "secret." As a result of examining these documents, we now understand much more than we did only a decade ago about how corporations operate and the many ways (in addition to promoting dangerous products like tobacco) they represent threats to public health.

We also understand more about the limits of "traditional" public health and health education approaches, which may promote ideas of disease causation that mask the responsibility of corporate entities, focusing overmuch on individual health behaviors and susceptibilities. What we are just now beginning to understand fully, through the tobacco industry's own documents, is the degree to which tobacco corporations—and other corporations which have drawn on their successes—appropriate and shape culture in ways that are socially destructive. The tobacco industry was the leader in showing other corporations how to link product branding with our very identity, for example, and how to exploit our most cherished ideals in ways that undermine the social contract. That is one reason why the statement from Durban is pathbreaking: it pierces through the "myth of cultural immutability" (Kottke & Hoffman, 2003) that has rendered corporate disease promotion almost invisible in public health education, research, and practice until recently (Freudenberg, 2005; Wiist, 2006).

This chapter provides an overview of the tobacco industry and the ways in which it has worked to preserve its profits at the expense of the health of its consumers. After some background information, including sources of information about the tobacco industry and the scope of tobacco as a public health problem, this chapter will outline some of the myriad ways in which the tobacco industry has undermined public health for decades, focusing on how the industry creates scientific "controversy," and how it shapes cultural understandings of smoking and of the industry itself through influencing nearly every sector of society. The chapter concludes with a call for citizens to hold their governments accountable for stopping corporate disease promotion.

Sources of Information

Because of whistleblower disclosures and several lawsuits against the tobacco industry, millions of pages of internal corporate documents have become available (MacKenzie et al., 2003; Malone & Balbach, 2000). The great majority of these documents were made public because of the Master Settlement Agreement (MSA) between the attorneys general of 46 U.S. states and major U.S. tobacco companies, settling lawsuits which sought to recover health care costs incurred by states for treatment of sick smokers (National Association of Attorneys General, 1998). These documents, which were acquired during the legal discovery process and released publicly only after considerable resistance from tobacco companies, were at first available only in two poorly indexed paper depositories operated by the industry in Minneapolis, Minnesota and Guildford, England. Examining the documents involved a tedious and very time consuming process of searching inadequate industry-supplied indexes for items of interest, filling out paper forms to request the boxes that held the documents, searching through the boxes to locate the documents, and filling out additional requests for photocopies of the documents, which were expensive and only forthcoming weeks to months later (Malone & Balbach, 2000). Undoubtedly, this is precisely the kind of laborious process tobacco corporations were counting on when they finally agreed to release the documents, calculating that, with such mountains of material in no particular order, by the time anyone found much of anything it would be old news.

What the industry perhaps did not anticipate was the rapid development of technology and funding resources that quickly allowed virtually the entire collection to be made electronically accessible. It is now available in an online, full-text searchable format within the Legacy Tobacco Documents Library, housed at the University of California, San Francisco (http://legacy.library.ucsf.edu). As a result, research drawing on these archives documents the activities, strategies, and tactics used by tobacco corporations across the decades of the past century. Additional documents continue to be released and archived, and the collection includes documents dating through April 2008, with the majority of the material dated from 1980 through 2000. Although some smaller collections of documents related to tobacco and other industries are available, there is perhaps no other comparable archive providing such rich access into the internal workings of corporations across an entire industry, including their coordinated activities with one another aimed at influencing science and thwarting regulations (Brandt, 2007; McDaniel et al., 2008).

Tobacco Products and Public Health

Cigarettes are the single most deadly consumer product ever made. While all forms of tobacco cause disease, commercial cigarettes have caused the premature deaths of millions since their introduction in the late 1800s. The aggressive and innovative marketing developed by tobacco companies contributed to an epidemic of diseases that took decades to comprehend—in large measure because tobacco corporations linked their products to pleasurable images and cultural values of every kind, and deliberately and systematically hid the truth about the disease consequences of using them.

Lung cancer is the disease most often associated with cigarette smoking. An extremely rare disease prior to the commercialization of cigarettes, lung cancer rapidly increased as cigarette use exploded across the past century (Kluger, 1997). However, tobacco use causes multiple other diseases, including cancers of the bladder, esophagus, larynx, pancreas, cervix, kidneys, and stomach. Smoking also causes aortic aneurysm, emphysema, leukemia, cataract, pneumonia, stroke, coronary heart disease, and congestive heart failure (U.S. Department of Health and Human Services, 2004). Smokers also have higher rates of pregnancy complications, stillbirth, and infant mortality. Secondhand smoke has been identified as a contributor to sudden infant death syndrome and many other diseases in nonsmokers, including lung cancer and heart disease (U.S. Department of Health and Human Services, 2004). Emerging evidence suggests that both active smoking and secondhand smoke independently contribute to breast cancer among premenopausal women (Slattery et al., 2008). Overall, cohort studies show that cigarettes kill about half their longtime users (Doll et al., 1994, 2004).

Tobacco costs borne by society include direct medical care, lost productivity, and neonatal care, costing the United States alone more than $157 billion a year (U.S. Department of Health and Human Services, 2004). (These costs exclude the pain and suffering of those with tobacco-caused diseases and the economic and emotional losses their families suffer due to the premature death of their loved ones.) Because cigarettes are also highly addictive, tobacco use contributes to poverty and childhood malnutrition as addicted smokers forego other basic needs in order to buy cigarettes (Armour et al., 2008; Best et al., 2008; John, 2008; Liu et al., 2006; Siahpush et al., 2003). Tobacco companies have also contributed to impoverishing farmers in developing countries through controlling the market for tobacco leaf (Otañez et al., 2007; Patel et al., 2007).

Tobacco has negative effects on public health and well-being more broadly. For example, tobacco cannot be economically grown without a range of pesticides, herbicides, fungicides, and other chemical products, which may contribute to water and soil contamination, air pollution, and damage worker health. Because they rely on these chemicals, tobacco companies have worked to weaken international pesticide regulations, using covert operatives to influence the policy development process (McDaniel et al., 2005; Zeltner et al., 2000). Tobacco growing contributes to deforestation as trees are felled to clear land for tobacco growing and to use as fuel for tobacco curing (Geist, 1999), and tobacco itself can be highly toxic to those who grow or handle it, causing nicotine poisoning or green tobacco sickness among workers (Arcury et al., 2008; Quandt et al., 2000).

Finally, cigarettes are a major contributor to litter and water pollution. In 2007, a shoreline cleanup day conducted by volunteers in 68 countries collected 1.9 million cigarettes and cigarette butts out of 7.7 million total items of debris collected worldwide (The Ocean Conservancy, 2007). Such materials constitute the largest source of litter by item. The nearly 370 billion filtered cigarettes smoked each year in the United States alone result in about 135 million pounds of nonbiodegradable butts littering the landscape, each saturated with multiple toxins (Lazarus, 2008).

That a product that is so destructive and so expensive to society remains on the market, sold in every convenience store and, until recently, in almost all pharmacies and hospital gift shops, is due to the ability of the tobacco industry to adapt to challenges, constantly repositioning itself in order to feed upon the social body as mosquitoes feed upon their victims. This chapter illustrates why the tobacco industry has been called the "vector" of the tobacco disease epidemic (LeGresley, 1999). However, this chapter also points to the failure of governments to protect public health from corporate predators.

The Tobacco Industry

The tobacco industry, broadly defined, includes not only major corporations that manufacture cigarettes and other products, but growers, distributors, lawyers, advertising and public relations firms working for the industry, retailers, and firms that supply manufacturers. Some of these constitute corporate entities in their own right, but a good number are smaller firms or networks that service the major tobacco corporations, and will not be addressed here.

This analysis focuses primarily on those tobacco corporations about which we have the most documentary evidence, namely Philip Morris USA and Philip Morris International, Reynolds American, Lorillard, and British American Tobacco, and their associated public relations and scientific entities. While the state-owned tobacco firms (such as China National Tobacco

Corporation) are also powerful industry actors, they are positioned differently in a structural sense than the for-profit corporations, and will not be addressed here. Excluding China National Tobacco, four tobacco corporations—PM International, *British American Tobacco* (BAT), Japan Tobacco, and Imperial—control 69% of the cigarette market (Yuk, 2008, June 9). Tobacco products are enormously profitable. For example, the Altria Group, Inc., parent company of Philip Morris USA and until 2008 of Philip Morris International, reported a net revenue of $73.8 billion in 2007 (Altria Group Inc., 2007). This has made the companies attractive to investors, some of whom include governments that must bear the costs of providing medical care for sick smokers.

Background: Generation of an Epidemic

While the full history of the development of the modern tobacco industry is beyond the scope of this chapter and has been detailed elsewhere (Brandt, 2007; Kluger, 1997), a brief historical overview sets the stage for understanding the following sections on tobacco industry activities. It is, first, essential to recognize that the global epidemic of tobacco-caused disease that we currently face is not merely the inevitable result of millions of bad individual behavior decisions. The epidemic was, in a most fundamental way, industrially created and is industrially sustained.

While tobacco has been used for centuries, it was used prior to the late 1800s mostly in pipe, cigar or chew forms, which involved minimal inhalation of smoke. It was the invention of the cigarette-rolling machine in 1880 and the rise of consumer culture in the United States that dramatically shifted the landscape of tobacco use. As commercial cigarettes became popular and cigarette smoking increased over the first part of the 20th century, concerns began to be raised about cigarettes' effects on health. A few studies in the early decades had linked cigarette smoking with disease, and some noted a rise in lung cancer, but a widespread scientific consensus had not yet emerged that cigarettes were the cause. Meanwhile, tobacco companies had developed innovative, now-legendary ways of marketing their products, linking them with images of freedom and health. During the 1930s and 1940s, for example, they developed advertising campaigns that featured reassuring nurses and doctors (Brandt, 2007). They also advertised cigarettes in the leading medical and nursing journals of the day (Malone, 2006). They continued these efforts in a slightly subtler form several decades later, creating ads designed to reassure concerned smokers that "light" cigarettes were safer than regular ones, even though they knew that as smoked by the consumer, they provided no health advantages (Anderson et al., 2006; Cataldo & Malone, 2008; Pollay, 2000).

It was *Reader's Digest*, a widely read magazine in the United States (and a publication that accepted no advertising) that shattered the tobacco companies' carefully constructed popular visions of cigarettes as benign, even healthful products. In a 1952 article entitled "Cancer by the Carton," the tobacco industry was accused of covering up the real dangers of smoking by reassuring customers about "mildness" and lack of throat irritation. The real danger, the article charged, was lung cancer (Brandt, 2007; Kluger, 1997). The article caused a sensation, and was followed by others that discussed research showing that cigarette smoke produced cancer.

In response, tobacco corporations began working intensively together in multiple public relations-oriented activities, discussed later, to create doubt and generate "controversy" about the scientific findings linking smoking with disease. It was not until 1999, nearly 50 years after the publication of the *Reader's Digest* article, that tobacco companies belatedly began admitting on websites that cigarettes cause disease (Meier, 1999; Smith & Malone, 2008). However, they continue to deny in court that their products have caused disease in individual cases (Friedman, 2007). And, even as they admit that cigarettes cause multiple diseases, they also continue, to this day, to aggressively promote their use.

Creating Scientific "Controversy": The Tobacco Companies' Conspiracy

Scientific rigor calls for replication of findings and consideration of alternative causal explanations; thus, scientists are typically cautious and tentative in drawing their conclusions. The tobacco companies exploited this tendency in their response to the lung cancer threat. With a strategy coordinated by the well-known Hill and Knowlton public relations firm, which counted among its clients the steel, oil, and aircraft industries, they sought to convey to the public and to smokers the idea that the industry was sincerely seeking the truth about the lung cancer issue (Brandt, 2007).

The major tobacco companies joined together to announce their creation of a new research organization, the Tobacco Industry Research Committee, purportedly charged with investigating the link between smoking and disease, but which in reality was but the first of a succession of industry-sponsored research organizations whose goal was to generate doubt about the scientific evidence that smoking and/or secondhand smoke caused disease. To publicize their plans, the companies sponsored the seminal corporate "issue" newspaper advertisement, the now-infamous "Frank Statement to Cigarette Smokers" of 1954 (see Figure 6.1) , in which the major U.S. tobacco companies claimed

A Frank Statement to Cigarette Smokers

RECENT REPORTS on experiments with mice have given wide publicity to a theory that cigarette smoking is in some way linked with lung cancer in human beings.

Although conducted by doctors of professional standing, these experiments are not regarded as conclusive in the field of cancer research. However, we do not believe that any serious medical research, even though its results are inconclusive should be disregarded or lightly dismissed.

At the same time, we feel it is in the public interest to call attention to the fact that eminent doctors and research scientists have publicly questioned the claimed significance of these experiments.

Distinguished authorities point out:

1. That medical research of recent years indicates many possible causes of lung cancer.
2. That there is no agreement among the authorities regarding what the cause is.
3. That there is no proof that cigarette smoking is one of the causes.
4. That statistics purporting to link cigarette smoking with the disease could apply with equal force to any one of many other aspects of modern life. Indeed the validity of the statistics themselves is questioned by numerous scientists.

We accept an interest in people's health as a basic responsibility, paramount to every other consideration in our business.

We believe the products we make are not injurious to health.

We always have and always will cooperate closely with those whose task it is to safeguard the public health.

For more than 300 years tobacco has given solace, relaxation, and enjoyment to mankind. At one time or another during those years critics have held it responsible for practically every disease of the human body. One by one these charges have been abandoned for lack of evidence.

Regardless of the record of the past, the fact that cigarette smoking today should even be suspected as a cause of a serious disease is a matter of deep concern to us.

Many people have asked us what we are doing to meet the public's concern aroused by the recent reports. Here is the answer:

1. We are pledging aid and assistance to the research effort into all phases of tobacco use and health. This joint financial aid will of course be in addition to that what is already being contributed by individual companies.
2. For this purpose we are establishing a joint industry group consisting initially of the undersigned. This group will be known as TOBACCO INDUSTRY RESEARCH COMMITTEE.
3. In charge of the research activities of the Committee will be a scientist of unimpeachable integrity and national repute. In addition there will be an Advisory Board of scientists disinterested in the cigarette industry. A group of distinguished men from medicine, science, and education will be invited to serve on this Board. These scientists will advise the Committee on its research activities.

This statement is being issued because we believe the people are entitled to know where we stand on this matter and what we intend to do about it.

TOBACCO INDUSTRY RESEARCH COMMITTEE

5400 EMPIRE STATE BUILDING, NEW YORK 1, N.Y.

SPONSORS:

THE AMERICAN TOBACCO COMPANY, INC.
Paul M. Hehn, President

BENSON & ILEDGES
Joseph F. Cullman, Jr., President

BRIGHT BELT WAREHOUSE ASSOCIATION
F. S. Royster, President

BROWN & WILLIAMSON TOBACCO CORPORATION
Timothy V. Hartnett, President

BURLEY AUCTION WAREHOUSE ASSOCIATION
Albert Clay, President

BURLEY TOBACCO GROWERS COOPERATIVE ASSOCIATION
John W. Jones, President

LARUS & BROTHER COMPANY, INC.
W. T. Reed, Jr., President

P. LORILLARD COMPANY
Herbert A. Kent, Chairman

MARYLAND TOBACCO GROWERS ASSOCIATION
Samuel C. Linton, General Manager

PHILIP MORRIS & CO., LTD., INC.
O. Parker McComas, President

R. J. REYNOLDS TOBACCO COMPANY
E. A. Darr, President

STEPHANO BROTHERS, INC.
C. S. Stephano, D'Sc., Director of Research

TOBACCO ASSOCIATES, INC.
(An organization of Pro-cured tobacco growers)
J. H. Hutson, president

UNITED STATES TOBACCO COMPANY
J. W. Peterson, President

FIGURE 6.1. The "Frank Statement" as published in 1954.

that they accepted "an interest in people's health as a basic responsibility, paramount to every other consideration in our business" (Brandt, 2007; Glantz et al., 1996; Tobacco Industry Research Committee, 1954). As Brandt (2007: 172) notes, however, at the time the Frank Statement was published in more than 400 newspapers, "the industry had yet to take even the first step toward creating a research program."

As we know now, this was a watershed moment, when these corporations had an opportunity to take their own words seriously and support genuinely independent research. Instead, the industry research bodies, once created, were controlled by public relations and legal staff, who ensured that the research funded was either (1) irrelevant to determining whether cigarettes caused lung cancer and other diseases; (2) designed explicitly to refute studies that suggested such an association; or (3) would otherwise increase the credibility of industry arguments (Barnes & Bero, 1996; Bero, 2005; Bero et al., 1994, 1995; Malone & Bero, 2003). Tobacco companies spent the next several decades perpetuating the idea that whether cigarettes caused cancer was still a matter of scientific "controversy."

The companies' concealment efforts, now well documented, included the manipulation of scientific findings to reflect the industry's public position that smoking was not a cause of disease; ghost authorship of studies (officially authored by seemingly independent scientists, but in reality primarily conducted by industry-affiliated scientists) that cast doubt on the links between smoking or secondhand smoke and disease; lawyer control over tobacco industry research funding and editing of scientific reports to ensure they did not contradict industry positions; attacking or attempting to have funding rescinded for scientists whose work was considered potentially threatening; and myriad other efforts aimed at casting doubt on scientific findings unfavorable to the industry (Barnes et al., 2006; Bero, 2005; Bero et al., 1995; Bitton et al., 2005; Chapman et al., 2003; Gruning et al., 2006; Hong & Bero, 2002; Landman & Glantz, 2009; Tong & Glantz, 2007; Tong et al., 2005; Trotter & Chapman, 2003).

The companies also concealed their product manipulation. Concerned that despite all their efforts to create "controversy," smokers were beginning to want to quit as the evidence against cigarettes mounted, tobacco companies engineered cigarettes in ways that maximized their addictiveness. An investigation by the Food and Drug Administration during the 1990s found that tobacco companies had sought dozens of patents for various means to enhance nicotine in cigarettes, including developing genetically modified tobacco plants with higher levels of nicotine and adding or enhancing transfer of nicotine through the manufacturing process (Connolly et al., 2007; Kessler, 2001).

Despite the fact that industry CEOs testified under oath before a Congressional hearing in the 1990s that they believed that nicotine was not addictive, internal company documents show that they had explicitly regarded it as such since at least the 1960s (Glantz et al., 1996). A now-infamous confidential Brown and Williamson document from 1963 baldly stated, "We are, then, in the business of selling nicotine, an addictive drug" (Brown and Williamson Tobacco Company, 1963). A 1984 memo from Philip Morris in Australia noted the declining market share of Marlboro and proposed altering the blend to conform with U.S. Marlboros, thus "making it harder for existing smokers to leave the product" (Webb, 1984, July 12). As industry documents later revealed, Marlboro's special attractiveness was related to ammonia technology, which increased freebase nicotine uptake (Stevenson & Proctor, 2008).

"Light" cigarettes, which when smoked by testing machines delivered lower levels of nicotine than regular cigarettes, were designed to deliver more nicotine as actually used by smokers, who, tobacco companies knew, "compensated" by smoking differently to get their nicotine dose (Hammond et al., 2006; Kozlowski & O'Connor, 2002; Wayne et al., 2006, 2008). "Lights" were supported by aggressive "lifestyle" marketing that implied health benefits (Assunta & Chapman, 2008; Cataldo & Malone, 2008; Kozlowski & Pillitteri, 2001), just as regular cigarettes had been marketed decades before. As Hammond and colleagues observed in reporting on their findings from internal industry documents, "the documents seem to reveal a product strategy intended to exploit the limitations of the testing protocols and to intentionally conceal from consumers and regulators the potential toxicity" of tobacco products that tobacco company research revealed (Hammond et al., 2006: 781).

In 2006, in a detailed, carefully annotated, 1600-page decision in *United States of America versus Philip Morris, et al.,* a massive federal case in which the tobacco companies were found guilty of fraud and racketeering, federal judge Gladys Kessler found of tobacco companies that:

> over the course of approximately fifty years ... in order to protect
> themselves from smoking and health related claims in litigation, and
> in order to avoid regulation which they viewed as harmful ... [defen-
> dant tobacco companies] suppressed, concealed, and terminated
> scientific research; they destroyed documents including scientific
> reports and studies ... (United States District Court for the District
> of Columbia, 2006: 4034).

This case (and earlier analyses of other sets of internal tobacco industry documents) revealed that tobacco companies had known, long before the health community—and worked actively to conceal—that cigarettes caused cancer, that secondhand smoke was harmful, that nicotine was addictive, and that so-called "light" cigarettes were just as harmful to health as regular ones (Barnes et al., 1995; Bero, 2003; Glantz et al., 1995; Hanauer et al., 1995; Slade et al., 1995). A 2003 review of the evidence at that time noted that "deception has been the *modus operandi* of the industry" (Bero, 2003: 271).

As secondhand smoke became a health policy issue during the 1980s, with concerns being raised about the health effects on nonsmokers of inhaling others' smoke from cigarettes, the industry replicated its "controversy" strategy. Working together, the major multinational tobacco companies developed multiple coordinated global strategies, using a massive international network (Francey & Chapman, 2000; McDaniel et al., 2008) to promote their assertions that there was still scientific "controversy" about the effects of secondhand smoke. This effort included establishing a worldwide "consultants" program in which scientists were paid through the industry's Washington, D.C.-based law firm, Covington and Burling, to develop and publish research supporting tobacco companies' assertions that secondhand smoke was not harmful (Assunta et al., 2004; Barnoya & Glantz, 2002, 2006; Hong & Bero, 2002; Tong & Glantz, 2007).

The industry also poured money into programs designed to convince policy makers and the public that the best solution to nonsmokers' concerns about inhaling secondhand smoke was "accommodation" of both smokers and nonsmokers in public places and that ventilation could address any discomfort nonsmokers experienced (Dearlove et al., 2002; Drope et al., 2004; Pilkington & Gilmore, 2004; Smith & Malone, 2008). Despite the fact that these solutions have been shown to be ineffective in protecting public health, tobacco companies continue even today to argue for them (Samet, 2008). In addition to influencing the policy debate with specious science, tobacco companies also sought to influence through both overt and covert means the International Standards Organization and other bodies involved in determining indoor air quality standards and the measurements of tar and nicotine yields (Bialous & Glantz, 2002; Bialous & Yach, 2001).

Working the Media

Tobacco corporations could not have conveyed the notion of "controversy" without aid from other institutions and organizations. The media were important players in tobacco industry efforts to claim that there were various "weaknesses" in the available scientific evidence that smoking and secondhand smoke caused disease, which allowed them to argue against effective tobacco control policies. For example, in the 1990s, in efforts to derail the U.S. Environmental Protection Agency's determination that secondhand smoke was a human carcinogen, Philip Morris recruited a network of journalists to generate media coverage critical of this decision, supported internships at a journalism school oriented toward conservative and market interests, and worked with journalists associated with public policy organizations to present industry positions in speeches. The plan was to "promote the 'care and feeding' of key journalists to develop a network sympathetic to Philip Morris concerns" (Muggli et al., 2004a: 574). Similar media strategies were used to try to generate media coverage that would derail the U.S. Occupational Safety and Health Administration's indoor air quality rule-making process (Bryan-Jones & Bero, 2003).

Contacts with media were carefully cultivated. In the Philip Morris Nordic Journalist Program, for example, selected journalists from Nordic countries were invited to Neuchatel, Switzerland to hear about the tobacco industry position on secondhand smoke, and their subsequent articles were appraised to determine whether they indicated that the journalists were "friendly" to the industry. Some apparently identified as such were provided with "consulting" contracts that appear linked to industry-favorable articles they wrote. Other journalists were provided with industry-paid junkets to the United States to attend programs similarly designed to offer tobacco company personnel the opportunity to get to know journalists and to communicate the tobacco industry's position (Hiilamo et al., 2008).

The tobacco industry also used paid "issue" advertising to communicate its policy positions, position itself as "concerned" about the problems, and convey the "controversy" messages. This served both to cultivate good relations with publications receiving the ad revenues and to convey the notion that the industry was sincerely seeking the truth in a situation in which the truth supposedly remained illusive. Decades after the appearance of the Frank Statement, an 1984 RJ Reynolds campaign suggested that "the case against smoking" was still open, launching a series of newspaper and magazine ads with titles like "Can we have an open debate about smoking?," "Passive smoking: an active controversy," and "Second-hand smoke: the myth and the reality" (R.J. Reynolds Tobacco Company, 1984b, 1984c, 1984d, 1985). Exploiting the media's interest in conflict, the campaign reportedly achieved prominent attention, with "virtually every daily newspaper in the country" and all of the major U.S. television networks covering it (Humber, 1984). Five months after the launch of the first ad, 250 articles on it had been published (R.J. Reynolds Tobacco Company, 1984a). No public health campaign could compete effectively with such media expenditures.

Creating a Culture in Which Smoking and
the Industry Were Accepted

In this chapter, culture is used in a generic sense to mean the wide variety
of activities, settings, practices, institutions, social rules, and taken-for-granted
understandings that, taken together, shape a comprehensible world. From
within a culture, certain kinds of practices "make sense" and others are
regarded as unthinkable. Across the last century, major tobacco corporations
successfully insinuated the cigarette into nearly every aspect and arena of
culture, worldwide, in order to keep smoking "normal" and the promotion of
deadly products acceptable.

Marketing Activities

In consumer societies, marketing plays a major role in shaping cultural understandings of objects of consumption and their makers. The industry's creative
marketing served as a model for many other companies, beginning in the
1920s with the father of public relations, Edward Bernays. Bernays arranged,
in an era when smoking by women was still frowned upon, to have prominent New York feminists and debutantes stroll on Fifth Avenue, smoking in
the Easter Parade and creating a sensation (Kluger, 1997). This was perhaps
the first of hundreds of campaigns designed to link cigarette smoking with
freedom, independence, and rebellion against traditional roles, and it proved
highly successful. Inhaling carcinogenic gas from a highly engineered burning paper tube 20 times a day would be seen as a form of liberation and also
as a testimony to the tobacco industry's prowess at tapping into social tensions
and exploiting cultural imagery. This linkage was replicated repeatedly across
the last century, from the Virginia Slims campaign (with its neo-feminist slogan "You've come a long way, baby") to the Marlboro Man, who hijacked the
imagery and cultural meaning (wide-open spaces of freedom) of the American
West (Hafez & Ling, 2005; West, 1996).

In recent years, the industry has developed a number of "youth nonsmoking programs" which also exploit this carefully crafted linkage between smoking and freedom/rebellion through "forbidden fruit" messages like "kids
shouldn't smoke" and "smoking is an adult choice" (Landman et al., 2002).
Research has shown that these industry-sponsored programs may actually
increase the likelihood that adolescents, who typically desire to be independent and rebel against parental authority, will be open to the idea of smoking
(Farrelly et al., 2002). One of the most successful youth nonsmoking programs

ever was the Florida (later American Legacy Foundation) "Truth" campaign, which featured messages suggesting that the industry wanted to manipulate youth into smoking (Farrelly et al., 2002, 2005; Hicks, 2001; Sly et al., 2001, 2002; Thrasher et al., 2004; Zucker et al., 2000). Tobacco companies attacked the program and later sued the Legacy Foundation in an attempt to stop the ads (Ibrahim & Glantz, 2006).

The shaping of cigarettes (and cigarette brands) as signifiers of particular social identities was done through a myriad of approaches, many of which were highly innovative. For example, tobacco companies may have been among the first to "segment" markets through psychographic studies that identified profiles within target groups (Ling & Glantz, 2002). They also were among the first to branch out from traditional billboards and print advertisements to incorporate music and activities into marketing. For example, the industry's interest in marketing menthol cigarettes to African Americans in low-income inner city areas led to the development of innovations like mobile rap music video vans. These were sometimes parked outside clubs and used to distribute free cigarettes in urban neighborhoods where employees were nervous about crime, shaping the racialized geography of today's health disparities (Yerger et al., 2007).

Cultural icons were linked with cigarette products by featuring them on cigarette packs, in advertisements, and in many other forms. Nothing was sacred—literally. In the Philippines, the Virgin Mary was featured on promotional calendars for Fortune Tobacco, the leading producer, which has had licensing agreements with R.J. Reynolds in the past (Alechnowicz & Chapman, 2004). In addition, while U.S. tobacco companies today deny engaging in paid product placement in movies, evidence shows that such placement was often arranged in the past, creating a whole generation of smoking movie icons (many of whom later died from tobacco-caused diseases) and featuring cigarette brands prominently even in movies aimed at young audiences. Movies aimed at young audiences continue to feature cigarettes and smoking, and seeing such films has been shown to increase the likelihood that youth will try smoking (Sargent et al., 2008; Song et al., 2007; Wills et al., 2008).

According to the Federal Trade Commission, $13.11 billion was spent in the United States alone on cigarette advertising and promotion in 2005, a decline from the record $15.15 billion reported by the major cigarette manufacturers in 2003, but still equivalent to almost $1.5 million an hour, 24 hours a day (Federal Trade Commission, 2007). The sheer scope of industry marketing is remarkable. While the once-ubiquitous outdoor billboards were eliminated in the United States by the 1998 Master Settlement Agreement, the industry continues to market cigarettes through bar promotions, self-published

"lifestyle" magazines, designer packs, web-based activities, point-of-sale gim-
micks, "viral" marketing, direct mail, and many other innovative approaches,
all aimed at convincing the young that its products are associated with vibrant
health, fun, sexiness, toughness, romance, coolness, and other desired social
attributes (Anderson & Ling, 2008; Hafez & Ling, 2006; Safran, 2000; Sepe
et al., 2002). To ensure favorable display, tobacco companies also pay retailers
special fees to prominently feature their products or signage (Feighery et al.,
2003).

However, the success of this toxic industry over so many decades cannot be attributed to overt product marketing alone. Tobacco companies also
extended their presence, products, and the idea of smoking into the culture in
dozens of much more subtle ways. For example, though now largely banned
in the United States, tobacco companies for many years sponsored sporting
events of all sorts, branding them with cigarette imagery; these practices
now continue as they move aggressively into developing country markets
(Alechnowicz & Chapman, 2004; Knight & Chapman, 2004). The industry
also provided sponsorship for major performing and visual arts organizations, community groups, festivals, and musical events. Sponsorships served
to associate tobacco with fun events and with healthy activities, portray the
company as a "good citizen" and friend of the community, and thereby market both the products and themselves as corporate entities (Rosenberg &
Siegel, 2001). They also serve to make tobacco seem a normal part of arts culture, sports culture, music culture, and youth culture in general (Knight &
Chapman, 2004).

Shaping the Culture of Policy making

For years, major tobacco corporations have exerted influence on the policy making process. This influence takes multiple forms: lobbying, campaign contributions, funding front groups to challenge tobacco control-related initiatives,
and bringing pressure to bear on government agencies through political allies
are just some of these. However, they may also simply write the policies themselves, as British American Tobacco (BAT) did in completely redesigning the
tobacco tax system in Uzbekistan during the privatization of the state-owned
tobacco monopoly there (Gilmore et al., 2007), and in Kenya, where it helped
draft legislation that advantaged BAT over its competitors (Patel et al., 2007).
The industry's policy-related activities have affected virtually every segment of
society, every level of political organization, and every societal arena in which
their corporate interests are at stake.

On the international level, the tobacco industry has used global agreements on trade to force open new markets, as it did in Thailand and other Asian markets in the late 1980s (Vateesatokit, 2003). Tobacco companies also aggressively sought to undermine the FCTC and, before its development, the work of the WHO Tobacco Free Initiative (Mamudu & Glantz, 2008; Mamudu et al., 2008; Zeltner et al., 2000). The Boca Raton Action Plan, for example, was developed as Philip Morris's Master Plan for 1989 to address perceived challenges to the tobacco business. It identified as its primary concern the WHO's tobacco control program, which it sought to "redirect" and "contain" through multiple avenues. These included the use of surrogates such as non-tobacco subsidiaries, business groups and supposedly independent journalists and consultants to exert pressure through other UN agencies, the media, international organizations, and governments. They may have included working to redirect funding for the tobacco control program toward other health areas. Paul Dietrich, a journalist who developed a reputation as "an independent critic of WHO," was apparently a key player in the "redirection" strategy, consulting for tobacco companies while suggesting to journalists and policy makers that WHO's tobacco control program was "misguided," drafting numerous articles critical of WHO, and addressing conferences, where he also claimed that the U.S. National Institutes of Health was suppressing research showing that tobacco did not cause disease (Zeltner et al., 2000).

At the federal level in the United States, the industry has exerted power for decades, primarily through powerful chairmanships held by tobacco-state Congressional allies who have been the recipients of tobacco industry contributions (Luke & Krauss, 2004). The industry worked with tobacco-state Congress members on the House and Senate Armed Services Committees to repeatedly thwart tobacco control initiatives, even those coming from within the U.S. military (Arvey & Malone, 2008; Smith et al., 2007). For example, the tobacco industry's Congressional allies quietly inserted into a defense authorization bill a provision that basically *requires* military stores to sell cigarettes and disallows commissary (military store) price increases unless explicitly approved by Congress (Smith et al., 2007). Since smoking negatively affects even short-term troop health and readiness, the military has made multiple efforts to institute tobacco control measures, but the industry has consistently worked to weaken or delay them. Even a modest partnership between an Air Force commissary and the American Cancer Society, in which antitobacco signs were displayed on the shelves of commissaries with relatively innocuous messages like "aim high—stop smoking," provoked the Tobacco Institute to enlist the aid of the House Armed Services Committee, which subsequently placed a hold on construction of two Air Force commissaries until after the signs were removed (Smith et al., 2007).

The tobacco industry typically works on multiple avenues to reach policy makers with its preferred messages; Philip Morris sought to create an "echo chamber" effect whereby members of Congress in the United States heard the same message from multiple sources or similar messages repeatedly from a single source (Landman & Glantz, 2009). These sources often included so-called "smoker's rights groups" based in multiple countries across Europe and in Australia, New Zealand, Hong Kong, and the United States (Lopipero & Bero, 2006; Smith & Malone, 2007). These groups, which were industry cre-ated, supported, and largely controlled, were used to conflate the legality of smoking with a "right to smoke," to suggest a groundswell of grassroots oppo-sition to policies prohibiting smoking in public places, including airplanes, and to sustain the social acceptability of smoking. While many of these groups were not particularly successful, some managed to delay the implementation of tobacco control policies and others were consulted by government bodies (Smith & Malone, 2007). Other industry front groups have included hotel, res-taurant, and retailer associations, and antitax organizations (Americans for Nonsmokers' Rights, 2008; Apollonio & Bero, 2007; Muggli & Hurt, 2003; Sweda & Daynard, 1996; Szilágyi & Chapman, 2004).

Many of the industry's outreach efforts are aimed at developing allies who will aid the industry in weakening or derailing tobacco control policy efforts. Sponsoring community groups created linkages that could be called upon when needed. Tobacco companies developed ties to multiple commu-nity organizations, inserting a tobacco presence particularly into organizations that worked on behalf of socially marginalized groups. For example, tobacco firms developed close ties with virtually every leadership organization in the U.S. African American community. These ties included shared board relation-ships, direct provision of funding, handling out free cigarettes at organiza-tional events, sponsorship of programs, and many other activities designed to position tobacco companies as "friends" to the black community (Yerger & Malone, 2002). Similar efforts were undertaken in other minority communi-ties; these developed allies who would support or provide cover for the indus-try's policy positions and/or helped defuse potential opposition (Offen et al., 2003, 2005; Yerger & Malone, 2002). Opinion leaders, suburban parents, "soc-cer moms," and other groups were also among those targeted by Philip Morris during recent years with an ad campaign designed to improve its public image, specifically because these groups were likely to be listened to by politicians (Szczypka et al., 2007; Tesler & Malone, 2008).

In addition to the legislative arena, the tobacco industry also exerts extraordinary influence over regulatory policy making. Among many examples illustrating the lengths to which corporations are prepared to go to respond to any perceived threat to their profits, when the U.S. National Center for Health Statistics in the 1990s published a new code that could have allowed physicians to classify secondhand smoke exposure as a contributor to disease, Philip Morris mobilized its Worldwide Regulatory Affairs office and enlisted business consulting and law firms to derail the measure (Cook et al., 2005). Working with a former federal official, Philip Morris first tried to prevent creation and adoption of the code, then challenged its validity on a Medicare billing form, and finally advocated for a new alternative coding system in order to prevent collection of health data on secondhand smoke (Cook et al., 2005).

In the 1990s, after Philip Morris failed to obtain raw data from National Institutes of Health-funded researchers by requesting it or suing them, it proposed legislation to change federal regulations governing the release of such data. PM sought support for its legislative proposals from business groups that were already challenging air quality regulations developed by the U.S. Environmental Protection Agency. The strategy involved working with the National Rifle Association, American Petroleum Institute, and the Electric Power Research Institute. The industry-backed legislative proposals were passed in 1998 and 2000, following which Philip Morris hired lobbyist Jim Tozzi to teach companies how to use the new regulations to their benefit (Baba et al., 2005). As Schick and colleagues noted in 2007, "the effects that the tobacco industry has on government regulatory process are still underestimated" (Schick et al., 2007: 898).

Tobacco companies have been equally active at the state level. There are dozens of examples of the industry's efforts to defeat state tobacco ballot initiatives and legislation, cut funding for state tobacco control programs, accuse tobacco control program personnel of illegal lobbying, overwhelm programs' relatively modest staffing with unreasonable demands for copies of program materials and correspondence, sue to stop program activities, and, when legislation appeared inevitable, pass weak laws that would preempt stronger local/city clean indoor air regulations (Aguinaga & Glantz, 1995; Aguinaga-Bialous et al., 2001; Glantz & Balbach, 2000; Ibrahim & Glantz, 2006; Nixon et al., 2004). It has shown itself capable of establishing improbable alliances when working on state policy. Notoriously, for example, the tobacco industry had extensive contacts with the California Medical Association and was successful in persuading it to withdraw its financial and political support from a tobacco tax initiative (Glantz & Balbach, 2000).

Lobbying and Philanthropy

While most corporations engage in direct lobbying activities, companies also lobby policy makers in less overt ways. An example is giving contributions to organizations that policy makers (or even their spouses) support and then arranging the check-presenting ceremonies so that company personnel get "face time" with legislators (Tesler & Malone, 2008). Philip Morris's corporate contributions during its late 1990s "PM21" (Philip Morris in the 21st Century) image-improvement campaign were carefully coordinated with its government relations office in order to allow PM lobbyists to meet with policy makers at events for their favored causes. The aim was to head off regulations such as increased excise taxes on cigarettes (which have been shown to reduce consumption). As the industry has expanded into low- and middle- income countries, it has utilized philanthropy in similarly strategic ways, sometimes through indirect channels (Chapman, 2008a, 2008b; MacKenzie & Collin, 2008).

These and other so-called "corporate social responsibility" (CSR) initiatives are aimed at preserving a favorable business climate, improving company image, staving off effective tobacco regulations, and undermining the tobacco control movement (Collin & Gilmore, 2002; Hirschhorn, 2004; Otañez et al., 2006; Yang & Malone, 2008). For this reason, the global FCTC includes provisions aimed at limiting such activities.

Financial Culture

Tobacco companies also have worked to influence universities, state public pension funds, and governments that, unfortunately, continue to provide capital to tobacco companies through stock investments in tobacco corporations. This has been characterized as a conflict of interest for public organizations concerned with social welfare, and public health activists have encouraged organizations to divest themselves of (sell off) tobacco company stockholdings. The tobacco industry is concerned about how such sell offs, if made public, might affect its stock prices, ability to raise capital, public image, and employee morale. Therefore, directly and through intermediaries, it has worked to thwart divestment, usually by arguing that organizations' fiduciary obligations require them to maximize value and that tobacco companies are good investments (Wander & Malone, 2004, 2006a). In one case, Philip Morris paid for preparation and distribution of a skewed consultants' report suggesting that funds indexed to exclude tobacco stocks underperformed when compared with funds that included them. The report was distributed to investment fund managers with a personal note by an ostensibly independent investment community representative, who reported to PM. The report was used to cast doubt on the claims of divestment advocates, who had argued, drawing on another report by the same consultant, that tobacco investments did not improve an institution's portfolio (Wander & Malone, 2006b).

Academic Culture

In addition to manipulating biological and epidemiological science and scientists, the tobacco industry has also employed networks of social scientists, including anthropologists, psychologists, sociologists, and economists. These hired consultants were used to enhance the social acceptability of smoking through promoting an industry-managed quasi-academic discourse (Landman et al., 2008; Smith, 2007). The consultants developed "reports" of "studies" which were never published in any peer-reviewed journal, claiming to have determined that smoking was one among many healthful "pleasures" and that quitting smoking could even be dangerous to health by increasing stress (Smith, 2007). Their work was disseminated widely in the media, creating yet another source of doubt about whether smoking was indeed as harmful as public health advocates claimed.

The industry's consultant-prepared economic reports typically argue that tobacco taxes are regressive and hurt the poor, and that smoke-free policies will harm business. In one now-infamous instance, Philip Morris touted an economic report on the Czech Republic which concluded that the early deaths of smokers were a net economic benefit for the country, since smokers who died prematurely utilized fewer resources than more long-lived people (Arthur D. Little International Inc., 2002; Dembart, 2001). In the face of the public outrage that ensued, the company quickly backed off, but the fact of a corporation arguing straight-faced that an early death was beneficial reveals the ethical vacuum at the core of the tobacco industry.

Influencing Legal Culture

In the legal arena, tobacco companies are known for denying and fighting against all claims of harm from their products. Since in many cases the effects of the products are not experienced for many years, as in the case of lung cancer, the industry argues to this day that their products did not cause disease in individual smokers, that smokers freely chose to smoke with full knowledge of the risks of disease, or makes procedural arguments and appeals that slow the case and require more resources from defendants (Balbach et al., 2006; Guardino & Daynard, 2007). Consequently, most defendants die before their cases are resolved.

Another strategy used by tobacco companies is to influence judicial decisions in product liability cases by gaining access to judges through "judicial education." Friedman (2006) documented Philip Morris's creation of the organization Libertad, Inc., which hosted vacation-destination seminars for judges (some of whom had pending tobacco litigation on their dockets) at which pro-industry legal arguments were discussed. As Friedman reports, Philip Morris denied that the company had any control over the organization, but a senior vice president of Philip Morris was president of the organization, which had the same address as Philip Morris headquarters, and Philip Morris was its sole funder. The seminars were also aimed at recruiting individuals to speak on behalf of the tobacco industry's agenda, which focused on the issues of commercial speech as well as product liability. The tobacco industry has also made large monetary contributions to university-based programs that are funded by multiple corporations and offer similar classes. Hundreds of judges have attended these expense-paid seminars and at least some attendees later ruled in favor of the tobacco industry (Friedman, 2006).

Tobacco companies now admit on their web sites that cigarettes cause disease (Smith & Malone, 2008). However, it appears that this belated provision of "information" is used offensively in court to suggest that individuals who smoke are solely responsible for diseases they develop from normal use of the product, and to deny responsibility for years of deceptive practices. When James Morgan, a former Philip Morris president and CEO, was pressed in a 1997 legal proceeding to clarify his company's position, which at the time included asserting that cigarettes were not addictive, he said that the company wanted consumers to

> know that that's what we believe and that they should take what we believe in the context of all the other information that they receive starting in first grade now and that they should make their own evaluation of where they come out. What we are stating is Philip Morris's position. And we want people to believe that's what Philip Morris believes ...

> LAWYER: And you want them to rely upon what you tell them, do you not?

MORGAN: No, I don't accept the word "rely." I want them to use what we believe in the context of all the information that they have available to them, and we want them to make their own decision.

LAWYER: So ... when Philip Morris makes a statement concerning its products, it does not really expect the consumer to believe them?

MORGAN: No, I'm not saying that ... I'm saying that we expect the consumer to understand that that's what we believe. And that to the degree they want to listen to what we believe in the context of all the other information they get from a whole variety of sources, we are telling them what we believe (cited in Balbach et al., 2006: iv40–iv41).

Direct Interference with Public Health Activities

In addition to manipulating science, media, marketing, the arts, philanthropy, politics, academia, and legal culture, the tobacco industry works to monitor and actively interfere with public health efforts at all levels (Saloojee & Dagli, 2000). Tobacco companies' extensive intelligence networks inform them of any potential activity that might constitute a threat to their business. These networks include tobacco retailers, third party consultants and public relations firms, advertising associations, business-friendly media contacts, funding recipients, including think tanks and policy organizations, "smokers' rights" groups, political allies, such as tobacco-state Congress members, and many others. There is literally no threat too small for them to bother with and nothing too big for them to tackle.

Many of the industry's efforts to disrupt public health have been described earlier; suffice to say that tobacco control efforts would undoubtedly have been much more successful in the absence of an active, engaged enemy of public health. Tobacco company spies have been identified at tobacco control meetings and conferences, where they may attend as "public relations specialists" (Malone, 2002) in order to ensure that the companies can counter any activities determined to be a threat. Tobacco companies have also sued local boards of health that have attempted to institute smoking bans (Dearlove & Glantz, 2002).

In the 1990s, the American Stop Smoking Intervention Study (ASSIST) was the largest and most comprehensive tobacco control intervention trial ever conducted in the United States (Bialous et al., 2001; White & Bero, 2004). The project provided state health departments with funding for three types of measures to reduce tobacco use, with a particular focus on tobacco control policies.

The Tobacco Institute mobilized a massive, industry-wide "plan of attack" on the program that included extraordinarily extensive Freedom of Information Act and open records document requests to national and state agencies and specious accusations that the programs were involved in illegal lobbying or other rule breaking. The industry also mobilized Congressional allies to call for an audit of all ASSIST contractors. Other measures included working to pass federal legislation that prohibited use of federal funds to lobby a local governmental body, thus making it harder for the coalitions formed through the programs to work toward policy implementation (Bialous et al., 2001; White & Bero, 2004).

Globally, industry documents show that the major multinational companies engaged in a decades-long conspiracy to deter regulation of advertising, taxation, smoking, and secondhand smoke (Francey & Chapman, 2000; McDaniel et al., 2008). Tobacco companies have also sought to disrupt and minimize media coverage of global tobacco control conferences by creating other competing health-related events. For example, a program to advocate children's vaccinations was created by the industry consultant Paul Dietrich and televised throughout Latin America during the 1992 World Conference on Tobacco or Health in Argentina (Muggli & Hurt, 2003). The World Health Organization compiled an extensive report on how the industry worked to undermine its efforts on tobacco (Zeltner et al., 2000) and recently published a second report on the industry's efforts to undermine tobacco control globally (World Health Organization, 2008b).

Illegal and Covert Activities

Raising taxes on cigarettes has been identified as one of the most effective measures to reduce tobacco consumption (Thompson, 2003). However, this measure can be undermined easily through sales of cheaper contraband cigarettes on which no tax is paid; thus, tobacco smuggling is a serious threat to public health (Joossens & Raw, 1998). An extensive body of work drawing on the internal industry documents and other sources shows that virtually all major multinational cigarette companies have long been involved with smuggling, referring to such shipments using coded language such as "in transit," "general trade," and "duty not paid" (Collin et al., 2004; Lee & Collin, 2006; Legresley et al., 2008; Nakkash & Lee, 2008; Wen et al., 2006).

Collin et al. (2004: ii105) report that the internal tobacco industry documents "provide remarkably detailed analyses of the suitability of specific regions, ports, islands and border crossings as transit routes, and also describe detailed monitoring of the availability of smuggled brands in key cities such as Bangkok or Ho Chi Minh City." Companies used distributors who purchased the cigarettes and then supplied them to "transiteers" for getting them across borders (Legresley et al., 2008). Smuggling benefited these corporations in multiple ways: it gave them increased leverage to argue against raising cigarette taxes and for opening new markets, helped them compete more effectively against one another, and allowed them to circumvent trade barriers that made legal market access difficult (Collin et al., 2004; Legresley et al., 2008). One analysis drawing on documents from British American Tobacco suggested that as much as one-quarter of the corporation's profits may come from such illegal trade (Lee & Collin, 2006).

Other areas of illegal or questionably legal activity include sponsorships and advertising in countries where such activities are prohibited. In Thailand, for example, British American Tobacco used sponsorship of major sports events to build demand for contraband products and circumvent an advertising ban (MacKenzie et al., 2007). The company embarked on a strategy of continuously testing the limits of the law.

The tobacco industry also engages in covert intelligence activities aimed at undermining public health—which it refers to as the "anti-tobacco industry" (McDaniel et al., 2006). Documents show that these include infiltrating public health groups, covert illegal audiotaping, and creating or exploiting conflicts within the tobacco control movement, such as by trying to enlist mainstream scientists and public health groups to "partner" with the industry (Carter, 2002; Malone, 2002; McDaniel et al., 2006; White & Bero, 2004). For example, Philip Morris's "Project Sunrise" explicitly sought to use intelligence to "build relationships" with tobacco control organizations the company regarded as "moderate" in order to collaborate on youth access legislation. The goal was to "create schisms" within the tobacco control movement, as other groups would find it unacceptable to partner with the industry (McDaniel et al., 2006).

The industry uses multiple means, often illegal or questionably legal, to conceal many of its activities (LeGresley et al., 2005). These include documents sent to home addresses or held at offsite or offshore locations, use of code names and acronyms, avoidance of written contact with certain individuals or organizations, bogus claims that certain documents are subject to legal privilege and thus not disclosable, and document alteration and destruction (LeGresley et al., 2005; Liberman, 2002; Muggli et al., 2004b). These efforts suggest that the full extent and implications of tobacco industry activities to undermine public health will never be known.

Conclusion

Within public health, some argue that the tobacco industry is unique in its destructiveness, and this is unquestionably true: millions of people have lost their health and lives who might otherwise have been persuaded to avoid or quit smoking were it not for the industry's deluge of deception. However, as other parts of this book suggest, the multiple ways in which the tobacco industry has manipulated almost every aspect of culture and social life and undermined public health are not unique to it. These chapters show that the nature of the corporate entity virtually requires companies to engage in activities that—while perhaps not as egregious as those of tobacco companies—are damaging to public health and well-being. This means that a key part of public health work must involve exposing and disrupting these activities, pressuring policy makers to protect the public by regulating the practices of corporations much more rigorously, and ultimately denormalizing the corporate entity as the ideal structure for the conduct of business (Callard & Collishaw, 2005).

The extensive activities of the tobacco industry described in this chapter are now being addressed at the global level within the FCTC, the world's first global public health treaty (World Health Organization, 2003). The FCTC builds upon the body of research exposing tobacco industry deceptions and directly addresses the role of the industry's efforts to undermine public health. Article 5.3 of the treaty specifies that "in setting and implementing their public health policies with respect to tobacco control, Parties shall act to protect these policies from commercial and other vested interests of the tobacco industry in accordance with national law" (World Health Organization, 2003: 7).

The treaty also calls on the countries that are parties to the treaty to undertake regulatory measures, including banning advertising, raising taxes on tobacco products, and mandating smoke-free spaces. Many have already begun to do so. However, the tobacco industry continues to resist and undermine such efforts.

We are not yet very far along in the work of calling into question whether the corporate entity as currently structured is really compatible with human health and societal well-being, and reducing corporate influence over policy making. However, the current economic crisis, which has reengaged citizens in pointing to the need for much more government involvement in supervising corporate activities, may open a window within which this may be discussed. Could other forms of structuring businesses, such as cooperatives, be more beneficial to society? Could different incentive structures allow corporations to modify destructive practices? What would be the gains and losses in terms of innovation, societal cohesiveness, and prices for needed goods? As others have discussed (Bakan, 2004), the obligation to produce profits for shareholders trumps all other obligations for corporations. Corporations are thus structured as enormously powerful economic and social actors without substantive moral obligations to the larger society. As corporations are currently being nationalized or subsidized by governments, citizens must demand that governments take a more proactive role in protecting the public.

The guidelines developed by the FCTC delegates at the convention hall in Durban cannot alone end the tobacco industry's destructive activities, but they are a hopeful sign that governments across the globe are recognizing the costs they and their citizens must pay for tobacco corporations' continued health. Just as other corporations have used the tobacco industry's strategies, other public health, environmental, and human rights movements can draw on the successes of the tobacco control movement. The tobacco control movement, and the FCTC itself, exemplify the kind of multidisciplinary, multicountry cooperation that will be needed to end corporate disease promotion.

Acknowledgments

Elizabeth Smith, Patricia McDaniel, Naphtali Offen, and Vera Harrell provided research assistance and invaluable comments on earlier drafts of this chapter.

REFERENCES

Aguinaga S, Glantz SA. The use of the public records acts to disrupt tobacco control. *Tob Control.* 1995;4:222–230.

Aguinaga-Bialous S, Fox BJ, Glantz S. Tobacco industry allegations of "illegal lobbying" and state tobacco control. *Am J Public Health.* 2001;91:62–67.

Alechnowicz K, Chapman S. The Philippine tobacco industry: "the strongest tobacco lobby in Asia." *Tob Control.* 2004;13(Suppl II):ii71–ii78.

Altria Group Inc. *2007 Annual Report.* Available at: http://www.altria.com/ annualreport/ar2007/2007ar_02_0100.aspx. Accessed December 5, 2008. Published 2007.

Americans for Nonsmokers' Rights. Get the facts: Front groups and allies. Available at: http://www.no-smoke.org/getthefacts.php?dp=d21|d23. Accessed December 4, 2008.

Anderson SJ, Ling PM. "And they told two friends...and so on": RJ Reynolds' viral marketing of eclipse and its potential to mislead the public. *Tob Control.* 2008;17:222–229.

Anderson SJ, Pollay RW, Ling PM. Taking ad-Vantage of lax advertising regulations: reassuring and distracting health-concerned smokers. *Soc Sci Med.* 2006;63(8):1973–1985.

Apollonio DE, Bero LA. The creation of industry front groups: the tobacco industry and "get government off our back." *Am J Public Health.* 2007;97(3):419–427.

Arcury TA, Vallejos QM, Schulz MR, et al. Green tobacco sickness and skin integrity among migrant Latino farmworkers. *Am J Ind Med.* 2008;21(3):195–203.

Armour BS, Pitts MM, Lee CW. Cigarette smoking and food insecurity among low-income families in the United States, 2001. *Am J Health Promot.* 2008;22(6):386–392.

Arthur D. Little International Inc. *Public Finance Balance of Smoking in the Czech Republic.* Available at: http://www.no-smoking.org/july01/07-27-01-2.html. Accessed December 4, 2008. Published 2002.

Arvey S, Malone RE. Advance and retreat: tobacco control policy in the U.S. military. *Mil Med.* 2008;173:985–991.

Assunta M, Chapman S. The lightest market in the world: light and mild cigarettes in Japan. *Nicotine Tob Res.* 2008;10(5):803–810.

Assunta M, Fields N, Knight J, Chapman S. "Care and feeding": the Asian environmental tobacco smoke consultants programme. *Tob Control.* 2004;13(Suppl 2):ii4–ii12.

Baba A, Cook DM, McGarity TO, Bero LA. Legislating "sound science": the role of the tobacco industry. *Am J Public Health.* July 2005;95(Suppl 1):S20–S27.

Bakan J. *The Corporation.* New York: Free Press; 2004.

Balbach ED, Smith EA, Malone RE. How the health belief model helps the tobacco industry: individuals, choice, and "information." *Tob Control.* 2006;15(Suppl 4): iv37–iv43.

Barnes D, Bero LA. Industry-funded research and conflict of interest: an analysis of research sponsored by the Tobacco Industry through the Center for Indoor Air Research. *J Health Polit Policy Law.* 1996;21(3):515–542.

Barnes DE, Hanauer P, Slade J, Bero LA, Glantz SA. Environmental tobacco smoke: the Brown and Williamson documents. *J Am Med Assoc.* 1995;274:248–253.

Barnes RL, Hammond SK, Glantz SA. The tobacco industry's role in the 16 Cities Study of secondhand tobacco smoke: do the data support the stated conclusions? *Environ Health Perspect.* 2006;114(12):1890–1897.

Barnoya J, Glantz S. Tobacco industry success in preventing regulation of secondhand smoke in Latin America: the "Latin Project." *Tob Control.* 2002;11(4):305–314.

Barnoya J, Glantz SA. The tobacco industry's worldwide ETS consultants project: European and Asian components. *Eur J Public Health.* 2006;16(1):69–77.

Bero L. Implications of the tobacco industry documents for public health and policy. *Annu Rev Public Health.* 2003;24:267–288.

Bero LA. Tobacco industry manipulation of research. *Public Health Rep.* 2005; 120(March-April):200–208.

Bero LA, Barnes DE, Hanauer P, Slade J, Glantz SA. Lawyer control of the tobacco industry's external research program: the Brown and Williamson documents. *J Am Med Assoc.* 1995;274:225–233.

Bero LA, Galbraith A, Rennie D. Sponsored symposia on environmental tobacco smoke. *J Am Med Assoc.* 1994;271:612–617.

Best CM, Sun K, de Pee S, Sari M, Bloem MW, Semba RD. Paternal smoking and increased risk of child malnutrition among families in rural Indonesia. *Tob Control.* 2008;17(1):38–45.

Bialous SA, Fox BJ, Glantz SA. Tobacco industry allegations of "illegal lobbying" and state tobacco control. *Am J Public Health.* 2001;91(1):62–67.

Bialous SA, Glantz SA. ASHRAE Standard 62: tobacco industry's influence over national ventilation standards. *Tob Control.* 2002;11(4):315–328.

Bialous SA, Yach D. Whose standard is it, anyway? How the tobacco industry determines the International Organization for Standardization (ISO) standards for tobacco and tobacco products. *Tob Control.* 2001;10(2):96–104.

Bitton A, Neuman MD, Barnoya J, Glantz SA. The p53 tumour suppressor gene and the tobacco industry: research, debate, and conflict of interest. *Lancet.* 2005;365(9458):531–540.

Brandt AM. *The Cigarette Century: The Rise, Fall, and Deadly Persistence of the Product that Defined America.* New York: Basic Books; 2007.

Brown and Williamson Tobacco Company. *Implications of Battelle Hippo I & II and the Griffith Filter.* Available at: http://www.legacy.library.ucsf.edu/tid/xrc72d00/pdf. Published 1963.

Bryan-Jones K, Bero LA. Tobacco industry efforts to defeat the occupational safety and health administration indoor air quality rule. *Am J Public Health.* 2003;93(4):585–592.

Callard C, Thompson D, Collishaw N. *Curing the Addiction to Profits: A Supply-side Approach to Phasing Out Tobacco.* Ottawa: Canadian Centre for Policy Alternatives; 2005.

Carter SM. Mongoven, Biscoe & Duchin: destroying tobacco control activism from the inside. *Tob Control.* 2002;11(2):112–118.

Cataldo J, Malone RE. False promises: the tobacco industry, low-tar cigarettes, and older smokers *J Am Geriatr Soc.* 2008;56:1716–1723.

Chapman S. Group Carso, health philanthropy, and tobacco. *Lancet.* 2008a;371(9620):1243.

Chapman S. International tobacco control should repudiate Jekyll and Hyde health philanthropy. *Tob Control.* 2008b;17(1):1.

Chapman S, Carter SM, Peters M. "A deep fragrance of academia": the Australian Tobacco Research Foundation. *Tob Control.* 2003;12(Suppl 3): iii38–iii44.

Collin J, Gilmore A. Corporate (anti) social (ir) responsibility: transnational tobacco companies and the attempted subversion of global health policy. *Global Social Policy.* 2002;2(3):354–360.

Collin J, Legresley E, MacKenzie R, Lawrence S, Lee K. Complicity in contraband: British American Tobacco and cigarette smuggling in Asia. *Tob Control.* 2004;13(Suppl 2):104–111.

Conference of the Parties to the WHO Framework Convention on Tobacco Control, *Decisions.* Available at: http://www.who.int/gb/fctc/PDF/cop3/FCTC_COP3_DIV3-en.pdf. Published 2009. Accessed February 26, 2009.

Connolly GN, Alpert HR, Wayne GF, Koh H. Trends in nicotine yield in smoke and its relationship with design characteristics among popular US cigarette brands, 1997–2005. *Tob Control*. 2007;16(5):e5.

Cook DM, Tong EK, Glantz SA, Bero LA. The power of paperwork: how Philip Morris neutralized the medical code for secondhand smoke. *Health Aff (Millwood)*. 2005;24(4):994–1004.

Dearlove JV, Bialous SA, Glantz SA. Tobacco industry manipulation of the hospitality industry to maintain smoking in public places. *Tob Control*. 2002;11(2):94–104.

Dearlove JV, Glantz SA. Boards of Health as venues for clean indoor air policy making. *Am J Public Health*. 2002;92(2):257–265.

Dembart L. Critics assail Philip Morris report on smoking; tobacco giant's analysis says premature deaths cut costs in pensions and health care. *International Herald Tribune*. July 18, 2001:N-4.

Doll R, Peto R, Boreham J, Sutherland I. Mortality in relation to smoking: 50 years' observations on male British doctors. *BMJ*. 2004;328:1519.

Doll R, Peto R, Wheatley K, Gray R, Sutherland I. Mortality in relation to smoking: 40 years' observations on male British doctors. *Br Med J*. 1994;309(6959):901–911.

Drope J, Bialous SA, Glantz SA. Tobacco industry efforts to present ventilation as an alternative to smoke-free environments in North America. *Tob Control*. 2004;13(Suppl 1):i41–i47.

Farrelly MC, Davis KC, Haviland ML, Messeri P, Healton CG. Evidence of a dose-response relationship between "truth" antismoking ads and youth smoking prevalence. *Am J Public Health*. 2005;95(3):425–431.

Farrelly MC, Healton CG, Davis KC, Messeri P, Hersey JC, Haviland ML. Getting to the truth: evaluating national tobacco countermarketing campaigns. *Am J Public Health*. 2002;92(6):901–907.

Federal Trade Commission. Cigarette report for 2004 and 2005. Washington D.C. Available at: http://www.ftc.gov/reports/tobacco/2007cigarette2004–2005.pdf. Published 2007.

Feighery EC, Ribisl KM, Clark PI, Haladjian HH. How tobacco companies ensure prime placement of their advertising and products in stores: interviews with retailers about tobacco company incentive programmes. *Tob Control*. 2003;12(2):184–188.

Francey N, Chapman S. Operation Berkshire: the international tobacco companies' conspiracy. *BMJ*. 2000;321:371–374.

Freudenberg N. Public health advocacy to change corporate practices: implications for health education practice and research. *Health Educ Behav*. 2005;32(3):298–319.

Friedman LC. Tobacco industry use of judicial seminars to influence rulings in products liability litigation. *Tob Control*. 2006;15(2):120–124.

Friedman LC. Philip Morris's website and television commercials use new language to mislead the public into believing it has changed its stance on smoking and disease. *Tob Control*. 2007;16(6):e9.

Geist H. Global assessment of deforestation related to tobacco farming. *Tob Control*. 1999;8:18–28.

Gilmore AB, Collin J, Townsend J. Transnational tobacco company influence on tax policy during privatization of a state monopoly: British American Tobacco and Uzbekistan. *Am J Public Health.* 2007;97(11):2001–2009.

Glantz S, Balbach E. *Tobacco War: Inside the California Battles.* Berkeley: University of California Press; 2000.

Glantz S, Slade J, Bero L, Hanauer P, Barnes D. *The Cigarette Papers.* Berkeley, CA: UC Press; 1996.

Glantz SA, Barnes DE, Bero LA, Hanauer P, Slade J. Looking through a keyhole at the tobacco industry: the Brown and Williamson documents. *J Am Med Assoc.* 1995;274:219–224.

Gruning T, Gilmore AB, McKee M. Tobacco industry influence on science and scientists in Germany. *Am J Public Health.* 2006;96(1):20–32.

Guardino SD, Daynard RA. Tobacco industry lawyers as "disease vectors." *Tob Control.* 2007;16(4):224–228.

Hafez N, Ling PM. How Philip Morris built Marlboro into a global brand for young adults: implications for international tobacco control. *Tob Control.* 2005;14(4):262–271.

Hafez N, Ling PM. Finding the Kool Mixx: how Brown & Williamson used music marketing to sell cigarettes. *Tob Control.* 2006;15(5):359–366.

Hammond D, Collishaw NE, Callard C. Secret science: tobacco industry research on smoking behaviour and cigarette toxicity. *Lancet.* 2006;367(9512): 781–787.

Hanauer P, Slade J, Barnes DE, Bero LA, Glantz SA. Lawyer control of internal scientific research to protect against products liability lawsuits: the Brown and Williamson documents. *J Am Med Assoc.* 1995;274:234–240.

Hicks JJ. The strategy behind Florida's "truth" campaign. *Tob Control.* 2001;10:3–5.

Hiilamo H, Kahl U, Lambe M. The Philip Morris Nordic journalist program: strategies, implementation and outcomes. *Health Policy.* 2009 January;89(1):84–96.

Hirschhorn N. Corporate social responsibility and the tobacco industry: hope or hype? *Tob Control.* 13(4):447–453.

Hong M, Bero L. How the tobacco industry responded to an influential study of the health effects of secondhand smoke. *Br Med J.* 325:1413–1416.

Humber T. *RJ Reynolds Issue Advertising.* Brown & Williamson, 1984: 690819538/690819553. Available at: http://legacy.library.ucsf.edu/tid/qzk01f00. Accessed September.

Ibrahim JK, Glantz SA. Tobacco industry litigation strategies to oppose tobacco control media campaigns. *Tob Control.* 2006;15:50–58.

John RM. Crowding out effect of tobacco expenditure and its implications on household resource allocation in India. *Soc Sci Med.* 2008;66(6):1356–1367.

Joossens L, Raw M. Cigarette smuggling in Europe: who really benefits? *Tob Control.* 1998;7(1):66–71.

Kessler D. *A Question of Intent: A Great American Battle with a Deadly Industry.* New York: Public Affairs; 2001.

Kluger R. *Ashes to Ashes: America's Hundred-Year Cigarette War, the Public Health, and the Unabashed Triumph of Philip Morris.* New York: Vintage Books; 1997.

Knight J, Chapman S. "Asian yuppies...are always looking for something new and different": creating a tobacco culture among young Asians. *Tob Control.* 13(Suppl 2):ii22–ii29.

Kottke TE, Hoffman BA. Confronting the myth of cultural immutability. *Am J Prev Med.* 2003;25(2):165–166.

Kozlowski LT, O'Connor RJ. Cigarette filter ventilation is a defective design because of misleading taste, bigger puffs, and blocked vents. *Tob Control.* 2002;11(Suppl 1):I40–I50.

Kozlowski LT, Pillitteri JL. Beliefs about "Light" and "Ultra Light" cigarettes and efforts to change those beliefs: an overview of early efforts and published research. *Tob Control.* 2001;10(Suppl 1):ii2–ii6.

Landman A, Cortese DK, Glantz S. Tobacco industry sociological programs to influence public beliefs about smoking. *Soc Sci Med.* 2008;66(4):970–981.

Landman A, Glantz SA. Tobacco industry efforts to undermine policy-relevant research. *Am J Public Health.* 2009;99(1).

Landman A, Ling PM, Glantz SA. Tobacco industry youth smoking prevention programs: protecting the industry and hurting tobacco control. *Am J Public Health.* 2002;92(6):908–916.

Lazarus D. Getting smokers to quit littering. *Los Angeles Times.* November 30, 2008.

Lee K, Collin J. "Key to the future": British American tobacco and cigarette smuggling in China. *PLoS Med.* 2006;3(7):e228.

Legresley E, Lee K, Muggli ME, Patel P, Collin J, Hurt RD. British American Tobacco and the "insidious impact of illicit trade" in cigarettes across Africa. *Tob Control.* 2008;17(5):339–346.

LeGresley EM, Muggli ME, Hurt RD. Playing hide-and-seek with the tobacco industry. *Nicotine Tob Res.* 2005;7(1):27–40.

LeGresley VE. A "vector analysis" of the tobacco epidemic. *Bulletin von Medicus Mundi Schweiz.* April 1999;72. http://www.medicusmundi.ch/mms/services/bulletin/bulletin199901/kapo1/03legresley.html. Accessed September 17 2009.

Liberman J. The shredding of BAT's defence: McCabe v British American Tobacco Australia. *Tob Control.* 2002;11(3):271–274.

Ling PM, Glantz SA. Using tobacco-industry marketing research to design more effective tobacco-control campaigns. *JAMA.* 2002;287(22):2983–2989.

Liu Y, Rao K, Hu TW, Sun Q, Mao Z. Cigarette smoking and poverty in China. *Soc Sci Med.* 2006;63(11):2784–2790.

Lopipero P, Bero LA. Tobacco interests or the public interest: 20 years of industry strategies to undermine airline smoking restrictions. *Tob Control.* 2006;15(4):323–332.

Luke DA, Krauss M. Where there's smoke there's money: tobacco industry campaign contributions and U.S. Congressional voting. *Am J Prev Med.* 2004;27(5):363–372.

MacKenzie R, Collin J. Philanthropy, politics and promotion: Philip Morris' "charitable contributions" in Thailand. *Tob Control.* 2008;17(4):284–285.

MacKenzie R, Collin J, Lee K. *Centre on Global Change and Health, London School of Hygiene & Tropical Medicine*. The tobacco industry documents: an introductory handbook and resource guide for researchers. Available at: http://www.lshtm. ac.uk/cgch/tobacco/Handbook%2008.07.03.pdf. Accessed December 22, 2008. Published 2003.

MacKenzie R, Collin J, Sriwongcharoen K. Thailand—lighting up a dark market: British American tobacco, sports sponsorship and the circumvention of legislation. *J Epidemiol Community Health*. 2007;61(1):28–33.

Malone RE. Tobacco industry surveillance of public health groups: the case of STAT (Stop Teenage Addiction to Tobacco) and INFACT (Infant Formula Action Coalition). *Am J Public Health*. 2002;92(6):955–960.

Malone RE. Nursing's involvement in tobacco control: historical perspective and vision for the future. *Nurs Res*. 2006;55(4S):S51–S57.

Malone RE, Balbach ED. Tobacco industry documents: treasure trove or quagmire? *Tob Control*. 2000;9:334–338.

Malone RE, Bero LA. Chasing the dollar: why scientists should decline tobacco industry funding. *J Epidemiol Community Health*. 2003;57(8):546–548.

Mamudu H, Glantz S. "Project Cerberus": tobacco industry strategy to create an alternative to the framework convention on tobacco control. *Am J Public Health*. 2008;98:1630–1642.

Mamudu HM, Hammond R, Glantz S. Tobacco industry attempts to counter the World Bank report Curbing the Epidemic and obstruct the WHO framework convention on tobacco control. *Soc Sci Med*. 2008;67(11):1690–1699.

McDaniel PA, Intinarelli G, Malone RE. Tobacco industry issues management organizations: creating a global corporate network to undermine public health. *Global Health*. 2008;4(2). Available at: http://www.globalizationandhealth.com/content/4/1/2 Accessed September 17, 2009.

McDaniel PA, Smith EA, Malone RE. Philip Morris's Project Sunrise: weakening tobacco control by working with it. *Tob Control*. 2006;15:215–223.

McDaniel PA, Solomon G, Malone RE. The tobacco industry and pesticide regulations: case studies from tobacco industry archives. *Environ Health Perspect*. 2005;113(12):1659–1665.

Meier B. Philip Morris admits evidence shows smoking causes cancer. *The New York Times*. October 13, 1999:A-1. Available at: http://query.nytimes.com/gst/fullpage. html?res=9404E1D91530F930A25753C1A96F958260. Accessed September 17, 2009.

Muggli ME, Hurt RD. Tobacco industry strategies to undermine the 8th World Conference on Tobacco or Health. *Tob Control*. 2003;12(2):195–202.

Muggli ME, Hurt RD, Becker LB. Turning free speech into corporate speech: Philip Morris' efforts to influence U.S. and European journalists regarding the U.S. EPA report on secondhand smoke. *Prev Med*. 2004a;39(3):568–580.

Muggli ME, LeGresley EM, Hurt RD. Big tobacco is watching: British American Tobacco's surveillance and information concealment at the Guildford depository. *Lancet*. 2004b;363(9423):1812–1819.

Nakkash R, Lee K. Smuggling as the "key to a combined market": British American Tobacco in Lebanon. *Tob Control*. 2008;17(5):324–331.

National Association of Attorneys General. Master Settlement Agreement. Available at: http://www.naag.org/backpages/naag/tobacco/msa/msa-pdf/1109185724_1032468605_cigmsa.pdf. Accessed December 3, 2008. Published 1998.

Nixon M, Mahmoud L, Glantz S. Tobacco industry litigation to deter local public health ordinances: the industry usually loses in court. *Tob Control*. 2004;13:65–73.

Offen N, Smith EA, Malone RE. From adversary to target market: the ACT-UP boycott of Philip Morris. *Tob Control*. 2003;12:203–207.

Offen N, Smith EA, Malone RE. The perimetric boycott: a tool for tobacco control advocacy. *Tob Control*. 2005;14:272–277.

Otañez MG, Mamudu H, Glantz SA. Global leaf companies control the tobacco market in Malawi. *Tob Control*. 2007;16(4):261–269.

Otañez MG, Muggli ME, Hurt RD, Glantz SA. Eliminating child labour in Malawi: a British American Tobacco corporate responsibility project to sidestep tobacco labour exploitation. *Tob Control*. 2006;15(3):224–230.

Patel P, Collin J, Gilmore AB. "The law was actually drafted by us but the Government is to be congratulated on its wise actions": British American Tobacco and public policy in Kenya. *Tob Control*. 2007;16:e1.

Pilkington P, Gilmore AB. The Living Tomorrow Project: how Philip Morris has used a Belgian tourist attraction to promote ventilation approaches to the control of second hand smoke. *Tob Control*. 2004;13(4):375–378.

Pollay RW. Targeting youth and concerned smokers: evidence from Canadian tobacco industry documents. *Tob Control*. 2000;9(2):136–147.

Quandt SA, Arcury TA, Preisser JS, Norton D, Austin C. Migrant farmworkers and green tobacco sickness: new issues for an understudied disease. *Am J Ind Med*. 2000;37(3):307–315.

R.J. Reynolds Tobacco Company. *Draft: Public Policy Committee Meeting*. 1984a. Available at: http://legacy.library.ucsf.edu/tid/fqu75d00. Accessed September 17, 2009.

R.J. Reynolds Tobacco Company. *Public Issues Campaign Ads. Second-hand Smoke: The Myth and the Reality*. RJ Reynolds; 1984b. Available at: http://legacy.library.ucsf.edu/tid/nbv87c00. Accessed September 17, 2009.

R.J. Reynolds Tobacco Company. *Public Issues Campaign. Executions and Reactions April 2, 1984: We Don't Advertise to Children*. RJ Reynolds; 1984c. Available at: http://legacy.library.ucsf.edu/tid/egz55d00. Accessed September 17, 2009.

R.J. Reynolds Tobacco Company. Wall Street Journal ad: can we have an open debate about smoking? Available at: http://legacy.library.ucsf.edu/tid/izn21f00. Accessed September 17, 2009. Published 1984d.

R.J. Reynolds Tobacco Company. *Public Issues Campaign. Passive Smoking: An Active Controversy*. RJ Reynolds; 1985. Available at: http://legacy.library.ucsf.edu/tid/grx87c00. Accessed September 17, 2009.

Rosenberg NJ, Siegel M. Use of corporate sponsorship as a tobacco marketing tool: a review of tobacco industry sponsorship in the USA, 1995–99. *Tob Control.* 2001;10(3):239–246.

Safran J. How I nearly became a Marlboro man. *Tob Control.* 2000;9(1):100–102.

Saloojee Y, Dagli E. Tobacco industry tactics for resisting public policy on health. *Bull World Health Organ.* 2000;78(7):902–910.

Samet JM. Secondhand smoke: facts and lies. *Salud Publica Mex.* 2008;50(5):428–434.

Sargent J, Gibson J, Heatherton T. Comparing the effects of entertainment media and tobacco marketing on youth smoking. *Tob Control.* 2008;18:47–53.

Schick SF, Bero LA, Cook DM. The tobacco industry and the Data Quality Act. *Science.* 2007;317(5840):898.

Sepe E, Ling PM, Glantz SA. Smooth moves: bar and nightclub tobacco promotions that target young adults. *Am J Public Health.* 2002;92(3):414–419.

Siahpush M, Borland R, Scollo M. Smoking and financial stress. *Tob Control.* 2003;12(1):60–66.

Slade J, Bero L, Hanauer P, Barnes DE, Glantz SA. Nicotine and addiction: the Brown and Williamson documents. *JAMA.* 1995;274(3):225–233.

Slattery ML, Curtin K, Giuliano AR, et al. Active and passive smoking, IL6, ESR1, and breast cancer risk. *Breast Cancer Res Treat.* 2008;109(1):101–111.

Sly DF, Hopkins RS, Trapido E, Ray S. Influence of a counteradvertising media campaign on initiation of smoking: the Florida "truth" campaign. *Am J Public Health.* 2001;91(2):233–238.

Sly DF, Trapido E, Ray S. Evidence of the dose effects of an antitobacco counteradvertising campaign. *Prev Med.* 2002;35(5):511–518.

Smith EA. "It's interesting how few people die from smoking": tobacco industry efforts to minimize risk and discredit health promotion. *Eur J Public Health.* 2007;17(2):162–170.

Smith EA, Blackman V, Malone RE. Death at a discount: how the tobacco industry thwarted tobacco control policies in U.S. military commissaries. *Tob Control.* 2007;16:38–46.

Smith EA, Malone RE. "We will speak as the smoker": the tobacco industry's smokers' rights groups. *Eur J Public Health.* 2007;17(3):306–313.

Smith EA, Malone RE. Philip Morris's health information web site appears responsible but undermines public health. *Public Health Nurs.* 2008;25(6):554–564.

Song AV, Ling PM, Neilands TB, Glantz SA. Smoking in movies and increased smoking among young adults. *Am J Prev Med.* 2007;33(5):396–403.

Stevenson T, Proctor RN. The secret and soul of Marlboro: Phillip Morris and the origins, spread, and denial of nicotine freebasing. *Am J Public Health.* 2008;98(7):1184–1194.

Sweda EL, Jr, Daynard RA. Tobacco industry tactics. *Br Med Bull.* 1996;52(1):183–192.

Szczypka G, Wakefield MA, Emery S, Terry-McElrath YM, Flay BR, Chaloupka FJ. Working to make an image: an analysis of three Philip Morris corporate image media campaigns. *Tob Control.* 2007;16(5):344–350.

Szilágyi T, Chapman S. Tobacco industry efforts to erode tobacco advertising controls in Hungary. *Cent Eur J Public Health.* 2004;12(4):190–196.

Tesler L, Malone RE. Corporate philanthropy, lobbying and public health policy. *Am J Public Health.* 2008;98(12):2123–2133.

The Ocean Conservancy. *International Coastal Cleanup Report 2007.* Available at: http://www.oceanconservancy.org/site/DocServer/ICC_AR07.pdf?docID=3741. Accessed December 8, 2008. Published 2007.

Thompson F. Cigarette smuggling and public health. *Int J Tuberc Lung Dis.* 2003;7(3):207.

Thrasher JF, Niederdeppe J, Farrelly MC, Davis KC, Ribisl KM, Haviland ML. The impact of anti-tobacco industry prevention messages in tobacco producing regions: evidence from the US truth campaign. *Tob Control.* 2004;13(3):283–288.

Tobacco Industry Research Committee. *A Frank Statement to Cigarette Smokers.* Available at: http://legacy.library.ucsf.edu/tid/qxp91e00. Accessed September 17, 2009 Published 1954.

Tong EK, England L, Glantz SA. Changing conclusions on secondhand smoke in a sudden infant death syndrome review funded by the tobacco industry. *Pediatrics.* 115(3):e356–e366.

Tong EK, Glantz SA. Tobacco industry efforts undermining evidence linking secondhand smoke with cardiovascular disease. *Circulation.* 2007;116(16):1845–1854.

Trotter L, Chapman S. "Conclusions about exposure to ETS and health that will be unhelpful to us": how the tobacco industry attempted to delay and discredit the 1997 Australian National Health and Medical Research Council report on passive smoking. *Tob Control.* 2003;12(Suppl 3):iii102–iii106.

U.S. Department of Health and Human Services. *The Health Consequences of Smoking: A Report of the Surgeon General.* USDHHS: Centers for Disease Control and Prevention, Office on Smoking and Health; 2004.

United States District Court for the District of Columbia. Final Opinion in United States of America v. Philip Morris, et al. Available at: http://www.tobaccolawcenter.org/doj-litigation.html. Accessed December 11, 2008. Published 2006.

Vateesatokit P. Tailoring tobacco control efforts to the country: the example of Thailand. In: deBeyer J, Brigden LW, eds. *Tobacco Control Policy: Strategies, Successes and Setbacks.* Washington DC: World Bank RITE; 2003:54–79.

Wander N, Malone RE. Selling off or selling out? Medical schools and ethical leadership in tobacco stock divestment. *Acad Med.* 2004;79(11):1017–1026.

Wander N, Malone RE. Fiscal vs. social responsibility: how Philip Morris shaped the public funds divestment debate. *Tob Control.* 2006a;15:231–241.

Wander N, Malone RE. Keeping public institutions invested in tobacco. *J Bus Ethics.* 73(2):161–176.

Wayne GF, Connolly GN, Henningfield JE. Brand differences of free-base nicotine delivery in cigarette smoke: the view of the tobacco industry documents. *Tob Control.* 2006;15(3):189–198.

Wayne GF, Connolly GN, Henningfield JE, Farone WA. Tobacco industry research and efforts to manipulate smoke particle size: implications for product regulation. *Nicotine Tob Res.* 2008;10(4):613–625.

Webb W. Status of Marlboro development program. Philip Morris. July 12, 1984. Available at: http://legacy.library.ucsf.edu/tid/gmr98e00. Accessed September 17, 2009.

Wen CP, Peterson RA, Cheng TY, Tsai SP, Eriksen MP, Chen T. Paradoxical increase in cigarette smuggling after the market opening in Taiwan. *Tob Control.* 2006;15(3):160–165.

West E. Selling the myth: western images in advertising. *Montana J West Hist.* 1996;46(2):36–49.

White J, Bero LA. Public health under attack: the American Stop Smoking Intervention Study (ASSIST) and the tobacco industry. *Am J Public Health.* 2004;94:240–250.

Wiist WH. Public health and the anticorporate movement: rationale and recommendations. *Am J Public Health.* 2006;96(8):1370–1375.

Wills TA, Sargent JD, Stoolmiller M, Gibbons FX, Gerrard M. Movie smoking exposure and smoking onset: a longitudinal study of mediation processes in a representative sample of U.S. adolescents. *Psychol Addict Behav.* 2008;22(2):269–277.

World Health Organization. *Framework Convention on Tobacco Control.* Geneva: World Health Organization; 2003. Available at: http://www.who.int/fctc/en/ Accessed September 17, 2009.

World Health Organization. *WHO Report on the Global Tobacco Epidemic, 2008: The MPOWER Package.* http://www.who.int/tobacco/mpower/gtcr_download/en/index.html. Accessed September 17, 2009. Published 2008a.

World Health Organization. *Tobacco Industry Interference with Tobacco Control.* Geneva: World Health Organization; 2008b. Available at: http://www.who.int/tobacco/resources/publications/tob_ind_int_cover_150/en/index.html. Accessed September 17, 2009.

Yang JS, Malone RE. "Working to shape what society's expectations of us should be": Philip Morris's societal alignment strategy. *Tob Control.* 2008; 17:391–398.

Yerger VB, Malone RE. African American leadership groups: smoking with the enemy. *Tob Control.* 2002;11:336–345.

Yerger VB, Przewoznik J, Malone RE. Racialized geography, corporate activity, and health disparities: tobacco industry targeting of inner cities. *J Health Care Poor Underserved.* 2007;18:10–38.

Yuk PK. Battleground for smokers lies in new markets. *Financial Times.* June 9, 2008. Available at: http://www.ft.com/cms/s/0/784456b6–33f6–11dd-869b-0000779fd2ac.html?nclick_check=1. Accessed September 17 2009.

Zeltner T, Kessler DA, Martiny A, Randera F. *Tobacco Company Strategies to Undermine Tobacco Control Activities at the World Health Organization.* Geneva: World Health Organization; 2000. Available at: http://www.who.int/tobacco/surveillance/ti_monitoring/publications/en/index.html Accessed September 17 2009.

Zucker D, Hopkins R, Sly D, Urich J, Kershaw J, Solari S. Florida's "truth" campaign: a counter-marketing, anti-tobacco media campaign. *J Public Health Manag Pract.* 2000;6(3):1–6.

7

The Pharmaceutical Industry, Disease Industry: A Prescription for Illness and Death

David Egilman and Emily Ardolino

Bob Ernst was a healthy, active 59-year-old man who lived happily with his wife Carol. Bob enjoyed swimming, rollerblading, and cycling. He ran 3–4 miles every day and collected finisher's medals for competing in the Dallas White Rock Marathon in 1995, 1996, and 1997. He and his wife often took long bike rides together, and in April 2001 they rode a tandem bike over 60 miles in the Beauty and the Beast bicycle tour of Tyler, Texas.

Bob's only physical limitation was an annoying and painful problem with arthritis in his hands. For his discomfort, Bob took Vioxx—a new nonsteroidal anti-inflammatory drug (NSAID) marketed as a safer and more powerful alternative to drugs like naproxen and aspirin.

Merck, the multibillion dollar pharmaceutical giant headquartered in Whitehouse Station, New Jersey, manufactured Vioxx. Merck developed Vioxx to perform the same anti-inflammatory function as other existing pain relievers, but with the added benefit that it caused fewer gastrointestinal (GI) bleeds than its competitors

Dr. Egilman has served as a paid consultant for patients suing Merck (Vioxx) Lilly (Zyprexa) and Pfizer (Neurontin). He also served as an unpaid consultant to the US Attorney investigating Lilly for Off-label marketing of Zyprexa.

(Bombardier et al., 2000).[1] The NSAID became one of Merck's most profitable and successful drugs with sales reaching $2.5 billion in the year before they withdrew it from the market (Cnnmoney, 2005).

Anticipating that Vioxx, a relatively specific Cox-2 enzyme inhibitor, might produce an increased risk of dangerous cardiovascular events, Merck's Vigor trial, their largest clinical trial of Vioxx, minimized the appearance of such side effects by selecting study participants who were unlikely to have heart attacks (Daniels, 1997; Krumholz, 2007).[2] Nonetheless, Vioxx use resulted in a five fold increase in heart attacks compared to naproxen (Bombardier et al., 2000). The Vigor data also showed that, although Vioxx patients suffered fewer GI bleeds, more patients on Vioxx *actually died* as a result of GI bleeding (Bombardier et al., 2000). Merck, however, combined fatal and trivial bleeds into one adverse event category and emphasized the fact that Vioxx patients suffered fewer *total number* of bleeds than patients on the comparator drug. Despite the fact that more Vioxx than control patients died because of GI bleeds, Merck used the Vigor results to gain Food and Drug Administration (FDA) approval to advertise that Vioxx was safer than traditional NSAIDs because it reduced the overall risk of bleeding (Bombardier et al., 2000).

Merck also designed a "seeding" trial they called Advantage. Unlike the Vigor trial, which was organized by Merck's research department, Advantage was orchestrated by the marketing department in order to expose doctors, many of whom were specifically targeted as key opinion leaders or otherwise influential figures in their fields, to Vioxx by giving them the chance to prescribe it to their patients for free for a period of several months. The trial was essentially a marketing ploy disguised as research; however, to Merck's chagrin, the results of the trial further implicated Vioxx as a risk increase for cardiovascular events.

Merck omitted some Vioxx-caused cardiovascular events from both the Vigor results they published in the *New England Journal of Medicine* (Curfman et al., 2005) and the published results of the Advantage trial (Egilman & Presler, 2006; Lisse et al., 2003). Faced with questions about cardiovascular risks, Merck misled doctors and the public by claiming during their marketing campaign that the Vigor trial "confirmed the cardiovascular safety of Vioxx" (Waxman, 2005).

Merck then promoted the "safety benefits" of Vioxx—the fact that it reduced the *overall* risk of GI bleeds—and marketed it to "blockbuster" status.[3] To achieve this level of sales, Merck spent hundreds of millions of dollars on direct-to-consumer (DTC) advertising involving television and magazine advertisements starring celebrities such as figure skater Dorothy Hamill and track athlete Bruce Jenner. In 2000, Merck spent more money ($160 million) advertising Vioxx to consumers, who could not even buy the drug without a prescription than PepsiCo spent advertising Pepsi ($125 million) and Budweiser spent advertising their signature beer ($146 million) (Anstice, 2005). The FDA sent Merck a formal warning letter noting that Merck's marketing minimized the serious cardiovascular findings of the VIGOR trial and "made unsubstantiated superiority claims" against other less expensive NSAIDs (Abrams, 2001).

Merck also spent hundreds of millions more on educational programs, free samples, gifts, meals, and vacations for prescribing physicians. They employed salespeople (detail representatives) who visited doctors in their offices to "educate" them about the benefits of Vioxx. Detail representatives were trained to dodge questions concerning drug side effects and mitigate doctors' concerns about the risks of Vioxx (Anstice, 2005; Horner et al., 2006).[4] Physicians received regular visits from Merck's detail representatives and had their questions and concerns about the new drug answered by individuals whose livelihoods depended on the number of Vioxx prescriptions that were written. Merck's aggressive and expensive marketing program for Vioxx embellished the drug's safety and efficacy in comparison to other commonly used drugs and omitted the company's knowledge of the fact that Vioxx-caused heart attacks and strokes.

Merck's DTC advertising convinced Ernst that Vioxx was a better medication and encouraged him to approach his physician, Dr. Wallace, to request to switch to Vioxx. Dr. Wallace, whose information about Vioxx came from Merck salespeople and adulterated medical literature saw no reason to deny him a prescription in place of the naproxen he had previously recommended. Ernst, a healthy, active man with no prior history or risk of heart disease, took Vioxx for 8 months before dying in his sleep of a heart attack.

Though Ernst's death and the trial that followed attracted substantial media attention, his story was just one of thousands. Over 20 million people had already taken Vioxx between its release in 1999 and its withdrawal from the market in 2004. Thousands of lawsuits were filed by the victims of Vioxx-induced heart attacks and strokes or by their surviving relatives. Because Vioxx caused such significant injuries and the company acted so recklessly, Merck agreed to pay $4.85 billion to settle the lawsuits (Berenson, 2008). But no amount of money will adequately compensate injured patients and the families who lost loved ones.

A Public Health Crisis

Hundreds of thousands of lives were devastated by Vioxx, and Vioxx is itself one of dozens of unsafe drugs inappropriately marketed by pharmaceutical companies. Millions of patients have become ill or needlessly lost their lives because of a breakdown in a system that has now grown into a public health crisis (Lazarou et al., 1998). Lazarou et al. (1998) estimated that adverse reactions to prescription and over-the-counter medications are the fourth leading cause of death in America. Between 1969 and 2002, over 75 drugs were removed from the market for safety reasons (Wysowski & Swartz, 2005). During that time period, special prescription requirements or restricted distribution programs have been instituted for at least 11 other pharmaceuticals on account of postapproval discovery of adverse events, and numerous other drug reactions have been "identified and added to the product labeling as boxed warnings, warnings, precautions, contraindications, and adverse reactions" (Wysowski & Swartz, 2005). This trend has continued over the past 5 years with several more black box warnings issued, label changes enforced, and drugs— including Vioxx—withdrawn from the market. New drugs are marketed without adequate testing and result in unnecessary death and disease. Every day, executives from corporations spanning the pharmaceutical and medical device industry, preoccupied with increasing profits and maintaining status as viable competitors in the industry, knowingly market unsafe or inadequately tested drugs and medical devices to raise their bottom line (Angell, 2005; Brody, 2007).

Over the past few years, a plethora of academics, economists, journalists, and public health professionals have rightly noted that the alarming tendency of medical products to hinder health (though they are supposedly designed to improve it) is not a series of random events (Angell, 2005, 2008, 2009a, 2009b; Angell & Relman, 1988; Brody, 2007; Carpenter, 2004; Dangerous Prescription, 2003; Hill et al., 2008; Krumholz, 2007; Lurie et al., 2006; Peterson, 2008; Wolfe, 2005; Wolfe et al., 2002/5; Wysowski & Swartz, 2005). These failures are the predictable consequence of an economic system that gauges success exclusively in terms of profits and has few, if any, real consequences for socially irresponsible behavior. Yet dangerous drugs and devices, unnecessary diagnostics, and inefficient interventions continue to flood the practice of medicine with relatively little challenge from policy makers, doctors, and patients.

Critics of the drug and device industries—or, more broadly, the disease industry[5]—have pointed to capitalism and corporate culture to explain how these tragedies occur. Joel Bakan describes the distorted morality of a corporation, a morality defined by law, which makes a corporation responsible only to its shareholders' monetary interests and prohibits it from sacrificing these interests for any reason.[6] He argues that all activities of a corporation are necessarily aimed at increasing profit. This means that all research and development, education and services provided by the disease industry to the medical profession and the general public are aimed at cutting production costs, edging out competitors, and selling more products to more customers. In this system, the quality of products, the corporation's impact on society, the interests of the corporation's employees, and those of its clients are prioritized only when they coincide with shareholders' interest in increased profits. Of course, a corporation's drive for profit often does coincide with the interests of employees, clients, and society as a whole. For example, employee benefits, higher pay, and increased flexibility for workers sustain morale in the workplace and may increase worker productivity and efficiency. Likewise, developing truly beneficial products can increase profits through sales to satisfied customers, and developing more energy-efficient processes can save money and attract positive attention from environmentally concerned customers. However, these interests are not a driving force behind corporate activity and are easily sacrificed in favor of higher profits. As Bakan writes:

> Unlike public institutions, whose only legitimate mandate is to serve the public good, corporations are legally required always to put their own interests above everyone else's. They may act in ways that promote the public good when it is to their advantage to do so, but they will just as quickly sacrifice it—it is their legal obligation to do so—when necessary to serve their own ends. (Bakan, 2004)

Economists refer to the effects of corporate activity focused on raising their bottom line as "externalities." While some economists, such as Milton Friedman, argue that corporations often produce positive externalities, such as creating new jobs or making useful, inexpensive products widely available, most think of externalities as the burdensome costs of production that corporations project, or "externalize," onto consumers, environment, and society. According to economist Robert Monks, a corporation "tends to be more profitable to the extent it can make other people pay the bills for its impact on society" (Monks & Minow, 1991). In other words, to the extent that corporations can shift costs to others they can increase profits. For example, if a factory saves $10 million in production costs by foregoing the installation of a smokestack emission control system, the company externalizes that cost onto the surrounding community and the environment in the form of pollution. The cost of the resultant industrial pollution may, and in the real world often does, far exceed the cost of preventing it (compare $10 million for pollution control to hundreds of millions of dollars in medical expenses for those who are injured by it), and the community, not the company, bears these costs.

Even though the amount of money saved by companies when they externalize costs may pale in comparison to the costs suffered by those onto whom they are externalized, incentives for companies to pay these costs themselves are virtually nonexistent, and externalization can be advantageous, if not necessary, to remain competitive in today's deregulated market economy. In the case of warnings and product safety, "ethical" companies are at a disadvantage. For example, if a drug manufacturer makes an antidepressant that is addictive and warns of this side effect adequately, they put themselves at a competitive disadvantage to other drug manufacturers that make similar antidepressants that are not advertised as addictive. Likewise, since FDA regulatory policies require minimal safety testing and do not require long-term studies before they approve drugs or devices, companies that perform premarketing or postmarketing tests for long-term adverse effects waste time and resources that could put them at a competitive disadvantage. Though failure to test and failure to warn adequately of product hazards may eventually result in legal liability and large amounts paid in compensation to those injured by the product, the penalties paid by the offending corporations generally do not come close enough to their profits to discourage them from externalizing costs.

A closer look at Merck's motives for aggressively marketing and selling Vioxx reveals the corporate survivalist, profit-seeking notions that governed their unethical behavior, and shows that patients' deaths were, in fact, an externalized cost of selling Vioxx. Merck is one of many pharmaceutical corporations struggling to keep afloat amongst a sea of powerful competitors. Like its competitors, Merck makes pharmaceuticals as cheaply as possible and sells them for as much as they can to as many customers as they can manage. The individuals pulling the strings at Merck are heavily rewarded for their ability to increase the company's bottom line. The ability to return large profits to shareholders defines success and results in professional advancement in this market.

In the late 1990s, Merck was a "successful" corporation; they made lots of money. However, some executives realized that their profits were in danger because the patents on six of their top-selling drugs were due to expire in the first years of the new millennium. This meant that Merck would lose exclusive rights to sell those drugs and prices of the drugs (and consequently Merck's revenue from them) would fall as other companies competed to sell them. If

Merck lost all of this revenue, its stock would plummet and the company might be subject to takeover by other, more powerful corporations. In order to stay afloat, Merck needed a lifesaver, and it needed one quick.

That lifesaver was Vioxx. Instead of taking the risk of putting their resources into discovering new drugs that might not turn enough profit for the company to survive, Merck took a conservative approach, putting over $1 billion into promoting one single drug they believed could become a blockbuster. From an economic standpoint, Vioxx was a good choice for several reasons. First, it was a drug to *alleviate pain* from a medical condition, not a drug that would *cure* a condition. This ensured that Vioxx would have continuous sales, unlike other drugs, such as antibiotics, that are used only for short periods of time to cure ailments. Second, the target sales market of patients suffering chronic pain from arthritis was very large. Third, Vioxx could be sold as a prescription drug, allowing Merck to charge many times more per pill than the cost of manufacture because consumers with insurance are not deterred by price.[7] Vioxx was thus an ideal drug for making money.

At the million-dollar private corporate launch party for Vioxx sales staff, Merck CEO, Ray Gilmartin, emphasized the importance of Vioxx sales:

> The major drugs going off patent in 2000 and 2001—VASOTEC, MEVACOR, PRINIVIL and PEPCID, plus our share of PRILOSEC— together represent a significant percentage of our sales. So producing replacement revenue through the launch of new products like VIOXX is very important for us (Vioxx Product Release Meeting Ray Gilmartin Dinner Speach Talking Points, 1999)

Merck's former top scientist, Ed Scolnick, wrote that Merck would be a "completely different company" if it could not make Vioxx a commercial success (Scolnick et al., 1997).

Needless to say, Merck did not inform the FDA, physicians, or patients of their priorities. Merck's public pronouncements conveyed that their product development was based on charitable motives, citing its founder's claim that "[the company is] driven by the idea that medicine is and always will be for the people and not for profits" (Working at Merck Frosst, 2008). Merck described their commitment to "the highest level of scientific excellence" and "improving human and animal health and the quality of life" while they simultaneously designed studies that exaggerated the efficacy of Vioxx and diminished its negative side effects (Working at Merck Frosst, 2008). The FDA noted a disconnect between Merck's conduct and its proclaimed objectives. In a 1999 letter, the agency expressed its concern that Merck's "promotional materials demonstrate[ed] a continuing pattern and practice of widespread corporate behavior to avoid compliance with regulations concerning disclosing risk information" (Baylor-Henry, 1999).

Following the completion of the Vigor trial in 2000, Merck entered into negotiations with the FDA to establish their right to advertise Vioxx as a "safer" pain reliever based on evidence that it reduced the overall incidence of GI bleeds. However, the data from Vigor and other trials such as Advantage confirmed the cardiovascular risks associated with Vioxx, and the FDA called for a revision of the Vioxx label that would include a warning about these side effects. Merck recognized the impact that a cardiovascular side effect warning would have on sales. Their 2002 Profit Plan calculated that Merck would lose $229 million in Vioxx sales if the label revisions were released in October 2001 instead of February 2002 (Profit Plan 2002 Merck A & A Franchise, 2002). During this time, Merck delayed the submission of unfavorable Advantage results and entered into 9 months of job negotiations with the FDA official who was responsible for overseeing the trial data submissions on which the warnings were to be based (Curriculum Vitae of Peter Honig, 2003; Scolnick, 1997, 2002). By the time the FDA approved the final version of the Vioxx label in 2002, which so understated the drug's cardiovascular side effects that Merck officials described it as a "miracle," it was too late for thousands of other Vioxx users who had already died (Scolnick, 2002).

The Vioxx debacle incited public outrage at the irresponsible behavior of pharmaceutical companies and the regulatory system that allowed this behavior to go unchecked. Jurors interviewed after the Ernst verdict said they were shocked that Merck had known of the dangers of Vioxx and sold the drug anyway. One juror declared, "That was the main thing that struck me at the time—they knew and they still put it out anyway" (Girion & Calvo, 2005). The jury awarded $229 million in punitive damages to reflect the "cost" that Merck externalized by delaying the label change.

The verdict was short-lived. Several months later, a Texas appellate court reversed the jury's decision. Though determinations about factual disputes among experts, such as whether Bob Ernst suffered a heart attack or not is the responsibility of the jury, the Texas Appellate Court decided that as a "matter of law," the impartial coroner and the other plaintiff experts who determined that Ernst had died of a heart attack had insufficient evidence to even present their opinions to the jury. Having dispensed with the plaintiff experts, the Court ruled that the jury could not find for the plaintiff.

Carol Ernst, who had already lost her husband, also lost her chance to assign responsibility to Merck. Merck, on the other hand, lost nothing, except for a momentary decline in stock price that steadily rebounded over the next year. Even after settling all pending Vioxx injury claims for $4.85 billion dollars, Merck still managed to make over $5 billion in profit from selling a drug that according to one estimate caused between 88,000 and 139,000 heart attacks out of which about one-third were fatal (Curtis, 2007; Graham, 2006; Graham et al., 2005). Despite Merck's unethical conduct and the price they paid for it, Vioxx still furthered their goal of providing high returns to shareholders and large payouts to its executives.[8]

The Problem Is Systematic. How Is the System Maintained?

Why do bad drugs and devices gain approval and continued use despite widespread recognition that their risks far outweigh their benefits? The disease industry problem implicates not just the corporate profit model, but also complex social and psychological factors that keep the system in place (Culp & Berry, 2007). These factors range from pervasive ideas and cultural assumptions about the nature of science and medicine to fraud and coercion carried out by corporations. Moreover, these phenomena are themselves interrelated: cultural assumptions often disguise or legitimize disease industry marketing while subtle marketing tactics framed as "research and development" and "medical education" covertly influence popular ideology. We have outlined these relations in a flow chart (Figure 7.1) that provides a framework for understanding the interactions between disease industry marketing, the practice of medicine, policy, and cultural understandings of health and disease.

Antonio Gramsci's theory of hegemony, which describes how ideology and cultural values influence or create a "common sense" that is reinforced through what he terms "civil society"—popular culture, media, schools, family, religion, and other institutions that are part of the everyday life experiences of individuals in a society, provides a useful framework for understanding how corporate externalities have worked their way into American society and why they so often go unchallenged. Gramsci's theory recognizes that the dominant social order's power derives not from force or overt manipulation but rather from the "consent" of the governed as determined and legitimized by a value system that appears to be "common sense." The theory of hegemony attributes political power to a ruling group's ability to conform to the values and ideology of those it rules, and, in practice, ruling groups use dominant ideology to legitimize their power and prevent consideration of other political orders (Jones, 2006). Gramsci used this theory to explain how agreement over fundamental

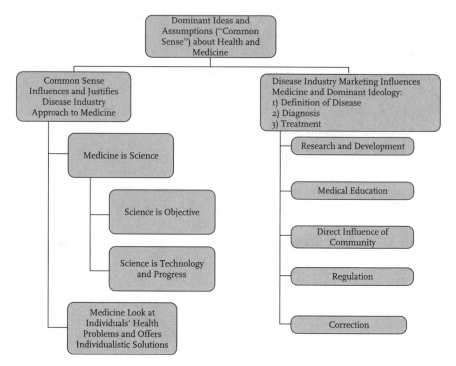

FIGURE 7.1. Hegemonic ideas that block reform and how they remain dominant.

values permitted the bourgeoisie to maintain political dominance over other classes. This chapter frames disease industry activity within the construct of hegemony to explain the persistence of corporate externalities. In this framework, we show how prevalent ideas and assumptions shape both popular and professional views in support of disease industry activity. We also show how the industry itself shapes these ideas covertly through research and marketing and also, at times, coercively through threats and reprisals. Ultimately, common sense notions about medicine and the role of disease industry products in health care create a certain blindness to and tolerance of disease industry externalities.

Common Sense about Health and Medicine

Common sense about health, disease, and medicine in America includes widespread assumptions about the nature of science and the practice of medicine.

Scientific inquiry is at the root of modern western allopathic medicine (Legal Status of Traditional Medicine and Complementary/Alternative Medicine: A Worldwide Review, 2001). Popular perceptions of medicine associate doctors with lab coats, experiments, biological mechanisms, and rationality while spirituality, culture, social organization, lifestyle, and politics are generally excluded from the domain of medicine. Though there are many definitions of science and various interpretations of what constitutes a "scientific endeavor," all agree that, in theory, science is characterized by observation, skepticism, and experimentation and that conclusions reached by scientific experiments must be replicable to have value (Latour, 1987). The public identifies science as a process that strives to avoid bias and pursues the truth. However, scientific processes are *not* inherently objective because they spring from human reasoning that is bound by culture (Feyerabend, 1975; Kuhn, 1962; Latour, 1987). As Gunnar Myrdal noted, "Prior to answers there must be questions. In the questions raised the viewpoint has (already) been chosen and the valuations implied" (Myrdal, 1978). Scientists determine which questions are asked, which observations are made, and how experiments are designed. These decisions are, for the most part, subjective and may depend on a variety of factors— such as funding, utility, prior knowledge of the issue, and incentives—that are independent of science itself (Latour, 1987). Popular conceptions of science, however, associate the field with objectivity and a dispassionate search for the truth. The public projects these notions onto medicine, which is considered to be scientific in this sense. Americans associate doctors with microscopes, laboratory tests, and high-tech equipment and believe that medical decisions and innovations are always based on thorough scientific investigation and knowledge of the biologic mechanisms of illness (Freidson, 1970).

While these assumptions are not entirely misguided, the practice of medicine, and even science itself, is nuanced and often uncertain. For example, it is common for surgeons to develop surgical techniques through trial and error, rather than through systematic investigation, and many treatments—such as aspirin for headaches—are commonly administered and effective even though doctors are uncertain of the exact biological mechanism that allows them to work. Gigerenzer et al. (2007) report regional differences in recommended medical interventions for the same disease signaling that factors independent of what has been "scientifically determined" play into the practice of medicine. The fact that allopathic medicine is not purely science based or objective in nature does not necessarily devalue its utility or effectiveness. Doctors make sound and beneficial clinical decisions everyday even though they are not based in or vetted by "science." However, the widespread perception that doctors depend solely on objective methods that are not influenced by their own biases or other circumstances can lend unmerited credibility to physician decision making and masks the influence of disease industry marketing and manipulation.

Furthermore, science and western medicine are associated with technology and innovation. The idea that "new" means "improved" and that "cutting-edge" implies "better" greatly affects the way in which Americans view medical interventions. While in many cases developments in medicine are, in fact, genuine improvements, new drugs and procedures are often unquestioningly promoted as preferable to previously employed interventions, and long-standing or "traditional" solutions are often overlooked. Phase III clinical trials for new pharmaceuticals rarely test drugs for more than a few months, and the study subjects rarely reflect the clinical profiles of the patient population to whom the drugs will be administered after marketing. Despite this, doctors rapidly adopt new drugs as "better" interventions (Graham, 2002; Rosenheck, 2005). Often, as was the case with Vioxx, new drugs and devices rapidly supplant inexpensive, established, and effective therapies. Hydrochlorothiazide is an example of a relatively safe, effective, and well-established treatment for hypertension that has been used for 50 years. Though it is economical and effective, doctors underutilize it in favor of more expensive, minimally tested patented alternatives (Knight et al., 2000). The preference for new treatments is derived from a value judgment that is inherent in the American conscious. New pills, devices, and tests developed in laboratories are treated with little or no skepticism and warrant nearly immediate acceptance because their newness is associated with improvement through "scientific methods." While some new products are genuine improvements, the rapid adoption of all things "new" is, at least in part, a cultural and marketing phenomenon because complete "scientific evidence" of efficacy and safety develops over time and is missing for new drugs (Rosenheck, 2005).

Faith in innovation and the objectivity of medicine leads patients and doctors alike to believe that the treatment they give or receive is the best there is to offer because it is based on cutting-edge, scientifically derived "truth" about biological systems. These assumptions are important in legitimizing disease industry activity because the preference for innovation gears Americans toward accepting products that have been minimally tested and allows manufacturers to redesign and remarket new versions of old products, practices that significantly reduce production costs and increase profits. The assumption of scientific objectivity not only increases trust and acceptance of disease industry products but also cloaks marketing strategies and manipulation of research in the guise of scientific truth.

A larger and, consequently, less apparent bias in today's medical industry is its focus on treating individuals with pharmaceuticals and devices and its exclusion of large-scale social changes that have been proven to improve health and quality of life—such as improving sanitation and food systems, educating and empowering citizens, and increasing community solidarity. The neglect of these other, less commonly acknowledged, approaches to healthcare—many of which are, ironically, supported by scientific research—indicates a bias toward the treatment of individual patients and the prevalent preference for intervention through drugs and devices in today's medical system (Bruhn & Wolf, 1979; Kass, 1970). This critique of western medicine should not suggest that the treatment of individuals with drugs and devices has no place or benefit but rather that this approach should be recognized as one of many possible interventions that can improve health. For example, interventions such as agricultural policies that decrease the use of pesticides on food, economic changes that make high caloric fast food less desirable, and school programs that encourage active lifestyles could be equally, if not more, effective at preventing death and disease than prescription drugs and surgeries. They would undoubtedly be less costly.

In most cases, the medical establishment continues to operate under the basic individualistic premise of "doctor treating patient." Increasingly, the medical profession is becoming so specialized that doctors no longer focus on treating whole patients but, instead, treat specific organs or body systems or even just particular symptoms or aspects of a disease. Large-scale social and policy changes are not considered formal medicine and are left to the "unscientific" and "subjective" realms of politics and social science regardless of the fact that many of these initiatives are backed by strong research findings. The common sense assumption that science is objective gives more value to medical procedures discovered in laboratories while deemphasizing the importance and potential of interventions that are not. Ironically, the most important health care breakthrough in the past 40 years in the United States was not a scientifically derived, innovative disease industry product; it was a tax on tobacco (Kristof, 2008).

As Marcuse noted, the success of the system is to make unthinkable the possibility of alternatives (Marcuse, 1964). The following section describes how the disease industry contributes to the formation and promotion of common sense notions about health and medicine and uses dominant ideology to advance their single-minded, profit-making objectives and externalize production costs onto individuals and society with the "consent" of the people.

Disease Industry Influences the Practice of Medicine
and Reinforces Popular Ideology

The disease industry did not invent medicine's individual treatment paradigm, create faith in the objectivity of science, or equate technology with progress. These dominant ideological constructs are sociocultural phenomena and are hegemonic in the American value system and way of life. However, as Gramsci put it, "common sense is not something rigid and immobile, but is continually transforming itself" as society evolves, agendas change, and different intellectual leaders come into prominence (Gurevitch, 1982). The root of hegemonic influence derives from an individual's interaction with "civil society"— the media, schools, churches, family, and other institutions—whose values and ideologies are explored and consecrated through everyday experience. The extent to which disease industry marketing, the cooption of academic researchers, and influence over government by the disease industrypermeates civil society determines the amount of influence that industry has on creating our collective common sense.

We interact with the disease industry through nearly all venues of civil society, especially the media and, most importantly, the medical establishment. The disease industry's relationship with the medical community is perhaps the single most important factor in its ability to exploit and influence hegemonic constructs that permit corporations to sell their products and externalize their costs while averting much skepticism and rebuke from society. Medical institutions, key opinion leaders, regulatory agencies like the FDA, and prescribing doctors serve as intermediaries between corporate, profit-driven manufacturers of pharmaceuticals and medical devices and the end users of their products. Corporations use their influence over the medical community to control ideas surrounding the definition of disease, the necessity of diagnostic tests, and treatment standards. More importantly, respected and trusted intermediaries (i.e., physicians, hospitals, medical universities, government agencies, medical journals, etc.) blur the distinction between disease industry marketing and professional judgment, giving legitimacy to disease industry propaganda and providing alternative explanations for their profit-driven failures.

The prominent caricaturist Al Hirshfeld was well known for hiding his daughter's name, *Nina*, in his cartoons. Though visible to the informed eye, uninformed readers focused on the figures, objects and political messages in the artwork; the image of her name only became apparent to those who were aware of the game and looked for it. In the same way, the disease industry's influence on thought and practice in the medical community is ever present, though often camouflaged. Essentially, all activities of a corporation are necessarily aimed at developing and marketing products and services that can be sold for a profit, and this holds true for products intended to treat patients. The activities, advertisements, education, research, and development sponsored by disease industry corporations are profit driven. However, what distinguishes medical product marketing from the marketing of commercial products such as clothing, cars, and snack foods is that much of it is conducted within the medical industry itself. In the case of hospitals, doctors and insurance companies stand between disease industry products (medical devices, diagnostics, and pharmaceuticals) and their end users (patients). The medical community, therefore, represents a crucial target market for disease industry products, and selling to this community requires that companies influence medical discourse in such a way as to ensure that there is the perception of a "need" for their products and that their products are regarded as filling that need. Alastair Matheson describes this discourse as the creation of a "drug narrative ... in which a drug typically provides the 'solution' to a 'problem'" (Matheson, 2008).

The disease industry influences popular as well as professional perceptions of health care by controlling the definition of disease, supplying methods for diagnosis of disease, and deciding what is acceptable and/or necessary treatment or intervention. Controlling the demarcation between health and disease allows drug companies and device manufacturers to determine the size of their markets. Lynn Payer named this phenomenon "disease mongering," which refers to the convergence of interests of doctors, drug companies, and media in exaggerating both the severity of illness and the efficacy of drugs:

> Since disease is such a fluid and political concept, the providers can essentially create their own demand by broadening the definitions of diseases in such a way as to include the greatest number of people, and by spinning out new disease (Payer, 1992).

According to Payer, disease mongering often involves the "medicalization" of what were previously considered normal laboratory results, behaviors, or feelings. Though cramping and mood swings during menstruation, loss of sexual stamina in males with age and flighty, energetic behavior in children are natural aspects of the everyday lives of millions, these normal variations have been redefined as "premenstrual dysphoric disorder," "erectile dysfunction," and "attention deficit hyperactivity disorder." Excessive retail spending and extreme shyness have been dubbed as "compulsive shopping disease" and "social anxiety disorder." Awareness campaigns backed by disease industry companies convince healthy people to consider the vagaries of everyday life as medical problems that can be solved by disease industry products. Pharmaceutical company-sponsored "awareness campaigns" are designed to convince healthy people that they are sick and sick people that they are very sick. The 1997 best seller *Listening to Prozac* gave voice to this fashion when its medical author asserted that selective serotonin reuptake inhibitors (SSRIs) could make people "better than well" (Kramer, 1997).

Henry Gadsden, president of Merck, explained the concept from a strategic perspective, stating that it is more advantageous for a pharmaceutical company to sell to everyone as opposed to being confined to selling to just sick people (Moynihan & Cassels, 2005). Vince Parry a marketing executive described the practice:

> The idea behind 'condition branding' is relatively simple: If you can define a particular condition and its associated symptoms in the minds of physicians and patients, you can also predicate the best treatment for that condition (Parry, 2003).

When disease industry companies establish the legitimacy or requirement for a diagnostic test, they bias medical practice toward "high-tech" solutions, conflate the idea of "prevention" with "early detection" and promote the idea that *earlier* treatment and *more* treatment is the most appropriate form of medical practice (Starfield et al., 2008). Diagnostic equipment manufacturers influence the choice of diagnostic equipment or tests that "should" be performed to diagnose diseases. Sometimes they promote the use of a test to diagnose an abnormality before there is any evidence that the "abnormality" should be treated. For example, computerized tomography (CT) scans detect cardiovascular variations in patients who are subsequently treated with cardiac bypasses or drugs; however, there is no evidence that these procedures prolong life or prevent disease in these patients (Redberg & Walsh, 2008). Regardless, CT scan manufacturers, along with the radiologists, cardiologists, and cardiac surgeons who make money from the scans, have aggressively promoted the use of CT for evaluation of heart disease. It is now a standard screening procedure for cardiovascular risks. Recently, the Centers for Medicare and Medicaid Services (CMS)—the organization that determines whether or not federal health insurance programs will pay for a particular procedure—proposed to disallow payment for CT scans because there was no evidence that the screenings improved health (Redberg & Walsh, 2008).

Deciding which interventions are "indicated treatments" as opposed to "quackery" allows the disease industry to advance the sale of its products as solutions to health problems and ensures demand for them by blocking out other alternatives. For example, drug companies fund researchers who write clinical practice guidelines (CPGs) which are written by groups of "expert" clinicians and usually endorsed by specialty societies. Doctors follow CPGs to determine diagnostic tests, devices, and drug treatments for various diseases. Choudhry et al. found that 87% of physicians who developed CPGs had received funding from drug companies whose drugs they were to evaluate. Fifty-eight percent had received financial support to perform research, 38% had served as employees or consultants for a pharmaceutical company, and 6% had equity interest in the pharmaceutical company (Choudhry et al., 2002).

Medicare and insurance companies pay for off-label (unapproved) uses for many drugs. They base their reimbursement decisions on "compendiums." The writers and editors of these private compendiums are not government employees. Medicare is essentially obliged to pay for any drug as long as at least one compendium approves it as treatment even if the FDA has specifically ruled that the drug should not be used for that disease. These compendiums have close financial ties to the drug industry and many conflicts of interest. Dr. Allan Korn, the chief medical officer for the Blue Cross and Blue Shield Association told the New York Times, "We have very little faith that those indications that make it into the compendia are safe, let alone effective." For example, the National Comprehensive Cancer Network guidelines and drug listings are written by experts, at least 47% of whom received more than $10,000 per year of drug company funding (http://www.nccn.org/disclosures/default.asp). A drug company can pay a $50,000 fee to the Foundation for Evidence-Based Medicine compendium to expedite review (but not guarantee inclusion) of their drug within 3 months (Abelson & Pollack, 2009).

In theory, establishing the medical community along with regulatory agencies as intermediaries in the sale of disease industry products to end users should protect patients by ensuring that qualified individuals (doctors) make informed decisions about health care with patients' best interests in mind. In many cases, this process works. The FDA keeps some dangerous drugs and devices off the market and doctors negotiate risks, benefits, and contraindications when prescribing a drug or recommending a procedure. This system works under the assumption that the medical establishment functions independently of the commercial pressures exerted by the disease industry and prioritizes patients' best interests. However, these sectors are *not* outside disease industry influence, and corporations utilize their influence over these intermediaries to justify the use of and lend credibility to their products. Disease industry corporations market their products by funding research and controlling discourse within the medical community, and many end users of their products, and often members of the medical community themselves, are blind to their influence (Matheson, 2008). Like the *Ninas* hidden in Hirschfeld's cartoons, disease industry marketing permeates the medical establishment yet remains hidden, unless you know what to look for.

In the following section, we highlight the specific methods employed by corporations to shape the discourse surrounding issues of health and health care, paying specific attention to the role of the medical community in accepting and perpetuating this influence and its effects on related policy and the popular conscious. Disease industry marketing flows to doctors, hospitals, and other caretakers through research and development, medical education, and increasingly to the general public through traditional and unconventional advertising.

Corporate Framing of Research Questions and Manipulation of Results

Since all activities of a corporation are driven by profits, the marketing of disease industry products begins with research and development. Corporations that make and sell pharmaceuticals and medical devices are usually the entities responsible for testing the appropriateness, efficacy, and safety of those products. Employment at a corporation or the receipt of corporate funding gives doctors and scientists conducting research a strong incentive to produce results that are favorable to a corporation's products. Contrary to popular belief about the objectivity of science, there are many ways to design scientific experiments that skew the data in a specific direction. These methods, which can be either intentional or unintentional, include designing the study with an inherent bias and reporting only favorable results (Greenland, 2009). Table 7.1 is a list of some of the specific techniques disease industry corporations employ that distort science and affect results.

Medical Education

In addition to influencing and subtly (or not so subtly) biasing research and development toward disease industry agendas, corporations also exert influence over the medical profession in the guise of medical education. Table 7.2 is a list of the main "educational venues" through which the disease industry asserts ideas and initiatives to control the hegemonic constructs that determine what is considered disease, proper methods of diagnosis, and expected treatments.

Direct Influence of Community Ideas about Health and Medicine

Direct influence of the community is the primary means through which the disease industry creates a consensus about medicine and disease and

TABLE 7.1. Chart of Methods Companies Use that Distort Results of Randomized Control Trials.

General Method	Specific Technique	How This Occurs	Examples
Design fails to examine expected adverse side effects	Choosing who gets studied	The chosen study subjects are less likely to show an adverse side effect than the populations most likely to use the drug or device.	In the Vioxx Vigor Trial, Merck scientists chose participants who were at low risk for cardiovascular events (i.e., 80% of participants were women, and the average age was 55 years) as opposed to older male and female patients who are most likely to be using the drug given its indication for arthritis (Morrison, 1997).
	Small studies	Studies are conducted on cohorts that are too small to demonstrate a side effect. For example, if a study has 1,000 participants and a side effect occurs once in every 5,000 patients, it is likely that no patient in the study will demonstrate the side effect. However, the effect might become serious when the drug is marketed and used by millions.	Merck conducted nine studies that constituted its new drug application for Vioxx to the Food and Drug Administration in 1998. None of these studies were large enough (50–250 patients) to properly evaluate cardiovascular risk which caused one extra heart attack for every 397 patients at low doses and one extra heart attack per year for every 75 patients at the high dose (Krumholz et al., 2007, Graham et al., 2005).
	Short-term studies	The majority of preapproval Phase III trials last between 6 weeks and 6 months, and there is no length requirement set by the FDA. This amount of time is rarely long enough for adverse side effect to appear, especially slow-developing cancers and other chronic diseases such as diabetes.	Eli Lilly's application and FDA's approval of Zyprexa for treatment of schizophrenia, a chronic condition, was based on short-term (4–6 week) studies (Physician's Desk Reference, 2000).The short-term trial data, which was provided to doctors, thus, did not show that Zyprexa use resulted in weight gain and hyperglycemia after months of use, though other data from longer trials—publication on which was delayed—showed this to be true (Zyprexa Highlights of Prescribing Information, 2009).

(*Continued*)

TABLE 7.1. Continued

General Method	Specific Technique	How This Occurs	Examples
Study shows exaggerated/ favorable results.	Selection of the study dose	High doses used for the drug to be tested and low doses for the competitor drug to show exaggerated effectiveness in comparison.	Drug companies sponsored multiple trials of their NSAID drugs in head to head comparisons with generics or competitor's drug. The sponsor's drug was administered in higher doses than the competing drug. The difference in effectiveness between cohorts was then used to support marketing claims that the sponsor's drug was more effective (Rochon et al., 1994).
Study uses an endpoint that does not predict efficacy for outcome of interest	Study evaluates surrogate outcomes	The effect of a drug is measured against a risk factor or other indicator/ symptom (surrogate) of a disease instead of against morbidity or mortality caused by the disease.	Nifedipine was tested and approved to treat high blood pressure, a risk factor for MIs and strokes; however, it was later found to increase the incidence of these events even though it effectively reduced blood pressure (Furberg et al., 1995).
Reporting results	Important side effects are lumped with unimportant side effects in a "composite endpoint."	Important side effects (such as heart attack deaths) combined with related, but less serious, side effects (such as hypertension or edema) to create a single outcome measure.	Ferreira-Gonzalez et al. reviewed over 90 studies and found that this practice was widespread and that as a result readers often overemphasized the drug's benefits. Outcomes, such as fatal MI and nonfatal MI are grouped and are reported as "reduces fatal and nonfatal MI" when almost all events are nonfatal" (Ferreira-Gonzalez et al., 2007).
Selective Publication	Results favorable to a product are more likely to be published	Drug and device manufacturers retain publication rights over the studies they fund. They often bias the medical literature by publishing favorable studies while burying those that are unfavorable.	Turner et al. (2008) reported that companies reported negative results on their antidepressant drugs to the FDA (as required by law) but correctly published 36 of 37 studies with favorable results, 3 of 25 negative trials and 11 other negative trials in a way that made them appear positive.

TABLE 7.2. Influencing Medicine by Masking Marketing as Education.

Form of "Education"	Explanation
Detailing	Product detail representatives, marketers from disease industry corporations, personally engage physicians through visits to their offices. Though these detail representatives are first and foremost salesmen and saleswomen whose primary goal is to influence doctors' prescribing habits toward their products, they are introduced to physicians as providers of important facts and information about disease industry products. Visits from detail representatives often involve incentives for physicians such as free drug samples, meals, tickets to shows or sports events, and in some extreme cases vacation getaways and outings to strip joints. Moreover, detail representatives are steeped in face-to-face marketing skills and trained in how to avoid answering critical questions about product safety and efficacy.
Peer-reviewed journals	Publication in peer-reviewed journals is the primary mode of establishing credibility and disseminating information throughout the medical community. Most medical professionals consider publication in a peer-reviewed scientific or medical journal a sign of credibility of study results. However, underlying data is infrequently audited, and publishing false results, a biased, ghostwritten, or otherwise defective study is a common occurrence (Hill et al., 2008).
Non-peer-reviewed journals	Publication of misleading scientific literature is even easier to accomplish in non-peer-reviewed journals. Although there is less credibility associated with non-peer-reviewed literature, many of these "throwaways" are distributed for free to physicians across the country without subscription.
Medical journal advertisements	Pharmaceuticals and medical devices are advertised through traditional paper advertisement schemes in medical journals with large physician readerships.
Product handouts and monographs	Companies distribute "information" or "educational" handouts that double as marketing materials for their products. The information on these handouts is not reviewed by anyone other than the companies themselves and may contain misleading information and/or ghostwritten supplements that appear to be legitimate including the creation of journals that were secretly conceived and funded by pharmaceutical companies.
Company-sponsored symposia, medical specialty meetings, and hospital lectures	Companies sponsor education programs at hospitals and medical schools, scientific research, publications, and professional meetings. At many medical professional organization conventions, the programs include promotional material about the sponsor's products. The Pharma-funded CME industry employs more than 30,000 people. Company advertising is the main source of income for the AMA. This is now true for most medical specialty organizations.
Continuing Medical Education (CME)	Practicing physicians are generally required to attend CME lectures or take CME courses online in order to refresh their medical knowledge and stay up–to-date on trends in their fields. Disease industry companies sponsor and design courses of study for many of these programs.

(Continued)

213

TABLE 7.2. Continued

Form of "Education"	Explanation
Gifts to physicians, medical students, and residents	Companies routinely provide doctors with breakfasts, lunches and "educational dinners" at expensive restaurants. Under the threat of a congressional ban in 2008, the pharmaceutical companies published a voluntarily guideline that banned small gifts like pens, pads, and mugs. The code did not limit the millions of dollars spent on speaking and consulting payments that drug makers have with tens of thousands of doctors.
Hiring physicians as consultants	Disease industry corporations hire practicing and research physicians as consultants, establishing financial ties between their interests and the interests of individuals in the medical community who are responsible for making medical decisions or influencing opinions. Consulting is often simply a way for companies to entice physicians financially under a guise of legitimacy, such as when detail representatives pay "consulting fees" to physicians for "preceptorships" in order to observe their patient examinations with the goal of having them use their company's drug.
Key opinion leaders (KOLs)	Disease industry corporations identify "key opinion leaders" in the medical profession, those physicians who are well known and respected in their field. They often hire them as consultants and pay them large sums of money to advocate for disease industry products by giving lectures, writing papers, or signing ghostwritten articles, and creating clinical practice guidelines. Companies will often share patent royalties with KOLs to give them incentive to support their products.

acceptance of their products outside of the medical profession. Table 7.3 is a partial compilation of the schemes companies use to influence individuals and entities that play a role in shaping medical and health policy, including the government and insurance companies.

Corporate Influence on Regulatory Processes

The FDA is the organization that oversees the approval of all medical drugs and devices. The agency is government sponsored and was designed to be an independent evaluator of the effectiveness and safety of disease industry products. However, the FDA is not, in actuality, isolated from corporate influence. Regulatory capture refers to the phenomenon where companies gain control over and/or influence agencies that are established to regulate their conduct. This aligns the regulatory agency's objectives with those of the corporations whose products they are vetting. As Graham put it:

TABLE 7.3. Ways Corporations Seek to Influence Public Constructs.

General Method	Specific Methods	Examples
Direct-to-consumer advertising	Television, radio, internet, and magazine advertisements	These are traditional marketing schemes and involve common advertising tricks such as sex appeal, bandwagon, celebrity endorsement, and others. Often DTC advertisements include lists of symptoms for self-diagnosis, which may further disease mongering by encouraging healthy people to identify normal variations in health (such as frequent urination, shyness, anxiety, or restless legs) as conditions that are treatable with medicine or medical devices (Angell, 2009a; Bell et al., 1999a, 1999b, 2000; Silverman, 2008).
Attempting to influence "independent" media and organizations	Paying media hosts	Corporations provided "speaker fees" of over one million dollars to the host of the "The Infinite Mind" radio program broadcast on public radio stations (Harris, 2008). This show legitimized "new disorders" like shoplifting and shyness and off-label use of drugs for these and other "medical disorders" (http://www.nccn.org/disclosures/default.asp).
Attempting to influence "independent" Non-profit Organizations	Disease-specific advocacy organizations	Disease industry corporations often sponsor or fund organizations that are viewed as independent and beneficent advocacy organizations. These "legitimate" organizations routinely promote new therapies and lobby the FDA to approve them (Carpenter, 2004; Front Groups, 2008).

The [FDA] culture also views industry as the client. They're serving industry rather than the public. In fact, when a former office director for the Office of Drug Safety criticized me and tried to get me to change a report I'd written on another drug—Arava—he said to me and to a colleague who was a coauthor on this report that 'industry is our client.' (Loudon, 2005)

The FDA, at its discretion, appoints "expert panels" to review new drug applications for controversial or innovative products. In 73% of FDA meetings, at least one advisory committee member reported a financial link to a drug's maker or a competitor (Lurie et al., 2006). There is much job transfer between middle and upper level management at the FDA and disease industry corporations (Revolving Door). For example, Merck entered into job discussions with the FDA Director of the Office of Post-Marketing Drug Risk Assessment that spanned approximately 9 months. During this period, the official (according to a memorandum) attended a meeting where the FDA discussed its position on the Vioxx label and met off-the-record with Merck representatives on FDA "Organizational changes and the status of regulatory documents and policies" (Memo from Goldmann B. to Dray M., Subj: Highlights of WRLG meeting with P. Honig MD, Director OPDRA, CDER, September 18, 2001). The official left the FDA and immediately took a position at Merck (Curriculum Vitae of Peter Honig, 2003; Rarick Honig FDA Label Meetings, 2001; Scolnick, 2002;). He later testified in the Vioxx civil litigation that he had "tried" to "distance" himself from Merck-related matters at the FDA while he was being considered for a position with the company (Deposition of Peter Honig, 2005).

Corporations hide adverse side effects and other unfavorable study results by submitting them to the FDA along with reams of unimportant information. Important data is often lost in the mix. Approval by the FDA, like endorsement by physicians, lends credibility to disease industry products that companies then use to dispute responsibility for injuries caused by their products.[9]

Corporate Use of Coercion

The disease industry controls the practice and acceptance of medicine primarily by "consent." Biasing research, disguising marketing as medical education, advertising directly to consumers, and meddling in regulatory processes masks industry influence and bolsters disease industry constructs of health and medicine through tacit influence of "civil society."[10] However, occasionally, consent cannot be maintained exclusively through normal civil society processes and corporations resort to direct coercion in order to gain approval for their views and products and prevent the consideration of noncommercial alternatives (see Table 7.4).

Conclusion

Companies in the disease industry are subject to the same incentives and structural constraints as all corporations, namely, the single-minded responsibility to provide high returns for their shareholders. In today's largely deregulated

TABLE 7.4. Examples of Alleged Coercive Acts.

Victim	Drug/Company	Story
Dr. David Graham	Vioxx/Merck (FDA)	FDA researcher Dr. David Graham conducted independent Vioxx trials that revealed Vioxx's cardiovascular risks. Upon complaint by Merck about his research, senior-level FDA managers allegedly orchestrated a campaign to discredit Dr. Graham by asking Lancet not to publish his work. They attempted to prevent Senator Grassley from calling him as a witness in a Vioxx investigation, and, according to Graham, the acting commissioner of the FDA offered him a promotion in order to "preempt" his testimony (Loudon, 2005).
Dr. John Buse	Avandia (rosiglita-zone)/SmithKline and Beecham	GlaxoSmithKline (GSK) called his department chair at the University of North Carolina and told him that Buse needed to retract his adverse comments on Avandia or they would sue the university for $4 billion in lost sales. GSK wrote a "retraction letter" for Buse to copy onto his own letterhead and sign, stating that he was wrong about his claims against Avandia. Buse eventually signed a letter that indicated he would not further discuss the issue (Glaxo CEO Knew Doc Was Intimidated, 2007).
Dr. Mary Money	Avandia (rosiglita-zone)/SmithKline and Beecham (which later merged to form GlaxoSmithKline)	Smith Kline employees visited her at her job to tell her that her conclusions were incorrect, stating that perhaps she was unable to read accurately echocardio-grams. SmithKline executives contacted Washington County's Chief of Staff and demanded that he make Dr. Money stop speaking out against Avandia (More on Pharma Intimidation of Doctors, 2008).

market, competition from other corporations and the prospect of mergers and hostile takeovers gives ample incentive for corporations to maintain competitive advantages by externalizing some of the costs of production onto consumers and society. Disease industry externalities are a special case of corporate externalizing behavior because of the direct effects they have on human health and well-being and, more importantly, because of the industry's ability to hide externalities within the context of the practice of medicine.

In accordance with Gramsci's theory of hegemony, the disease industry exercises influence and avoids criticism by exploiting common sense notions about health, medicine, and the role of disease industry products in everyday life. They further their profit-oriented agendas with public "consent" that derives from apparent endorsement by the media, the medical profession, and regulatory agencies. Moreover, these institutions, especially the medical community and the government, lend credibility to disease industry goals and ideas to an exceptional degree because they give the appearance of legitimacy.

The disease industry exploits the ideas that science is objective, that technological advances are more valuable than long-standing therapies, and that keeping people healthy involves treating individuals in order to create the perception that their products are needed and represent the best medical solutions. However, they violate the tenets of the "common sense" they rely on by intentionally biasing and manipulating scientific research, creating "new" technologies that are no better or worse than old ones and creating consensus around medical diagnostic and treatment options that are wasteful and expensive when more cost-effective alternatives exist. The second part of this chapter shed light on some of the specific techniques disease industry corporations use to infiltrate "civil society" and influence common sense.

The disease industry exploits existing ideologies and cultural assumptions while simultaneously reinforcing and recreating them through the guise of legitimacy afforded to them by medical, regulatory, and public interest intermediaries. This cyclical reinforcement is what allows disease industry externalities to go effectively unchallenged, if not unnoticed (like the *Ninas* hidden in Hirschfeld's cartoons), by patients and society who bear the exaggerated costs of corporate misconduct.

NOTES

1 We ascribe actions and knowledge to the corporation as a whole, which under US law, is a "person."

2 Most NSAID pain relievers, like aspirin and ibuprofen, work by inhibiting both Cox-2 and Cox-1 enzymes. Inhibition of Cox-1 increases the risk of GI bleeding and protects against heart attacks. Vioxx primarily inhibits the Cox-2 enzyme and, thus, produced fewer cases of GI bleeds and ulcers. However, the Cox-2 enzyme is required for GI healing, so by blocking it, Vioxx increased the likelihood that a bleed would be severe if it occurred (Wright, 2002).

3 "Blockbuster" is a Wall Street term reflecting a drug or device with more than one billion dollars in annual sales.

4 Merck trained their representatives with a game they called "Dodge Ball" which involved practicing methods to avoid answering questions about Vioxx side effects

including heart attacks. In this training game, prospective detail representatives could only move onto the next round if they gave Merck-approved answers to possible doctor's questions about Vioxx safety or dodged such questions altogether.

5 We use the term "disease industry" to refer collectively to those companies that sell products and services designed to diagnose, treat and prevent disease such as pharmaceuticals, medical devices and diagnostic equipment.

6 Legal precedent gives corporations the status of persons under the law under the premise that corporations procure important benefits for society. However, the justification for this right is faulty. Unlike human beings who have moral responsibilities to other individuals and society that are enforced by both society and the law, corporations, legally, have no responsibility to society or individuals other than their shareholders, and—as we will develop in this chapter—the law and society rarely hold them accountable for their trespasses. There is growing evidence that some executives act in their own and not shareholder interest (Dennis, 2004).

7 The price of Vioxx was as much as $3 per pill. Comparatively, generic versions of other equally effective (and safer) arthritis pain medications retailed for around $0.06 per pill (Vioxx, 2008)..

8 Former CEO Raymond Gilmartin earned $54 million during the five year period of Vioxx sales. By 2001 he had over $181 million dollars in unexercised stock options and had more than 102 million in pension benefits (Bebchuk and Jackson, 2005).

9 In February 2008, the United States Supreme Court issued a 6–3 ruling against a pharmaceutical manufacturer's right to claim preemption from liability for a defective product under the premise that the product had been approved by the FDA. Though the court ruled against preemption, FDA approval remains an attempted legal defense strategy in litigation.

10 In Gramsci's discussion of hegemony, he distinguishes government from civil society. However, when we apply the theory of hegemony to the disease industry, it is important to note that the government (i.e., the FDA and governmental health policy) actually becomes part of civil society along with the medical profession, popular media, etc. because it is a supposedly independent institution through which ideas about health and medicine are perpetuated in ways that affect the everyday lives of citizens.

REFERENCES

Abelson R, Pollack A. Medicare widens drugs it accepts for cancer. *New York Times.* January 26, 2009.

Abrams TW. Food and Drug Administration, Division of Drug Marketing, Advertising and Communications Warning Letter re: NDA 21-042 Vioxx (rofecoxib) tablets Warning Letter to Gilmartin, R. 2001. http://www.fda.gov/CDER/warn/2001/9456.pdf. Accessed March 29, 2009.

Angell M. Drug companies & doctors: a story of corruption. *The New York Review of Books.* January 15, 2009a.

Angell M. Drug companies & doctors: a story of corruption. *The New York Review of Books.* 2009b;56.

Angell M. Industry-sponsored clinical research: a broken system. *JAMA.* 2008;300:1069–1071.

Angell M. *The Truth About the Drug Companies: How They Deceive Us and What to Do About It.* New York: Random House Trade Paperbacks; 2005.

Angell M, Relman AS. Fraud in biomedical research: a time for congressional restraint. *N Engl J Med.* 1988;318:1462–1463.

Anstice D. Testimony in Ernst v. Merck Vioxx Litigation in the District Court of Brazoria County, Texas Case No. 619 3/18/2005. 2005.

Bakan J. *The Corporation: The Pathological Pursuit of Profit and Power.* New York: Free Press; 2004.

Baylor-Henry M. FDA Warning Letter to Anstice D., 1999. http://dida.library.ucsf. edu/pdf/oxx12q10. Accessed March 29, 2009.

Bebchuk LA, Jackson RJ Jr. Executive pensions. *J Corp Law.* 2005;30:32.

Bell RA, Kravitz RL, Wilkes MS. Direct-to-consumer prescription drug advertising and the public. *J Gen Intern Med.* 1999;14:651–657.

Bell RA, Wilkes MS, Kravitz RL. Advertisement-induced prescription drug requests: patients' anticipated reactions to a physician who refuses. *J Fam Pract.* 1999;48:446–452.

Bell RA, Wilkes MS, Kravitz RL. The educational value of consumer-targeted prescription drug print advertising. *J Fam Pract.* 2000;49:1092–1098.

Berenson A. Courts reject two major Vioxx verdicts. *The New York Times.* May 8, 2008.

Bombardier C, Laine L, Reicin A, et al. Comparison of upper gastrointestinal toxicity of rofecoxib and naproxen in patients with rheumatoid arthritis. *N Engl J Med.* 2000;343:1520–1528.

Bombardier C, Laine L, Reicin A, et al. Comparison of upper gastrointestinal toxicity of rofecoxib and naproxen in patients with rheumatoid arthritis. VIGOR Study Group. *N Engl J Med.* 2000;343:8.

Bradford WD, Kleit AN, Nietert PJ, Steyer T, McIlwain T, Ornstein S. How direct-to-consumer television advertising for osteoarthritis drugs affects physicians' prescribing behavior. *Health Aff (Millwood).* 2006;25:1371–1377.

Brody H. *Hooked: Ethics, the Medical Profession, and the Pharmaceutical Industry.* New York: Rowman & Littlefield Publishers, Inc.; 2007.

Bruhn JG, Wolf S. *The Roseto Story: An Anatomy of Health.* Norman: University of Oklahoma; 1979.

Carpenter D. The political economy of FDA drug review: processing, politics, and lessons for policy. *Health Aff.* 2004;23:52–63.

Choudhry NK, Stelfox HT, Detsky AS. Relationships between authors of clinical practice guidelines and the pharmaceutical industry. *JAMA.* 2002;287:612–617.

Culp D, Berry I. Merck and the Vioxx Debacle: deadly loyalty. *St John J Legal Comment*. 2007;22:34.

Curfman GD, Morrissey S, Drazen JM. Expression of Concern: Bombardier et al., "Comparison of Upper Gastrointestinal Toxicity of Rofecoxib and Naproxen in Patients with Rheumatoid Arthritis. *N Engl J Med*. 2000;343:1520–1528. *N Engl J Med*. 2005: NEJMe058314.

Curriculum Vitae of Peter Honig MD. 2003. Available at: http://vioxxdocuments. com/Documents/Oxford/Honig%20CV.pdf. Accessed March 29, 2009.

Curtis G. Merck's Vioxx Settlement a Relief for Investors. 2007. Available at: http:// research.investopedia.com/news/IA/2007/Mercks_Vioxx_Settlement_A_Relief_ For_Investors_MRK.aspx?ad=IA_RSS_11142007&partner=rss-advisor. Accessed March 16, 2009.

Dangerous Prescription. 2003. Available at: http://www.pbs.org/wgbh/pages/ frontline/shows/prescription/. Accessed March 29, 2009.

Daniels B. Email to Simon, T, Ehrich, E., Morrison, B., Reicin, A., re: GI Outcomes trial protocol. 1997. Available at: http://dida.library.ucsf.edu/pdf/oxx03f10. Accessed March 29, 2009.

Dennis A. What's next in corporate pay practices? *J Account*. 2004;198.

Deposition of Peter Honig, M.D., In re Vioxx Litigation, Case No. 619, Superior Court of New Jersey, Atlantic Count, August 8, 2005:69–72.

Egilman DS, Presler AH. Report of specific cardiovascular outcomes of the ADVANTAGE trial. *Ann Intern Med*. 2006;144:781.

Families USA Publication, Off the Charts: Pay, Profits and Spending by Drug Companies. 2001. Available at: https://www.policyarchive.org/bitstream/ handle/10207/6386/offthecharts6475.pdf?sequence=1. Accessed March 30, 2009.

Ferreira-Gonzalez I, Busse JW, Heels-Ansdell D, et al. Problems with use of composite end points in cardiovascular trials: systematic review of randomised controlled trials. *BMJ*. 2007;334:786.

Feyerabend P. *Against Method: Outline of an Anarchistic Theory of Knowledge*. London: Humanities Press; 1975.

Freidson E. Profession of medicine: a study of the sociology of applied knowledge. New York: Dodd, Mead; 1970.

Front Groups. 2008. Available at: http://www.sourcewatch.org/index. php?title=Front_group. Accessed September 11, 2009.

Furberg CD, Psaty BM, Meyer JV. Nifedipine: dose-related increase in mortality in patients with coronary heart disease. *Circulation*. 1995;92:1326–1331.

Gigerenzer G, Gaissmaier W, Kurz-Milcke E, Schwartz L, Woloshin S. Helping doctors and patients make sense of health statistics. *Psychol Sci Public Inter*. 2007;8:43.

Girion L, Calvo D. Merck Loses Vioxx Case. *Los Angeles Times*. 2005. August 20, 2005;Sect. A-1.

Glaxo CEO Knew Doc Was Intimidated. 2007. Available at: http://www.pharmalot. com/2007/09/avandiagate-jp-knew-doctor-was-intimidated/. Accessed December 22, 2008.

Graham DJ, Campen D, Hui R, et al. Risk of acute myocardial infarction and sudden cardiac death in patients treated with cyclo-oxygenase 2 selective and non-selective non-steroidal anti-inflammatory drugs: nested case-control study. *Lancet.* 2005;365:475–4781.

Graham DJ. COX-2 inhibitors, other NSAIDs, and cardiovascular risk: the seduction of common sense. *JAMA.* 2006;296:1653–1656.

Graham GK. Postmarketing surveillance and black box warnings. *JAMA.* 2002;288:955–956; author reply 8–9.

Greenland S. Accounting for uncertainty about investigator bias: disclosure is informative: How could disclosure of interests work better in medicine, epidemiology and public health? *J Epidemiol Community Health.* 2009;63: 593–598.

Gurevitch M. *Culture, Society, and the Media.* London, New York: Methuen; 1982.

Harris G. Radio host has drug company ties. 2008. *New York Times*, November 21, 2008.

Hill KP, Ross JS, Egilman DS, Krumholz HM. The ADVANTAGE seeding trial: a review of internal documents. *Ann Intern Med.* 2008;149:251–258.

Horner B, Hartwell M, Levin A. "DODGEBALL." The Pharmaceutical Companies' Direct Marketing to Doctors and the Impact on Health Care Costs and Patient Safety. 2006.

Jones S. *Antonio Gramsci.* London: Rutledge; 2006.

Kass EH. Infectious diseases and social change. *Antimicrob Agents Chemother (Bethesda).* 1970;10:1–5.

Knight EL, Glynn RJ, Levin R, Ganz DA, Avorn J. Failure of evidence-based medicine in the treatment of hypertension in older patients. *J Gen Intern Med.* 2000;15:702–709.

Kramer P. *Listening to Prozac.* New York: Penguin; 1997.

Kristof N. Miracle tax diet. *New York Times.* December 8, 2008.

Krumholz HM, Ross JS, Presler AH, Egilman DS. What have we learnt from Vioxx? *BMJ.* 2007;334:120–123.

Kuhn TS. *The Structure of Scientific Revolutions.* 1st ed. Chicago: University of Chicago Press; 1962.

Latour B. *Science in Action.* Cambridge, MA: Harvard University Press; 1987.

Lazarou J, Pomeranz BH, Corey PN. Incidence of adverse drug reactions in hospitalized patients: a meta-analysis of prospective studies. *JAMA.* 1998;279:1200–1205.

Legal Status of Traditional Medicine and Complementary/Alternative Medicine: A Worldwide Review 2001. Available at: http://whqlibdoc.who.int/hq/2001/WHO_EDM_TRM_2001.2.pdf.

Lisse JR, Perlman M, Johansson G, et al. Gastrointestinal tolerability and effectiveness of rofecoxib versus naproxen in the treatment of osteoarthritis: a randomized, controlled trial. *Ann Intern Med.* 2003;139:539–546.

Loudon M. The FDA Exposed: An Interview With Dr. David Graham, the Vioxx Whistleblower. 2005. Available at: http://www.naturalnews.com/011401.html. Accessed March 19, 2009.

Lurie P, Almeida CM, Stine N, Stine AR, Wolfe SM. Financial conflict of interest disclosure and voting patterns at Food and Drug Administration Drug Advisory Committee meetings. *JAMA*. 2006;295:1921–1928.

Marcuse H. *One-dimensional Man: Studies in the Ideology of Advanced Industrial Society*. Boston: Beacon Press; 1964.

Matheson A. Corporate science and the husbandry of scientific and medical knowledge by the pharmaceutical industry. *BioSocieties*. 2008;3:355–382.

Monks R, Minow N. *Power and Accountability*. New York: HarperCollins; 1991.

More on Pharma Intimidation of Doctors. 2008. Available at: http://www. healthyskepticism.org./library/ref.php?id=15421. Accessed November 19, 2008.

Morrison B. Email to Simon T, et al Gi Outcomes Trial Protocol.2/25/1997. Available at: http://dida.library.ucsf.edu/pdf/oxx03f10. Accessed September 12, 2009.

Moynihan R, Cassels A. *Selling Sickness: How the World's Biggest Pharmaceutical Companies Are Turning Us All into Patients*. New York, NY: Nation Books; 2005.

Myrdal G. Institutional economics. *J Econ Iss*. 1978;12:771–783.

National Comprehensive Cancer Network, (NCCN), Identification and Disclosure of Relationships with External Entities. Available at: http://www.nccn.org/ disclosures/default.asp. Accessed July 7, 2009.

Parry V. The art of branding a condition. Medical Marketing and Media.pgs 42–49 May, 2003. Available at: http://findarticles.com/p/articles/mi_qa5351/ is_200305/ai_n21330426/ accessed September 12, 2009.

Payer L. *Disease-Mongers: How Doctors, Drug Companies, and Insurers Are Making You Feel Sick*. New York: J. Wiley; 1992.

Peterson M. *Our Daily Meds*. New York: Sarah Crichton Books; 2008.

Physician's Desk Reference. *Montvale, NJ: Medical Economics*. 2000:1973–1978.

Profit Plan 2002 Merck A & A Franchise. 2002. Available at: http://dida.library.ucsf. edu/tid/o/x/x/oxx08w10/original.pdf. Accessed March 29, 2009.

Pauls L., Meeting Minutes Regulatory Briefing minutes Subject: Safety Profile of Cox 2 Drugs, 9/21/2001. Available at: http://dida.library.ucsf.edu/pdf/oxx18d10. Accessed September 12, 2001.

Redberg RF, Walsh J. Pay now, benefits may follow—the case of cardiac computed tomographic angiography. *N Engl J Med*. 2008;359:2309–2311.

Rochon PA, Gurwitz JH, Simms RW, et al. A study of manufacturer-supported trials of nonsteroidal anti-inflammatory drugs in the treatment of arthritis. *Arch Intern Med*. 1994;154:157–163.

Rosenheck R. The growth of psychopharmacology in the 1990s: evidence-based practice or irrational exuberance. *Int J Law Psychiatry*. 2005;28:467–483.

Scolnick E. Email to Goldmann, B., Greene, D., Kim, P., Re: Vioxx Label. 2002. Available at: http://dida.library.ucsf.edu/pdf/oxx12a10. Accessed March 13, 2009.

Scolnick E. Email to Blois, D, Goldmann, B., Slater, E,. Perlmutter, R., Subject: Vioxx Vs circular Exhibit 5 Deposition Testimony Ernst v Merck 2005. 1997. Available at: http://vioxxdocuments.com/Documents/Oxford/Exhibits5%20 -completely%20different%20company.pdf. Accessed March 29, 2009.

Silverman, ed. dtc-ads-were-the-worst-decision-roche-exec. 2008. Available at: http://www.pharmalot.com/2008/12/dtc-ads-were-the-worst-decision-roche-exec/. Accessed March 29, 2009.

Starfield B, Hyde J, Gervas J, Heath I. The concept of prevention: a good idea gone astray? *J Epidemiol Community Health.* 2008;62:580–583.

Swartz M. Texas tort reform: Hurt? Injured? Need a Lawyer? Too bad! . In: Texas Monthly: Caperton v A.T. Massey Coal Company, Inc., October 2005.

Turner EH, Matthews AM, Linardatos E, Tell RA, Rosenthal R. Selective publication of antidepressant trials and its influence on apparent efficacy. *N Engl J Med.* 2008;358:252–260.

Vioxx Lawsuits Snowballed in 2Q. Cnnmoney, 2005. Available at: http://money.cnn. com/2005/07/21/news/fortune500/merck_lawsuits/index.htm. Accessed March 29, 2009.

Vioxx Product Release Meeting Ray Gilmartin Dinner Speach Talking Points. 1999. Available at: http://dida.library.ucsf.edu/tid/o/x/x/oxx05t10/original.pdf. Accessed March 15, 2009.

Vioxx. 2008. Available at: http://www.prescriptionaccess.org/lawsuitssettlements/ current_lawsuits?id=0028. Accessed September 11, 2009.

Waxman HA. The lessons of Vioxx—drug safety and sales. *N Engl J Med.* 2005;352:2576–2578.

Wolfe F, Flowers N, Burke TA, Arguelles LM, Pettitt D. Increase in lifetime adverse drug reactions, service utilization, and disease severity among patients who will start COX-2 specific inhibitors: quantitative assessment of channeling bias and confounding by indication in 6689 patients with rheumatoid arthritis and osteoarthritis. *J Rheumatol.* 2002/5;29:1015–1022.

Wolfe SM. *Worst Pills, Best Pills: A Consumer's Guide to Avoiding Drug-Induced Death or Illness.* New York: Pocket Books; 2005.

Working at Merck Frosst. 2008. Available at: http://www.merckfrosst.ca/mfcl/en/ corporate/careers/workatmerck/discover_our_culture.html. Accessed December 31, 2008.

Wright JM. The double-edged sword of COX-2 selective NSAIDs. *Can Med Assoc J.* 2002;167:1131–1137.

Wysowski DK, Swartz L. Adverse drug event surveillance and drug withdrawals in the United States, 1969–2002: the importance of reporting suspected reactions. *Arch Intern Med.* 2005;165:1363–1369.

Zyprexa Highlights of Prescribing Information. Warnings and Precautions: 5.4 and 5.5. Updated March 2009. Available at: http://pi.lilly.com/us/zyprexa-pi.pdf. Accessed September 11, 2009.

8

Motor Vehicle Industry

Leon S. Robertson

In the late 19th century, inventors began attaching motors to carriages that were formerly pulled by animals. Inventors and manufacturers experimented with steam and electric motors; some sold to the public, but internal combustion engines burning gasoline or diesel oil soon became the motors used by most of the manufacturers that survived. Since then, the exponential growth in sales of motorized vehicles is among the most important transitions in transportation history. As early as 1925, motor vehicle manufacturing was estimated as the largest industry in the United States (Eastman, 1984).

The growth of adverse public health effects was also rapid. In 1926, "accidents" involving motor vehicles first made the list of the top 10 causes of deaths in the United States. (National Center for Health Statistics, 2008). The deaths from cancers and pulmonary diseases caused by years of exposure to vehicle exhausts are yet to be separated by specific numbers in official statistics, largely because the causes of chronic conditions are difficult to isolate after the fact.

Although the timing of major effects on public health of global warming, substantially exacerbated by carbon dioxide from vehicle exhausts, is in dispute, the scientific community is near consensus that the risk of such effects is growing rapidly and will have a major impact on future generations (Broome, 2008).

In his seminal work on the history of the motor vehicle industry's behavior relative to vehicle-related injury, Joel Eastman (1984) wrote:

> A scientific approach to the design of a motorcar would have required the establishment of definite criteria for the construction and operation of road vehicles, the evaluation of various alternative designs in light of these criteria, and the selection of a single, standardized design. The general goal of such an approach would be to develop a vehicle, which would operate as efficiently as possible within the highway system, and thus, a balance would have to be struck between speed, economy, and safety. Because of the laws of physics, the point of diminishing returns to an increase in the motive power and potential top speed of a vehicle is soon reached. Each increase in the power of the engine brings a decline in economy and a rise in exhaust emissions and requires an increase in the strength of the chassis and body and a modification of the weight distribution and suspension. Each increase in the maximum speed, likewise, necessitates a stronger construction to handle higher stress and to protect occupants in the event of a collision and larger brakes to bring the vehicle to a halt. Increments in power and speed also bring an increase in the demands on the human operator and a decrease in his margin of error. When these observations are considered along with the fact that the highways, themselves, have to be designed for specific operating speeds, it is obvious that maximum speeds should not be especially high.

Although it would have been unwise to adopt a "single, standardized design" that would inhibit innovation to further maximize efficiency and safety or minimize pollution, these general goals and how to balance them should have been considered early on. In fact, for more than 50 years, most of the corporations in the motor vehicle industry promoted safety as solely a driver problem, ignored emissions, and engaged in destructive horsepower races that made vehicles capable of speeds far above those advisable on even the best designed roads. The industry lobbied federal and state governments for taxes to publicly subsidize roads and against governmentally imposed standards to make vehicles safer. In 1949, General Motors, Firestone Tire, and Standard Oil, along with transit companies they had financed, were convicted of, in the juries words, "conspiracy to monopolize the transit business for their own oil, tires and busses." They bought 42 local electric trolley systems, dismantled them and substituted busses (Black, 2006). Despite the oil supply shocks of the 1970s, when U.S. oil production peaked and began its decline, the precursor of a world decline was expected early in the 21st century (Deffeyes, 2005), virtually every corporation in the motor vehicle industry promoted heavy, high-powered vehicles that consumed inordinate amounts of oil well into the 21st century.

The adverse consequences of primary dependence on motor vehicles for transportation, and in many cases the more destructive types of vehicles, occurred because of corporate greed, failure of government, and a gullible public. Corporations that were primarily invested in the production, care and feeding of motor vehicles focused only on immediate profits and opposed virtually all efforts to improve safety and fuel economy. Ironically, they experienced huge capital losses as oil prices spiked in 2005–2008 partly as a result of their inattention to fuel economy. Governments often failed to provide the infrastructure for alternative means of transportation and to set timely standards for motor vehicles to minimize human damage and conserve fuel. And most vehicle buyers failed to understand that their emotions were being manipulated by advertising and other marketing ploys. Less motorized countries seem to be repeating many of these mistakes in their rush to put motor vehicles in the hands of their citizens.

Infrastructure

Operation of motor vehicles at speeds substantially beyond those achievable by walking or on horseback requires smooth roads to accommodate them. Countries with limited road systems have the choice of building alternatives such as tracks for mass transit of people and goods among population, farming and business hubs, with local roads only for taxis, rental vehicles, busses and trucks to distribute passengers and goods to and from local points. Countries with highly developed road systems could use the roadbeds to lay tracks for a similar result. Once the car culture is predominant, however, dismantling it will likely occur only when the cost of operating motor vehicles is out of reach of a vast majority of the population. The ecological and economic consequences of such a process, all of which impacts the public's health, will be dire (Broome, 2008).

In the United States, road construction has a huge lobby, called the "Road Gang" by its opponents (http://www.highbeam.com/doc/1G1-54754434.html, accessed July 1, 2008). Corporations that produce gravel, asphalt, and concrete for roadbeds join with steel manufacturers who build bridge superstructure, construction companies, vehicle enthusiast groups, and vehicle manufacturers to maximize the allocation of public tax monies to road construction and maintenance (Kelley, 1971). Other forms of ground transportation (e.g., rail and bicycles) have their corporate interests and enthusiasts but they are poorly financed and are given a pittance in subsidies by federal, state, and local governing bodies compared to the road interests.

Federal and state departments of transportation occasionally do studies of the relative costs and benefits of various changes in transportation infrastructure. The benefits are often measured only in travel times with little or no consideration of effects on safety, air pollution, and depletion of fuel supplies. The latter is relevant to the cost side as well because increasing gasoline prices as the world's oil supply diminishes are not factored into the equation. Given these limitations, it is not surprising that light rail appears in these studies as less cost-beneficial than other approaches such as special road lanes for cars and light trucks based on vehicle occupancy or purchased licenses to drive in the fast lane (e.g., http://www.azdot.gov/TPD/ATRC/Publications/project_reports/PDF/AZ582.pdf, accessed July 1, 2008).

Injury Risk Reduction

The risk of injury and death on roads can be achieved by changing road characteristics, vehicle characteristics, and driver behavior. The earlier quote from Eastman indicates these factors are not independent. The effect of vehicle speeds on safety partly depends on road characteristics and conditions as well as adjacent environments. These, in turn, influence limits on vehicle crashworthiness and driver perceptions. For example, crashing into a rigid roadside pole concentrates energy on occupants of a vehicle far more than broad energy-absorbing surfaces. Signs on those poles that distract rather than inform drivers are a hazard.

To reduce death and injury on roads, road and vehicle builders historically emphasized changing drivers by education, admonition, and law enforcement. Occasionally, when there was a profit to be made on road or vehicle safety equipment, or in rare instances of ethical consciousness, the "Road Gang" and vehicle manufacturers opted for the road and vehicle modifications. In general, modification of vehicles and roads is more effective in reducing injury and death than attempts at changing drivers.

Even after decades of vehicle improvements, partly in response to governmental safety standards, many vehicles could be made much safer. An analysis of death risk among 114 makes and models of cars, vans, and sports utility vehicles manufactured during 1999–2005 in the United States indicated that 60–80% of deaths in those vehicles or to people struck by them would have been prevented if they had electronic stability control systems, good performance on crash tests, and improved static stability (Robertson, 2007a).

Part of the failure to adopt life-preserving technology is based on an unproductive argument about causation. The point of an analysis that indicates that deaths are largely preventable by vehicle modifications is not that the vehicles cause the deaths to that extent. Causation is far more complex than that. The point is simply that the deaths were preventable by vehicle modifications despite the complex combinations of driver, vehicle, and road factors that increased the risk of a crashes or their severity. The industry tacitly acknowledges the effect of vehicle crashworthiness when it advertises that it does well on Insurance Institute or government crash tests. Yet a physicist employed at General Motors made a career of claiming that the safety problem is primarily behavioral (Evans, 1991) or the relative weights of vehicles in crashes (Robertson, 2006). His employer made a disproportionate number of the heaviest vehicles sold.

While it is not surprising that the original inventors and manufacturers of motor vehicles did not consider the health and safety consequences of their products, the strategy of primarily blaming driver behavior was long lasting and concerted. Eastman presents numerous statements by corporate officers of vehicle manufacturers to the effect that the vehicles are as safe as they can be and that bad drivers cause the injury problem.

Beginning in 1924, the U.S. government occasionally organized conferences on road safety. These were mostly devoted to uniform traffic laws and driver behavior but also addressed issues such as placement of throttle and brake pedals, vehicle headlamps, and brakes (First National Conference on Street and Highway Safety, 1924). In the 1930s, the industry began major involvement in safety organizations that emphasized changing driver behavior. In response to Reader's Digest articles on deaths and the consequences of serious nonfatal injuries in 1935, the Automobile Manufacturers Association recommended that the industry provide grants to safety organizations. The Automotive Safety Foundation was formed to dispense grants related to licensing, record keeping, driver education, enforcement, training, research, and engineering. Engineering was confined to traffic flow, not motor vehicle safety features or crashworthiness (Eastman, 1984). Death rates were declining during this period but there is no way to know whether or to what extent specific safety efforts contributed. Economic depression in the 1930s, World War II, and the increasing density of vehicles in urban areas were no doubt a factor. Deaths rates are lower where crash rates are higher because the volume of vehicles per mile of road that usually occurs with urbanization reduces speed but increases fender benders.

Although a few writers at the time warned that driver education in high schools could make matters worse rather than better, it would be 40 years before the adverse effect would be documented definitively. Early critics noted that the major interest of manufacturers in such programs was to produce more drivers in order to increase sales (Eastman, 1984). That proved to be the adverse effect. High school driver education increases the numbers of 16–17-year-old drivers without making them better drivers, thus increasing the crash rates of teenaged drivers per population (Robertson, 1980; Shaoul, 1975).

While supposedly promoting safety through foundation grants, the industry participated to a far greater extent in efforts that contributed to design changes and speeding with injurious consequences. The emphasis on yearly model changes was initiated to appeal to the "keep up with the Joneses" (or really stay ahead of the Joneses) folkways among the U.S. middle and upper classes. Huge resources were expended each year for engineering, retooling, and marketing of superficial changes in sheet metal and glass. Sometimes safety was sacrificed to such designs, such as their effect on driver's field of vision or points and edges on interior and exterior surfaces that increased severity of injury to occupants and pedestrians respectively. In years when a major design change was not done, an increase in horsepower of the engine was often emphasized as a must-have item, initiating horsepower races among competitors (Eastman, 1985).

Speed and horsepower were also promoted by the industry's participation in stock car racing. Manufacturers apparently think that racing sells, given the huge budgets appropriated to company racing teams, even when the companies are losing money. Ford Motor Company lost $12.7 billion in 2006 but spent an estimated $20 million on racing. (http://www.nytimes.com/2007/02/17/sports/othersports/17nascar.html?scp=6&sq=Nascar+General+Motors+racin g&st=nyt accessed July 1, 2008).

The New York Times reported

> Despite reporting a record $38.7 billion loss in 2007, General Motors said it had no plans to eliminate its support of Nascar. General Motors has dominated the series in recent years, with Chevrolet drivers having won the last three championships. "Obviously, the last racing we would drop in the racing that we're in would be

Nascar right now, because it's still got the best return for us," said John Middlebrook, the vice president for global sales and marketing for General Motors. (http://www.nytimes.com/2008/02/18/sports/othersports/18autos.html?_r=1&scp=2&sq=Nascar+General+Motors+racing&st=nyt&oref=slogin accessed July 1, 2008).

The effects of racing on sales of more powerful vehicles and their speeds in use by ordinary drivers on U.S. roads would be difficult to research but it is interesting that death rates are higher in southern states where such racing is more popular. One joke circulated on the Internet says: "When voice monitors were placed in vehicles to record precrash driver utterances, New England drivers usually said 'Oh, my God' while Southern drivers were often heard saying, 'Watch this'." Although the U.S. federal government was given authority to set standards for vehicle safety in the 1960s, speed capability of vehicles sold to the general public has not been regulated. Some governmental and corporate fleets are equipped with speed governors. The national 55 mile-per-hour maximum speed limit, imposed by Congress during the 1970s fuel crisis, was repealed despite the reductions in deaths and fuel use realized in the interim (Altshuler et al., 1984).

Prior to the regulatory period, manufacturers occasionally flirted with preventing injury severity by modifying their vehicles. For example, shatter-resistant glass was developed in the first years of the 20th century and was adopted by a couple of now defunct companies. Ford adopted the technology after one of its design engineers was badly cut in a crash but it did not become standard equipment for all manufacturers until numerous states passed laws requiring it in the 1930s (Eastman, 1984).

Collaboration among outside physicians and researchers and automotive engineers sometimes influenced vehicle modifications. In the 1930s, Detroit plastic surgeon Claire L. Straith installed padded dashboards and shatter-resistant glass in his vehicle and promoted them to manufacturers. In the 1940s, after suffering severe injuries in a plane crash, Hugh DeHaven began studies of injuries in falls from heights relative to surfaces contacted and the effect on injury of configuration of seat belts and other passenger compartment features. He formed a group at Cornell Medical Center in New York to continue the studies and wrote articles for engineering and medical journals emphasizing that the physical principles of mechanical forces and human tolerance to those forces were no different in falls, aircraft crashes, or road crashes. DeHaven visited and consulted with state police and University researchers who collaborated to initiate automotive crash injury research (ACIR) projects in Indiana and later elsewhere that have influenced such field studies ever since. General

Motors and, later, other manufacturers began paying attention to DeHaven's work. In 1952, he convened a conference of what would nowadays be called stakeholders—vehicle manufacturers, insurance companies, safety organizations, and medical and other researchers. The auto manufacturers requested that they be kept informed of DeHaven's and ACIR results. In the 1950s, the automakers started some crash testing using dummies as a result of ACIR findings (Eastman, 1984).

Also in the 1950s Air Force Col. John Stapp turned his attention from crashworthiness of airplanes to automobiles. He put belted monkeys and then humans, including himself, on deceleration sleds to establish human limits to deceleration forces if the energy was spread over the surfaces of the belts. Accompanied by other engineers, he approached the Society of Automotive Engineers to establish an annual conference on vehicle crashworthiness and biomechanics issues that continues to this day as the Stapp Car Crash Conference. After military budgets for injury research were cut, one of Stapp's contractors, James J. Ryan at the University of Minnesota, obtained funding from the U.S. Health Department for 2 years, one of the earliest recognitions by public health authorities that injuries are a public health problem (Eastman, 1984).

In 1951, the insurance industry became involved in sponsorship of research when Liberty Mutual employed Cornell's Aeronautical Laboratory to study vehicle crashworthiness issues. Liberty Mutual subsequently established its own research facility that still operates in Hopkinton, MA. The industry established the Insurance Institute for Highway Safety, which, after reorganization in the early 1970s, has conducted and sponsored key research projects and crash tests ever since.

When Chevrolet introduced a new 8-cylinder engine in the mid-1950s, its sales outpaced Ford's. Ford's Assistant General Manager, Robert S. McNamara, fought the great resistance of his corporation's leaders to counter with a safety package (improved padding and energy-absorbing steering wheels, safety door locks and seat belts). Although demand for seat belts outpaced supplies, the continued greater sales of Chevrolets led to a slogan in the industry, "Safety doesn't sell" (Eastman, 1984). Whether it does or not, that is no excuse to exclude safety features as standard equipment on vehicles. For example, research indicates that electronic stability control in modern vehicles reduces the risk of death about 42% (Farmer, 2006). Yet in 2008 models, it was standard equipment on only 65% of cars and light trucks. (http://www.iihs.org/ratings/esc/esc.aspx, accessed 7/1/2008).

When auto engineers began talking with outsiders about vehicle safety and participating in standard setting in the Society for Automotive Engineering, corporate executives were pooh-poohing the idea. In 1961, General Motors President dismissed "a foolproof and crash proof car" as "unrealistic" (Eastman, 1984). Obviously, but to refuse to do what one could on such grounds was foolish.

Other than the setting up of periodic vehicle inspection in certain states and the adoption of a few consensus standards, such as for headlamps, legislators did not seriously consider regulation of injury-producing characteristics of motor vehicles until the sixth decade of their widespread use. Congressional hearings were held in the 1950s on the developing research knowledge but no legislation was enacted. A few state governments required the installation of lap belts in the front outboard seats of new cars sold in their states in the early 1960s.

By 1964, 14 states required lap belts and manufacturers began installing them in all cars as standard equipment (U.S. Department of Transportation, 1972). Also in 1964, Congress authorized the General Services Administration (GSA), the federal government's management and purchasing agency, to specify safety standards for vehicles sold to the federal government. Requirements for equipment such as energy-absorbing steering assemblies to reduce penetration or crushing of chests in frontal crashes and high penetration-resistant windshields to reduce ejections and severe lacerations were adopted, applicable to 1966 and subsequent model years. The manufacturers responded by providing the equipment somewhat earlier in some cases and as standard equipment in high-volume models sold to the public as well as to the government.

In 1966, Congress enacted and President Lyndon B. Johnson signed the National Traffic and Motor Vehicle Safety Act (Public Law 89-563) along with the separate Highway Safety Act (Public Law 89-564), the latter to establish standards for state programs and assistance in their implementation. The Motor Vehicle Safety Act directed the establishment of a National Traffic Safety Agency in the Commerce Department, which later evolved into the National Highway Traffic Safety Administration (NHTSA) in a newly created Department of Transportation. The act specified that "initial standards" for manufacture of new cars be in effect, based on existing safety standards available at the time, on a prompt schedule by January, 1968. Existing safety standards were mainly those adopted previously for government vehicles and some adopted by the Society of Automotive Engineers. Also, research and development by the new government agency was to begin toward the initiation of subsequent standards. Provision for required notice to owners by manufacturers regarding vehicle defects was also included in the act and subsequently resulted in recall of tens of millions of vehicles.

The process by which such important legislation often comes into being in the United States is instructive. Similar to previously enacted legislation to regulate food and drugs, scandal was the catalyst for the enactment of the laws. In 1965, hearings by the Senate Subcommittee on Executive Reorganization were held on federal government efforts to reduce motor vehicle injuries. The committee's chair, Senator Abraham Ribicoff, during his tenure as Governor of Connecticut became interested in highway injury and gained publicity from a crackdown on speeding. He saw a New York Times article in late 1964 on Haddon, Suchman, and Klein's book, Accident Research, and was intrigued by the point that injuries could be reduced by increasing crashworthiness of vehicles in addition to efforts at "accident prevention." He decided to call upon auto executives to testify about their activities on the issue. During the hearings, the committee staff learned that a lawyer advising them was under surveillance by a private detective hired by General Motors Corporation in an apparent attempt to find information to discredit him. When the committee made this maneuver public, the resulting uproar led the chairman of the board of GM to apologize to the committee and the lawyer. After that, the passage of legislation was only a matter of working out the details among the appropriate congressional committees and the administration. All of the ingredients for action were in place: the scientific evidence, an activist government, and a juicy scandal to bring the issue to the public's attention (McCarry, 1972). The young lawyer that GM had investigated was Ralph Nader, who used his newfound celebrity status and money from a lawsuit against GM and his book, Unsafe at Any Speed, to form organizations active in the passage of other consumer product, safety, and health legislation in the late 1960s and early 1970s. Nader and his raiders, as they were called, were highly critical of the newly formed or upgraded agencies that emerged during the period, as well as of the older regulatory agencies (Sethi, 1977). While scientists sometimes are appalled at the quality of evidence used by so-called citizens' lobbies, whether the pro-regulation types or more recently formed antiregulation types, these lobby-ists have become a part of the political spectrum that must be considered in attempts to modify public health policy.

Among the initial standards issued by the new motor vehicle agency were crash avoidance standards, including reduced glare in drivers' eyes, redundant braking systems, side marker lights, and tire performance and loading. Standards to reduce the severity of injury during a crash specified performance of energy-absorbing steering assemblies, seat belts, windshields, head restraints, and other interior structures as well as performance of door locks and doors to reduce injection or penetration. Post crash, the reduction of fire was the primary focus.

Evaluation of the effectiveness of these standards has produced some contradictory conclusions, but the overwhelming evidence suggests about 40% fewer occupant deaths in cars meeting the standards (trucks were exempted until long thereafter) and some reductions in injuries to persons struck by regulated vehicles (Robertson, 2007b).

After the initial standards were put in effect in 1968, the pace of standards development slowed, at least partly because of a change in U.S. government. When Richard Nixon became President, the first head of the agency, William Haddon, Jr., was not reappointed and was hired by the insurance industry to reorganize the Insurance Institute for Highway Safety into a scientific research organization. The Institute initiated a crash test program and produced a film, In the Crash, showing how its and other organizations tests indicated that far more could be done to modify vehicles to reduce injury severity and property damage. The film, including slow motion air bag test footage, was premiered at a conference of stakeholders convened by the Institute in 1970 (Wixom, 1970). The government did some crash testing but it was mainly focused on compliance with extant standards. Even compliance testing was slowed by administration actions such as impounding of funds intended to build a government crash test facility (Insurance Institute for Highway Safety, 1973).

The most controversial proposed motor vehicle safety regulation in the 1970s was the so-called air bag standard. The first patent for an automatically inflatable bag that would absorb crash forces in severe frontal crashes and spread the forces over larger body surfaces than padding or seat belts was obtained in 1952. In the succeeding years, several companies worked on developing the concept into a workable system. Major motor vehicle manufacturers and suppliers kept the newly formed National Highway Safety Bureau informed of some of the developments. When scientists in the agency were convinced that the system was sufficiently developed, a new standard was proposed. The agency issued an advanced notice of proposed rule making in 1969 to become effective January 1, 1972 (Insurance Institute for Highway Safety, 1977). This original proposal set performance requirements for an "inflatable occupant restraint system" that, after various comments were received, was changed to a more general performance standard specifying automatic provision for minimum crash forces on the head, chest, and knees of a test dummy in a 30-mile-per-hour front and front-angle crash into a rigid test barrier. The standard could then be met by automatic wraparound seat belts as well as air bags (Warner, 1982).

The auto industry argued during the comment period that the technology was not sufficiently developed, was too costly, and that it did not allow sufficient lead-time. These were not new arguments, having been used in opposition to several of the initial standards for 1968 models (Sobel, 1976). Failing to budge the agency beyond a 1-year delay, Henry Ford II and Lee Iacocca, then of Ford Motor Company, met with President Richard M. Nixon and John Ehrlichman in the White House and attempted to convince the president to delay the safety rule making as well as that for emissions and fuel economy. Like other of the transcripts of the White House tapes, there are many unintelligible passages, but the president can be heard directing Mr. Ehrlichman to look into the matter (White House Tapes, 1982). Subsequently, the agency was ordered, over its strong opposition, to accept the buzzer and interlock devices in an attempt to increase seat belt use as an alternative to airbags. Developed by Ford Motor Company, those systems buzzed at drivers, and a later version would not allow the vehicle to start, unless belts were extended from their stowed positions. Many in the public hated the "belt reminder" systems and wrote to Congress objecting to them. Mr. Iacocca subsequently used their unpopularity as an example of the follies of pernicious regulators (Robertson, 1979). In fact, it was one of Ford's worse ideas and the company apparently knew it. Ford ran television ads in 1970 describing the interlock that said, "You probably won't even like it." (Insurance Institute for Highway Safety, 1977). Congress subsequently banned it.

National Highway Traffic Safety Administration's (NHTSA) administrator, and later the Secretary of Transportation, held hearings on the passive restraint rule in 1975 and 1976, respectively. The Secretary found that the benefits of either air bags or automatic belts would greatly exceed the costs but dropped the rule—despite his finding that something more than 12,000 deaths would be prevented each year if all vehicles had air bags—in favor of a "demonstration project" in collaboration with the auto industry. He said his choice was based on concern over public acceptance (U.S. Department of Transportation, 1976), ignoring the public opinion surveys favoring increased automatic crash protection presented in the hearing. The original estimate of the secretary that the demonstration project would involve approximately one-half million automobiles was reduced to less than 70,000 in the actual, nonbinding statements of intent from the auto companies a few months later. Following the election of Jimmy Carter as President, a new Secretary of Transportation announced hearings on the issue. The auto companies then backed out of the previous agreement for a demonstration project. The 1977 hearings produced no new evidence but a different decision was rendered. The new rule required passive restraints in large 1981 models, compact to mid-sized 1982 models, and all 1983 models. Groups both for and against went to court, the former to step up the timetable for the standard and the latter to kill it. The court let it stand.

After the 1980 election, President Reagan appointed a new administrator of the NHTSA, who soon announced a 1-year delay in implementation in 1981 and, after additional hearings, rescinded the standard. The automakers testified that they would use only automatic belts that could be easily detached, and the administrator said that he doubted that the public would use such belts, ignoring any change in the rule that would reduce the likelihood of nonuse or an alternative approach (Warner, 1982).

Various insurance companies and citizens' action groups again appealed to the courts. In a sharply stated opinion, the United States Court of Appeals for the District of Columbia Circuit agreed with the petitioners that the dumping of the standard was "arbitrary, capricious, an abuse of discretion, a violation of law as defined by Section 10 of the Administrative Procedure Act" (State Farm Mutual Insurance Co. et al. v U.S. Department of Transportation, 1982). The court ordered the standard to be reinstated. The government, as well as domestic and foreign automobile manufacturers, appealed the decision but the Supreme Court refused to hear the case, letting the "air bag decision" stand. After moving to Chrysler and learning that two drivers walked away from a head-on crash of Chrysler-made vehicles equipped with air bags, Lee Iaccoca, by then President of Chrysler, became a late convert to support air bags.

As air bags became standard equipment on new passenger cars in the late 1980s, the industry ramped up its introduction of new models of so-called sport utility vehicles (SUVs) and pickup trucks despite evidence that they had a high rollover propensity than passenger cars. In 1978, Professor Richard Snyder and colleagues of the University of Michigan prepared an extensive study of rollover for the Insurance Institute for Highway Safety. He noted that rollover propensity of a vehicle is primarily a function of the width between the center of the tires (T) divided by twice the height of center of gravity from the ground (H), expressed in a simple formula, T/2H. This was called the stability ratio. The ratio measures the force equivalent of gravity needed to tip the vehicle on its side while sitting still. If a vehicle has weight higher off the ground, but has the same width as another vehicle, it will overturn more frequently in turning maneuvers at the same speed. The turning maneuver creates the gravity equivalent lateral force, called centrifugal force.

The Snyder team collected statistics that showed higher rollover rates among vehicles with lower values of T/2H. He found that all vehicles with a stability ratio less than 1.2 had inordinately high rollover rates. The worst among these was the Jeep CJ5, a vehicle much like the staff vehicle used by the military during World War II and thereafter, but sold to the public for use as a utility vehicle (Snyder et al., 1980).

The Insurance Institute for Highway Safety tested the Jeep CJ5 and a slightly more stable CJ7 in turns at various speeds, driven by remote control. In a 90-degree turn, the CJ5 overturned at 22 miles per hour. In a slalom-like avoidance maneuver, the CJ5 rolled over at 32 miles per hour. The Insurance Institute's tests were broadcast on the popular TV news program *60 Minutes* in 1981. Statistical studies at the University of North Carolina (Reinfurt et al., 1984) and the NHTSA (Smith, 1982) found high rollover rates and/or rollover death rates per registered vehicle among sports utility vehicles in comparison with cars.

A colleague and I updated the data in the mid-1980s and found a strong correlation between T/2H and rollover among vehicles with T/2H less than 1.2 (Robertson & Kelley, 1989). Soon after our rollover paper was completed in 1986, my coauthor, Ben Kelley, sent a copy, along with other studies, to then Congressman Timothy Wirth. Mr. Wirth submitted a petition to the NHTSA requesting consideration that a minimum stability of T/2H = 1.2 be required for new vehicles sold in the United States for passenger use and that recall of Jeep CJs be considered.

Although the federal regulatory agencies were by then run by antiregulation ideologues, some members of the staff at the NHTSA welcomed the stimulus to study the issue further. Two of the agency's staff, Anna Harwin and Keith Brewer, collected center of gravity data on a larger set of vehicles than we had examined. They correlated T/2H with total rollover rates, not just fatal, in several states. They found an even stronger correlation of T/2H and total rollover rates than we had found in the fatality data. The study was published eventually, but was initially suppressed by the government (Harwin & Brewer, 1990).

Years later, after she left the government, Anna Harwin told me that people involved in the investigation were behaving like the results were a state secret. She and Brewer wanted to present the results of their study at a meeting of the Society of Automotive Engineers but were not allowed to do so because of opposition from the office of the Chief Counsel. In a memorandum to Michael Finkelstein, who was Harwin and Brewer's boss, Steven Wood wrote: "The very first sentence of the abstract states that statistical confirmation of the relationship between rollover stability and rollover risk has been established. Such a statement is the basis explicitly set forth in the Wirth petition for the requested rulemaking and defect investigation on vehicle rollover." After noting some disagreement in the agency on the issue, Wood wrote: "After the agency has resolved this internal disagreement and published its response to the Wirth petition, you may wish to revise this paper to reflect the agency position on the issue." In other words, one of the top lawyers in the federal safety agency wanted a scientific paper revised to support a political decision.

The agency sent the Harwin-Brewer data to be analyzed by researchers at the Transportation Systems Center in Cambridge, MA. The government researchers there used a different statistical technique, but the conclusion was nevertheless the same: "The previous results of Kelley/Robertson and Harwin/ Brewer in finding the stability factor important for predicting rollover rate have been confirmed and strengthened by these results" (Mengert et al., 1989).

Several senior staff in the agency recommended in memoranda to Barry Felrice, Associate Administrator for Rulemaking, that a rollover standard be adopted but the standard was rejected at the direction of Diane Steed, the Reagan-appointed Administrator of the agency. Steed had no prior education or experience in motor vehicle safety. She was obviously an administration watchdog who was appointed to the job to quash regulation. The justification for the rejection, written by Felrice, is a tortured, self-contradictory document (Felrice, 1987). In a memorandum on a draft of the rejection circulated before its publication, Michael Finkelstein wrote to Felrice, "It is clear, however, that the inclusion of analyses in this draft has been very selective, and was designed to support a certain rulemaking position." Later Finkelstein again wrote Felrice objecting to false statements put in the Federal Register: "The statement 'while a vehicle's stability factor has some relation to its rollover propensity, etc.', is misleading and grossly understates the high degree of correlation that has been found between Rollover frequency and Rollover Stability Factor." ... "We see no new data, analysis, or arguments in this document which would change our previously stated view that this petition should be granted." Nevertheless, the standard was not adopted and, not long thereafter, in April 1988, George Parker, Associate Administrator for Enforcement, denied Wirth's petition for a defect investigation of the Jeep CJs.

I was invited to give a presentation at the Society of Automotive Engineers Government-Industry meeting in Washington the following month. Using the data on static stability gathered by the government during consideration of the Wirth petition, I expanded the sample of vehicles to include more recently marketed Bronco IIs, Samurais, and small Blazer-Jimmys. The results were the same. On average, as the stability ratio increased, the fatal rollover rates declined precipitously up to $T/2H = 1.2$. During 1982 through 1987, the Jeep CJ5 had a rollover death rate 19 times that of passenger cars. The Jeep CJ7, pre-1978 Bronco, and Bronco II rolled over about 10 to 12 times the car rate. The Suzuki Samurai, made infamous by Consumer's Union finding of "unacceptable" in Consumer Reports, was actually somewhat more stable than the Jeep and Ford vehicles, but was bad enough to roll at 6 times the rate for passenger cars (Robertson, 1989). During my presentation, a few auto engineers argued that the effect of static stability could be offset somewhat by suspension systems. When I asked whether it could be totally offset, none said that it could.

The Consumer Reports article, based on tests showing the Samurari's lack of rollover resistance in a slalom course, caused a media feeding frenzy. Consumer Reports later carried an article pointing to the stability problems of the Bronco II, but it did not call it "unacceptable."

Texas enacted a law that allowed courts to release "court protected" industry documents if a compelling reason to protect public health was indicated. Russ Cook, a Houston attorney, petitioned a court to release Ford's Bronco II history. The court granted the petition. Among the documents was a memorandum regarding a meeting between Ford executives and the staff of Consumer's Union. The memo said that the Ford team thought they had clouded the minds of the CU staff. Cloudy mind or no, Consumers Union, the Insurance Institute for Highway Safety, and individual citizens continued to submit petitions to the government for a stability standard and the recall of vehicles such as the Jeep CJs, the Suzuki Samurai, and the Ford Bronco II. All of these petitions were rejected in the first Bush and Clinton administrations.

The Ford memo on its visit to Consumer's Union is only one of many internal documents that would reveal corporate attempts to hide problems. Often such evidence is found in discovery proceedings in lawsuits but is protected by the courts, allegedly because documents include "trade secrets" that would be advantageous to competitors if revealed. These include descriptions of crash tests revealing fire hazards, rollover propensity, rooftop failures in rollovers, and the like (Robertson, 2000). Trial lawyers for the injured often agree to such protection in exchange for substantial settlements for their clients.

After her government tenure, Diane Steed headed a lobbying group called Coalition for Vehicle Choice funded largely by vehicle manufacturers. She testified in a court case that the main focus of the lobbying was in opposition to fuel economy standards. In 1991–1992, her organization took in $6 million for such work. When newspaper articles critical of sports utility vehicles appeared, Steed wrote letters to the editors defending the vehicles with half-truths. In the Hartford Courant she wrote, "Data from the National Highway Traffic Safety Administration and the Insurance Institute for Highway Safety show light trucks (SUVs, pickups, and minivans), especially the large SUVs, have among the lowest fatality record on the road" (Steed, 1998). In fact, the Insurance Institute for Highway Safety's newsletter, Status Report, reported data indicating that pickup trucks and SUVs in the same weight class as cars had consistently higher occupant death rates than the cars in that weight class. While it is true that the nonrollover occupant death rates of some of the larger utility vehicles were relatively low compared to smaller vehicles, they were low because their weight resulted in a huge energy transfer to occupants of other vehicles in crashes (Insurance Institute for Highway Safety, 1998). In collisions with other motor vehicles, the heaviest pickups and SUVs, of which there are no comparable cars in weight, kill people in the other vehicles more frequently and kill more pedestrians and bicyclists. Their higher bumpers override the side door beams of passenger cars and they strike pedestrians in vital organs rather than the legs. Not counted in that analysis is the greater frequency that vehicles with high center of gravity run over children while backing up in home driveways. The visibility to the rear from the position of a higher seated driver is poorer than that from passenger cars.

Several others among the NHTSA's political appointees and career bureaucrats, after retirement, went to work for the motor vehicle industry or its defenders. The Motor Vehicle Manufacturer's Association hired Barry Felrice, who wrote the Federal Register entries rejecting all of the petitions for a rollover standard prior to 1998. George Parker, who rejected most of the CJ, Samurai, and Bronco II defect petitions, retired to work for the Association of International Vehicle Manufacturers. Usually, when the media took note of the rollover problem, Felrice or Parker was trotted out by the industry to claim that the problem is behavioral rather than vehicular. In 1998, Parker told Dateline NBC, "But I think if you look at the facts from the large scale accident data, you come to the same conclusion that NHTSA does ... I think there's a myth that taking avoidance maneuvers for obstacles in the roadway is going to cause the vehicle to roll over. That's just not the case. The person driving that vehicle did something to lose control of that vehicle. What they are mostly doing is driving on curvy rural roads with high alcohol use."

In fact, NHTSA said nothing of the sort. For example, in the June 28, 1994 Federal Register, the agency noted that only 23% of the differences among vehicles in rollover was explained by driver and environmental factors. "The results of both the logistic and linear regression analyses performed by the agency suggest that a vehicle stability metric alone can account for approximately 50 percent of the variability in rollover risk in single vehicle accidents, for the population of make/models studied. While ideally it would be desirable to have these variables explain 100 percent of the remaining variability, such statistical correlations are almost never achieved" (Felrice, 1994). And many of the rollovers of unstable vehicles do occur in avoidance maneuvers—the vehicle rolls when the driver turns sharply in an attempt to protect animals as well as human pedestrians, or to keep from hitting other vehicles or objects in the road. Despite this kind of evidence, the government had not set a standard for static stability as of mid-2008.

The special lobbying group developed by Diane Steed as well as the older trade associations for whom Barry Felrice and George Parker worked after leaving the government are part of the extensive lobbying presence in Washington, D.C. and state capitols maintained by the motor vehicle industry. Federal lobbying expenditures for the motor vehicle manufacturers more than doubled in the first 7 years after the turn of the 21st century, reaching approximately $58 million in 2007 (http://www.opensecrets.org/lobby/induscode. php?lname=T2100&year=2008, accessed July 26, 2008). Corporations are also the major sponsors of "think tanks" devoted primarily to promoting antigovernment "scholars," "tort reform," and other policies favorable to corporations (http://www.washingtonmonthly.com/features/1999/9911.callahan.think. html; http://www.corporateeurope.org/ThinkTankSurvey2006.html, accessed August 5, 2008).

The adverse effect of huge SUVs and pickup trucks was not just higher rollover rates. Because of their excess weights, they had larger, more powerful engines that emitted more pollutants and consumed more fuel per mile, on average, than cars. Although industry-based scientists claimed that increased weight increased safety, the net effect of excess weight, after accounting for other vehicle characteristics, is adverse to safety as well as fuel economy and emissions (Robertson, 2006).

Reduction of Risk from Emissions

Motor vehicles have an environmental impact ranging from the extraction and processing of the materials to make them, the extraction of the oil and refining process to run them, the emissions of combustion by-products, and the return of materials to the environment from junked vehicles (Melosi, 2004). Most of the wars of the 20th century, as well as the Iraq War beginning in 2003, involved issues related to the control of oil reserves (Hiro, 2007). Many of the effects of extraction and refining oil are more local but the emissions from burning gasoline and diesel oil have spread worldwide.

A high concentration of registered vehicles per population and the effect of heat inversions in the Los Angeles basin made vehicle pollution evident earlier in California than in other areas of the world. That state has led the United

States for decades in attempts to reduce pollution by regulation, its rules often adopted eventually for the United States as a whole.

The first major public recognition of air pollution in California occurred during a heat inversion in the summer of 1943 in Los Angeles. Many corporations, including motor vehicle manufacturers and oil interests, recognized that it was in their interest to support pollution control technology rather than have to deal with limits on population and vehicle growth (Gonzalez, 2005). In 1947, the state government enacted an Air Pollution Control Act that provided for monitoring of air pollution. In 1952, nitrogen oxides and hydrocarbons, major components of vehicle emissions, were found to create smog when exposed to ultraviolet radiation from the sun. The Federal Air Pollution Control Act of 1955 authorized support for research and technical assistance but not standards. California legislators directed the State Health Department to set air quality standards, including vehicle emissions. The Positive Crankcase Ventilation (PCV) valve was required on vehicles sold in California in 1961. The PCV entry in Wikipedia says that General Motors perfected the valve, licensed it free to other manufacturers and it was placed voluntarily on vehicles in California but the California governmental history states that it was required (http://www.arb.ca.gov/html/brochure/history.htm accessed July 1, 2008). Planting of false claims favorable to corporations or adverse to its critics on the Internet may be a relatively new industry tactic difficult to document. The originators of much of the material on the great misinformation superhighway are anonymous.

The first Federal Clean Air Act was enacted in 1963 followed by the Motor Vehicle Air Pollution Control Act of 1965. This legislation gave the Secretary of Health, Education and Welfare the authority to study air pollution and issue standards to reduce it. California adopted standards for tailpipe emissions of hydrocarbons and carbon monoxide in 1966. Legislation consolidating the clean air provisions and creating the U.S. Environmental Protection Agency (EPA) to administer those and other environmental standards were enacted in 1970. California continued to regulate in advance of the federal government and sometimes in conflict with the U.S. government as well as industry.

In 1972, the EPA turned down California's State Implementation Plan. Nevertheless, California standards resulted in the motor vehicle industry's use of catalytic converters that reduce the toxicity of nitrogen oxides and hydrocarbons. An important benefit of the adoption of the catalytic converter was the banning of lead additives in gasoline because it destroyed the effectiveness of the converter. EPA adopted the California standards as national standards in 1975. One of the by-products of the catalytic converter, however, is carbon dioxide, now known as a substantial factor in global warming.

Lead diminishes brain function and is related to a variety of behavioral problems in children. Dr. Herbert Needleman, who did pioneering research on the health effects of lead (Needleman et al., 1979), was badgered by the lead industry and charged by its paid consultants with falsifying evidence. The scientific community ultimately exonerated Needleman but his work suffered from the distraction. More recently, governmental scientists warning of global warming have had their work edited to water it down by their superiors and both sides in the debate have complained of harassment (Eilperin, 2006; Lindgren, 2006).

By the mid-1980s, the air in U.S. cities was noticeably cleaner to anyone who was there in the 1960s and environmental scientists declared it healthier but the continuous increase in numbers of vehicles partly offsets the gains (Ayres et al., 2006). Although the motor vehicle industry argued in the 1970s that it would be ruined by the combination of safety, fuel economy and pollution standards, even threatening to shut down, it thrived through most of the 1980s and 1990s until the stock market and housing market bubbles burst and oil price rose exponentially after the turn of the century.

Lessons for Public Health

This chapter has presented numerous instances in which corporations making motor vehicles and their allies in supportive industries have attempted to divert attention from the harmful effects of their products and prevent governmental intervention to reduce harm. Their major strategies are: (1) Deny responsibility (claim that the driver is the cause); (2) lobby against legislation and specific proposed federal and state rules to regulate safety, pollution and fuel economy; and (3) support trade associations, think tanks and ad hoc issue groups to produce material for public media in support of the first two strategies.

Public health policy relative to effects of corporate actions evolves in the context of national history, prevalent ideology regarding the proper role of government in protecting the public's health, more or less scientific certainty regarding the health effects of specific acts or negligence in corporate behavior, and the power of corporations to influence government and public debate. Despite the nation's history of economic enterprise largely unfettered by governmental influence, prevalent antiregulation ideology by several U.S. Presidents, substantial lack of scientific interest in practical health issues relative to "basic science," and antiregulation rhetoric and lobbying by some of the most powerful corporations in the world, motor vehicles sold in the United States are far less likely to maim or poison their users and others exposed to them than they were in the first 65 years of their use. Yet much that is known to minimize risk is not yet fully applied.

This chapter has noted several approaches to influence corporate behavior that have had at least some success.

Scientists whose findings conflict with corporate claims may influence industry by publicizing the findings. Advocates may also use the information to create an aura of scandal. A periodic conference of stakeholders to review scientific evidence has sometimes changed corporate behavior. Scientific societies where independent scientists and corporate scientists and technicians exchange information may be useful. In stakeholder meetings and scientific societies, however, scientists and others must be cautious that cooperation does not become co-optation.

Revelation of scandal has been a potent force for adoption of new rules for health and safety. One way to reveal scandal is to search files of registered lobbyists and research their backgrounds. For example, is a retired or active member of Congress who benefited from industry connected campaign contributions fronting for the industry?

When federal agencies are co-opted by antiregulation ideologues and corporate lobbyists, persuading state governments to adopt standards may lead to universal adoption by corporations. Support for research and advocacy may be obtained from corporations hurt by the actions or negligence of other corporations.

REFERENCES

Altshuler AA, et al. *55: A Decade of Experience*. Washington, DC: National Research Council; 1984.

Ayres J, Maynard R, Richards R, eds. *Air Pollution and Health*. London: Imperial College Press; 2006.

Black E. *Internal Combustion: How Corporations and Governments Addicted the World to Oil and Derailed the Alternatives*. New York: St. Martin's Press; 2006.

Broome J. The ethics of climate change. *Sci Am.* 2008;298:96–102.

Deffeyes KS. *Beyond Oil: The View from Hubbert's Peak*. New York: Hill and Wang; 2005.

Eastman JW. *Styling vs. Safety: The American Automobile Industry and the Development of Automotive Safety*. Lanham, MD: University Press of America; 1984.

Eilperin J. Climate researchers feeling heat from White House. Available at: http://www.washingtonpost.com/wp-dyn/content/article/2006/04/05/AR2006040502150.html. Published 2006. Accessed July 28, 2008.

Evans L. *Traffic Safety and the Driver.* New York: Van Nostrand Reinhold; 1991.

Farmer CM. Effects of electronic stability control: an update. *Traffic Inj Prev.* 2006;7:319–324.

Felrice B. Denial of petition for rulemaking. *Fed Regist.* 1987;52:49033–49038.

Felrice B. Consumer information regulations; Federal Motor Vehicle Safety Standards; rollover prevention. *Fed Regist.* 1994;59:33254–33271.

First National Conference on Street and Highway Safety. Washington, DC: U.S. Department of Commerce; 1924.

Gonzales GA. *The Politics of Air Pollution.* Albany: State University of New York Press; 2005.

Harwin EA, Brewer HK. Analysis of the relationship between vehicle rollover stability and rollover risk using the NHTSA CARDfile Accident Database. *J Traffic Med.* 1990;18:109.

Hiro D. *Blood of the Earth: The Battle for the World's Vanishing Oil Resources.* New York: Nation Books; 2007.

Insurance Institute for Highway Safety. President Nixon impounds safety funds. *Status Report.* 1973;8(4):1.

Insurance Institute for Highway Safety. *Background Manual on the Passive Restraint Issue.* Washington, DC: Insurance Institute for Highway Safety; 1977.

Insurance Institute for Highway Safety. Crash compatibility: How vehicle type, weight affect outcomes. *Status Report.* 1998:33.

Kelley AB. *The Pavers and the Paved.* New York: Donald W. Brown, Inc; 1971.

Lindgren R. Climate of fear. Available at: http://www.opinionjournal.com/extra/?id=110008220. Published 2006. Accessed July 28, 2008.

McCarry C. *Citizen Nader.* New York: Saturday Review Press; 1972.

Melosi, MV. The Automobile and the Environment in American History. Available at: http://www.autolife.umd.umich.edu/Environment/E_Overview/E_Overview4.htm. Published 2004. Accessed July 1, 2008.

Mengert P, Salvatore S, DiSario R, Walter R. *Statistical Estimation of Rollover Risk.* Transportation Systems Center, U.S. Department of Transportation; 1989.

National Center for Health Statistics. *Leading Causes of Death 1900–1998.* Atlanta, GA: Centers for Disease Control; 2008.

Needleman HL, Gunnoe C, Leviton A, et al. Deficits in psychologic and classroom performance of children with elevated dentine lead levels. *N Engl J Med.* 1979;300:689–732.

Reinfurt DW, Stutts JC, Hamilton EG. *A Further Look at Utility Vehicle Rollovers.* University of North Carolina Highway Safety Research Center; 1984.

Robertson LS. Gimcrack from Ford? *Wall St J.* October 15, 1979.

Robertson LS. Crash involvement of teenaged drivers when driver education is eliminated from high school. *Am J Public Health.* 1980;70:599–603.

Robertson LS. Risk of fatal rollover in utility vehicles relative to static stability. *Am J Public Health.* 1989;79:300–303.

Robertson LS. *The Expert Witness Scam.* 2000. www.lulu.com.

Robertson LS. Motor vehicle deaths: failed policy analysis and neglected policy. *J Public Health Policy.* 2006;27:182–189.

Robertson LS. Prevention of motor-vehicle deaths by changing vehicle factors. *Inj Prev.* 2007a;13:307–310.

Robertson LS. *Injury Epidemiology (Appendix 13-1).* New York: Oxford University Press; 2007b.

Robertson LS, Kelley AB. Static stability as a predictor of rollover in fatal motor vehicle crashes. *J Trauma.* 1989;29:313.

Sethi SP. Corporations and the citizens at large. In: Sethi SP, ed. *Up Against the Corporate Wall: Modern Corporations and Social Issues of the Seventies.* Englewood Cliffs, NJ: Prentice-Hall; 1977.

Shaoul J. *The Use of Accidents and Traffic Offenses as Criteria for Evaluating Courses in Driver Education Salford.* England: University of Salford; 1975.

Smith SR. *Analysis of Fatal Rollover Accidents in Utility Vehicles.* Washington, DC: National Highway Traffic Safety Administration; 1982.

Snyder RG, McDole TL, Ladd WM, Minahan DJ. *On-road Crash Experience of Utility Vehicles.* Ann Arbor: University of Michigan Highway Safety Research Center; 1980.

Sobel LA. Safety and other problems. In: Sobel LA, ed. *Consumer Protection.* New York: Facts On File, Inc.; 1976.

State Farm Mutual Insurance Co., et al., v. Department of Transportation, No. 81-2220 and National Association of Independent Insurers, Automobile Owners Action Council, et al., v. National Highway Traffic Safety Administration, No. 81-2221. Washington, DC: United States Court of Appeal for the District of Columbia; 1982.

Steed DK. Misguided criticism of SUVs. *Hartford Courant* March 21, 1998:A8.

U.S. Department of Transportation. Laws requiring seat belts. *Traffic Laws Commentary.* 1972;1:1.

U.S. Department of Transportation. *The Secretary's Decision Concerning Motor Vehicle Occupant Protection.* Washington, DC: U.S. Department of Transportation; 1976.

Warner KW. *Mandatory Passive Restraint Systems in Automobiles: Issues and Evidence.* Washington, DC: U.S. Congress Office of Technology Assessment; 1982.

White House Tapes. Part of a Conversation Among President Nixon, Lide Anthony Iacocca, Henry Ford II and John D. Ehrlichman in the Oval Office on April 27, 1971, between 11:08 and 11:43 A.M. *Automotive Litigation Reporter.* November 18, 1982:1784–1798.

Wixom C, ed. *Key Issues in Highway Safety.* Washington, DC: Insurance Institute for Highway Safety; 1970.

9

Alcohol Industry Interests, Global Trade Agreements, and Their Impact on Public Health

Donald W. Zeigler

Global Impact of Alcohol, No Ordinary Commodity in
Trade Agreements

Alcohol is deeply embedded in many societies and cultures.
Harmful use of alcohol is one of the main factors contributing to
premature deaths and avoidable disease burden worldwide (WHO,
2008). There are causal relationships between alcohol consumption
and more than 60 types of disease and injury, including traffic
fatalities. Alarmingly, 4% of the total global burden of disease is
attributable to alcohol, about as much death and disability globally as
tobacco or hypertension (Room et al., 2005).

Alcohol consumption is the leading risk factor for disease
burden in low-mortality developing countries and the third largest
risk factor in developed nations. Beyond the numerous chronic
and acute health effects, alcohol use is associated with widespread
social, mental, and emotional consequences (WHO, 2004). Growing
scientific evidence has demonstrated the harmful effects of
consumption prior to adulthood on the brains, mental, cognitive, and
social functioning of youth and increased likelihood of adult alcohol
dependence and alcohol-related problems among those who drink
before full physiological maturity. Alcohol is a drug that causes
substantial medical, psychological, and social harm by means of

physical toxicity, intoxication, and dependence. The global burden related to alcohol consumption, both in terms of morbidity and mortality, has a major impact on public health (Zeigler et al., 2005).

Decades of hard-fought advocacy and research have identified evidence-based strategies that reduce alcohol-related problems in society. An expert international panel sponsored by the World Health Organization identified "best practices": addressing minimum legal purchasing age, government monopoly of retail sales, restrictions on hours or days of sale, outlet density restrictions, and alcohol taxes (Babor et al., 2003). However, the alcohol industry generally opposes such measures in favor of less effective measures that are less threatening to their bottom line. Industry-promoted alternative measures include alcohol education, corporate self-regulation, and drinkers taking personal responsibility (Anderson 2003; Yoast 2004).

Alcohol is a global commodity. While beer is primarily produced locally by or under licensure from multinational corporations, branded spirits and wines are exported widely. Spirits account for the largest global sales followed by European-style beer (Room et al., 2002). Agreements between countries facilitate commerce, including the transport and sale of alcohol products. This chapter addresses ways the alcohol industry is involved in international trade agreements and how such agreements affect and even undercut alcohol control measures that seek to reduce overall consumption and thereby reduce the harmful consequences of alcohol use and overuse. This dichotomy demonstrates the fundamental conflict between unfettered free trade in alcohol and public health (Forut, 2007).

Global Trade Agreements: Background

Globalization involves the integration of national economies into a single market for goods and services and for the flow of capital and investment. The past two decades have witnessed the emergence and consolidation of a global economic paradigm focused on the removal of barriers to trade and finance, including domestic deregulations (Cornia, 2001). A leader of the World Economic Forum, of which SABMiller brewing company is an industry partner, cynically defined "globalization as the freedom of our corporation to invest where and when we want, to produce what we want, to buy and to sell where we want, and to keep all the restrictions through labor law or other political regulations as slight as possible" (Herfeldt, 2002).

As with any other globally traded commodity, policies dealing with alcohol fall under legal obligations that nations make with each other within the body of international treaties that have grown up since the end of World War II. This section provides somewhat technical background on trade agreements beginning with the World Trade Organization (WTO) and then to regional or bilateral agreement. This orientation is important for understanding the tools available to the alcohol industry to expand trade of its products and to disregard or weaken domestic alcohol control policy (Anderson & Baumberg, 2006).

World Trade Organization

International agreements establishing rules for trade among signatory countries have formalized the process of world trade, foreign investment, and reduced government regulations. The WTO, currently with 153 member countries, is the major player in this global trading process. The WTO presumes that stimulating trade will produce significant benefits through enhanced competition and efficiency, lower prices, and better quality and wider consumer choice of products and services. Moreover, increased domestic and foreign investment will lead to economic growth, a higher standard of living, and improved health for all societies, particularly the developing countries (Zeigler, 2009).

Under the General Agreement on Trades and Tariffs (GATT) and multilateral treaties from the 1940s to the formation of the WTO in 1995, trade agreements focused on trade in *goods* and, specifically, reducing tariffs, and taxes (Campaign, 2002). Import tariffs increase the price of imported products and thus have the effect of lessening demand and consumption of the particular product. Since consumers pay more for the foreign products, domestic producers face less outside competition and have less incentive to advertise or to improve the quality and variety of their products (Secretariat, 2005). However, these consequences of tariffs are consistent with alcohol control policies since higher prices, less marketing, and lower quality tend to reduce alcohol consumption and related problems (Babor et al., 2003; World Bank, 2003).

The WTO General Agreement on Trade in Services (GATS) is the first and only set of multilateral rules governing international trade in *services* and "constitutes one of the most important trade agreements from the perspective of health" (Fidler et al., 2005; WTO, 1999). GATS covers a broad range of service sectors, every possible means of supplying a service, and might include the production, transportation of grain to the brewery or distillery, alcohol production, bottling, distribution, marketing, advertising and serving of alcohol (Grieshaber-Otto & Schacter, 2002; Fidler et al., 2005; Secretariat, 2005).

World Trade Organization (WTO) member voluntarily nations make specific commitments to open particular service sectors and specify conditions of trade. However, nations are also obligated to "engage in successive rounds of negotiations with a view to achieving progressively a higher level of liberalization in trade in services" (Fidler et al., 2005). While Canada has totally declined to make any commitments on alcohol (Ontario, 2003), the United States has not yet made broad commitments covering alcohol distribution. But, if WTO members achieve the GATS objective to eventually including all services, these limits on open markets by the United States will be temporary (Shaffer, Waitzkin et al., 2005). Moreover, nations can request that other countries open their borders to trade in particular service sectors. For example, the *European Union* and United States seek market access on alcohol in all countries (Gould, 2005).

Since the purpose is expansion of trade, agreements can only constrain or proscribe—rather than strengthen—government regulation of alcohol, for example, advertising and even policies that are clearly nondiscriminatory to foreign interests (Gould, 2005). Moreover, under GATS, no government action, whatever its purpose, is in principle beyond scrutiny and challenge, including measures taken by "central, regional or local governments and authorities; and non-governmental bodies" in the exercise of government-related powers. Thus, trade agreements made by national governments preempt measures by local governments to control alcohol problems (Sinclair & Grieshaber-Otto, 2002).

Some obligations imposed by GATS are analogous to constitutional obligations, as they restrict exercise of domestic legislative power in matters of fundamental importance (such as health), in ways that are difficult to undo (Belsky et al., 2004). Countries that modify or withdraw commitments are liable for requests for punitive trade sanctions or compensation from other affected countries (Sinclair, 2005). Later in this chapter, we shall discuss an example of when a case brought by Antigua shocked the United States and reverberates with significant public health ramifications.

It is important to note that trade agreements bind national governments but not corporations (Grieshaber-Otto & Schacter, 2002). Moreover, trade agreements are notorious for extending to corporations the rights of individuals, including freedom of (commercial) speech, and protection against government actions that might impair a corporation's future ability to profit from its investments (Jernigan, 2001).

Regional and Bilateral Agreements

Regional trade agreements (RTAs) have become a very prominent feature of the multilateral trading system in recent years with close to 400 RTAs scheduled to be implemented by 2010 (WTO, 2008b). The United States and *European Union* are leading this expansion of RTAs and bilateral agreements with the hope that a multitude of these agreements, covering enough of the globe, will have changed international norms and terms of trade. Bypassing the WTO, RTAs offer flexibility to pursue "trade-expanding policies not addressed well in [WTO] global trading rules" (Newfarmer, 2005). RTAs "increasingly touch upon policy areas uncharted by ... [WTO] agreements [and] may place developing countries, in particular, in a weaker position" with stronger trade partners that are attempting to open markets (Fidler et al., 2005; Weissman, 2003).

While WTO rules have relatively weak protections for investors, new RTAs contain greater enforcement provisions favoring corporations (Shaffer and Brenner et al., 2005). The North American Free Trade Agreement (NAFTA) includes the first investor rights clause in RTAs and contains very strong investment provisions, including allowing investors to bring law suits against a government without making any distinction between socially beneficial or harmful investments. Since any new domestic regulation is bound to have an economic impact on some private interests, this doctrine is a formula to limit the authority of government and cripple the regulatory state (Greider, 2001; Weissman, 2003). The U.S. model Bilateral Investment Treaty includes this investor-state provision and is now a common feature in U.S. regional and bilateral treaties (USTR, 2004).

Since foreign investors can directly challenge a government for alleged breaches of the treaty (Taylor et al., 2000), the investor-state dispute mechanism bypasses domestic laws and juridical authority that protect the public's health and general welfare and shortcut ways that governments normally resolve disputes between themselves (Greider, 2002). Since corporations can challenge government regulations as barriers to free trade or even expropriating their assets, this may have a chilling effect on governments seeking to formulate appropriate health legislation, including domestic regulation of alcohol (Baumberg & Anderson 2008; Gould, 2005; Shaffer et al., 2005).

While many nongovernmental, public health and antiglobalization groups are concerned about the rapid development and draconian features of regional and bilateral agreements, it might surprise many that even the WTO has a special Committee on Regional Trade Agreements (RTAs), set up in 1996, to monitor and assess whether regional trade agreements help or hinder the overall WTO (WTO, 2005b). Of concern to the WTO has been the "regulatory regimes which increasingly touch upon policy areas uncharted by multilateral [i.e., WTO] trade agreements [that] may place developing countries, in particular, in a weaker position with stronger trading partners attempting to open their markets than under the multilateral [i.e. WTO] framework" (Crawford & Fiorentino, 2005).

Goals of Industry in Trade Agreements—Immediate, Long
Term, Potential

The alcohol industry is a complex, international group of business entities
with great economic and political power and influence at all levels of society
and around the globe. Even though segments within the overall industry may
conflict over particular issues and fight for market share, the alcohol industry
seeks to maximize its profits and create a policy and legislative environment
favorable to its operations with as few controls as possible. As a whole, the
industry seeks to build, maintain, and expand product and brand loyalty and
sales, and to obscure its role as anything other than a good corporate citizen.
While marketing and promotion foster consumption and sales through an
image of alcohol's connections with all the good things in life (and none of the
bad), the goal of the industry is to act to increase profits and sales, to maintain
and enlarge its consumer base, and to create a political, economic, cultural
environment conducive to reaching these goals. It is not interested in reducing its scale, consumption of its product, or its abilities to operate as it sees fit
(Callard et al., 2001; Yoast, 2004).

Unfettered free trade enhances the likelihood that industry will achieve
its goals. Without exception, free trade agreements treat alcohol products as
conventional "goods" and assume that expanding commerce in these products is beneficial (Babor et al., 2003; Campaign, 2001; World Bank, 2003).
Consequently and quite deliberately, liberalization of trade increases availability and access, lowers prices through reduced taxation and tariffs, and increases
promotion and advertising of alcohol (Andreasson et al., 2006; Secretariat,
2005; World Bank, 2003). The net result is increased sale and consumption
of alcohol.

It therefore follows that the industry "enthusiastically supports the
work of the World Trade Organization." In April, 2006, the Distilled Spirits
Council of the United States (DISCUS) reported that since the "conclusion
of the Uruguay Round of WTO in 1994, U.S. exports of distilled spirits
have increased 86%, growing to $743 million in 2005" (DISCUS, 2006a).
According to the European Spirits Organization (commonly referred to as
CEPS), the "EU is the world's leading producer of spirit drinks, exporting
to some 200 world markets and generating more than €5 billion a year to
the EU's balance of payments. Given such large export interests, it is hardly
surprising that ... CEPS is so heavily involved in international trade matters."
The sector contributes more than €4 billion to the *European Union's* (EU's)
balance of trade and represents Europe's most exported foodstuff (European
Spirits News, 2006).

Prior to the 2005 WTO Hong Kong Ministerial meeting, the World Spirits Alliance reported that while ending tariffs is its "foremost priority ... tariffs have been driven down progressively within the GATT ... so the *importance of non-tariff barriers as impediments to market access has increased significantly.*" (emphasis added). Moreover, it "is clear that the services negotiating mandate [of WTO] includes those areas of particular interest to the industry, namely distribution and advertising services" (World Spirits Alliance, 2005). The industry realizes that tariffs are less an ongoing issue and that they will increasingly target "service" sector barriers that affect their bottom line.

Similarly, during the WTO Doha Round, the European Spirits Coalition described its sector's priorities as follows:

1. improved access to third country markets;
2. reduction, and where possible, elimination of tariffs imposed by WTO members on imports of distilled spirits, with particular emphasis on "peak tariffs";
3. liberalization, and where possible, elimination of nontariff barriers to access for imported spirits;
4. better protection of spirits with geographical indications, most notably through the creation of a legally binding registry for wines and spirits; and
5. an ambitious agreement on trade facilitation (European Spirits Organization, 2008d).

In addition, the World Spirits Alliance set a priority to liberalize services related to "restrictions on marketing, including elimination of discriminatory advertising measures" (DISCUS, 2001b; World Spirits Alliance, 2005). According to DISCUS, the World Spirits Alliance had called for a "unified trade negotiating strategy" covering *nontariff measures* (import quotas and licensing, state trading, product standards, and labeling requirements) and *services* (restrictions on marketing and advertising, distribution and retailing) (DISCUS, 2003b). If accomplished, trade agreements would liberalize "restrictions on distribution rights and advertising freedoms as essential components of market access" (World Spirits Alliance, 2005). Similarly, an objective of DISCUS had been "elimination of discriminatory restrictions in the advertising and distribution of imported spirits" (DISCUS, 2006a). Such measures, unless addressed in trade agreements, may restrict promotion and sale of alcohol and reduce consumption and corporate profits.

Moreover and legitimately, the industry placed high priority on the Trade Related Aspects of Intellectual Property Rights (TRIPS) Agreement and its special provisions to protect geographic indications for wines and spirits, for example, Champagne, Scotch, Bourbon, and Tennessee Whiskey as distinctive U.S. products, Chablis, and Burgundy (DISCUS, 2001b, 2003c, 2003d; European Spirits Organization, 2005; WTO, 2005b).

Historically, public monopolies of alcohol retail outlets have been effective means of regulating the sale of alcohol. Government monopolies can restrict the physical availability of alcohol by limiting the number of retail outlets and their hours of sale. Government monopolies are common in Scandinavia, Canada, and parts of the United States so "that economic incentives for maximum sales were eliminated and policies supporting moderate consumption were put in place" (Babor et al., 2003; Callard et al., 2005; Campaign, 2002; National Association, 2008; Ontario, 2006).

However, industry groups seek to privatize government-run enterprises. The World Spirits Alliance met with WTO Director General in 2000 to call for changes in "state trading enterprises that hold monopoly importation and distribution rights and which unfairly discriminate between substitutable and directly competing products" (World Spirits Alliance, 2000). DISCUS urged that the proposed Free Trade Agreement of the Americas (FTAA) eliminate "non competitive practices by state monopolies regarding production or sale of goods" (DISCUS, 2003b). However, elimination of government off-premise (i.e., package sale) monopolies has been shown to increase total alcohol consumption. When Finland went from government-owned stores to private outlets, consumption rose by 46% in 1 year and experienced an increase in alcohol problems, including drinking among 13–17-year-olds. Sweden also witnessed higher consumption when higher strength beer became available in grocery stores rather than state monopoly stores (Babor et al., 03).

How the Alcohol Industry Influences Trade Agreements

The following assessment draws from publicly available materials in English, sources far limited compared to the tobacco industry documents made public by legal cases and the U.S. Master Settlement Agreement. What we find, however, is that the means used by the alcohol industry to influence trade policy is similar to that of other corporate interests. According to European researchers, formal corporate involvement includes submission of position papers, "expert" testimony at public hearings, and participation in consultation meetings that open communication between decision makers and industry. Moreover, major corporate groups are often informally involved in the direct work of the decision-making body, for example, through participation in advisory groups, regular contact with high-level bureaucrats and politicians, drafting proposals, and assisting in setting agendas for policy making (Trade, Societies 2004).

While the WTO does not allow active participation or voting by representatives of industry or public interest organizations, it allows their participation as observers in selected meetings at Ministerial Conferences. Outside of Ministerial Conferences, civil society has no formal access to the WTO committees or working groups charged with daily operations, either as observers or for the purpose of distributing information. Even though formal participation in the WTO is closed to public interest and industry groups, industry or corporate access and influence at the *national* level has a significant impact on the decisions taken in the WTO (Trade, Societies 2004).

Governments negotiate trade agreements primarily in secret, often under pressure from and/or in close consultation with business interests. The alcohol industry is increasingly active in the policy arena and "[i]n some countries, the industry is the dominant non-governmental presence at the policy making table" (Babor et al., 2003). Available resources demonstrate that the alcohol industry, particularly the distilled spirits interests, has been active in trying to influence trade policy (Deardorff & Hall, 1997).

Lobbying/Insider Influence

Industry lobbyists follow ongoing issues and advocate at every opportunity. It has been well documented that trade lawyers move in and out of U.S. government service, writing the official texts and laws they later use as tools on behalf of future corporate clients (Greider, 2001). For example, Deborah Lamb served for 10 years on the staff of the U.S. Senate Finance Committee and helped formulate permanent normal the United States and China trade relations. Ms. Lamb left government service and became Vice President for International Issues and Trade of DISCUS which "seeks to promote and protect the spirits industry's interests in multilateral, regional and bilateral trade agreements and to monitor and address wide-ranging regulatory developments that affect worldwide exports of U.S.-produced distilled spirits" (DISCUS, 2001b, 2008e). The Bush administration named her to the U.S. Trade Representative's (USTR) transition advisory team where she gave advice on market access and bilateral and multilateral trade (DISCUS, 2001a). Currently, she represents American spirits interests as Vice Chair of the USTR's Trade Advisory Committee on Consumer Goods (USTR, 2008).

Beginning in 2001, the Doha Round of WTO negotiations to open specific service sectors to trade was to end in 2007 (Wallach, 2005). Hoping to influence policy, DISCUS and the World Spirits Alliance were among nongov-ernmental organizations (NGOs) at the WTO Ministerial meetings in Cancun (2003) and Hong Kong (2005). Not only from an NGO, Ms Lamb was "an advi-sor to the U.S. government delegation" at Cancun where she urged negotiators to agree to a "plan for aggressive trade liberalization" (Discus Tariffs, 2003c).

The Industry as Formal Trade Advisor

U.S. law requires consultation with the private sector in the development of trade proposals. Accordingly, the USTR established 14 trade advisory com-mittees. Currently, five alcohol industry representatives serve on Consumer Goods, Distribution Services, and Intellectual Property (USTR, 2008). As an example of their role, the Consumer Goods Committee that included Deborah Lamb of DISCUS, Marcus Smith of Brown-Forman Corporation, and chaired by Donald Nelson of Altria, endorsed the U.S.-Bahrain Free Trade Agreement (FTA) (Nelson, 2004). If passed, tariffs on all alcohol and tobacco products were to be eliminated on imports from the United States even though "[a]lco-hol and tobacco were sensitive for [Muslim] Bahrain for cultural and public health reasons" (USTR, 2005).

Noting that industries dominant the trade advisory committees, the U.S. Government Accountability Office reported that public health input into U.S. trade policy has been extremely limited (U.S. Government, 2007). Currently, there is a movement among American public health and environmental groups to acquire permanent input in trade negotiations even though this effort has met resistance from the Bush administration (Center, 2006; Shaffer & Waitzkin et al., 2005).

Alcohol Industry Coalitions

u.s. coalitions. Another means of corporate influence is through coalitions of sister companies. For example, American brewers drew upon the WTO Technical Barriers to Trade Agreement (TBT) to reduce nontariff barriers in a challenge of an Ontario law taxing disposable containers, arguing that the policy benefited Canadian brewers who used more glass bottles (Grossman, 2000). Moreover, Canadian health advocates warned that the TBT could also threaten public health measures related to alcohol production and sale, alcohol licensing restrictions, and sales in stadiums or other venues (Grieshaber-Otto & Sinclair et al., 2000).

Distilled Spirits Council of the United States (DISCUS) is the national trade association that represents American producers, marketers, and exporters of distilled spirits products. Member companies include Bacardi USA, Barton, Brown-Forman, Cruzan International, Diageo, Future Brands, Luxco, McCormick Distilling, Moet Hennessy USA, Pernod Ricard USA, Remy Cointreau USA, Sidney Frank Importing, and Suntory International (DISCUS, 2008a).

DISCUS took credit for the reduction of Romanian tariffs on U.S. Bourbon. In 2003, the spirits lobby petitioned the U.S. Government to suspend preferential duty-free treatment (extended to developing countries) until Romania reduced its tariff on U.S. spirits to the level imposed on EU products (DISCUS, 2003a). DISCUS also lobbied for passage of the U.S.-Central American-Dominican Republic FTA (CAFTA-DR) to reduce alcohol tariffs that "will have a direct and immediate impact on the sale of U.S. made spirits products" (DISCUS, 2005).

Dr. Peter Cressy, DISCUS President, retired U.S. Navy Rear Admiral and former Chancellor of the University of Massachusetts at Dartmouth, testified in 2003 before a U.S. Congressional hearing on the proposed U.S.-Chile FTA. According to Cressy, the FTA would eliminate most tariffs and enable American products to compete in Chile "on an equal footing with spirits from Mexico, Canada and the European Union" (Cressy, 2003; DISCUS, 2008d). Since lowering tariffs reduces the price of imported items, consumers of alcoholic beverages respond to changes in prices, and heavy or problem drinkers appear to be no exception to this rule (Babor et al., 2003).

DISCUS issued a statement of disappointment upon the suspension of the Doha Round in 2006 due to disputes over EU and U.S. agricultural subsidies (DISCUS, 2006b). During 2008 meetings in Geneva, the WTO failed again to reach a compromise in negotiations to open agricultural and manufacturing markets, trade in services, expanded intellectual property regulation and or to achieve the objective of making trade rules fairer for developing countries.

U.S. business interests supported Vietnam's entry into the WTO. For example, Anheuser-Busch and Diageo served as corporate cochairs of the U.S.-Vietnam WTO Coalition which also had DISCUS among its 157 general members (U.S.-Vietnam, 2006). According to Deborah Lamb,"Vietnam's membership in the WTO has been a top priority for the U.S. distilled spirits industry." DISCUS saw that Vietnam's WTO accession would benefit the distilled spirits industry. Vietnam would lower its tariffs on imported spirits from 65% to 45%; within 3 years of accession; Vietnam would reform its discriminatory excise tax regime for spirits, which was structured to assess significantly higher taxes on imported spirits than on domestic spirits; import trading rights for distilled spirits would be granted in 2007; and U.S. spirits companies would be able o engage in wholesale and retail businesses 3 years after Vietnam joins the WTO (DISCUS, 2006c). All of these measures would stimulate alcohol sales and consumption and exacerbate alcohol problems in Vietnam.

EUROPEAN COALITIONS. The European Spirits Organisation (CEPS) consists of 38 national associations from 29 countries, as well as a group of leading spirits producing companies (European Spirits Alliance, 2008a). CEPS was a "steadfast supporter of the ... [WTO] since its formation in 1995 and ... has participated in a wide-range dialogue with officials from key national delegations and the WTO Secretariat in Geneva, aimed at furthering trade liberalization in world markets." CEPS monitors the notifications relevant to its interests and provides the EU and third country authorities with technical expertise on their products and markets (European Spirits Organization, 2008d).

Anticipating the possibility that the WTO 2005 Hong Kong Ministerial might "fail to deliver the hoped-for progress in the Round, thus making a swift conclusion unlikely ... CEPS believes that the EU should consider using alternative means of securing improved market access for EU exports in key overseas markets, through mechanisms such as bilateral and regional Free Trade Agreements" (European Spirits Organization, 2005).

The European Spirits Organisation reported that it had "a particularly busy time" up to and following 2006 collapse of the WTO negotiations. "While disappointed with the overall outcome from Hong Kong, the EU spirits industry remains committed to pursuing its trade agenda on a multilateral basis via the WTO with the help of its partner associations in the World Spirits Alliance, and is optimistic that the ... [Doha] talks may yet resolve some of the problems currently facing EU spirits in key markets" (European Spirits News, 2006).

Frustrated at the slow progress of WTO negotiations, in October 2006, the European Commission undertook a new generation of bilateral trade agreements allegedly to complement its commitment to the WTO. At the time, CEPS indicated that "specific initiatives must be considered in order to improve the industry's competitiveness on the world market. In combination with an active multilateral [i.e., WTO] agenda, the spirits trade welcomes the positive approach for a new generation of ... FTAs and fully supports the opening of negotiations with South Korea, ASEAN, India and Russia, all of which show extremely promising growth for exports" (European Spirits Organization, 2006).

When Vietnam became a member of the WTO in 2007, EU spirits producers sought full implementation of Vietnam's WTO commitments, most notably, in tariff reduction, a WTO consistent excise rate regime for spirits, and liberalized import and distribution rights in order to increase sale and consumption of alcohol products in this rapidly developing Asian nation.

Moreover, former communist nations were opening their markets and were attempting to join the multilateral trading community. The European spirits organization expressed great interest in the accession negotiations of these countries into the WTO. CEPS considers Russia, which in discussions for entry into the WTO, to be a key market for the EU spirits industry and called for the prompt removal of a number of its alleged trade irritants. Before Ukraine joined the WTO in 2008, the industry was keen to secure better protection of intellectual property rights and a reduction in what they considered nuisance tariffs in the forthcoming FTA negotiations (European Spirits Organization, 2008b).

GLOBAL INDUSTRY COALITIONS. In order to be active observers and influencers of policy, the distilled spirits groups have obtained status as NGOs at WTO Ministerial conferences. For example, the following spirits groups were NGOs at WTO meetings in Cancun (2003) and Hong Kong (2005): European Spirits Organization; Confederation of the Food and Drink Industry of the EU; DISCUS; Federation des Exportateurs de Vins et Spiritueax de France; Federation Internationale des Vins et Spiritueax; Federation of the German Food and Drink Industries; Foreign Spirits Producers Association (of Hong Kong and China); International Federation of Wines & Spirits; Liquor, Australian Hospitality & Miscellaneous Union; UK's Scotch Whiskey Association; and the World Spirits Alliance (WTO, 2005d).

The World Spirits Alliance, of which CEPS is a founding member, comprises national associations from Australia, Canada, the Caribbean, Europe, Japan, Mexico, New Zealand, South Africa and the United States (European Spirits News, 2006). Prior to the 2005 WTO Hong Kong Ministerial meeting, the Alliance called for "elimination of non-tariff barriers and other procedural/regulatory obstacles to trade but warned that if the [Doha Round] negotiations on trade in services do not succeed, the industry will seek action through the Triennial Review of the agreement on Technical Barriers to Trade" (World Spirits Alliance, 2005).

Alcohol Industry Involvement on Other Business Coalitions

The industry has also been active with other business coalitions that promote free trade agreements. For example, DISCUS and Diageo served on the U.S.-Thailand FTA Business Coalition (U.S.-Thailand, 2004). Moreover, Brown-Forman, Diageo, and DISCUS served on the Comprehensive Market Access Coalition to pass the Central American-Dominican Republic FTA (Comprehensive Market, 2006a). DISCUS also participated on the National

Pork Producers Council in support of the Peru Trade Promotion Agreement and on the U.S.-Middle East Free Trade Coalition (National Pork, 2006; U.S.-Middle East, 2006).

The alcohol industry, most notably distilled spirits, has lobbied with other nonalcohol businesses for passage of regional and bilateral agreements. For example, DISCUS supported negotiations of NAFTA, the Free Trade Agreement of the Americas (FTAA), and Chile's accession to the WTO by providing position papers at meetings of the Business Forum of the Americas (Columbia 1996, Brazil 1997, and Costa Rica, 1998) (Free Trade, 1998). During ongoing negotiations for the FTAA, at the 2003 Miami meeting of the Forum's Working Group on Market Access, DISCUS recommended the elimination of all tariffs and discriminatory internal tax systems that protect domestic industries and which inhibit importation of American liquor (DISCUS, 2003d). Adoption of these proposed agreements would have opened Western Hemisphere's huge markets to cheaper American hard liquor, its hard marketing campaigns, and enhanced political and economic influence.

In 2005, the broad-based Business Roundtable (which included DISCUS and Diageo North America) lobbied the U.S. Senate to quickly approve Robert Portman as the new U.S. Trade Representative so that he could address pending votes and ongoing trade negotiations that were making 2005 one of the busiest ever for the U.S. trade agenda. Upcoming votes included the CAFTA-DR and the U.S.-Bahrain FTAs, possible votes on continued participation in the WTO, and renewal of the President's authority to negotiate agreements that the Congress can only approve or disapprove but cannot amend or filibuster, ongoing multilateral negotiations in the WTO, and regional negotiations under the FTAA. In addition, bilateral FTA negotiations with Thailand, Panama, the Andean Countries, and the United Arab Emirates required strong USTR leadership (Business Roundtable, 2005).

Prior to the 2005, WTO Hong Kong Ministerial the American Business Coalition for Doha (ABCDoha) brought together leading U.S. companies, associations, and other organizations dedicated to achieving ambitious results from the ongoing WTO Doha Round of multilateral trade negotiations. The Coalition lobbied Congress to maintain "leadership role in shaping an international trading system that allows American commerce to thrive and grow well into the future." DISCUS and Diageo North America were among the 200 signatories with a Call to Action to the WTO Trade Ministers "to maintain a high overall level of ambition for the Doha Round which must deliver significant new commercial opportunities for agriculture, manufacturers, and service providers alike" (American Business, 2005a, 2005b).

Concerned that alcohol or tobacco might be singled out, in March 2006, Diageo, DISCUS, and Altria (Philip Morris) joined 73 diverse businesses to pressure the USTR not to exclude any product, service, or sector in the agreement with South Korea (Comprehensive Market, 2006b). Similarly, DISCUS urged negotiators of the Doha Round to include "[d]isciplines on the designation of 'special products' and 'sensitive products' so that these do not become market access escape routes" (DISCUS, 2006a). Despite alcohol being a drug that causes substantial medical, psychological, and social harm by means of physical toxicity, intoxication, and dependence, the industry wanted to assure that its products are treated no less favorably than other commodities in order to have maximal market penetration.

Governments' Trade Policies Support Alcohol Industry Expansion

Following the prevailing neoliberal free trade ideology, governments tend to prioritize trade with little or no consideration of the health implications and often work "hand-in-glove" with corporations to "pry open key markets" (Anderson & Baumberg, 2005; Callard et al., 2001). Trade agreements between governments treat alcohol products as conventional "goods" (like butter or bread) under the assumption that expanding commerce in these products is beneficial (Babor et al., 2003; Campaign, 2002; World Bank, 2003).

NATIONAL GOVERNMENTS. Governments tend to promote the interests and rights of their major industries and producers and take every advantage of opportunities to foster these interests. For example, WTO member governments adopted TRIPS, the first multilateral agreement on intellectual property rights, which covers trademarks, product logos, brand names, and trade secrets and could affect trademark protection and disclosure of product information considered confidential by producers (Campaign, 2002; Secretariat, 2005; WHO & WTO, 2002). TRIPS addresses a high priority for the alcohol industry with special provisions which protect geographic indications for wines, beers, and spirits, for example, Champagne, Scotch, Tennessee Whiskey (DISCUS, 2001b, 2003b, 2003d; European Spirits Organization, 2005; WTO, 2005b). In 2005, the EU and United States, with strong backing of the Wine Institute, agreed to remove barriers to wine trade and recognized geographic names of products from U.S. states and wine growing regions to prevent counterfeiting (USTR, 2007; Wine Institute, 2006). From a public health perspective, this has a lesser impact on alcohol control measures and is probably legitimate and reasonable protection of the rights of corporations.

Another example of national government support for industry objectives occurred when several countries filed complaints that taxes in Chile and South Korea favored their indigenous products over imported spirits with higher alcohol content. In 1998, a WTO panel concurred. The trade document revealed unusual candor when Chile's representatives expressed shock to the point of asking whether WTO membership was worth having to be forced to overturn domestic legislation. Chile gave in and reduced its tariffs on *pisco*, it's most important spirits export (Gould & Schacter, 2002). When the United States and Chile completed negotiations on a bilateral agreement in 2002, DISCUS praised the USTR and indicated that the "agreement signifies a victory for U.S. spirit producers and American business in general …. Chile is one of South America's most vibrant economies and represents a developing market for U.S. goods with outstanding upside potential" (DISCS, 2002).

In addition, participating national governments, in the Hong Kong Ministerial Declaration, directed groups of members to start presenting requests on various services sectors to other members (WTO, 2006). Subsequently, the EU, United States, and other delegations issued plurilateral (or collective) requests pertaining to distribution services (which includes alcohol unless otherwise negotiated and specified county-by-country) (WTO, 2008a). Having the potential to undermine the most effective health-based approaches to alcohol regulation, the United States and the EU are pressuring other nations, particularly developing countries, to make full commitments "with no limitations." Making this concession would make it more difficult for governments to adopt the very policies that evidence shows to be among the most effective in reducing the serious harm caused by alcohol in society. For example, applying GATS market access rules according to the US–EU request would conflict with monopoly control of retail alcohol sales, constrain governments' regulatory ability, and subject important internal public health decisions involving alcohol to WTO oversight and control (Ontario, 2006).

Moreover, applying the US–EU plurilateral request would achieve another industry objective compromising a government's ability to establish a minimum price designed to restrain alcohol consumption and harm. The request could also overturn taxes on beverages according to their alcohol content as a means to encourage the consumption of beverages with less alcohol. Moreover, governments may no longer be able to tax imported "alcopops" (flavored alcoholic beverages that are particularly attractive to youth) at disproportionately high rates. Retaining and implementing these tax policies could delay the onset of drinking and reduce alcohol consumption among young people (Ontario, 2006).

In the 1990s, the EU Commission sought harmonization of alcohol taxes by challenging Britain, Ireland, and the Nordic countries to lower and not raise alcohol taxes (Camerra-Rowe, 2005; Gould, 2004; Room et al., 2002). Following a U.S. challenge, Canada lowered its minimum prices and allowed access for cheaper U.S.-produced beer into Ontario's monopoly beer retail system (Ferris et al., 1993). Moreover, the United States, Canada, and the EU leveraged WTO rules to eliminate Japan's higher taxes on imported spirits than on the traditional *shochu* (Secretariat, 2005). Japan subsequently opened its market to vodka, gin, rum, brandy, whiskey, and other imported spirits (Fidler et al., 2005; Grieshaber-Otto, 2000). This was an important victory for the U.S. distilled spirits industry and, by 2007, Japan had grown to the fourth largest export market for U.S. spirits (DISCUS, 2008b; Stern, 1998).

In global trade agreements, the EU has consistently challenged its trading partners to end government monopolies. In its request of Canada, the "EU equates the Canadian Liquor Boards with monopolies, and perceives these monopolies as imposing restrictions on European imports" (Alavaikko, 2002). Achieving privatization facilitates wider promotion and sale of alcohol even though its also deprives governments of revenue while, at the same time, increasing problems associated with increased consumption (Andreasson et al., 2006; Chaloupka & Nair 2000; Gould, 2004; Grieshaber-Otto et al., 2000).

Given the slow progress in the Doha Round, the EU has sought new ways to secure better trading conditions and market penetration in third countries, principally through a series of bilateral trade negotiations with a wide range of countries and blocs: MERCOSUR (Argentina, Brazil, Paraguay, and Uruguay), Korea, India, the ASEAN countries, Central America, and the Andean Community. The EU spirits producers, seeing huge potential markets for sales, communicated to the European Commission specific objectives that these proposed agreements should achieve (European Spirits Organization, 2008b).

GLOBAL (WTO). According to the 2005 Hong Kong Ministerial Declaration, members "must intensify their efforts to conclude the negotiations on rule-making" under GATS and new "disciplines" on domestic regulation that would require governments to take the least burdensome approach when regulating services and constrain both the content and process for democratic lawmaking. The Declaration called for "use of relevant international standards" that would empower national governments to preempt local standards that are less burdensome (Forum, 2005, 2006; Wallach, 2005a; WTO, 2005a, 2005c). Following these principles, governments would become even more business friendly and not resist the opening of their markets or insist on domestic regulations to curtail sales or consumption. Industries, moreover, could propose that its ineffective codes of self-regulation and weak public educational campaigns (e.g., "drink responsibly") become the least burdensome "international standards" adopted in trade negotiations.

The WTO exerts significant pressure to open trade through its periodic Trade Policy Reviews of member nations. These reports identify barriers to trade that are inconsistent with WTO goals—and presumed to be detrimental to trade. For example, the 2004 report on Norway pointed out that cross-boarder shopping to Sweden increased due to Norway's high levels of excise duties on alcohol and tobacco (Gould & Schacter, 2002). Similarly, the 2003 WTO Trade Policy Review pressured Canada to liberalize its monopoly system (WTO, 2003). If Norway or Canada adopted these "suggestions," the outcome would surely be increased alcohol consumption and related problems.

The European Commission, the United States, and Australia requested formal WTO consultations with India over certain Indian state-level taxation and retail rules discriminating against imports of wines and spirits. According to Deborah Lamb, DISCUS and member of a U.S. trade advisory committee, "India's exorbitant tariffs have made it nearly impossible for U.S. products—primarily Bourbon and Tennessee Whiskey—to break into the Indian market" (DISCUS, 2007a). "The Distilled Spirits Council and its members strongly support the Administration's decision" (DISCUS, 2007b). The EU wine and spirits producers also welcomed this move to create a more level playing field in the huge Indian market. Once decided, the U.S. trade publication, Wine and Spirit, declared "[v]ictory in India for the spirits and wine biz today. The World Trade Organization (WTO) has just reversed an earlier ruling that Indian duties on U.S. alcohol imports are not discriminatory (much to the dismay of companies like Beam Global and Brown-Forman) in response to the Bush administration's appeal." (Wine & Spirit, 2008).

When a country is referred to the WTO for consultation (as was India), parties undergo a formal 60-day dialogue. In cases when parties reach no agreement, the WTO may establish a Dispute Settlement Panel to make recommendations on how the disputed measure can conform to WTO rules (European Spirits Org, 2008a; USTR, 2007). Following U.S. and EU complaints, the WTO established U.S.-India Wine and Spirits Dispute Panel which forced India to remove the additional import tax on liquor, wine, and beer (White & Case, 2007). India represents a huge and growing market.

As we have seen, GATS has become "the world's first multilateral agreement on investments and covers cross-border trade and every possible means of supplying a service, including the right to set up commercial presence in the export market" (WTO, 1999). However, in 1998, WTO Director-General

Ruggiero predicted the unexpected since "GATS provides guarantees ... into areas never before recognized as trade policy. I suspect that neither governments nor industries have yet appreciated the full scope of these guarantees or the full value of existing commitments" (Ruggiero, 1998). It is highly probable, however, that industries are appreciating the full scope of GATS more than governments or other sectors of civil society.

A dramatic example of the potential and unintended (or maybe intended) consequences of GATS is how even the powerful United States has felt the blunt force of these international trade agreements. Arguing GATS principles, the Caribbean nation of Antigua challenged the United States since several States have laws prohibiting internet gambling, even though the United States had made no commitment related to gambling. However, the Appellate Body found that the United States violated GATS market access rules since gambling could be understood to be part of commitments the United States made on recreational services (Fidler et al., 2005). Rather than change its States' laws to comply, the United States withdrew its commitments on recreation. However, according to WTO regulations, when members withdraw a service commitment in one sector, they are obligated to provide compensation with substitute commitments in other service sectors. Since the EU is one of the parties in negotiation with the United States, European alcohol companies used this unusual opportunity to pressure the United States into further opening alcohol distribution. If successful, European negotiators and corporations could achieve their long goal of undermining U.S. control state monopolies (Inside U.S. Trade, 2007). There would follow greatly enhanced promotion and availability of alcohol through more sales outlets, provide additional economic incentives to maximize sales, and exacerbate availability of alcohol to minors and adults drinkers who might over use. In fact, this gambling decision has significant implications for all domestic policies (State, 2005; Wallach, 2005b). In other words, forcing the United States to open up markets in these 18 States could overturn complete bans on sales or advertising of alcohol.

"Perfect Storm" for Greater Global Health Problems Related to Alcohol

Increased promotion, availability, and accessibility of alcoholic beverages are changing drinking patterns across the world. As if forewarned by astute weather forecasts, we note a confluence of factors that, if not addressed, will likely lead to what Caetano and Laranjeira described as a "perfect storm" of alcohol-related problems. Expanding globalization brings economic growth and the capability of more people to purchase alcohol. The product is more widely available and relatively inexpensive. Multinational corporations increasingly target potential markets. Slick marketing appeals to the growing youth population in developing countries. Widespread mass communication and media penetration more often can not portray alcohol in highly positive ways. In most of the world, there is weak and/or threatened alcohol control policy and lack an adequate prevention infrastructure. Moreover, business-friendly trade agreements, as currently written, will only add fuel to the gathering storm (Caetano & Laranjeira, 2006; Callard et al., 2001; Secretariat, 2004).

To date, most of the focus of corporations in the trade arena has been to expand market access by reductions in tariffs and protection of geographic indications for their products—the low hanging fruit. Achievements in these areas led DISCUS to report in 2008 that "[s]ince the conclusion of the Uruguay Round of WTO negotiations in 1994, US exports of distilled spirits have increased by 253%, growing to $1.01 billion in 2007" (DISCUS, 2008c).

This writer points back to WTO Director-General Ruggiero's 1998 prediction (and what should be a warning) that GATS "provides guarantees ... into areas never before recognized as trade policy. I suspect that neither governments nor industries have yet appreciated the full scope of these guarantees or the full value of existing commitments" (Ruggiero, 1998). From what we report in this chapter, it appears that alcohol industries more fully appreciate the full scope of GATS and other agreements—certainly more than leaders of public health and civil society. Alcohol industries, seeking always to maximize profits, are increasingly aware of the tools available to them in trade agreements to eliminate what they consider are barriers to trade. GATS, Technical Barriers to Trade, TRIPS, and even stronger regional and bilateral agreements are now available to industry and their business-friendly governments to promote trade. Table 9.1 outlines specific trade law obligations that companies and/or their governments can apply to expand global alcohol consumption and constrain effective alcohol control.

Efforts to Address Alcohol Problems

Unfortunately, weak civil society and public health policy and slowly developing global strategies through the World Health Organization suggests greater challenges in confronting the growing global burden of disease and social problems linked to high-risk alcohol consumption throughout the world. Moreover, unless constrained, corporations will use their influence and invoke

TABLE 9.1. How Trade Law Obligations Constrain Policy Options for Alcohol Control.

Policy Interventions for Alcohol Control	Provisions Relevant to Policy Interventions	Key Factors Influencing Vulnerability to Trade Disputes
Best Practices Minimum legal purchase age Government monopoly of retail sales Restrictions on hours or days of sale Server liability Outlet density restrictions Taxation and pricing Sobriety check points Lowered BAC limits Administrative license suspension Graduate licensing for novice drivers Brief interventions for hazardous drinkers Other less effective policies Different availability by alcohol strength Education and persuasion Warning labels Advertising bans Advertising content controls	Alcohol advertising • GATS Art. II: nondiscrimination among foreign providers; Art. III: transparency of regulations; Art. VI: administration of domestic regulations* • GATT Arts. I and III: nondiscrimination among foreign products, between domestic and foreign products Taxation • GATT Arts. I and III: nondiscrimination among foreign products, between domestic and foreign products Regulation of product characteristics • GATT Arts. I and III: nondiscrimination among foreign products, between domestic and foreign products • TBT Art. 2: nondiscrimination, least trade-restrictive measures, international standards Import bans, quotas, or tariffs • GATT Arts. II, XI, XIII: tariff binding; general prohibition on quantitative restrictions Regulating retail outlets • GATS Art. II: nondiscrimination among foreign providers; Art. III: transparency of regulations; Art. VI: administration of domestic regulations* • NAFTA Ch. 11: expropriation of foreign investments Alcohol labeling and packaging • GATT Arts. I and III: nondiscrimination among foreign products, between domestic and foreign products • TBT Art. 2: nondiscrimination, least trade-restrictive measures, international standards • TRIPS Art. 20: unjustifiable interference with trademarks	Exceptions for the protection of human health , enforcement of domestic regulations (GATT, GATS) • Are measures necessary for the protection of health? • Are measures necessary to prevent misleading or deceptive advertising? • Would other reasonably available measures that do not restrict trade provide the same degree of protection? • Are measures a disguised restriction on trade, or arbitrary or unjustifiable discrimination? Least trade-restrictive measures (TBT) • Do measures restrict trade more than necessary to achieve a legitimate public health objective? International standards (TBT) • Are measures based on or in accordance with international standards? Discrimination among foreign products or between foreign and domestic products (GATT, GATS, TBT) • Do regulations or taxes have a discriminatory intent or effect? • Are "like" products being treated differently?

Source: Adapted with permission from Von Tigerstrom 2008.

trade agreements to circumvent government regulation, control of sale and distribution, or other measures that would restrict consumption.

As we have described, the alcohol industry is a complex, international industry with great economic and political power and impacts at all levels of society and around the globe. While extremely powerful, it is not invincible and not always united. It seeks to keep everyone's focus on what may be desirable and pleasant about the product and its purported positive economic and health benefits. But it also knows it has a major source of weakness: alcohol itself and the dangers, risks, and great harm to life, health and community well-being that it engenders (Yoast, 2004).

In order to address the storm of alcohol-related problems, governments and public health groups should take several steps. An appropriate dictum for alcohol policy as it relates to trade policy is to follow the "precautionary principle." According to this principle, it is prudent to take preventive action even in the face of uncertainty; to shift the burden of proof to the proponents of a potentially harmful activity; to offer alternatives to harmful actions; and to increase public involvement in decision making (Center, 2006; Gram, 2007; Kriebel & Tickner, 2001; National Conference, 2007). Trade policy almost never considers health or social implications—only increased trade. However, decision making in areas like international trade agreements should also assume the likelihood of public risk, rather than have government policy guided solely by potential for profit and economic considerations of the few.

Accordingly, introduce and support stringent alcohol policies wherever possible in order to counteract the effect of liberalization that is taking place. Be diligent of corporate involvement in coalitions. Counter industry "experts" in public hearings and in legislative campaigns. Public health voices must advocate for a significant role in trade deliberations and demand consideration of the health and social impact of trade policies. Where possible, governments should avoid making any further commitments related to alcohol in the future in order to avoid negative effects of liberalization per se. Advocate for greater openness and transparency in trade negotiations so that terms that are detrimental to health are foreseen. Insist that there be no preemption features since agreements must allow for adoption of new alcohol control interventions when there is further evidence of problems and when research demonstrates innovative and effective strategies.

In order to protect and advance alcohol control, give consideration of alcohol as no ordinary commodity in trade negotiations. Measures affecting the supply, distribution, sale, advertising, promotion, or investment in alcoholic beverages should be excluded (carving alcohol out) from trade agreements without balancing not only the economic impact with health and social consequences (American Medical, 2008; Babor, et al., 2003; World Medical, 2005).

Policy makers should design policy explicitly to maximize health impact with minimal amount of economic disruption. Policy makers should base policy entirely on evidence of effectiveness, ethics, and politics, in ways that are as "trade-unobtrusive as possible," rather than being concerned about questions of legality or whether it will stand the test of WTO. Lastly, establishment of a Framework Convention on Alcohol Policy, similar to the Framework Convention on Tobacco Control, could provide an international community of support for alcohol policy and add weight in defense of alcohol policies in trade disputes (Baumberg & Anderson, 2008).

REFERENCES

Alavaikko M. Nordic alcohol policies and the liberalization of international trade. *Nordic Stud Alcohol Drugs.* 2002;19(Eng Suppl):69–75.

American Business Coalition for Doha. Letter to members of the United States Congress. Available at: http://www.nopa.org/content/newsroom/2005/dec/120505_lettertocongress_fromabcd_rehongkong.pdf. Published 2005a. Accessed November 14, 2008.

American Business Coalition for Doha. U.S. Business Leaders Issue "Call to Action" in Hong Kong. Available at: http://www.abcdoha.org/news/press_release/20051213_call.html. Published 2005b. Accessed November 14, 2008.

American Medical Association. Exclusion of Tobacco and Alcohol from Trade Agreements. Available at: http://www.ama-assn.org/ama1/pub/upload/mm/467/414.doc. Published 2007. Accessed November 23, 2008.

Anderson P. The beverage alcohol industry's social aspects organizations: A public health warning. *Eurocare.* Available at: http://cc.msnscache.com/cache.aspx?q=%22eurocare+org%22+the+beverage+alcohol+%22industry+s%22+social+aspects+organizations+a+public+health+warning&d=75196585614733&mkt=en-US&setlang=en-US&w=c7618936,9183971. Published 2003. Accessed January 5, 2009.

Anderson P, Baumberg B. *Stakeholders' Views of Alcohol Policy.* London: Institute of Alcohol Studies; 2005.

Anderson P, Baumberg B. *Alcohol in Europe.* London: Institute of Alcohol Studies; 2006.

Andreasson S, Holder HD, Norstrom T, Osterber E, Rossow I. Estimates of harm associated with changes in Swedish alcohol policy: results from past and present estimates. *Addiction.* 2006;101:1095–1105.

Babor T, Caetano R, Casswell S, et al. *Alcohol: No Ordinary Commodity.* New York: Oxford University Press; 2003.

Baumberg B, Anderson P. Trade and health: how World Trade Organization (WTO) law affects alcohol and public health. *Addiction.* 2008;103(12):1952–1958.

Belsky L, Lie R, Mattoo A, Emanuel EJ, Sreenivasan G. The general agreement on trade in services: implications for health policymakers. *Health Aff.* 2004;23(3):137–145.

Business Roundtable. Business Leaders Urge Quick Approval of Portman at USTR. Available at: http://trade.businessroundtable.org/news/brt_urges_portman.html. Published 2005. Accessed December 26, 2008.

Caetano R, Laranjeira R. A "perfect storm" in developing countries: economic growth and the alcohol industry. *Addiction.* 2006;101:149–152.

Callard C, Thompson D, Collishaw N. *Curing the Addiction to Profits: A Supply-side Approach to Phasing Out Tobacco.* Ottawa, ON: Canadian Centre for Policy Alternatives; 2005.

Callard E, Chitanonondhm J, Weissman R. Why trade and investment liberalization may threaten effective tobacco control efforts. *Tob Control.* 2001;10:68–70.

Camerra-Rowe P. Trouble brewing? EU and member-state public health policy and their European beer industry. Policy Paper No. 10. University of Pittsburgh Center for West European Studies; November 2005.

Campaign for Tobacco-Free Kids. *Public Health and International Trade. Vol II: Tariffs and Privatization.* Washington, DC: Campaign for Tobacco-Free Kids; 2002.

Center for Policy Analysis on Trade and Health. *Campaign for Public Health Representation in Trade Policy.* San Francisco, CA: Center for Policy Analysis on Trade and Health; 2008. Available at: http://www.cpath.org/id4.html. Accessed November 15, 2008.

Chaloupka FJ, Nair R. International issues in the supply of tobacco: Recent changes and implications for alcohol. *Addiction.* 2000; Suppl 4:S477–S489.

Comprehensive Market Access Coalition. *Membership List.* Available at: http://web.archive.org/web/20060304201150/http://www.marketaccesscoalition.com/. Published 2006a. Accessed October 19, 2008.

Comprehensive Market Access Coalition. *Written Comments on the U.S.- Republic of Korea Free Trade Agreement.* Available at: http://web.archive.org/web/20061130082342/http://www.marketaccesscoalition.com/. Published 2006b. Accessed November 22, 2008.

Cornia GA. Globalization and health: results and options. *Bull World Health Organ.* 2001;79:834–841.

Crawford JA, Fiorentino RV. *The Changing Landscape of Regional Trade Agreements. Discussion Paper No. 8.* Geneva, Switzerland: World Trade Organization; 2005.

Cressy PH. *Statement of Peter H. Cressy, Distilled Spirits Council of the United States, Inc. to the House Committee on Ways and Means.* Available at: http://waysandmeans.house.gov/hearings.asp?formmode=printfriendly&id=1096. Published June 10, 2003. Accessed November 14, 2008.

Deardorff A, Hall R. *Explaining the Role of Interest Groups in United States Trade Policy. Research Seminar in International Economics. Discussion paper No. 415.* Ann Arbor, MI: University of Michigan. Available at: http://web.archive.org/web/20060927050755/http://ideas.repec.org/p/fth/michin/415.html. Published November 11, 1997. Accessed November 14, 2008.

Distilled Spirits Council of the United States. *Distilled Spirits Trade Expert Named to USTR Transition Team.* Available at: http://web.archive.org/ web/20020821150126/http://www.discus.org/mediaroom/2001/pr1301.htm. Published 2001a. Accessed September 20, 2009.

Distilled Spirits Council of the United States. *WTO Agreement Launches New Global Trade Negotiations Expanded Markets for Distilled Spirits Exports Sought.* Available at: http://www.discus.org/media/press/article.asp?NEWS_ID=14. Published 2001b. Accessed November 14, 2008.

Distilled Spirits Council of the United States. *US–Chile Free Trade Agreement Completed Tariffs to End on Distilled Spirits.* Available at: http://www.discus.org/ media/press/article.asp?NEWS_ID=68. Published 2002. Accessed December 7, 2008.

Distilled Spirits Council of the United States. *Distilled Spirits Council: Romania Cuts Tariff on Bourbon.* Available at: http://www.discus.org/media/press/article. asp?NEWS_ID=89. Published 2003a. Accessed November 14, 2008.

Distilled Spirits Council of the United States. *World Spirits Alliance Agrees to Unified Trade Stance.* Available at: http://www.discus.org/media/press/article. asp?NEWS_ID=107. Published 2003b. Accessed October 31, 2006.

Distilled Spirits Council of the United States. *Distilled Spirits Council Calls for Reduced Tariffs, Open Markets at Cancun WTO Ministerial.* Available at: http://www. discus.org/media/press/article.asp?NEWS_ID=115. Published 2003c. Accessed October 29, 2006.

Distilled Spirits Council of the United States. *Recommendations of the US Distilled Spirits Industry. VIII Americas Business Forum: Working Group on Market Access. Miami. FL.* Available at: www.sice.oas.org/ftaa/miami/ABF/papers/miabf-e.asp. Published 2003d. Accessed October 14, 2006.

Distilled Spirits Council of the United States. *Distillers Praise Congress for Passing DR-CAFTA: Free Trade Pact Eliminates Tariffs on American Spirits.* Available at: http://www.discus.org/media/press/article.asp?NEWS_ID=223. Published 2005. Accessed November 14, 2008.

Distilled Spirits Council of the United States. *World Trade Organization—Doha Development Agenda. Objectives of the U.S. Spirits Industry.* Available at: http:// www.discus.org/pdf/Attachment6.pdf. Published 2006a. Accessed November 14, 2008.

Distilled Spirits Council of the United States. *Distilled Spirits Council Disappointed Over Suspended WTO Trade Negotiations.* Distilled Spirits Council of the United States; 27 July 2006. Available at: http://www.discus.org/media/ press/international/article.asp?NEWS_ID=292. Published 2006b. Accessed September 1, 2006.

Distilled Spirits Council of the United States. *Vietnam's WTO Membership Will Significantly Reduce Spirits Tariffs: Distilled Spirits Council urges Congress to Grant PNTR Status.* Available at: http://www.discus.org/media/press/article. asp?NEWS_ID=401. Published 2006c. Accessed December 5, 2008.

Distilled Spirits Council of the United States. *US Decision to Challenge India's Discriminatory Liquor Tariffs Applauded by Distilled Spirits Council.* Available at: http://www.discus.org/media/press/article.asp?NEWS_ID=440. Published 2007a. Accessed November 23, 2008.

Distilled Spirits Council of the United States. *US Spirits Producers Cheer Elimination of India's Extra Duties on Spirits.* Available at: http://www.discus.org/media/press/article.asp?NEWS_ID=443. Published 2007b. Accessed November 23, 2008.

Distilled Spirits Council of the United States. *Member Companies.* Available at: http://www.discus.org/about/members.asp. Published 2008a. Accessed November 14, 2008.

Distilled Spirits Council of the United States. *Distilled Spirits Council 2007 Industry Review.* Available at: http://www.discus.org/pdf/2007Review-Brief. Published 2008b. Accessed September 20, 2009.

Distilled Spirits Council of the United States. *World Trade Organization—Doha Development Agenda Objectives of the U.S. Spirits Industry.* Available at: http://www.discus.org/pdf/DISCUSDohaobjectivespaperNov2008.pdf. Published 2008c. Accessed December 6, 2008.

Distilled Spirits Council of the United States. *President's Bio.* Available at: http://www.discus.org/about/bio.asp. Published 2008d. Accessed December 7, 2008.

Distilled Spirits of the United States. *International Issues: Free Trade Agreements.* Available at: http://www.discus.org/issues/international.asp. Published 2008e. Accessed November 14, 2008.

European Spirits News. *Trade Update.* Available at: http://www.europeanspirits.org/documents/european_spirits_news_-_july_2006_en.pdf. Published 2006. Accessed November 14, 2008.

European Spirits Organisation. *The EU Spirits Industry's Trade Priorities for the 6th WTO Ministerial Conference in Hong Kong.* Available at: http://www.europeanspirits.org/documents/hong_kong_Conf.pdf. Published 2005. Accessed October 14, 2006.

European Spirits Organisation (CEPS). CEPS welcomes a modernized EU trade policy. Available at: http://www.europeanspirits.org/documents/press_release_on_global_europe__final.pdf. Published 2006. Accessed November 14, 2008.

European Spirits Organisation. *About Us. Members.* Available at: http://www.europeanspirits.org/feedback/members.asp. Published 2008a. Accessed November 14, 2008.

European Spirits Organisation. *Annual 2007–2008.* Available at: http://www.europeanspirits.org/documents/AnnualReport20072008.pdf. Published 2008b. Accessed November 14, 2008.

European Spirits Organisation. EU wine and spirits producers welcome WTO talks on Indian state taxes. Available at: http://www.europeanspirits.org/documents/pr-003-2008.pdf. Published 2008c. Accessed November 23, 2008.

European Spirits Organisation. *The Issues: The World Trade Organisation*. Available at: www.eruopeanspirits.org/TheChallenge/WTO.asp. Published 2008d. Accessed November 14, 2008.

Ferris J, Room R. Public health interests in trade agreements on alcoholic beverages in North America. *Alcohol Health Res World*. 1993;17(3):235–241.

Fidler DP, Correa C, Agniam O. Legal Review of the General Agreement on Trade in Services (GATS) from a Health Policy Perspective. WTO GATS Legal Review Team. Available at: http://www.who.int/trade/resource/GATS_Legal_Review_15_12_05_01.pdf. Published 2005. Accessed October 29, 2006.

Forum on Democracy & Trade. *The WTO Moves on Domestic Regulation*. Available at: http://www.forumdemocracy.net/trade_negotiations/forum_news_domestic_regulation_intro_111805.html. Published 2005. Accessed November 3, 2006.

Forum on Democracy & Trade. *Assessing the WTO Hong Kong Ministerial*. Available at: http://www.forumdemocracy.net/trade_negotiations/assessing_hongkong_ministerial.html. Accessed November 3, 2006.

Forut. *WTO/GATS, Alcohol and Development*. Available at: http://web3.custompublish.com/getfile.php/390299.994.baeuuvyywt/Fact+Sheet+WTO+GATS,+alcohol+and+development.pdf?return=www.add-resources.org. Published 2007. Accessed January 6, 2008.

Free Trade Area of the Americas. Available at: http://web.archive.org/web/20040626191726/www.sice.org/ftaa/costa/forum/workshops/papers/ppwks1e.asp. Accessed November 14, 2008.

Gould E. Negotiating under the influence: the WTO and corporate interests. *Nordic Stud Alcohol Policy*. 2004;21(English Suppl):111–117.

Gould E. Trade treaties and alcohol advertising policy. *J Public Health Policy*. 2005;26:359–376.

Gould E, Schacter N. Trade liberalization and its impacts on alcohol policy. *SAIS Rev*. 2002;22(1):119–139.

Gram D. International trade tribunals seen trumping state laws. *The Boston Globe*. December 2, 2007. Available at: www.boston.com/news/local/vermont/articles/2007/12/02/international_trade_tribunals_seen_trumping_state_laws. Accessed September 15, 2008.

Greider W. The right and US trade law: Invalidating the 20th century. *The Nation*, 2001. Available at: www.thenation.com/docprint.mhtml?i=20011015&s=greider. Accessed March 3, 2006.

Greider W. Brakes on fast track. *The Nation*, 2002. Available at: http://www.thenation.com/docprem.mhtml?i=20020527&s=greider. Accessed October 31, 2006.

Grieshaber-Otto J. Trade agreements. *The Globe. Special Ed. Proceedings of the Global Alcohol Policy Advocacy Conference*. Syracuse, NY, USA; 2000:62–65.

Grieshaber-Otto J, Schacter N. The GATS: impacts of the international "services" treaty on health-based alcohol regulation. *Nordic Studies of Alcohol & Drugs*. 2002;19(Eng Suppl):50–68.

Grieshaber-Otto J, Sinclair S, Schacter N. Impacts of international trade, services and investments on alcohol regulation. *Addiction.* 2000;95(Suppl 4):S491–S504.

Grossman P. Corporate interest and trade liberalization. *Organization & Environment.* March 2000;13(1):61–85.

Herfeldt M. Corporate-driven globalization: the role of the world economic forum. *Earth Times,* 2002. Available at: http://www.earthtimes.org/jan/ngoopinioncorporatejan28_02.htm. Accessed December 5, 2008.

Inside U.S. Trade. U.S. extends gambling negotiations on compensation with claimants. Available at: www.InsideTrade.com. Accessed October 26, 2007.

Jernigan D. Alcohol marketers find compassion in Bush's Conservatism: reports on recent developments in the USA. *The Globe.* 2001(New Series 1):19–20.

Koivusalo M. World Trade Organisation and trade-creep in health and social policies. GASPP Occasional Papers, No 4. Helsinki, Finland: *Stakes,* 1999. Available at: http://gaspp.stakes.fi/NR/rdonlyres/C984F2C1-6D13-4219-AE9A-D971E178B77D/0/gaspp41999.pdf. Accessed November 2, 2006.

Kriebel D, Tickner J. Reenergizing public health through precaution. *Am J Public Health.* 2001;91:1351–1355.

National Alcohol Beverage Control Association *Historical Overview.* Available at: http://www.nabca.org/cms/index.php?pid=65/. Accessed December 27, 2008.

National Conference of State Legislatures. *Free Trade and Federalism.* Available at http://www.ncsl.org/standcomm/sclaborecon/sclaborecon_Policies.htm#FreeTrade. Accessed February 27, 2008. Published 2007.

National Pork Producers Council. *Ag Coalition for US-Peru trade Launches Efforts to Promote Congressional Passage of the PTPA.* Available at: http://www.nppc.org/News/PressRelease.aspx?DocumentID=22279. Accessed November 14, 2008. Published 2006.

Nelson D. *Report of the Industry Trade Advisory Committee on Consumer Goods on the US-Bahrain Free Trade Agreement.* Available at: http://www.ustr.gov/assets/Trade_Agreements/Bilateral/Bahrain_FTA/Reports/asset_upload_file985_5517.pdf?ht=. Accessed November 14, 2008. Published July 8, 2004.

Newfarmer R. Regional trade agreements and development: upside potential and downside risks. *World Bank Group.* 2005;Trade Note 24.

Ontario Public Health Association. *Public Health Issues Involving Alcohol in GATS and FTAA Treaty Negotiations. Letter to The Honourable Pierre Pettigrew, Minister for International Trade.* Available at: http://www.opha.on.ca/advocacy/letters/alcohol-gats-sept03.html. Published 2003. Accessed October 31, 2006.

Ontario Public Health Association. *U.S./EU "Plurilateral" GATS Request on Alcohol Distribution Services. Letter to Susan C. Schwab (U.S. Trade Representative) and Peter Mandelson (European Commissioner for Trade).* Available at: http://www.opha.on.ca/our_voice/letters/GATSandAlcohol-27Nov06.pdf. Published 2006. Accessed December 5, 2008.

Room R, Babor T, Rehm J. Alcohol and public health: a review. *Lancet.* February 2005;365:5519–5530.

Room R, Jernigan D, Carlini-Marlatt B, et al. Alcohol and the developing world: a public health perspective. *Finnish Foundation for Alcohol Studies.* 2002;46:75.

Ruggiero R. "Towards GATS 2000—a European strategy": Address to the conference on trade in services, organized by the European Commission, in Brussels. *WTO News*, June 2, 1998. Available at: http://www.wto.org/english/news_e/sprr_e/brussi_e.htm. Accessed October 31, 2006.

Secretariat of the Pacific Countries. *Tobacco and Alcohol in the Pacific Island Countries Trade Agreement: Impact on Population*. Noumea, New Caledonia: Secretariat of the Pacific Community; 2005.

Shaffer E, Brenner J, Houston T. International trade agreements: a threat to tobacco control policy. *Tob Control*. 2005;14(suppl II):ii19–ii25.

Shaffer E, Waitzkin H, Brenner J, Jasso-Aguilar R. Global trade and public health. *Am J Public Health*. 2005;95(1):23–34.

Sinclair S. *The GATS and South Africa's National Health Act: A Cautionary Tale*. Canadian Centre for Policy Alternatives. Ottawa, Ontario. Available at: http://www.policyalternatives.ca/documents/National_Office_Pubs/2005/South_Africa_and_GATS.pdf. Accessed November 14, 2008. Published November 2005.

Sinclair S, Grieshaber-Otto J. *Facing the Facts: A Guide to the GATS Debate*. Ottawa, ON: Canadian Centre for Policy Alternatives; 2002.

State Attorneys General. *A Communication from the Chief Legal Officers of 29 States. Letter to Ambassador Rob Portman, US Trade Representative*. Available at: http://www.citizen.org/documents/29AGs_GATS_May2005.pdf. Accessed November 3, 2006. Published 2005.

Stern RM. *The WTO Trade Policy Review of the United States, 1996. Discussion Paper No. 424*. Research Seminar in International Economics. School of Public Policy, The University of Michigan: Ann Arbor, Michigan; 1998. Available at: http://www.fordschool.umich.edu/rsie/workingpapers/Papers401-425/r424.pdf. Accessed December 26, 2008.

Taylor A, Chaloupka FJ, Guindon E, et. al. The impact of trade liberalization on tobacco consumption. In: Prahbhat J, Chaloupka F, eds. *Tobacco Control in Developing Countries* (pp. 343–364). Washington, DC: World Bank; 2000.

Trade, Societies and Sustainable Development SUSTRA Network. *Vested Interests and Trade Policy Reforms: Policy Brief Paper Based on the Conclusions of the SUSTRA Seminar on "Vested Interests and Trade Policy Reforms."* London (UK): Field; 2004. Available at: http://www.agro-montpellier.fr/sustra/publications/policy_briefs/policy-brief-VI.pdf. Accessed December 6, 2008.

United States Government Accountability Office. *Intellectual Property: U.S. Trade Policy Guidance on WTO Declaration on Access to Medicines May Need Clarification*. Available at: http://www.gao.gov/highlights/d071198high.pdf. Accessed January 5, 2009.

United States Trade Representative. *2004 Model BIT: Treaty between the Government of the United States of America and the Government of [country] Concerning the Encouragement and Reciprocal Protection of Investment*. Available at: http://www.ustr.gov/assets/Trade_Sectors/Investment/Model_BIT/asset_upload_file847_6897.pdf. Published 2004. Accessed November 14, 2008.

United States Trade Representative. *Trade Facts: U.S.—Bahrain Trade Agreement: FTA Creates Opportunities for Agricultural Exports*. Available at: http://www.ustr. gov/assets/Trade_Agreements/Bilateral/Bahrain_FTA/Briefing_Book/asset_ upload_file752_8092.pdf?ht=. Published 2005. Accessed November 14, 2008.

United States Trade Representative. *United States and European Community Reach Agreement on Trade in Wine*. Available at: http://www.ustr.gov/Document_ Library/Press_Releases/2006/March/United_States_European_Community_ Reach_Agreement_on_Trade_in_Wine.html. Published March 10, 2006. Accessed October 29, 2006.

United States Trade Representative. *United States Files WTO Case Against India Challenging Excessive Duties on US Wine and Spirits*. Available at: http://www. ustr.gov/Document_Library/Press_Releases/2007/March/United_States_Files_ WTO_Case_Against_India_Challenging_Excessive_Duties_on_US_Wine_ Spirits.html. Published 2007. Accessed November 23, 2008.

United States Trade Representative. *List of USTR Advisory Committees*. Available at: http://www.ustr.gov/Who_We_Are/List_of_USTR_Advisory_Committees. html?ht=. Accessed November 14, 2008.

US-Middle East Free Trade Coalition. *Coalition Members*. Available at: http://www. nftc.org/default/trade/mefta/MEFTA%20Coalition%20Company%20List.pdf. Published 2006. Accessed November 14, 2008.

US-Thailand FTA Business Coalition. *Written testimony to US International Trade Commission*. Available at: http://www.us-asean.org/us-thai-fta/ITC.pdf. Published 2004. Accessed November 14, 2008.

US-Vietnam WTO Coalition. *Corporate Co-chairs*. Available at: http://www.usvtc. org/trade/wto/coalition/CoalitionMembers.pdf. Published 2006. Accessed December 5, 2008.

Von Tigerstrom B. *Do Trade Law Obligations Constrain Policy Options for Obesity Prevention*. San Diego, CA: American Public Health Association Annual Meeting; 2008.

Wallach L. *Annotated Version of the Hong Kong Ministerial Declaration*. Available at: http://www.citizen.org/documents/Annotated_Ministerial_Text.pdf. Published 2005a. Accessed November 23, 2008.

Wallach L. *Testimony of Lori Wallach, Public Citizen's Global Trade Watch. European Union Parliament, Committee on International Trade Hearing on the "Doha Development Agenda."* Available at: http://www.citizen.org/documents/FINAL_ LORI_EU_TESTIMONY.pdf. Published 2005b. Accessed November 14, 2008.

Weissman R. *International Trade Agreements and Tobacco Control: Threats to Public Health and the Case for Excluding Tobacco from Trade Agreements*. Washington, DC: Essential Action; 2003:2.0.

White & Case. *Japan External Trade Organization WTO and Regional Trade Agreements Monthly Report: 1-43*. Available at: https://www.jetro.go.jp/theme/ wto-fta/news/pdf/w_c_monthly_report-2007_July.pdf. Published July 2007. Accessed November 23, 2008.

Wine & Spirit Daily. *WTO Reverses Decision on Indian Tariffs*. Available at: http://
www.winespiritsdaily.com/2008/10/wto-reverses-decision-on-indian-tariffs.
html. Accessed December 5, 2008.

Wine Institute. *Signing of US-EC Trade Agreement Expands Opportunities for
Wine*. Available at: http://www.wineinstitute.org/communications/statistics/
US-ECTradeSigning.html. Accessed October 29, 2006.

World Bank. *Alcohol at a Glance*. Available at: http://siteresources.worldbank.org/
INTPHAAG/Resources/AAGAlcohol1103.pdf. Published 2003. Accessed January
6, 2008.

World Health Organization. *Global Status Report on Alcohol 2004*. Geneva: World
Health Organization; 2004.

World Health Organization. *Strategies to Reduce the Harmful Use of Alcohol*. EB122/10.
Geneva: World Health Organization; 2008.

World Health Organization and World Trade Organization. *WTO Agreements & Public
Health: A Joint Study by the WHO and the WTO Secretariat*. Geneva, Switzerland:
WTO Secretariat; 2002.

World Medical Association. *Statement on Reducing the Global Impact of Alcohol on
Health and Society. 56th WMA General Assembly. Santiago, Chile*. Available at:
http://www.wma.net/e/policy/a22.htm. Published 2005. Accessed November 3,
2006.

World Spirits Alliance. *Global Spirits Industry Meets WTO Director General
September 28, 2000*. http://www.canadiandistillers.com/eng/WhoWeAre/
newsreleases/000928.cfm?pg=#pg. Published 2000. Accessed November 14,
2008.

World Spirits Alliance. *The DOHA Development Agenda: Position and Priority
Objectives of the International Spirits Industry*. Available at: http://www.wto.org/
english/forums_e/ngo_e/posp54_wsa_e.doc. Published October 2005. Accessed
November 14, 2008.

World Trade Organization. *WTO Business Guide to the General Agreement on Trade
in Services International Trade Center*. UNCTAC/WTO. Geneva: World Trade
Organization; 1999.

World Trade Organization. *Trade Policy Review: Canada, 2003*. Geneva: World Trade
Organization {19 March 2003 (03-1598) WT/TPR/S/112/Rev.1]; 2003.

World Trade Organization. *DOHA Work Programme. Ministerial Declaration Adopted
on 18 December 2005. Ministerial Conference, 60th Session. Hong Kong, December
13–18, 2005*. WT/MIN(05)/DEC 22 December 2005. Geneva: World Trade
Organization; 2005a.

World Trade Organization. *Understanding the WTO*. Geneva, Switzerland: World
Trade Organization; 2005b.

World Trade Organization. *Attachment 1: Illustrative List of Possible Elements for
Article VI:4 Disciplines. Report of the Chairman of the Working Party on Domestic
Regulation to the Special Session of the Council for Trade in Services. JOB(05)/280*
15. Geneva: World Trade Organization; 2005c.

World Trade Organization. *NGOs Attendance to the WTO Sixth Ministerial Conference, Hong Kong, China, December 13–18, 2005*. Available at: http://www.wto.org/english/thewto_e/minist_e/min05_e/list_ngo_hk05_e.pdf. Published 2005d. Accessed November 14, 2008.

World Trade Organization. *News Items: Services. Plurilateral Negotiations in Services Start. February 28, 2006*. Available at: http://www.wto.org/english/news_e/news06_e/serv_28feb06_e.htm. Published 2006. Accessed October 23, 2008.

World Trade Organization. *Collective Request on Distribution Services*. Available at: http://www.tradeobservatory.org/library.cfm?RefID=79991. Published 2008a. Accessed November 23, 2008.

World Trade Organization. *Regional Trade Agreements*. Available at: http://www.wto.org/english/tratop_e/region_e/region_e.htm. Published 2008b. Accessed January 6, 2008.

Yoast R. *Alcohol Industry101: Its Structure and Organization*. Chicago: American Medical Association; 2004.

Zeigler DW. International trade agreements challenge tobacco and alcohol control policies. *Drug Alcohol Rev.* 2003;25(6):567–579.

Zeigler DW. The alcohol industry and trade agreements: a preliminary assessment. *Addiction.* 2009;104(Suppl. 1):13–26.

Zeigler DW, Wang CC, Yoast RA, et al. The neuro-cognitive effects of alcohol on adolescents and college students. *Prev Med.* 2005;40(1):23–32.

IO

Food and Agriculture Industry

Judith A. Pojda

Introduction

The discipline of public health cannot be considered in isolation from the continuum represented by the multiplicity of agricultural, environmental, economic, and social factors which influence human health. This is evident by two facts: (1) that over the last 25 years, approximately 20% of the citizens in 45 of the 50 United States are obese (Centers for Disease Control and Prevention, National Center for Health Statistics, 2004) and at least nine million children over the age of six (Institute of Medicine of the National Academies, 2004) are considered obese; and (2) almost one billion persons in developing countries are undernourished (FAO, 2006). Overweight and obese individuals are at increased risk of chronic health conditions such as hypertension, heart disease, type-2 diabetes, and some cancers; obesity for children translates into high risk for premature morbidity and mortality during adulthood. This also translates into high economic risk for taxpayers as Medicaid and Medicare paid approximately $50 billion in 1998 for direct and indirect obesity-related diseases—an indication that obesity disproportionately affects the working class and poverty-stricken communities. In 1998, total medical expenses related to obesity accounted for almost 10% of all U.S. medical expenditures (Brownell, 2008). Public health professionals can do much to promote development of sound lifestyle and eating habits, however, unless various sector specialists begin to overlap their areas of expertise, knowledge, and information will lead only to a narrow set of interventions. With these interventions comes the inability to ascertain what actions and resources are really required to address the root causes of these problems. For instance, the ways that agribusiness markets food from farm-to-plate now contributes to unhealthy outcomes and behaviors.

Modern agribusiness corporations are legally beholden only to their shareholders who are interested in the "bottom line." In our dominant agri-food system, food is seen as a commodity where labor and natural resources are secured from the cheapest source and products sold where they bring the highest price. Agribusinesses seek to maximize production and continually create new products—usually highly processed foods—that end up being sold at fast food outlets. The fact that these products contribute to the current obesity epidemic, and damage the environment (using 7 kg of grain to produce 1 kg of beef) is unimportant to the "bottom line." The fact that food is different, and people always need to eat, and the right to food is guaranteed by international law does not figure into the equation. Food cannot be left to the marketplace of supply and demand.

This chapter touches on agribusiness strategies within the context of public health as it relates to: agribusiness concentration throughout the agricultural supply chain; agricultural concentration and the environment; genetically modified seeds, crops, and biodiversity; intellectual property rights and patents; trade; alternatives to industrialized agriculture; and agribusiness influence in public policy, the government and influencing science, health and nutrition professionals and their organizations.

Agribusiness Concentration

Global mergers and acquisitions accounted for almost 80% of all global foreign direct investment in 1996. Agrochemical/pharmaceutical companies have control of small plant breeders and regional companies: the 10 largest agrochemical corporations accounted for 82% of sales in 1996; less than five agrochemical companies controlled 85% of the global market and 99.99% of the entire global genetically modified seed market (McLaughlin, 2002). The dominance of an ever smaller number of large, powerful companies—concentration—is a defining trend across our entire global agri-food system. As a rule of thumb, if concentration levels exceed 40% by more than four companies (CR4—concentration ratio 4), that industry is viewed as highly consolidated.

The greater the horizontal concentration (e.g., only a few companies dominate a given point in a production chain: the seed companies), the fewer purchasing choices for farmers, processors, and consumers.

Presently, beef, pork, and chicken companies are all consolidated at a range of CR4 58.5% (chickens: Pilgrim's Pride, Tyson, Perdue, Sanderson) to CR4 83.5% (beef: Tyson, Cargill, JBS/Swift & Co., National Beef Packing Co.); CR4 64% of the pork processing is done by Smithfield Foods, Tyson Foods, Swift & Co. and Cargill (Hendrickson & Heffernan, 2005); the three top dairy companies are Dean, Kraft, and Land O' Lakes (Hendrickson et al., 2001); DuPont and Monsanto own 58% of the U.S. corn seed market (CR2); more than 60% of the global grain handling being done by Cargill, Archer Daniels Midland (ADM) and Bunge (CR3); Cargill, ADM, and Bunge also control 80% of oilseed processing (CR3) (Hendrickson et al., 2008).

Within the past decade, the agri-food system has also been integrated vertically: meaning the same company dominates several points along the supply chain: is likely to own the seeds, the farmland, the fertilizer, pesticide, processing plant, and ultimately the food product that gets packaged and sent to the supermarkets or restaurants.

Concentration has also occurred at the retail food level. Nearly 50% of U.S. retail food sales are controlled by five firms: Kroger's (which also owns Fred Meyer and other stores); Albertson's (also Shaw's, Star Market, Acme, American Stores, and others); Safeway; Ahold USA (a subsidiary of a Dutch company and owner of Stop and Shop, Giant, Pea Pod, and others); and Wal-Mart (also owner of Sam's Club in the United States and supermarket giants ASDA in the United Kingdom and Mycal in Japan, among many others) (Kaufman, 2000). Because supermarkets have a dual role: selling locally to consumers and buying from farmers, processors, manufacturers, and so forth, the power they exert as economic actors in communities has long-reaching effects. It is the retailers—the supermarkets—who now dictate wage structure, benefits, working conditions, food prices, and store locations (usually not in urban centers but in outlying suburban centers). Although the perception by consumers is "the larger the supermarket, the cheaper the food prices," the reality does not bear out. Studies have shown that such retail concentration actually leads to higher prices and even though the supermarkets are buying at lower prices, they are not passing any of those savings on to consumers (Cartensen, 2000; Cotterill, 1999; Lamm, 1981; Marion & Basiley, 1993; Weiss, 1989). The immense power of supermarkets to manipulate the prices or quantities of the products they sell has led to what some might call, unfair practices. Supermarkets now set the terms by which they will purchase products, and even give preference to certain suppliers. When suppliers are paid lower prices by the supermarkets, farmers and ranchers get paid less for their products. At the same time seeds, fertilizers, fuel, and equipment prices are rising for the producers. As farmers are squeezed, farmworkers and food processing laborers suffer due to a drop in work hours and/or wages.

So what does all this concentration in the agribusiness sector mean for public health professionals? As these mega-supermarkets dictate wages and benefits, a large number of their employees end up qualifying for federal benefits. For instance, a superstore with 200 employees being paid low wages will cost taxpayers $36,000/year for free and reduced lunches for just 50 of the families; $100,000/year for additional Title I expenses (assuming 50 families with two children each); $108,000/year for additional federal health care costs of moving into state children's health insurance programs (assuming 30 employees with two children each); and other costs related to the employee or their family's health and welfare, all adding up to approximately $420,750/year for 200 employees (Democratic Staff of the Committee on Education and the Workforce, U.S. House of Representatives, 2004).

Agribusiness and the Environment: Externalizing Costs

Passing health and welfare costs onto taxpayers is only one of the hidden costs of agribusiness concentration. Another more pressing and hidden problem for public health professionals is related to the damage an industrialized, fossil fuel-based agricultural system does to the environment. And by environment we need to consider such issues as soil health and conservation, water quality and ownership, wildlife protection, healthy livestock conditions, and biodiversity.

Livestock: During the past 30 years, our livestock production has moved from farms to confined animal feeding operations (CAFOs). The public health impact of CAFOs cannot be understated as air, surface and ground water pollution, odor, and antibiotic resistance compromise not only the health of the communities where they are located, but the health of all of us. For instance, 55% of the U.S. hog inventory is housed in 110 of the largest operations, with each CAFO containing over 50,000 hogs (Donham et al., 2007). Most CAFOs store livestock waste in massive lagoons that hold millions of gallons of liquid manure. Raw manure can contain up to 100 million fecal coliform bacteria per gram, as well as ammonia, phosphorus, and other nutrients and microbes that contaminate soil and water in high concentrations (Cole et al., 2000). High concentration of nitrates found in many wells used for drinking have caused fatal respiratory illnesses in babies and some evidence indicates its contribution to developmental defects in fetuses or miscarriages (Cole et al., 2000). *E. Coli* bacteria have been found in the manure of at least 25% of the beef cattle

CAFOs (Wallinga, 2004). Careful management and removal of these large amounts of waste is crucial to preserving environmental and human health. Many CAFOs spray the liquid manure on fields as fertilizer. This sends dust particles into the air which contain toxic gases such as ammonia and hydrogen sulfide which may cause loss of consciousness, coma, or death at high exposure levels (Wallinga, 2004). Studies have shown that manure lagoons can leach antibiotic-resistant bacteria into ground and surface water (Osterberg & Wallinga, 2004). Antibiotic resistance is a serious concern for public health professionals as a growing number of illnesses no longer respond to antibiotic treatment, resulting in prolonged illness or death in patients with resistant strains of illness (Keep Antibiotics Working, 2007). This industrialized model of raising livestock also continues to promote a fossil fuel-based system of agriculture. It uses petroleum-based fertilizers, pesticides, and hormones; it has environmental costs in the form of greenhouse gases from semitrailer trucks carrying feed to CAFOs and shipping calves to feedlots. At the heart of all CAFOs are agribusiness corporations who have likely received large tax relief packages, low-interest finance, and limited liability agreements from state or local governments, much to the despair of the community upon whom the external costs of CAFOs have been foisted (Johnsen, 2003).

Genetically Modified Seeds, Crops, and Biodiversity

In July 2008, against the backdrop of the current world food crisis, several agribusiness corporations have formed an "Alliance for Abundant Food and Energy" which makes claims that it will meet the global demand for food and energy through the use of new technologies (biotechnology, genetic engineering) and agrofuel production. The companies include Monsanto, DuPont, ADM, Deere & Company, and Renewable Fuels Association (RFA). These companies are not new to the claim that "biotechnology will feed the world." The debate about genetically modified (GM) crops has raged for several years about whether it will increase yields and nutritional content, how it will affect human health and ecological biodiversity, and what impact its introduction will have on the ownership of land and food production/distribution systems. To date, the biotechnology industry has conducted its research primarily in commodities such as soybeans, corn, canola, and cotton to improve yields and insect resistance. Little research has been conducted on staple foods important to developing countries, or on sustainable applications that could support small holder farmers who farm in hostile geographical areas (e.g., high salinity, arid, low-nitrogen soils). There are few researchers who would disagree that genetically engineered crops hold great potential in relation to the global food supply, however, serious concerns have been expressed about the use of this technology. These concerns include the following:

Environmental risk of genetic engineering (GE)

The primary environmental risks are genetic drift (when GE seeds or pollen are blown onto another farm or into the wild), loss of biodiversity (the impact of widespread monoculture of GE crops), weed resistance, and insect resistance to GE pest-resistant crops. The long-term behavior of GE crops is not well understood, and long-term cumulative impact, field, and ecosystem studies have not been done (Muir & Howard, 2001). There is ongoing debate as to whether or not the release of GE pollen into nature constitutes an ecological hazard. Several scientists hypothesize that GE pollen or seeds might threaten the survival of similar wild plant varieties (Regal, 1987; Tiedje et al., 1989), while others believe that any risks are minimal (Knibb, 1997).

Loss of biodiversity and large spread monoculture

Promotion of industrial agricultural models alters social and economic relationships within societies as farmers are induced to use high input methods and/or develop a continuing dependence on multinational corporations which concentrate power and control over the food chain in the hands of a few. Presently, GE crops are predominantly commodity crops, with a high percentage intended for export. The trend toward monocropping was set during the Green Revolution, and as vertical and horizontal integration of agribusiness increases, this trend has become the industry standard for success. The UN's Food and Agriculture Organization (FAO) reported that the spread of modern commercial agriculture has led to dependency on too few crops and that biodiversity, in the form of thousands of genetic varieties, has been lost in the process (FAO, 1996). It has been reported that some farmers in developing countries have rich pools of genetic landrace material (saved seed) into which the biotechnology industry has dipped in order to establish profitable genebanks. The industry claims that these genebanks will provide them with all the material they need to feed the world for the next 200 years (Yiching, 1998).

Health risks

Health risks of GE foods are really food safety issues, and food safety concerns would be a natural consequence of the implementation of the human right to food and food sovereignty. Although there have been no direct reports of illness to date associated with human consumption of GE foods, that does not prove illness cannot be caused by these products. Ethical and human rights issues pertaining to health should direct policy makers to include thorough health assessments regarding biotechnology in food. The concept of substantial equivalence (when a new product is not created; a familiar product is only genetically altered or engineered) is not rigorous enough to assess health risk. There are questions of alterations in immune competence, allergies, antibiotic resistance, carcinogenesis, endocrine function, fertility, degenerative conditions, behavioral changes, and other metabolic changes which must be addressed. Testing methods should include biochemical, microbial, nutritional, and genetic assessments of plants and seeds for several generations, as well as testing the edible portions of crops when raw, boiled, roasted, and so forth (Aluwihare, 2005).

In an interview with the BBC in 2002, Richard Horton, then editor of the highly respected medical journal *The Lancet* stated: "There is a great deal of potential research investment in the UK that could come from food technology industries, and any concerns about the safety of these foods could jeopardize this huge investment. So I can understand why [some] scientists would be very anxious about jeopardizing that investment."

Biopatents and Intellectual Property Rights

A patent is considered the most powerful tool in the intellectual property system. It allows the patent holder to exclude anyone from making, using, or selling that invention in the country that granted the patent right, or importing it into that country for approximately 20 years. Plant breeders' rights are another form of property protection for plants which allows the holder (usually agribusiness corporations) to have a legal monopoly over commercialization of that plant variety for a prescribed length of time. Copyrights are important for biotechnology companies because the databases that hold information about plant genes can now be copyrighted, although they are not as strong a protection as patents. Contracts also provide corporations with protection to extend or establish property rights. Contracts include "material transfer agreements" between the developer and a third party which limit the transfer and use of materials. "Bag label" contracts between manufacturers and buyers of seed may further limit uses of the purchased material. "Technology use agreements" between technology suppliers and farmers to control the right to plant a given seed on a specific area of land for a certain period of time. Licensing agreements between patent holders and buyers negotiate some or all of the holder's rights (Pardy et al., 2001). Pharmaceutical/biotechnology companies and agribusiness corporations have been the main investor in patents (about $2.5 billion annually) because the level of protection is significant. For example, GlaxoSmith-Kline obtained 374 patents in 2000 (compared to 208 patents for the entire prior 5 years); Monsanto obtained 349; Merck 265; AstraZeneca (now Syngenta) 204. The legal cost of obtaining a patent application is $10,000; to litigate a patent generally costs $3 million; startup companies budget at least as much for patent litigation as they do for research (Erosion, Technology and Concentration Group, 2001). Although corporations continue to obtain patents at dizzying rates, many of these corporations are beginning to adopt new strategies that effectively bypass the entire IP system, such as GURTs (genetic use restriction technology) which is less expensive than obtaining a patent and imposes technical limits on farmers' use of seeds.

It was a 1980 U.S. Supreme Court ruling (*Diamond vs. Chakrabarty* 447 U.S. 303) that ultimately granted that living things are patentable. This meant that animals (except humans), seeds, and seed-grown plants are patentable and that biotechnology companies have 20 years of monopolistic protection for these patents. It is thought that this U.S. Supreme Court decision has diminished the concept of the "common good." Many small-scale farmer and civil society organizations advocate limiting patenting law to technical processes rather than patenting of genes, gene sequences, or genetically engineered species; and to add protection of small farmers' rights to biological resources and sovereignty of indigenous knowledge.

Agricultural Trade

It is important to note that less than 10% of total global trade is accounted for by agriculture, with 60% of that being food and 40% being cotton, other fibers, horticulture, tobacco, and rubber (McLaughlin, 2002). Even so, this represents billions of dollars. Tariffs on industrial goods are about 4% but can be more than 60% on agricultural goods. One of the realities of trade is that while "Member States" or governments appear to be the contract negotiators, the actual negotiating positions are largely determined by corporate influence over public policy. This influence is exerted through lobbying efforts, influencing bilateral and multilateral trade agreements, and exchange of favors with government officials. It is important to remember that the actual trading does not occur between countries, but among corporations, or groups of corporations. A report of development, relief, and social service organizations from 198 countries stated that *"reducing poverty in a significant way cannot be achieved without trade policies and rules which give the South additional advantages and opportunities together with the ability to protect themselves against unfair trade."* The report went on to note the defects of Northern corporate agricultural interests (including agricultural biotechnology conglomerates) which threaten the livelihoods of small farmers in the South, and assert that although some developing countries have undergone trade liberalization, "the predicted social benefits of importing food at lower world prices have failed to accrue to consumers" and that it is the concentration of market power, in particular the companies in the distribution chain, who reap the profits (Murphy, 2001).

Alternatives to Industrialized Agriculture

The dominant thinking is that subsistence agriculture encourages misuse of resources and damages the environment and that countries should produce what they produce best, and trade (Remarks by Whitney MacMillan, 1992). For agribusinesses who supply inputs, buy, trade, and process commodities, the rationale is that *"Breaking the poverty cycle means shifting from subsistence agriculture to commercialized agriculture. Subsistence agriculture locks peasants out of income growth; it leaves populations outside the food-trading system and therefore more vulnerable to crop disasters, and it harms the environment through overuse of fragile land resources"* (Cargill Vice President Robbin Johnson to the USDA Outlook '93 Conference, 1993). These views differ considerably from the recent International Assessment of Agricultural Science and Technology for Development (IAASTD) report which was sponsored by the United National Environmental Program (UNEP), UNESCO, WHO, FAO, World Bank, and other global agencies to assess the potential of agricultural science and technology to contribute to reducing poverty, eliminating hunger and ensuring sustainable rural livelihoods for everyone. Contributions from 400 experts were synthesized and the report concluded that *"... the way the world grows its food will have to change radically to better serve the poor and hungry if the world is to cope with growing population and climate change while avoiding social breakdown and environmental collapse"* (IAASTD Report, 2008). The UN Conference on Trade and Development (UNCTAD) and the UNEP report "Organic Agriculture and Food Security in Africa 2008" stated that *"Progress in agriculture has reaped very unequal benefits and has come at a high social and environmental cost."* and that *"... food producers should try using natural processes like crop rotation and use of organic fertilizers ..."* (UNCTAD and UNEP Report, 2008). The popularity of farmers markets, community sustainable agriculture cooperatives, community gardens, and the growth of local and organic food markets is sending a signal that the dominant model of agriculture is indeed changing to a healthier, more sustainable, earth-friendly model.

Agribusiness Influence

Food companies influence key decisions governing everything from food safety to subsidies to competition policy. They shape food policy and limit regulatory oversight through generous political campaign contributions, persistent lobbying, participation on government advisory committees (such as the Food & Nutrition Board, Meat and Poultry Inspection Committee, the Agricultural Policy Advisory Committee on Trade to name a few), and get themselves appointed to high-level positions at the USDA, FDA, and other official agencies. This corporate influence shapes nutrition guidelines, labeling laws, and content disclosure. Strong lobbying efforts by the American Soybean Association resulted in the passage of the "Bumpers Amendment" by the U.S. Congress in 1986 to guide the agricultural research of the U.S. Agency for International Development. The amendment states that *"none of the funds to be appropriated to carry out Chapter 1 of the Foreign Assistance Act of 1981 may be available for any testing or breeding, feasibility study, variety improvement or introduction, consultancy, publication, or training in connection with growth or production in a foreign country for export if such export would compete in world markets with a similar commodity grown or produced in the United States."* This Amendment also ensured that U.S. funds for agricultural research would not be used for any projects involving palm or coconut oil—in order not to compete with U.S. produced soy oil (Manicad, 1995). Soy oil had been a cheap way to "add value" to processed foods through partial hydrogenation. This chemical process turns the oil into a solid that improves texture and provides longer shelf life for most baked goods. This process also converts the polyunsaturated fat in soy oil into trans fatty acids which act similar to saturated fats and can raise the cholesterol level in human beings, thus increasing the risk of heart disease. Food companies have known about the unhealthy effects of trans fatty acids for at least 20 years and, after lobbying vigorously to oppose nutrition labeling of trans fatty acids, it is only within the past few years that food companies have been forced to comply with nutrition labeling laws.

Armed with very large marketing budgets, agribusinesses influence how the general public eats. Top food companies (Altria Group, ConAgra, Nestle, Sarah Lee Corp, Campbell Soup Co., General Mills, and Mars, Inc.) spend over $6 billion per year to advertise "unhealthy" products. The nutrition education budget of the USDA hovers around $300 million (Gallo, 1999). "Empty" calorie foods are regularly advertised to children on television, contracts are negotiated with school systems to sell soft drinks and snack foods, and restaurants are encouraged to "supersize" their products. Food companies also participate in the Women, Infants and Children (WIC) program by contracting with the U.S. government to promote their artificial breast milk substitutes (formula). The free milk substitutes and accompanying literature undermines breastfeeding—and exclusive breastfeeding—that has been shown to be the desired public health behavior. Wanting to be seen as good citizens, many agribusiness companies support food banks, and donate food/grain to nongovernmental organizations working on hunger (hunger that is usually caused by the very policies the companies created), all the while understanding that this behavior will likely result in a larger market share, thus in a greater ability to wield influence at many levels.

Agribusiness also has great influence in determining what type of research is conducted. Public research dollars have shrunk over the past decade and agribusiness firms have stepped up to fill the gap. Of particular note is the evolving role of the public and private sector regarding biotechnology. Since the mid- to late-1980s "a relationship was established in the United States between the private sector entities and all of those elements of the agriculture and seed industry that were needed to commercialize these new crop products. These partnerships have taken many forms, driven largely the nature of the seed systems and of the products to be commercialized, and by national and commercial considerations. The public sector participants have included national seed companies, universities and other research entities, and provincial, state and national governments" (Barry & Horsch, 2000).

Corporations also exert influence as they sponsor meetings and conferences for many medical and health professional health societies. For instance, it is not unusual to attend an annual meeting of the American Dietetics Association and find highly processed, sugary foods, beverages, and candy being offered by various food companies. Fast food companies sponsor public health and nutritional education materials that give double messages to the consumer. A video called "What's On Your Plate?" (Society for Nutrition Education, 1993) made by the Society for Nutrition Education in partnership with McDonald's Family Restaurants featured the importance of eating vegetables; however, the McDonald golden arches on three sides of the packaging, on the video, and at the beginning and end of the video sends a subliminal message to the viewers, especially since the intended audience is very young children. Even when public opinion pools show increasing trends to favor restricting children's food advertising (73%), to favor soft drink/snack food bans in schools (69%), and to favor required calorie labeling in restaurants (80%), companies can easily ignore them (Brownell, 2008). If we look at these spheres of influence corporations hold over professional organizations—the partnerships, relationships, associations—is really about power, money, and influence; as a society it is troubling when our public health decisions, decisions about the common good, are made on a playing field that is obviously not level. Again, for agribusiness, health and environment are not high priorities; maximizing production and creating new products without adding costs are.

Conclusions

It is clear that identifying the cause of public health problems is key to mounting effective action to address it. Ignorance of what are the determinants of poor health and an inability to ascertain what resources and actions are needed to alleviate the situation are part of the explanation why agriculturalists or other sector specialists are not making significant progress—despite all of the knowledge that has been accumulated to date. Changes in agricultural policy, technology, markets, and associated changes in food consumption patterns affect the cross-sector nature of food, agriculture, and health. If our global society continues to embrace market-oriented agricultural policies, it will mean that agribusiness will continue its heavy-handedness in determining food prices, rural incomes, and the amount of land that can be devoted to subsistence farming. It may go even further to explicitly determine who will eat what kind of food (depending upon the amount of money earned), and even determine who will eat at all.

Formal public policies should explicitly define what is considered to be the common good for all citizens of a nation, and these policies should outline exactly how the government intends to prioritize its actions. At many high-level meetings, civil society organizations present their recommendations for improving health outcomes for all stakeholders including hungry persons, farmers, labor, consumers, and environmentalists. Some recommendations from various declarations include the following:

- Recognize people's basic right to food
- Realize people's food sovereignty as the framework for food production and distribution and for national and international trade and investment policies
- Promote and support biodiversity based on agroecological food production methods
- Promote community-based seed and grain stores/banks
- Develop local food markets, strengthen public procurement, distribution, and stock reserve systems for food

- Ensure that food production and consumption are more equitable and beneficial for women and girls
- Stop indiscriminate agricultural land use: stop the change from food crops to agrofuel crops and other global commodities
- Control speculative trading and stop futures contract trading.

In the United States, public health professionals can emphasize the links between food, farm policy, and public health, and build stronger collaborations between the sectors. Public health advocates can actively engage in mobilizing communities to address local, state, and federal issues related to agriculture and public health. The sectors can build alternatives to the present agri-food system.

Lastly, we rarely consider the obvious fact that humans are also an essential part of the environment, and an integral part of our agricultural sector (especially in our role as eaters). Because of this fact we must go beyond examining how we, as a global society, treat our farmers and those who harvest, process, package, distribute, and eat food, and examine—or reexamine—our values about food. Some principles to support thinking about alternative food systems might include the following: that all persons have the right to nutritious, safe, and culturally appropriate food; food should be healthy and affordable; food should be produced in a manner that supports fair wages and healthy working conditions; food systems should support the humane treatment of animals; diets should be sustainable and conserve natural resources, including limiting "food miles"; and that local purchasing and local food production should be supported.

REFERENCES

Aluwihare A. Global issues and health interactions: Reflexions from the south. In: Gunn S, Mansourian P, Davies A, Piel A, Sayers B, eds. *Understanding the Global Dimensions of Health* (pp. 241–251). Springer Science & Business Media; 2005.

Barry G, Horsch R. Evolving role of the public and private sector in agricultural biotechnology for developing countries. In: Persley G, Lantin M, eds. *Agricultural Biotechnology and the Poor* (pp. 183–185). Washington DC: CGIAR and US NAS; 2000.

Brownell K. *Obesity, Politics and Economics.* Rudd Center for Food Policy and Obesity. Connecticut: Yale University; 2008.

Cargill Vice President Robbin Johnson to the USDA Outlook '93 Conference, M&B December 22, 1993.

Cartensen P. Concentration and the destruction of competition in agricultural markets: the case for change in public policy. *Wis L Rev.* 2000;Spring:531.

Centers for Disease Control and Prevention, National Center for Health Statistics. 2004. Available at: http://www.cdc.gov/nchs/fastats/overwt.htm. Accessed Septmeber 2006.

Cole D, Tood L, Wing S Concentrated swine feeding operations and public health: a review of occupational and community health effects. *Environ Health Perspect.* 2000;108(8):685–699.

Cotterill R. Measuring market power in the Demetz quality critique in the retail food industry. *Agribusiness.* 1999;15(1):101–118.

Democratic Staff of the Committee on Education and the Workforce, U.S. House of Representatives. Everyday low wages: the hidden price we all pay for Wal-Mart. Available at: http://www.mindfully.org/Industry/2004/Wal-Mart-Labor-record 16feb04.htm. Published 2004.

Donham K, Wing D, Osterberg D, et al. Community health and socioeconomic issues surrounding concentrated animal feeding operations. *Environ Health Perspect.* 2007;115(2):317–320.

Erosion, Technology and Concentration Group (ETC). *New Enclosures: Alternative Mechanisms to Enhance Corporate Monopoly and Bioserfdom in the 21st Century.* ETC Communique, Issue #73, Winnipeg, CA; November–December 2001.

FAO. *State of Food Insecurity in the World.* Rome: FAO; 1996.

FAO (Food and Agriculture Organization of the United Nations). *The State of Food Insecurity in the World 2006.* Rome, Italy: FAO; 2006.

Gallo A. Food advertising in the United States. In: Frazao E, ed. *America's Eating Habits: Changes and Consequences* (pp. 173–180). Washington DC: USDA ERS; 1999.

Hendrickson M, Heffernan W. *Concentration of Agricultural Markets.* Columbia, MO: Department of Rural Sociology, University of Missouri; 2005.

Hendrickson M, Heffernan W, Howard P, Heffernan J. *Consolidation in Food Retailing and Dairy: Implications for Farmers and Consumers in a Global Food System.* Columbia, MO: National Farmers Union; 2001.

Hendrickson M, Wilkinson J, Heffernan W, Gronski P. *The Global Food System and Nodes of Power.* Available at: http://papers.ssrn.com/sol3/papers. Published 2008.

IAASTD Report. www.agassessment.org. Published 2008.

Institute of Medicine of the National Academies. *Preventing Childhood Obesity: Health in the Balance.* September 2004.

Johnsen C. *Raising a Stink: The Struggle over Factory Hog Farms in Nebraska.* Lincoln, NE: University of Nebraska Press.

Kaufman P. Consolidation in food retailing: prospects for consumers and grocery suppliers. *Agricultural Outlook* USDA/ERS: 18-22; Washington, DC; 2000.

Keep Antibiotics Working. *Antibiotic Resistance: An Emerging Public Health Crisis.* Washington, DC: KAW; 2007.

Knibb W. Risk from genetically engineered and modified marine fish. *Transgenic Research.* 1997;6:59–67.

Lamm. Prices and concentration in the food retailing industry. *J Ind Econ.* 1981;30(1):67–78.

Manicad G. Agricultural biotechnology projects within USAID. *Biotechnol Dev Monit.* 1995;24:810.

Marion H, Heimforth K, Bailey W. Strategic groups, competition and retail food prices. In: Cotterill R, ed. *Competitive Strategy Analysis in the Food System* (pp. 179–202). Boulder, CO: Westview Press; 1993.

McLaughlin M. *World Food Security.* Bladensburg, MD: Homart Press; 2002.

Muir W, Howard R. Fitness components and ecological risk of transgenic release: a model using Japanese Medaka. *Am Nat.* 2001;158(1):1–16.

Murphy S. *Food Security and the WTO.* Brussels: CIDSE and Caritas Internationalis; 2001.

Remarks by Whitney MacMillan (then President of Cargill) before the Columbus [Ohio] Council on World Affairs, December 15, 1992.

Osterberg D, Wallinga D. Addressing externalities from swine production to reduce public health and environmental impacts. *Am J Public Health.* 2004;94(10):1703–1709.

Pardy P, Wright B, Nottenburg C. *A Primer on Intellectual Property Rights and Agricultural Biotechnology.* Washington, DC: IFPRI; 2001.

Regal P. Models of genetically engineered organisms and their ecological impact. *Recomb DNA Tech Bull.* 1987;10:67–85.

Society for Nutrition Education. *What's On Your Plate?* Oak Brook, IL: Video produced by McDonald's Nutrition Information Center; 1993.

Tiedje J, Colwell R, Grossman Y, et al. The planned introduction of genetically engineered organisms: ecological considerations and recommendations. *Ecology.* 1989;70:298–315.

UNCTAD and UNEP Report. *Organic Agriculture and Food Security in Africa.* Geneva: UNCTAD; 2008.

Wallinga D. *Concentrated Animal Feeding Operations: Health Risks from Air Pollution.* Minneapolis, MN: Institute for Agriculture and Trade Policy, Food and Health Program; 2004.

Weiss L, ed. *Concentration and Price.* Cambridge, MA: MIT Press; 1989.

Yiching S. Feminization of maize agricultural production in Southwest Chine. *Biotechnology and Development Monitor.* 37:6–9

PART III

Tactics to Counter the Corporation

II

Using Charters to Redesign Corporations in the Public Interest

Charlie Cray

Introduction: Why Corporate Redesign?

Lax regulatory enforcement and unchallenged laissez-faire dogma under both Democratic and Republican administrations has resulted in a consolidation of corporate power over many areas of public life, undermining the accountability mechanisms advanced by our political system, threatening the sustainability of our environment, and threatening the stability of a society that thrived upon a strong foundation of middle-class prosperity for decades.

Over the past few decades we've seen:

- the U.S. economy consumed by an epic corporate merger and consolidation movement, especially in critical sectors such as agriculture (to the detriment of family farms), the news media, energy and other sectors;
- a precipitous decline in the strength of organized labor, with its ability to keep corporations in check as a countervailing power severely weakened;
- an epidemic of corporate crime, including financial fraud, accounting chicanery, war profiteering and the spread of life-threatening defective products;
- unprecedented threats to public health and the environment, including global warming,

- the spread of commercial values and corporate influence throughout traditionally "off-limits" areas of society, including colleges and universities (Washburn, 2006);
- the unprecedented influence of corporations over regulatory, judicial, legislative and electoral processes.

Other developments have fed into the growing power of corporations, including the growth of corporate-driven globalization.

Where it still exists to keep corporations in check, the best regulation is limited in scope and often weakly enforced. New regulations are usually only enacted as half-measures, in response to a newly revealed crisis. In fact, most of the weak regulations we have today were originally sought by corporations themselves as a way to forestall meaningful regulation (McCaw, 1984).

The trajectory of corporate power has become such that we have become virtually colonized by corporations. Not only our economy, but our system of laws, our culture, and our politics are dominated by corporate interests. Thus, after a century of regulatory experimentation, our task remains the same as it was in Teddy Roosevelt's day, when he suggested: "The citizens of the United States must effectively control the mighty commercial forces which they have themselves called into being."

What would Roosevelt do today to control "the mighty commercial forces" that are now more powerful than ever?

In this chapter, we present a summary of several strategies to elevate the public interest and hold corporations accountable. Then we turn to a way in which many of these strategies can be combined into a coherent regulatory framework: federal chartering. Next, we examine how such a chartering framework might be applied to certain specific industrial sectors. Finally, we explore some additional ways that the current hegemony of corporate power either are or should be challenged.

Examples of Commonly Recommended Corporate Reforms

While acknowledging that there is no simple solution to so complex and systemic a problem, there are several proposals that lawmakers, business people, academics and activists commonly agree would improve our economic system and strengthen our democracy. Some of the more familiar include:

- Restrain corporate control over public life. Get corporations out of politics. Restrict corporations from any form of involvement in elections. If necessary, overturn those corporate-friendly doctrines that equate money with speech and establish full public funding of elections.
- Reclaim and expand public spaces (the commons) and restrict commercial interests from turning essential services (e.g., water) into

commodities. Ban advertising in public space and other incursions that degrade the quality of community life.

- Regulate markets to protect them from reckless corporate conduct. Strengthen the enforcement of antitrust laws. Limit cross-sector ownership structures that facilitate anticompetitive behavior or which lead to inherent conflicts of interest (Weissman, 2002). Cut corporate welfare (Nader, 2000).

- Democratize the governance of corporations themselves to make them more responsible to the society that sustains them. Give shareholders and other stakeholders more say in how they are governed through increased proxy access and by making certain votes binding on management. Restructure corporate boards and committee structures to include relevant stakeholders and add public interest directors (Stone, 1975). Expand the liability of preferred stockholders to reduce the incentive for shortsighted planning and destructive behavior.

- Cap CEO pay and restore a progressive income tax, especially on accumulated wealth, and raise the income floor through a national living wage or guaranteed income.

- Challenge unsound corporate claims to constitutional rights, such as the doctrine of corporate "personhood" and corporate claims to "speech" rights that undermine the common good.

- Improve corporate transparency and public reporting of corporate taxes, subsidies, and overseas operations.

- Restrict corporate ownership of other corporations (so as to eliminate the structural evasion of accountability, tax avoidance, etc.).[1]

- Create public stock ownership structures that provide taxpayers benefits in return for the subsidies they give corporations. Keep valuable goods, such as medicines developed through taxpayer-funded research, patent-free, and in the public domain (Weissman, 2007).

Although we could add many additional reforms to this list, including many designed for particular business sectors, our purpose here is not to be exhaustive but to point out how many potential steps can be taken.

Using Charters to Streamline Redesign and Create an Effective Framework for Corporate Policy

Perhaps just as important as any specific reform is the challenge of organizing the various reforms into a coherent whole. Currently, there is no single body responsible for the regulation of corporations—that task is shared by a variety of state and federal agencies. Yet if we wish to redesign corporations themselves so that they clearly serve some public purpose, then we will need to establish a means of doing so. Establishing an authority that not only has the relevant expertise and legal authority, but also a certain independence from political pressure which might dilute its effectiveness—has great appeal.

"Corporations are constructs of the law," legal scholar Harry Glasbeek explained in his book Wealth by Stealth. "They are not natural phenomena" (Glassbeek, 2002: 7) Any attempt to redesign them, therefore, rests upon the recognition that it is the people's right, through their government, to alter a corporation's design.

We have rarely chosen to exercise that authority. After two centuries of economic, technological, and historical evolution, we haven't fundamentally changed the system of laws that create corporations.

The U.S. constitution omits any mention of corporations, in effect leaving their creation and status under the law to the state governments. Consequently, state governments continue to hold significant chartering authority today. The people of the state of Delaware (where nearly 60% of the Fortune 500 are incorporated)—a population of less than one million people—effectively define the responsibilities, privileges, and rights of most giant corporations (including limited liability). And after an historical "race to the bottom" that led corporations to reincorporate to New Jersey and other states before landing in Delaware, corporations are used to having minimal interference with internal decisions. Delaware law also gives executive managers control at the expense of the company's owners (the shareholders) (Greenwood, 2002). Absent a federal framework for governing the incorporation process, Delaware corporate law has served as the de facto national corporate law for over a century.

Moreover, because fundamental decisions governing a corporation's structure and design are regulated by the state of origin, the internal affairs doctrine suggests that no other states can exceed their authority and intrude upon such matters. The result is an almost total failure of corporate law to address broader societal concerns (Greenfield, 2007). In effect, it results in a failure of accountability to the society that fosters their very existence. As the U.S. Government Accountability Office stated in a recent report to Congress, "Most states do not [even] require ownership information at the time a company is formed" (GAO, 2006).

As many historians have explained (Dodd, 1954; Nace, 2005), this was not always the case.

Lessons from the History of Corporate Chartering

"What we take for granted today was hotly debated as the eighteenth century turned into the nineteenth," writes Charles Perrow. "Citizens and elites recognized at the time that permitting the existence of large organizations that were primarily responsive only to owners, and not to the public, was a fateful act" (Perrow, 2005: 32).

Early state legislators vociferously debated the creation of corporations and their implications, often writing specific structural constraints into the blueprint of the corporations they chartered. Rules were established on capitalization, debt, landholdings, and sometimes profits. States limited corporate charters to a set number of years, forcing their review and renewal when the charter expired. And unless a legislature renewed a charter, the corporation was dissolved and its assets divided among shareholders. Legal rules also limited the issuance of stock, clarified shareholder voting rules, and determined procedures for record-keeping and disclosure of corporate information (Perrow, 2005: 32).

Much of what we attempt today through external regulations on corporate behavior was originally accomplished through the chartering process, which defined a corporation's purpose. When a corporation violated its charter—that is, operated ultra vires (outside the powers bestowed)—it could be dissolved by an act of the legislature that created it (Greenfield, 2007).

Although the ability of state legislatures to control corporations through their charters was undermined over the course of the 19th century through a series of court decisions and legislative developments (Nace, 2005), fierce debates over the power of corporations continued to erupt over the course of the 20th century. Although it was never adopted, proposals to establish a federal corporate chartering framework were often seen as the solution.

For example, Teddy Roosevelt established a new Bureau of Corporations within his new Commerce Department to take on the trusts, but the Bureau's work was a disappointment. It had no formal connection to antitrust enforcement and its function was largely "advisory" and "experimental." Opponents of monopolization soon began to advocate for federal chartering. "Between 1903 and 1914, Presidents Roosevelt, Taft, and Wilson all voiced support for a federal incorporation or licensing scheme in their annual messages to Congress. President Taft had his attorney general, George Wickersham, draft a federal licensing bill and propose it to Congress in 1910." The proposal was even endorsed by the *Wall Street Journal* in 1908 (Nader et al., 1977: 67).

Different federal corporate charter proposals were included in the 1904 Democratic Platform, the 1908 Republican Platform, and the 1912 Democratic Platform. Between 1915 and 1932, at least eight bills related to federal chartering were introduced in Congress.

Decades later, populist Senator Joseph O'Mahoney of Wyoming concluded the most comprehensive examination of corporate power in the American economy to date by suggesting that the country needed "National Charters for National Business." In his concluding statement to the Temporal National Economic Committee (TNEC) on March 11, 1941, O'Mahoney suggested that to ensure business responsibility, it would be necessary to have "national charters for national business" (TNEC, 1941: 681).

O'Mahoney's proposal would have required corporations with assets in excess of $100,000 to obtain a federal license to engage in interstate business. His proposal would have forbidden stock ownership by one corporation in another and the diversification of a corporation's business beyond the provisions of its charter. O'Mahoney threatened corporations that violated child labor and collective bargaining laws with the loss of their license to engage interstate business.

After Watergate, scandalous revelations about multinational corporations including ITT led to deeper congressional investigations (including one by Senator Frank Church's committee), and new challenges to corporate power. New laws were passed to deal with the multinationals (e.g., the Foreign Corrupt Practices Act of 1976, which made corporate bribery illegal).

Federal chartering proposals are more often discarded as a result of fierce industry resistance. After the OPEC oil embargo, for instance, Senator Henry Jackson of the Senate Subcommittee on Investigations proposed the "federal chartering" of the "Seven Sister" big oil companies, allowing the appointment of a government nominee on each board to ensure that they acted in the public interest, and Senators Adlai Stevenson III and John Moss introduced a bill that would have created the Federal Oil and Gas Corporation, a federal government-owned corporation that would develop and sell natural gas and oil from federal lands, a proposal that Ralph Nader called "a constructive and lasting solution to the monopolistic grip that the giant oil companies have on the nation, small businesses and consumers" (Juhasz, 2008: 98). Although both proposals failed, they put corporate chartering at the center of the national security and energy debate. Meanwhile, Nader and his colleagues issued a comprehensive examination of the federal chartering option in their book, Taming the Giant Corporation, in which they suggested that all businesses with more than $250 million in annual sales or more than 10,000 employees be required to obtain a federal charter. Under their proposal, federal charters would provide a framework for introducing corporate governance reforms (e.g., requiring corporations to hire full-time outside directors), requiring the disclosure of certain facts about business operations (e.g., workplace conditions and tax returns) of importance to consumers, shareholders, taxpayers and communities, and placing structural restraints on cross-sector ownership and monopolistic practices (Nader et al., 1977).

Although the proposal went nowhere as the conservative movement began to take hold and corporate lobbyists sought to outmaneuver Nader and his allies, the concept of federal chartering received consideration.

Federal chartering creates a potential vehicle for public policymaking that could extend far beyond the aforementioned examples where it served to fill a vacuum left by markets. In fact, federal chartering may be the most coherent unused tool we have for reforming corporate behavior and addressing the problems unique to specific industrial sectors, especially when other regulatory measures fall short.

As the U.S. Department of Justice's Law Enforcement Assistance Administration concluded in 1979, although a system of federal charters "alone would not in itself necessarily offer a solution to all corporate law violations; it would offer simply a better situation for accountability. The provisions of the charter would still have to be enforced by government agencies. Yet, the more uniform framework of a federal charter might offer greater coordination than is now provided by the SEC, the FTC, and other agencies that try independently to regulate illegal activities and secure disclosure, often without adequate legal weapons."

The 2008 Wall Street crisis and the federal government's response illustrates another way that federal chartering can serve as a model for fundamental changes in public policy and corporate regulation. As banks and other corporations come begging to the taxpayers for a bailout, not only have rigid arguments for market-based solutions been exposed as inadequate, but these failures have created new opportunities to redesign the structural flaws of such businesses alongside reforms in the regulations that govern their behavior.

Other examples where corporations can be redesigned as a means of protecting the public interest include:

- Industries which principally rely upon public resources (including taxpayer-funded contracts) or the commons for their very existence (essential services like water; the broadcast media; extractive industries). In such cases public claims upon the corporation can be made either through direct ownership or concessions bargained for in exchange for the benefits received (whether that come in the form of financial support, a license, patent on expropriated good, etc.). When public resources are involved, they should be used by the private sector in a way that spreads their benefits equitably throughout the broader community, and with respect for the interests of future generations;
- Industries that serve a compelling national interest (e.g., weapons manufacturers and other contractors whose primary income is derived from federal defense, intelligence and/or homeland security contracts) should be required to operate at least in part under public ownership. (See discussion of defense contractors, below.)

- Other industries (e.g., energy and transportation) with a key role in national security debates and perceived collective emergencies should be required to operate under federal charters that, by design, serve the national interest rather than the interest of a few shareholders, especially since they benefit from taxpayer or other forms of public support.
- Industries that provide an inherently public function should be structured in a way that protects the broader economy. A good example of this is the Big Four auditing firms which have been pressing for a liability cap under the argument that they are "too big to fail." At a minimum these firms should be required to fully divest themselves of any remaining operations (e.g., tax consulting) that create inherent conflicts of interest. ("Tax work requires you to be an advocate for the client," suggests one industry expert critical of the tax consulting loophole in Sarbanes-Oxley. "That is not compatible with audit work" (Michaels, 2003)). Another option, proposed by Reagan-era SEC commissioner Bevis Longstreth would be to put the SEC in charge of auditing public companies—the way that bank examiners audit banks—a proposal that was actually included in the original draft of the legislation creating the SEC (Corporate Crime Reporter, 2007).
- Industries whose control is critical to achieving public health goals (see tobacco example below).
- Industries where the pressures of "short-termism" cannot be alleviated by conventional reforms such as changes in executive compensation policies, corporate governance, or an emphasis on strategic planning (Tonello, 2006).
- Recidivist corporations and criminogenic industries that repeatedly break the law, where structural remedies are needed to isolate and/or eliminate the source of such behavior. As Justice Department criminologists have suggested, "The size and the complex interrelationships of large corporations make it extremely onerous for government agencies to exercise any effective social control ... Consequently, a partial solution would be to break up the power of the large corporations by forcing them to deconcentrate and to divest themselves of certain product lines or subsidiaries" (U.S. Department of Justice, 1979).

Until we actually have a system of federal chartering like the one proposed by Nader and his colleagues, the federal government's ability to alter a corporation's charter can be exercised in other ways, such as under bankruptcy rules. Under the SEC's proceeding against WorldCom, for example, a court-appointed corporate monitor issued 78 recommendations designed to address explicit abuses that were instrumental in the company's collapse, including a "maximum wage" for the new CEO (Breeden, 2003). Similarly, many economists and policymakers have recently suggested, the Wall Street banks and other corporations bailed out under the Bush Administration's $700 billion Troubled Asset Relief Fund (TARP) program or elsewhere should, at minimum, be required to abide by caps on executive pay, restrictions on lobbying activity, and (in the case of the Big Three auto companies) a requirement that they develop a long-term business plan.

State governments also have the authority to assert their control over corporations: Nearly every state has a statute that provides for the revocation of corporate charters (CELDF, n.d.). This authority, exercised pursuant to a legal procedure known as quo warranto, remains woefully underused (Yaron, 2000). In 1998 a coalition of California citizens filed a 127-page petition with their attorney general to revoke the charter of Union Oil Company of California (Unocal), based on its many environmental violations and complicity in "unspeakable" human rights violations, such as its work with brutal governments in Afghanistan and Burma (Unocal Petition, 1998). The petition explained the attorney general's authority for doing so, along with a history of corporate charter revocation (Benson, 1999).

While charter revocation has most often been exercised in recent years against small corporations, in the past it was viewed as the most appropriate response to extreme corporate abuses—even by the most powerful corporations. In 1892, for example, the Supreme Court of Ohio ruled that the most powerful corporation of its time—John D. Rockefeller's Standard Oil Trust—was "organized for a purpose contrary to the policy of our laws" and therefore "void." The Ohio court found that the Ohio-chartered company had gone beyond its charter by entering into a trust. "The act so done is ultra vires [i.e., beyond the powers] of the corporation and against public policy," the court held, and ordered the trust's dissolution (Nader et al., 1977). But before the state could enforce the order, Standard Oil was reorganized as a New Jersey corporation. It took two more decades for the U.S. Justice Department to convince the Supreme Court to break the company up under federal antitrust laws.

Although California Attorney General Dan Lungren rejected the petition against Unocal with a terse, three-sentence letter (Benson, 1998), a state Senator followed up by introducing a Corporate Three Strikes bill that would require his office to revoke any corporation's charter if it is convicted of three major felonies (defined as felonies with a fine of $1 million or more or that result in a human death) within a 10-year period. For corporations not incorporated in the state, the attorney general could revoke the corporations' rights to conduct business in the state (SB 335, 2003). If and when corporations flout obligations to obey the law, and become a danger to society, the governments that give the right to do business are not powerless to act, but rather have the authority—and the means—to dismantle them, rather than assess penalties that too often amount to "the cost of doing business."

As Robert Benson, author of the Unocal petition, explained, "The people mistakenly assume that we have to try to control these giant corporate repeat offenders one toxic spill at a time, one layoff at a time, one human rights violation at a time. But the law has always allowed the attorney general to go to court to simply dissolve a corporation for wrongdoing and sell its assets to others who will operate in the public interest" (Unocal Petition, 1998). The failure of public officials to act accordingly suggests how atrophied the use of corporate law in service of the public interest has become.

It might be helpful if we were to examine specific industrial sectors, to explore how they might be redesigned in the public interest. By doing so we can see how public policy mandates can be used to reshape today's dominant corporations to function more like public institutions.

Example One: Big Tobacco

In 2003 a new tobacco company called "Licensed to Kill, Inc." was incorporated in Virginia. The company's purpose, as set out in its articles of incorporation, was "the manufacture and marketing of tobacco products in a way that each year kills over 400,000 Americans and 4.5 million other persons worldwide" (http://www.licensedtokill.biz).

Without questioning the officers or directors of the new company, the Virginia Secretary of State's office simply collected a modest incorporation fee ($130), filed the paperwork, and voila—Licensed to Kill, Inc. was free to conduct business.

Although Licensed to Kill was incorporated by antitobacco activists as a parody, the exercise served to illustrate how weak corporate law has become for purposes of directing corporations to serve the public interest. License to Kill's treatment under the law is in fact not that much different from the way the law treats the giant tobacco multinationals like Altria (formerly Philip Morris) and RJ Reynolds—real corporations with a track record of selling deadly products to millions of consumers, often through deceptive means. These giant tobacco companies similarly hold corporate charters granted by state governments: RJ Reynolds is incorporated in Delaware and Altria is incorporated in Virginia. As public health restrictions have begun to constrict their behavior in the United States, these companies have been free to restructure themselves in order to elude accountability: In early 2008, Philip Morris restructured its operations so that while Philip Morris USA still sells Marlboros in the United States, its operations elsewhere around the rest of the world are no longer affiliated with Altria, but rather organized through Philip Morris International, a Swiss corporation. Tobacco control activists see this move as a way of subverting global and national tobacco control laws: Shortly before Altria made the announcement it introduced new tobacco products such as "wides," which it expects to market successfully in rapidly expanding markets like China unhindered by United States or European marketing restrictions (Weissman, 2008).

Failed attempts to regulate the tobacco industry in the past have led experienced policymakers to suggest the need for a new approach. Toward the end of his FDA memoirs, David Kessler, the head of the Food and Drug Administration from 1990 to 1997, concluded that regulating the tobacco industry in the traditional sense would not adequately achieve national public health objectives:

> My understanding of the industry's power finally forced me to see
> that, in the long term, the solution to the smoking problem rests
> with the bottom line, prohibiting the tobacco companies from
> continuing to profit from the sale of a deadly, addictive drug. These
> profits are inevitably used to promote that same addictive product
> and to generate more sales. If public health is to be the centerpiece of
> tobacco control—if our goal is to halt this manmade epidemic—the
> tobacco industry, as currently configured, needs to be dismantled . . . .
> [T]he industry cannot be left to peacefully reap billions of dollars in
> profits . . . (Kessler, 2002: 392).

Instead of attempting to regulate the industry's behavior, market by market and product by product, Kessler proposed that the tobacco companies themselves be redesigned, forced to be spun off from their corporate parents. Kessler recommended that Congress "charter a tightly regulated corporation, one from which no one profits, to take over manufacturing and sales" (Kessler, 2002: 392).

Kessler's solution to the tobacco problem is a bold public health policy proposal along the lines discussed here: Through Congressional action, the public would exercise fundamental control over the very corporations that its laws have created. In this case, those corporations whose business mission is in direct conflict with public health would not simply have their behavior regulated, but their operations would be restructured in a way that they could no longer induce new customers to begin smoking (through direct restrictions on advertising in their charter).

Tobacco has long been recognized as a public health threat. The Centers for Disease Control and Prevention estimates that in addition to causing 440,000 premature deaths each year, smoking costs the nation $167 billion a year in health care costs and lost productivity—well over seven dollars for each pack of cigarettes purchased by consumers (CDC, 2005).

Although Kessler's tobacco proposal might seem politically impractical to some, it reminds us of a way that, as Roosevelt put it, we can "control the mighty commercial forces that" we ourselves allow to exist.

Example Two: The Chemical Industry

A similar approach to that suggested by Kessler's could also be used to control other industries that use inherently dangerous technologies which pose a threat to public health.

The chemical industry, for example, is at the center of the spread of certain persistent toxic pollutants (e.g., dioxin, PCBs, and DDT and other pesticides) recognized to cause a wide range of serious human health and environmental effects—the vast majority of them based on the production use and disposal of one particular class of chemicals: organochlorines (Thornton, 2000). Various organizations including the American Public Health Association, the United States/Canadian International Joint Commission on the Great Lakes, and numerous environmental groups, have called for a planned phaseout of the industrial production and use of chlorine-based chemicals—a class that includes 11,000 individual chemicals. In 1994, the Environmental Protection Agency (EPA) proposed to study the viability of a national strategy to "prohibit, substitute, or reduce" the use of chlorine in four key industrial sectors (PVC, solvents, pulp bleaching, and water treatment), but a powerful response from the Chlorine Chemistry Council defeated the EPA's proposal (Thornton, 2000: 362).

Since then, evidence of the global impacts of chlorine-based chemicals led to the Stockholm Convention on Persistent Organic Pollutants, which recognizes the global threat from dioxins and other chemicals produced throughout the production, use and disposal of chlorine-based chemicals. In addition, homeland security experts have raised national security concerns about the terrorist threat of chlorine transportation and storage near populated areas around the country (Homeland Security, 2004).

A chlorine phaseout could be achieved through an industrial policy strategy similar to Kessler's proposal for controlling Big Tobacco. Under such a policy, corporations like Dow and Occidental that produce and use large amounts of chlorine could be required to adhere to a phaseout timetable or required to spin off the associated subsidiaries for public ownership, as part of a planned phaseout that takes into account the interests of communities and workers (Thornton, 2000: 368).

Example Three: The Defense Industry

"The Big Defense Firms Are Really Public Firms and Should be Nationalized."

This was the title of a feature article published John Kenneth Galbraith in the New York Times Magazine in 1969 (Galbraith, 1975).

If anything, the reasons Galbraith cited have become more evident and urgent today, decades after President Eisenhower sounded the alarm about the "military-industrial complex." In some respects, it is hard to imagine an industrial sector better suited for federal chartering than the nation's defense and security contracting firms. As Galbraith suggested, the existence of these firms is predicated upon federal policy goals, with the largest receiving major income streams through federal contracts. Lockheed Martin, for example, the Pentagon's primary contractor, received $21.9 billion in 2003 from the Pentagon out of its total sales of $32 billion (Weiner, 2004). Yet Lockheed and other big national defense corporations are chartered under state law, where they enjoy the same weaknesses of state control that benefit other corporations.

When for-profit firms are allowed to influence defense policies, national security objectives can be deeply distorted toward their interests. As Admiral Hyman Rickover stated in his farewell testimony to Congress, "Many large corporations, because of their economic power and influence, have ready access to higher level government officials who, although not always familiar with the subtleties of the issues presented to them all too often act without consulting their subordinates. This undermines the subordinates and does not always protect the interests of the taxpayer. Some large defense contractors know this and exploit it" (Rickover, 1982: 14).

Examples of private contractors defining the government's defense policy in ways that undermine national security objectives are disturbingly frequent—as exemplified by unworkable and unnecessary weapons systems or the wholesale privatization of military and intelligence functions of government (Shorrock, 2007). The outsourcing and privatization of government goods and services has accelerated to an unprecedented extent in recent years, with federal contractors receiving a new high of $412 billion in 2006. Overall, the federal government now spends over 40 cents of every discretionary dollar on contracts with private companies (Waxman, 2007).

John Kenneth Galbraith presciently recognized that big defense companies, which do all but a fraction of their business with the government, are really public firms and should be nationalized: "By no known definition of private enterprise can these specialized firms or subsidiaries be classified as private corporations," Galbraith wrote at a time where the firms were nowhere near as large as they are now. He also noted that much of the fixed capital of these firms is owned by the government and that as a highly concentrated industry, the defense firms were effectively protected from competition. There is still no market between the firm and the government. (Over half of the contracts awarded in 2006 were given out through no-bid and limited competition contracts.) Instead, members of two public bureaucracies work out agreements for supplying weapons and other war technologies.

"The process of converting the defense firms from de facto to de jure public enterprises would not be especially complicated," Galbraith suggested, outlining a strategy for doing so: If a company or subsidiary exceeded a certain size and degree of specialization in the weapons business, its common stock would be valued at market rates well antedating the takeover, and the stock and the debt would be assumed by the Treasury in exchange for Government bonds. Stockholders would thus be protected from any loss resulting from the conversion of these firms.

Converting the companies to publicly controlled, nonprofit status would also introduce a key change: it would reduce the entities' impetus for aggressive lobbying and campaign contributions. Chartering the defense contractors at the federal level would in effect allow Congress to ban such activities outright, thereby controlling an industry that is now a driving force rather than a servant of foreign policy objectives. As public firms, they would certainly continue to lend their expertise to the relevant policy for a designed to determine the nation's national security and defense technology needs, and as such would certainly help drive its development, but the profit-driven impetus to control the process in order to best serve corporate shareholders would be significantly reduced, if not eliminated. By turning defense and security firms into full public corporations, we would make it possible to replace quarterly earnings targets with other criteria more consistent with the national interest.

Example Four: The Media

One industrial sector where corporations owe an obvious debt to the public is the broadcast news media. Broadcast corporations pay nothing for use of the public's airwaves, the most valuable resource of the information economy, with an estimated commercial value of over $750 billion (Calabrese, 2005). The U.S. Supreme Court in Red Lion Broadcasting v. FCC (1969) concluded that broadcasters who receive licenses to operate on the public airwaves free of charge must serve the public interest. Given a license to operate, they are entrusted with the "privilege of using scarce community broadcast frequencies, and are therefore obligated to give suitable time and attention to matters of great public concern" (*Red Lion Broadcasting v. FCC*, 395 US 367 (1969)).

Yet corporate broadcasters are currently required to meet only minimal public interest standards as a condition of their local station licenses. Industry observers have repeatedly observed the broadcast industry's poor performance in fulfilling these public obligations, especially when it comes to serving local communities (Benton Foundation, 2005).

As media policy analysts Michael Calabrese and Matt Barranca suggest, "Public airwaves that are exclusively licensed and sold off to the highest industry bidder, or given away without commanding any sort of compensation for their use—represent an immense waste of human and civic potential beyond any economic calculation" (Calabrese, 2005).

The handful of huge media conglomerates that dominate today's media— including Viacom, Time Warner, Rupert Murdoch's News Corporation, General Electric, and Disney—and emerging second-tier conglomerates, use top-down approaches to determine the information an average American receives. Media analysts link this concentrated corporate ownership of the media to biased news reporting and a decline in the dissemination of community, cultural, and political perspectives (Donahue, 1989; McChesney, 2004).

Criticism of the obstacles to diverse access to the airwaves that corporate control of the media has created occurs across the political spectrum, and even from industry insiders. Ted Turner argued that had he started his career in broadcast ownership in 2003, when the FCC proposed to further loosen media ownership rules, he would not have been able to launch CNN: "Large media companies are more profit-focused and risk-averse. They sometimes confuse short-term profits and long-term value. They kill local programming because it's expensive, and they push national programming because it's cheap—even if it runs counter to local interests and community values" (Turner, 2003).

"The concentration of power—political, corporate, media, cultural— should be anathema to conservatives," *New York Times* columnist William Safire observed as he joined critics of the media oligopoly in their opposition to the FCC's new ownership rules. "The diffusion of power through local control, thereby encouraging individual participation, is the essence of federalism and the greatest expression of democracy" (Safire, 2003).

The media reform movement has developed strategies to reclaim the public airwaves, protect public broadcasting, and hold news corporations accountable to their public interest obligations (McChesney, 2004; Nader, 1988). These strategies include challenges to renewals of station broadcast licenses, demands for limits on commercial advertising, and the creation of free municipally controlled wireless communication networks (http://www.freepress.net).

FCC Commissioner Michael J. Copps—who dissented from his fellow commissioners' proposal to loosen corporate media ownership rules during the Bush administration—has called for changes in FCC rules that would bolster public responsibilities in the broadcast industry. He wants a "comprehensive proceeding on the public-interest obligations of digital television broadcasters," licensing of low-power FM stations to local community-based organizations, and broader license renewal obligations that force radio stations to take their public interest obligations more seriously or lose their licenses (Copps, 2005).

"The widest possible dissemination of information from diverse and antagonistic sources is essential to the welfare of the public," the U.S. Supreme Court declared in Associated Press v. United States (326 U.S. 1, 20 (1945)), and that "[i]t is the purpose of the First Amendment to preserve an uninhibited marketplace of ideas in which truth will ultimately prevail, rather than to countenance monopolization of that market, whether it be by the government itself or a private licensee" (*Red Lion Broadcasting v. FCC*, 295 US 367 (1969)).

In addition to some of the reforms already described, certain structural limits should be placed on news corporations through their charters. Meanwhile, we should declare parts of the broadcast spectrum off-limits to for-profit private corporations and require that the fairness doctrine be reinstated as a quid pro quo for use of the remaining parts.

Example Five: Essential Services

Using charters to redesign corporations to better serve the public interest, while important, should be viewed as only one, but a key, part of a larger strategy for balancing corporate power with the public interest. In some cases the question is not how we should design corporations to serve the public interest, but rather how certain parts of the community or public sphere should be made off-limits to corporations entirely. In order to protect the natural, cultural or political commons, for example, we may need to support other kinds of institutions that are designed to better serve the community—including trusts, cooperatives, and publicly owned utilities.

When it comes to delivering essential services (water, electricity, transportation) in an equitable manner, for example, the public interest is often best protected by resisting any form of privatization.

Municipally controlled corporations (e.g., water, electricity, and transportation utilities) are usually more responsive to the communities they serve; more able to respect the environments in which they operate, and less subject to outside disturbances (i.e., electricity blackouts, terrorist attacks, market manipulation) than conglomerate-controlled corporations. The 2000–2001 California electricity crisis did not affect everyone in the state, because some cities and municipalities (e.g., Sacramento and Los Angeles) that controlled their own utilities were insulated from Enron and other companies' predations. Thus, while inherent technological requirements and structural efficiencies make such essential services as electricity and water "natural monopolies" (Slocum, 2001), local ownership can keep them under community control.

Across the country, 2,100 municipalities own their own utilities, and there are an additional 900 energy cooperatives. In 1999, the Department of Energy found that, on average, customers who owned their utilities paid 18% less than customers of investor-owned utilities (Morris, 2001). The New Rules Project explains, "Because customer-owned utilities are democratically and locally controlled, and service rather than profit oriented, we should encourage their formation. In today's topsy-turvy electricity world, states should encourage the formation not only of customer-owned distribution utilities, but public transmission utilities as well" (New Rules).

Local control creates additional benefits. As the big northeastern blackout of August 2003 demonstrated, a nationally- or regionally integrated grid system is potentially vulnerable to a failure in one location. Recognizing that vulnerability, beginning in the early 1980s, Pentagon analysts and energy efficiency experts made the case that a decentralized system of energy and electricity would improve our national security (Lovins, 1982). Smaller, locally owned utilities rarely build giant power plants that are costlier to the environment and prime targets for terrorist attacks (Nuclear Control Institute, 2002). Additionally, municipal control facilitates the introduction of locally appropriate and ecologically sustainable technologies (New Rules Project, 2002).

Past experiments with privatization demonstrate why municipal services perform better under public control than when privatized. According to historian Clifton Hood, New York City's subway system was first operated in 1904 by the Interborough Rapid Transit Company and with the Brooklyn Rapid Transit Company in 1913. Rising inflation after World War I caused both companies to teeter in and out of bankruptcy, and in 1933, the city started its own subway network. The Independent Subway System competed with the private lines, which delivered poor service, and in 1940, the city created a unified, municipally run system (Hood, 2004).

Firefighting is another example. Although many remote communities have experimented with private firefighting services, often the results have often been disastrous. In 1985, the Salem, Arkansas Fire Corporation arrived at a fire and let the home burn because the owner had not paid the $20 annual subscription fee. "Once we verified that there was no life in danger, and no immediate danger to a (subscriber's) property, then according to our rules we had no choice but to back off," the fire corporation's chief explained (Tolchin, 1985).

In recent years, there has been a quiet explosion of community-oriented economic institutions that, as author Gar Alperovitz has suggested, collectively posit an alternative to the current corporate-dominated political economy. The tens of thousands of cooperatives, community-based trusts and development corporations and other mission-oriented nonprofits operating in communities across the country have begun to sew the seeds of a broader economic trans-formation and "nurture the conditions of democracy with a small d in everyday life." Spurred on as they have been in recent years by new fiscal constraints— these new institutions have emerged as a potential alternative for communities across the country, regardless of partisan interests (Alperovitz, 2005). Their success in the face of the political advantages that corporations enjoy at the state and federal level is a testament to their efficiency and greater ability to serve the needs of their communities—whether it's community supported agriculture and food production centers, Employee-Owned Enterprises and worker-controlled coops, housing development trusts, community banks, and so forth—these economic institutions are the new engines of local employ-ment, the provision of services (e.g., housing, food) to those most in need, enhanced community awareness and cohesion, and a greater incentive to respect and care for the local environmental commons.

As Alperovitz suggests, efforts like these will inevitably instill a deeper political probing and "much more fundamental institutional exploration and development," as communities once again serve as the traditional "laborato-ries" of democracy.

The potential for a new democratic economic paradigm to emerge could increase as these alternative institutional designs are fortified by new tax incentives and other policies that help them challenge the current corporate domination of federal policymaking.

Meanwhile, with each successive wave of corporate failure and scandal widespread disgust with the power of large corporations and financial institu-tions will only continue to spread.

Indeed populist sentiments against corporations have peaked year after year, as poll after poll has revealed. A year before Enron collapsed into bankruptcy, for example, Business Week published a poll which revealed that the vast majority of Americans think corporations have too much power and influence over public life (Bernstein, 2000).

Rather than retreating into facile cynicism, the failure of the current corporate-dominated system should encourage people to understand the fundamental importance of exercising democratic control over corporations. If we accept that corporations are fundamentally public institutions—created under a process in which ultimate authority is vested in the citizenry—then it is clear that corporations do not intrinsically bear any rights or privileges except those that citizens choose to confer on them.

Today virtually no public benefits or obligations are bargained for in exchange for the advantages (e.g., limited liability) conferred through the corporate form. Yet, as we have seen in public reaction to the Wall Street bailout, that could change quickly.

Conclusion: A Rapidly Changing World

Once faith is restored in the power of collective self-governance and government accountability, rapid transitions are possible. It is possible to control corporations in key areas of public life where they currently wield significant and often illegitimate influence, including elections, essential services, and other inherently governmental functions.

The use of charters as instruments of corporate accountability is only possible if corporations and their ideological allies are no longer able to forestall the demands of an engaged citizenry.

Although deep changes in the political and regulatory frame of mind may already be underway, the role of corporations and the structure of specific industrial sectors must be placed squarely at the center of the debate. As we have suggested here, the use of a federal chartering system—or its equivalent under bankruptcy reform and other rules—could play a key role in advancing public health objectives within industrial policymaking.

NOTE

1 A narrower version would prohibit offshore tax haven subsidiaries and related structures.

REFERENCES

Alperovitz G. *America Beyond Capitalism*. New York: Wiley; 2005.

Benson B. Complaint lodged with the Attorney General of California under California Code of Civil Procedure § 803, California Corporations Code § 801, to Revoke the Corporate Charter of the Union Oil Company of California September 10. In: *Challenging Corporate Rule*. New York: Apex Press; 1999.

Benton Foundation. Citizen's Guide to the Public Interest Obligations of Digital Television Broadcasters. Washington, DC: Benton Foundation; 2005.

Bernstein, A. *Too Much Corporate Power?* New York: Business Week, September 11, 2000.

Breeden R. *Restoring the Trust*. Report to The Hon. Jed S. Rakoff, U.S. District Court for the Southern District of New York, August 2003.

Calabrese M. Reclaiming the public airwaves. In: McChesney R, ed. *The Future of the Media* (pp. 207–218). New York: Seven Stories; 2005.

CDC. Smoking Deaths Cost Nation $ 92 Billion in Lost Productivity Annually (press release), June 30, 2005. Available at: http://www.cdc.gov/media/pressrel/ r050630.htm Accessed September 12, 2009. ; Smoking Costs Nation $150 billion Each Year in Health Costs, Lost Productivity, April 12, 2002. Available at: http://www.cdc.gov/media/pressrel/r020412.htm. Accessed September 12, 2009.

Community Environmental Legal Defense Fund. *A Citizen's Guide to Corporate Charter Revocation Under State Law* (n.d.). Available a at: http://www.celdf.org/ ProgramAreas/CorporationsDemocracy/CorporationsDemocracyIndex/tabid/108/ ctl/Edit/mid/429/CorporationsDemocracy/ACitizensGuidetoCorporateCharter/ tabid/104/Default.aspx. Accessed September 12, 2009.

Copps M. Where is the public interest in media consolidation? In: McChesney R, et al., eds. *The Future of the Media* (pp. 117–125). New York: Seven Stories; 2005.

Corporate Crime Reporter. Lynn Turner Says Unless Big Four Change, Bring on SEC as Public Auditor. February 17, 2007.

Dodd E. *American Business Corporations Until 1860*. Cambridge, MA: Harvard University Press; 1954.

Donahue J. *Shortchanging the Viewers: Broadcasters' Neglect of Public Interest Programming*. Washington, D.C.: Essential Information; 1989.

Galbraith JK. *The Big Defense Firms Are Really Public Firms and Should be Nationalized*. New York: New York Times Magazine; November 16, 1969.

GAO. *Company Formations: Minimal Ownership Information is Collected and Available*. Washington, D.C.: GAO-06-376; April 2006.

Glasbeek H. *Wealth by Stealth*. Toronto: Between the Lines; 2002.

Greenfield K. *The Failure of Corporate Law*. Chicago: University of Chicago Press; 2007.

Greenwood, D. *Democracy and Delaware: The Puzzle of Corporate Law*. George Washington University Law School, Public Law & Legal Theory Working Paper # 55; 2002. Available at http://people.hofstra.edu/Daniel_J_Greenwood.

Homeland Security Council. *Planning Scenarios, Executive Summaries: Created for Use in National, Federal, State, and Local Homeland Security Preparedness*

Activities. 8-1–8-3; 2004. Available at: www.globalsecurity.org/security/library/report/2004/hsc-planning-scenarios-jul04_exec-sum.pdf.

Hood, C. *722 Miles: The Building of the Subways and How They Transformed New York.* Baltimore: The Johns Hopkins University Press; 2004.

Juhasz J. *The Tyranny of Oil: The World's Most Powerful Industry—And What We Must Do to Stop It.* New York: William Morrow/HarperCollins; 2008.

Kessler, D. *A Question of Intent: A Great American Battle with a Deadly Industry.* New York: New York: Public Affairs Press, 2002.

Lovins A. *Brittle Power: Energy Strategy for National Security.* Andover, MA: Brick House; 1982.

McCaw T. *Prophets of Regulation.* Cambridge, MA: Harvard University Press; 1984.

McChesney R. *The Problem of the Media.* New York: Monthly Review; 2004.

Michaels A. Accounting journal joins tax debate. London: *Financial Times*, September 1, 2003.

Morris D. *Solutions to Electricity Crisis* (op ed). Oakland: Oakland Tribune, June 5, 2001.

Nace T. *Gangs of America* (revised). San Francisco: Berrett-Koehler; 2005.

Nader. Oh, say can you see: a broadcast network for the audience. Virginia: *University of Virginia Journal of Law & Politics*, Fall 1988.

Nader R. *Cutting Corporate Welfare.* New York: Seven Stories Press; 2000.

Nader R, Green M., Seligman J. *Taming the Giant Corporation.* New York: W.W. Norton; 1977.

New Rules Project. *Customer-Owned Electric Utilities: Generation, Transmission and Distribution.* Available at: http://www.newrules.org/electricity/customerowned.html. Published 2002. Accessed September 12, 2009.

Nuclear Control Institute (NCI). *Nuclear Regulatory Commission memo warning of terror attacks.* January 31, 2002. Memo and related news stories available at www.nci.org.

Perrow C. *Organizing America: Wealth, Power and the Origins of Corporate Capitalism.* New Jersey: Princeton University Press; 2005.

Rickover H. *No Holds Barred: Final Congressional Testimony.* Washington, DC: Center for Study of Responsive Law; 1982.

Safire W. *The Great Media Gulp* (op ed). New York: *New York Times*; December 10, 2003.

S.B. 335. Senate Bill 335 § 4003(2), Reg. Sess. (Cal. 2003).

Shorrock T. The corporate takeover of U.S. intelligence. *Salon* June 1, 2007.

Slocum T. Electric utility deregulation and the myths of the energy crisis. London: *Bulletin of Science, Technology and Society.* December 2001;21(6):473.

Stone C. *Where the Law Ends.* New York: HarperCollins; 1975.

Thornton J. *Pandora's Poison: Chlorine, Health and a New Environmental Strategy.* Boston: MIT Press; 2000.

TNEC. National charters for national business, March 11, 1941. In: *Final Report and Recommendations of the Temporary National Economic Committee*, Document No. 35.

Tolchin M. Localities shift to private firefighters. New York: *New York Times*; July 27, 1985.

Tonello, M. *Revisiting Stock Market Short-Termism*. New York: The Conference Board. April, 2006.

Turner T. *Monopoly or Democracy* (op ed). Washington, D.C.: Washington Post, May 30, 2003.

Unocal Petition. *Environmental, Human Rights, Women's and Pro-Democracy Groups Petition Attorney General of California to Revoke Unocal's Charter* (press release). September 10, 1998.

U.S. Department of Justice. Illegal corporate behavior. Washington, D.C.: *DoJ Law Enforcement Assistance Administration*, October 1979.

U.S. Supreme Court, *RED LION BROADCASTING CO. v. FCC*, 395 U.S. 367 (1969) 395 U.S. 367. *RED LION BROADCASTING CO., INC., ET AL. v. FEDERAL COMMUNICATIONS COMMISSION ET AL*. CERTIORARI TO THE UNITED STATES COURT OF APPEALS FOR THE DISTRICT OF COLUMBIA CIRCUIT. No. 2. Argued April 2-3, 1969. Decided June 9, 1969. Text of the case available from Findlaw at http://caselaw.lp.findlaw.com/scripts/printer_friendly.pl?page=us/395/367.html.

Washburn J. *University, Inc.: The Corruption of Higher Education*. New York: Basic Books; 2006.

Waxman H. (D-CA). More dollars, less sense. Staff report of the House Comm. on Oversight and Gov. Reform, June 2007. Available at: http://oversight.house.gov/features/moredollars/. Accessed September 12, 2009.

Weiner T. *Lockheed and the Future of Warfare*. New York: *New York Times*; November 28, 2004.

Weissman R. *Divide and Conquer: Restraining Vertical Integration and Cross-Industry Ownership*. Washington, D.C.: Multinational Monitor, October/November 2002.

Weissman R. *The Role of Federally-Funded University Research in the Patent System*. Testimony before the Committee on the Judiciary, U.S. Senate, October 24, 2007.

Weissman R. *Philip Morris Intl Commences New Plans to Spread Death and Disease*. Washington, D.C.: Multinational Monitor (editor's blog), March 31, 2008.

Yaron G. Awakening Sleeping Beauty: Reviving Lost Remedies and Discourses to Revoke Corporate Charters, Masters Thesis. Vancouver: Univ. British Columbia Law School. Available at: http://www.aurora.ca/info/revoke.pdf. Accessed July 25, 2005.

12

A New Democracy in Action

Mari Margil

For 7 years, residents of the small, rural Town of Nottingham, New Hampshire, fought to keep USA Springs, Inc. from withdrawing over 300,000 gallons of water a day from their local aquifer to bottle and sell commercially.

Communities across New England are facing the privatization of their water by water bottling corporations such as USA Springs and Nestle. Corporate water withdrawals—siphoning off hundreds of thousands of gallons a day from local aquifers—impact both surface and groundwater resources. They can deplete drinking water and contaminate aquifers and wells. In addition, withdrawals may dry up streams, wetlands, and rivers, as well as reduce lake levels, damaging habitat and harming wildlife.

Nottingham's fight cost hundreds of thousands of dollars and countless hours as residents tried to block the corporation's plans. For years, they filed lawsuits, appealed permits, held signs, circulated petitions, lobbied the state legislature, and kept their neighbors informed and organized in an effort to protect their water.

Residents of the neighboring Town of Barnstead watched Nottingham carefully and vowed not to be caught in the same fight. They educated themselves as to why the residents of Nottingham were unable to simply say "No" to USA Springs, and why their government that they looked to for help to stop the water project, was in fact legally permitting it.

At their March 2006 Town Meeting, Barnstead residents voted 135-1 to adopt the first-in-the-nation law banning corporations from engaging in water withdrawals in the community. In addition, the Barnstead law eliminates certain corporate constitutional "rights" that corporations use to undermine community efforts to protect the local environment and public health.

Nottingham residents looked to Barnstead's example. They formed the *Nottingham Tea Party* to put forward a version of the Barnstead law to the town for a vote. In so doing, they were challenging nearly 200 years of law and jurisprudence that puts the interests of commerce and property—that is, corporations—over the interests of people, communities, and nature. At their Town Meeting on March 15, 2008, Nottingham residents voted to adopt the new law.

What's the Problem?

At first glance, it may seem that the residents of Nottingham were simply following in the footsteps of thousands of communities before them that have fought to stop an unwanted incinerator, nuclear power plant, or other corporate threat. But what the residents of Nottingham, Barnstead, and over 100 communities across the country have now done is recognize that *the system of law gives more rights to corporations than the communities where they seek to do business.* Further, they understood that their state government preempted the community from protecting its water under laws giving corporations the legal authority to take their water.

The residents of Nottingham concluded that the state and federal government was not there to protect and secure their rights, but the rights of corporations. And, thus, that the problem they faced wasn't simply about water—but that *they did not have the ability to decide* what could happen with their water, corporations did. Thus they "reframed" the problem from one of *water* to one of *democracy.*

One Person/One Vote = Democracy?

The "national self-image" of the United States, notes historian Alexander Keyssar, is that America is "the standard bearer of democratic values on the stage of world history" (Keyssar, 2000). Central to this, he explains, is our belief in our right to vote. "(I)n popular usage, the term *democracy* implies that everyone, or nearly everyone, has the right to participate in elections; the

image of a democratic United States is that of a nation with universal suf-
frage" (Keyssar, 2000). Ferdinand Lundberg writes that elections are considered "the hallmark of democracy" (Lundberg, 1989). Even as the drafters of the
U.S. Constitution gathered in Philadelphia in 1787, "(I)t was established that
democracy consisted of popular voting pure and simple ..." (Lundberg, 1989).

Indeed, for most Americans, the practice of democracy comes every few
years at election time. We stand in line at the local elementary school or town
hall to cast our ballot for candidates that we hope will represent our interests whether in city hall, the state legislature, or Congress. But what happens when they get to Washington or the state house? We want and expect
our elected officials to protect us, our families, and our communities from
threats to our health, safety, and welfare. But what if they can't because our
"democracy"—as the residents of Nottingham found—puts the interests of
private corporations over the interests of the people who voted them into
office?

A Democracy Problem?

The people in Nottingham and in communities around the country are struggling every day as they seek to protect their environment and public health
from threats that they don't seem to be able to stop. They are coming to the conclusion that our system of law and governance seems to give a small handful
of corporate directors the power to override decisions of whole communities.
They and thousands of communities and activists like them are wrestling with
the problem that our system of law and governance—vaunted as the greatest
democracy in the world—isn't so *democratic* after all.

Many are coming to the conclusion that we have a "democracy problem"
in this country.

A host of advocacy and nonprofit organizations have defined this problem
as one of *access to democracy* and are focused on removing the barriers that
stand in the way of people exercising democracy. By this they mean voting, and
thus they seek to improve access to voting and who we can vote for.

Many of these efforts are aimed at increasing voter registration and boosting turnout on Election Day. For example, the nonpartisan *Southwest Voter
Registration Education Project* focuses its efforts on registering Latino voters
in places with high Latino populations such as Los Angeles, Denver, Santa
Fe, and Dallas. *Project Vote* launched a voter registration drive ahead of the
2008 presidential election, registering over one million new voters in the
process (Project Vote, 2008). Organizations such as *ACORN* and the national

Republican and *Democratic Parties* also engage in large-scale voter registration drives and get-out-the-vote efforts to increase voter turnout at the polls.

Other organizations are focused on ensuring all eligible voters can vote and that their ballots are accurately counted. *Common Cause's* project *Protect the Vote* monitors voting across the United States. The nonpartisan coalition *Election Protection* provides legal support for voters who are prevented from voting and operates a "1–800" telephone number to track voting irregularities on Election Day.

In response to the significant concerns raised about voter access to the polls and proper counting of ballots in the wake of the 2000 presidential election, the *League of Women Voters* launched its *Democracy Agenda* project to improve access to voting and integrity in the voting system. The League provides nonpartisan information to voters on candidates and ballot measures. Likewise, *Project Vote Smart* created the *Voter's Self-Defense System* to provide voters unbiased information about candidates and ballot measures. In addition, to bring greater transparency to the role of big business in the electoral process, the *Center for Responsive Politics* runs the *Open Secrets* project to track corporate spending on federal candidate races.

Organizations such as *Public Campaign, Public Citizen,* and *Fair Elections* advocate on issues related to who voters are able to vote for. For example, through its *Clean Money, Clean Elections* initiative, Public Campaign advocates for publicly funding elections at the state and local level. The goal is to open up access to running for office to all eligible candidates, not just those with large campaign treasure chests. Beginning with Maine in 1998, seven states now have in place laws establishing publicly funded campaign programs for certain elected offices. These voluntary programs establish specific amounts of public funds that candidates may receive to campaign for office.

In addition to publicly funded or "voter-owned" elections, many organizations are focused on passing campaign finance reform legislation at the federal, state, and local level to limit corporate money in elections. The *Brennan Center,* part of the New York University School of Law, assists state and local efforts to put campaign finance laws in place and defends existing campaign finance laws. As well, the nonpartisan *Democracy 21* organization seeks to make "democracy work for all Americans" by advocating for campaign finance reform measures (Democracy 21, 2008).

Is It Enough?

Will these efforts—publicly financing candidate elections, increasing voter registration and turnout, campaign finance reform—solve our "democracy problem?" Do they address the core problem or have the possibility of ending what Charlie Cray and Lee Drutman describe as the "corporate stranglehold on the electoral process?" (Cray & Drutman, 2004). It's this corporate vice grip on elections, they say that drowns "out citizen voices and explains why legislation coming out of Washington often reads like it was ripped straight out of a playbook written by the Business Roundtable" (Cray & Drutman, 2004).

Consider the 2002 federal Bipartisan Campaign Reform Act. Known as McCain-Feingold for its chief sponsors U.S. Senators John McCain and Russ Feingold, the law was the first major piece of campaign finance legislation to pass since the Federal Election Campaign Act of 1971. Yet, even with its ban on corporate "soft money" donations to political parties, the 2008 federal candidate campaigns were the most expensive in history with corporate dollars leading the way (Center for Responsive Politics, 2008).

Why won't campaign finance reform or increasing voter turnout or publicly funding elections solve our "democracy problem?" It is because when we advocate for these measures, we are only able to address the symptoms of the problem, not the problem itself. Because the problem isn't simply that there's too much corporate money in the electoral system. Or that there are simply not enough people engaged in the electoral process that boosting voter registration and turnout will solve. Or even that corporations have too much lobbying power on Capitol Hill. Rather, this "democracy problem" is far more complex and goes to the roots of our country's founding. It goes to the question of who our system of law and governance works for and why. And ultimately, the critical question of "Who decides?"

Analyzing the Democracy Problem

Our "democracy problem" dates back to before the U.S. Constitution a document that was drafted by a small handful of wealthy white men who developed a form of government that was inherently undemocratic. As Lundberg writes "Democracy was not highly rated by the writers of the Constitution" (Lundberg, 1989).

This is seen throughout the Constitution's seven articles. They include, and still do, indirect election of the president. They include, and still do, indirect appointment of the U.S. Supreme Court. They included, and did so until amended in 1913, indirect election of the U.S. Senate. They created a form of government under which the only people allowed to vote were the people considered people—white men of wealth and property. This left out everyone else—including women, African Americans, Native Americans, and poor white men.

The Constitution, we find, protects and forwards the interests of the few over the many; it is undemocratic both in form and substance.

Such thinking challenges our national sense of self, Howard Zinn writes, because we are "inculcated from childhood by pledges of allegiance, national anthems, waving flags, and militaristic rhetoric ..." (Zinn, 2004). He explains:

> The Preamble to the United States Constitution, which declares
> that "we the people" wrote this document, is a great deception. The
> Constitution was written in 1787 by fifty-five rich white men—slave
> owners, bondholders, merchants—who established a strong central
> government that would serve their class intentions.
>
> That use of government for class purposes, to serve the needs of the
> wealthy and powerful, has continued throughout American history,
> down to the present day. It is disguised by language that suggests
> all of us, rich and poor and middle class, have a common language.
> (Zinn, 2004)

The drafters themselves spoke clearly of their intentions at the Constitutional Convention and during ratification. James Madison, known as the architect of the Constitution, averred that the Constitution "ought to be so constituted as to protect the minority of the opulent against the majority" (Elliot, 1836). Alexander Hamilton declared that the people of the new nation were "tired of an excess of democracy" (Elliot, 1836). Edmund Randolph, a delegate from Virginia, argued for the new constitution by observing that "the general object was to provide a cure for the evils under which the U.S. labored; that in tracing these evils to their origin every man had found it in the turbulence and follies of democracy ..." (Madison, 1987).

Following ratification, the interests of this minority were greatly advanced with the aid of the new centralized, federal government and Constitution. We see this throughout the 1800s, as corporations—the key vehicle used by the privileged few—grew not only in number but also in power. By the end of the century, corporations had gained constitutional rights and protections with the generous and facilitative hand of those who were in and allowed to hold judicial and elected positions. So successful were they that corporations were recognized as having constitutional rights decades before women were.

A Corporate State

It is with these rights and protections that corporations are able to *legally* insert themselves into our electoral and political processes, wielding tremendous power and influence over law making and governance.

This is described by many, such as former New York Times reporter Chris Hedges, as *a corporate state run by a corporate government* (Hedges, 2008). Author David Sirota observes that "government and big business are one and the same" (Sirota, 2006). And David Korten adds that corporations are now "the dominant governance institutions on the planet ..." (Korten, 1995). In fact, it was President Rutherford B. Hayes who won the White House in 1877 in a corporate dominated election, who said that "this is a government of the people, by the people and for the people no longer. It is a government of corporations, by corporations, and for corporations" (Korten, 1995).

What Does the Corporate State Look Like?

Prior chapters paint a clear picture of the corporate state in action, where decisions are made not by and for "We the People," but by and for corporate interests.

The money alone that is spent by corporations on lobbying and elections is in the billions of dollars each year. And the influence doesn't stop on Election Day or at the Capitol Hill steps—corporations today are involved in every aspect of governance.

Consider the federal Food and Drug Administration (FDA). There are countless reports of FDA panels stacked with pharmaceutical industry representatives approving new drugs and medical devices. The case of Vioxx is just one recent example. Even after significant concerns were raised that the pain killer increased risk of heart attacks, 10 members of an FDA panel convened in 2005 to consider whether to continue the sale of Vioxx had financial ties to the drugs' manufacturer Merck. The panel approved continued sale of the drug even as Merck was being sued by thousands of patients who'd experienced cardiac problems while taking Vioxx (Center for Science in the Public Interest, 2005).

In 2006, the National Research Center for Women & Families released a study of the pharmaceutical industry's participation on FDA panels considering their products, finding that the vast majority of drug advisory panels had at least one member with a financial conflict of interest. The report references a study published in the *Journal of the American Medical Association* that "found that at 73% of FDA drug advisory committee meetings from 2001 through 2004, the FDA announced that at least one voting member had a financial conflict of interest; at 22% of the meetings, more than half the advisory committee members had such conflicts" (National Research Center for Women & Families, 2006).

The study also found that nearly 80% of drugs considered by FDA panels were recommended for approval and concluded that when a panel member with financial ties to the drug manufacturer was "very enthusiastic about a product, that enthusiasm will be contagious, and if he or she is the first to recommend approval, the product would likely be recommended for approval, probably unanimously" (National Research Center for Women & Families, 2006).

The U.S. Department of Agriculture (USDA) similarly works hand in hand with corporations. The agency's efforts to protect the meatpacking industry following the finding of bovine spongiform encephalopathy (mad cow disease) in U.S. cows was revealing. The following year, when Creekstone Farms Premium Beef announced that it planned to test all of its cows for the disease, the USDA fought against the testing arguing that it would "harm the U.S. meat industry" (Associated Press, 2007). Harm to the public health did not appear to be a concern despite nearly 50 countries shutting their doors to U.S. beef due to a lack of testing for mad cow.

Corporations are similarly able to guide policy and law making on Capitol Hill. For two decades the auto industry successfully blocked efforts to increase federal fuel efficiency, or Corporate Average Fuel Economy (CAFE), standards for cars and light trucks. Since 1990, campaign contributions by the auto industry to congressional candidates have exceeded $125 million. Since then, the industry has spent over four times that on lobbying those same candidates, now holding office in the U.S. House and Senate, to block increases in CAFE standards (Center for Responsive Politics, 2008). It's no wonder then that corporations, with their multimillions of dollars, have "only their views ... heard" (Morris, 2001).

We also see corporations using the courts as tools of governance. For example, in 1994, Vermont enacted a law requiring labeling of products from cows injected with artificial recombinant bovine growth hormone or rBGH. The law was adopted in response to concerns about the possible public health impacts from rBGH. The International Ice Cream Association, Grocery Manufacturers of America, and other industry groups sued the state claiming that the law violated corporations' First Amendment free speech rights. The court agreed, ruling that the labeling requirement violated their First Amendment right *not* to speak and threw out the law (*International Dairy Foods Association v. Amestoy*, 1996).

So What Do We Do?

This small sampling provides but a glimpse into how corporate governance occurs. Our activism is stuck inside this system, a box whose shape and contours are not defined by us.

So instead of putting our time and energy into protecting the public health, for example, we are instead forced to fight endlessly about how much harm to the public health corporations can inflict. Instead of requiring corporations to follow the Precautionary Principle to ensure that the public health is protected from possible threats from corporate activities, we can't, because to do so would violate corporate constitutional rights and protections. Rather than our government requiring all cows be tested for mad cow, it instead advocates against universal testing arguing that it will hurt the meat industry. And the list goes on.

Because we're so busy fighting inside this box—that is labeled "democracy" but is in fact the "corporate state"—we're not able to see the box for the trap that it is and figure out how to break out of it.

Breaking Out of the Box

The tiny Town of Halifax, with less than 2,000 people, is located in southern Virginia's piedmont near the North Carolina border. With its rolling hills and farmland, the town is the county seat of Halifax County.

In the fall of 2007, residents learned of a massive new uranium mine proposed for Pittsylvania County, the neighboring county to the west. A quarter of a century after the Virginia General Assembly approved a statewide moratorium on uranium mining—coinciding with a bottoming out of the market for uranium—it was now considering overturning the moratorium and creating a permitting process to allow the mining to go forward.

The radioactive history of uranium mining in the United States and around the world is devastating for the environment and public health. Knowing this, communities across the region began to organize to oppose the mine. The public health community also weighed in with the Danville Pittsylvania County Academy of Medicine calling for a continuation of the moratorium on mining, along with a similar call from the Medical Society of Virginia, with its membership of over 8,500 physicians across the state.

On February 7, 2008, the Halifax Town Council voted unanimously to adopt a new law to ban mining. Known as the "Town of Halifax Corporate Mining, Bodily Trespass and Community Self-Government Ordinance," the law challenges the fundamental system of law that prohibits communities from being able to decide whether the mining can take place.

Halifax reframed the problem as being about democracy, not mining. Thus the law puts in the hands of the people of Halifax the ability to decide what can happen in their community. The law prohibits corporations from conducting mining and any activities that cause chemical and radioactive bodily trespass. In addition, it eliminates certain corporate constitutional rights and protections within the jurisdiction.

The people of Halifax simply wanted to say "No" to the mining, so they didn't pass a new law to regulate uranium mining better. The residents of Nottingham and Barnstead, in New Hampshire, trying to protect their water from being privatized, took similar steps. Rather than passing laws to improve how corporations siphoned off their water, they said that they didn't want their water taken at all. Like Halifax, they adopted local ordinances that challenge the existing system of law that empowers corporations, not the community, to decide what can happen with their water.

In so doing, these communities join over a hundred others in not merely bucking the system—but rather challenging nearly 200 years of law and jurisprudence that puts the interests of corporations over the interests of people, the public health, communities, and the environment.

Building a Democracy Movement: From the Ground Up

The Pennsylvania-based *Community Environmental Legal Defense Fund* is pioneering this work with communities—such as Nottingham, Barnstead, and Halifax—whose experience shows them that the system of law allows a minority (corporations) to override majority (community) decision making. Thomas Linzey, a founder of the Legal Defense Fund explains, "We work with communities who have come to the conclusion that we don't live in a democracy in this country" (Linzey, 2008).

Through this work, the Legal Defense Fund assists communities to examine and address the fundamental question "Why?" Why does it seem that corporations have more rights than us? Why are coal corporations able to come into our town when their mining operations will knowingly destroy rivers, streams, houses, and farmland? Why can't we stop Nestle from coming in and siphoning off our water to bottle and sell overseas? And why, when nowhere in the world has uranium mining been done safely, are we prohibited from saying "No" to it in our community?

Such questions first led the Legal Defense Fund to launch the *Daniel Pennock Democracy Schools* in 2003 to help communities in Pennsylvania and across the country—their residents and their local elected officials—gain a foothold on "Why?"

Created by the Legal Defense Fund and historian Richard Grossman, nearly 200 Democracy Schools have now been taught across the United States. Over the course of a weekend, Democracy School participants take a close look at the system of law in the United States, analyzing who it works for and why, and how communities are beginning to frontally challenge this system to try to change it.

The Democracy Schools grassroots organizing model grew out of the work of the Legal Defense Fund that began in the late 1990s, as the organization began to work with rural townships in Pennsylvania seeking to stop factory farms from locating in their communities. Factory farms now dominate food production in the United States. Known as "confined animal feeding operations" or CAFOs, agribusiness corporations such as Smithfield and Hatfield Foods warehouse millions of pigs, cows, and chickens in factory like settings where the animals are unable to turn around or go outside for the entirety of their lives.

There are a wide range of reasons why communities may not want a factory farm to come to town. These include the fact that the rise of the agribusiness industry has caused hundreds of thousands of family and independent farms to go out of business. In addition, the severe odor and water pollution generated by CAFOs has significant public health and environment impacts.

Communities approached the Legal Defense Fund for help to stop the factory farms from coming in. Recognizing that communities don't have the legal authority to say "No" to factory farms, the Legal Defense Fund worked with them to do something fundamentally different. The results were the first "Anti-Corporate Farming Ordinances" that ban corporations from engaging in farming in their communities.

From factory farms, the Legal Defense Fund began to assist communities facing the land application of sewage sludge. The Democracy Schools are named for Danny Pennock, a Pennsylvania boy who died after exposure to sludge. Sludge includes anything that is "flushed, poured, or dumped into our nation's wastewater system—a vast, toxic mix of wastes collected from countless sources, from homes to chemical industries to hospitals" (Center for Food

Safety, 2008). The Legal Defense Fund has assisted over 75 municipalities in Pennsylvania to draft and adopt first-in-the-nation laws banning corporations from engaging in the land application of sewage sludge. Like the laws on factory farms, these laws challenge the fundamental system of law that gives corporations the ability to override community decision making and prohibit communities from saying "No."

The work of the Legal Defense Fund has since expanded into other places and issues as communities from across the country seek help to stop the privatization of their water, uranium mining, coal mining, oil and gas drilling, and a range of other threats. The Legal Defense Fund works with these communities to reframe these seemingly single issues, to address the core problem that people and their communities don't have the power to decide what happens in their community.

A critical piece of the over 300 page Democracy School curriculum comes early in the schools. Known as the "Regulatory Triangles," participants examine how the system of law works. Democracy School lecturers—made up of Legal Defense Fund staff, community organizers, and partners—will often use the example of factory farms to describe how the system works. The curriculum includes a graphic of an upside down triangle to demonstrate how even though communities have a wide range of reasons why they don't want a factory farm to come to town (representing the broad base of the triangle at the top of the page), all of their energy and activism is funneled down to the narrow point at the bottom of the upside down triangle. That narrow point represents the "regulatory point"—the laws that regulate an activity such as factory farming.

In Pennsylvania, the regulatory point is represented by the state's Nutrient Management Act—under which the state issues permits to corporations seeking to operate factory farms. Under the Act, communities are only able to seek to modify a permit on the basis of a narrowly tailored set of regulations and laws that the agribusiness corporations themselves helped draft. In this case, the primary issue is manure—how much will be generated and where it will be deposited. Concern about factory farms driving family farms out of business is not considered by the state in issuing the permit. Concern about whether it is appropriate for the community is not considered. Nor does the state weigh whether the people in the community even have the ability to decide whether the factory farm is actually something they want in their township. None of these concerns are considered relevant under the system of law. Rather, the only thing that is considered relevant is manure—that narrow regulatory point at the bottom of the triangle. So the question isn't whether the factory farm can come in or not, it's where are they going to put all the shit.

This is how, as described in the Democracy Schools, the system of law works. Most any corporate threat can be run through the triangles. Consider a community facing a Wal-Mart or other big box store. Under law, communities can't say "No" to Wal-Mart, rather they can only fight about issues such as traffic or building façades—not the economic, environmental, and other impacts from these giant stores. So while there are any number of reasons hundreds of communities across the United States have fought to stop Wal-Mart—the system of law channels them down to a narrow point where they can only argue about stop lights or signage. This is why when a community is facing the privatization of its water that it's only able to fight a corporate water permit on issues related to the number of trucks that can go in and out of the facility each day or similar issues—not whether the facility can be sited at all. Those questions have already been decided by corporations working with state legislatures— wielding their constitutional rights and protections to draft legislation, lobby for its passage, contribute to the elected officials who are voting on it, and threaten to sue a state or community if it is not enforced in their interests.

The work of the Legal Defense Fund with communities has evolved from ordinances through which communities seize their local self governing authority to say "No" to corporations, to now actually eliminating the constitutional rights and protections that corporations wield against communities.

One example we find in Western Pennsylvania coal country. In 2006, Blaine Township, Washington County, facing underground longwall coal mining, worked with the Legal Defense Fund to draft and adopt ordinances that ban corporations from engaging in mining and eliminate corporate constitutional rights. Below is an excerpt from the "Blaine Township Democratic Self-Government and Local Control Ordinance":

> This Ordinance is adopted and enacted pursuant to the inherent
> authority of the residents of Blaine Township to self-government,
> and to authority granted to Blaine Township by all relevant state and
> federal Constitutions and laws, including, but not limited to ...
>
> The Declaration of Independence, which declares that the people of
> Blaine Township are born with "certain unalienable rights" and that
> governments are instituted among people to secure those rights ...
>
> The Pennsylvania Constitution...which declares that "all power is
> inherent in the people and all free governments are instituted for
> their peace, safety, and happiness ...

Democracy means government by the majority, with citizen rights secured to all ...

Usurpation of the democratic process by corporations—and the few who run them—denies the rights of human persons to participate in their democracy in Blaine Township and enjoy a republican form of government therein ...

The ability of citizens of Blaine Township to adopt laws to protect the health, safety, and welfare of township residents has been denied by the wielding of constitutional "rights" by corporations. (Blaine Township, 2006)

Lessons from Past People's Movements

Participants in the Democracy Schools examine how past people's movements, when faced with a system of law that was fundamentally undemocratic and failed to provide remedy for people under the law, took on that system to try to change it.

The Abolitionists, for example, ran up against a system of law that legalized slavery, protecting the interests of the slaveholder over the slave. They fought for decades to change the U.S. Constitution, even though their antislavery activism was considered treasonous. The Suffragists would vote on Election Day even though it was illegal for women to do so and they could end up in jail. And similarly, Rosa Parks and members of the Civil Rights Movement sat on busses and at lunch counters, refusing to accept the system as it was.

Past people's movements fought to expand rights—moving slaves, women, and others from being considered *property* under the law to being *rights-bearing people*. Today, local communities are, in essence, the private property of states whichtellthe communitieswhat can and cannot happen there. Under a legal doctrine known as "Dillon's Rule"—the relationship between states and municipalities has been determined to be that of a parent to a child. Under this doctrine, developed in the late 1800s by Iowa Supreme Court Justice and former railroad lawyer John Dillon, municipal governments only have powers explicitly given to them by the state. Much in the way slaves and women were stuck inside a legal structure where they could only do what they were told, communities today are similarly stuck. And like past people's movements, they are beginning to break out of this structure, to challenge and change it.

Rights of Nature: Pioneering a New Form of Law

The Abolitionists, Suffragists, and other people's movements focused on recognizing and legally protecting the rights of natural people—people previously treated as property under the law.

During slavery, slaves were property that a slave owner could legally harm at will. Today, nature is treated similarly, such that owners of property may harm or destroy it as they wish. Nature has no rights under law.

By most every measure, the environment today is in worse shape than when the major U.S. environmental laws were adopted over 30 years ago. Since then, countries around the world have sought to replicate these laws. Yet, species decline worldwide is increasing exponentially, global warming is far more accelerated than previously believed, deforestation continues unabated around the world, and overfishing in the world's oceans is pushing many fisheries to collapse.

The Legal Defense Fund is working with communities that recognize that environmental protection cannot be attained under a structure of law that treats natural communities and ecosystems as *property*.

These laws—including the federal Clean Air Act and the Clean Water Act—legalize environmental harms by regulating how much pollution or destruction of nature can occur under law. They were passed under the Commerce Clause of the U.S. Constitution that grants exclusive authority over "interstate commerce" to Congress. Treating nature as commerce has meant that all existing environmental law frameworks in the United States are anchored in the concept of nature as property (Linzey, 2008).

The Legal Defense Fund has assisted communities in Pennsylvania, New Hampshire, Maine, and Virginia to craft and adopt new laws that change the status of natural communities and ecosystems from being regarded as *property* under the law to being recognized and protected as *rights-bearing entities*. Those laws recognize that natural communities and ecosystems possess an inalienable and fundamental right to exist and flourish, and that residents of those communities possess the legal authority to enforce those rights on behalf of ecosystems. Thus, when Nottingham, NH, adopted its "Anti-Corporate Water Withdrawal Ordinance" in 2008 to ban water privatization, not only were the people in the community granted rights to enforce the new law, ecosystems within that community were also recognized as having rights. Residents can now confront corporations with the rights of both people living in the community as well as the rights of natural communities harmed by the corporation.

In addition, because corporate constitutional rights are regularly wielded to harm and destroy ecosystems, efforts to change the status of ecosystems under the law inevitably proceed hand in hand with efforts to eliminate corporate rights. Thus, this struggle for ecosystem rights has also become a struggle to eliminate corporate rights.

In 2008, the Legal Defense Fund assisted Delegates to the Ecuador Constituent Assembly to draft Rights of Nature provisions for the country's new constitution. It was approved by an overwhelming margin through a national referendum on September 28, 2008. With that vote, Ecuador became the first country in the world to codify a new system of environmental protection based on rights.

Conclusion

There are communities in the United States such as Nottingham, Halifax, and Blaine that are beginning to recognize and address the problem that we don't live in a democracy. In so doing, they are forced to reveal that which is so readily camouflaged by our government and culture. It is unpopular and many—government, corporations, and others—seek to stop them. Yet, like past people's movements before them, they are determined, understanding that they must do what is difficult to achieve what is necessary.

REFERENCES

Associated Press. *Feds Fight Broad Testing for Mad Cow Disease: False Positives Could Harm Meat Industry, USDA Argues.* MSNBC Website, available at: http://www.msnbc.msn.com/id/18924801. Accessed May 29, 2007.
Blaine Township, Washington County, PA. *Blaine Township Democratic Self-Government and Local Control Ordinance.* 2006.
Center for Food Safety. Available at: http://www.centerforfoodsafety.org/sewage_slu.cfm. Accessed November 8, 2008.
Center for Responsive Politics, Press Release. U.S. Election Will Cost $5.3 Billion, Center for Responsive Politics Predicts. October 22, 2008.
Center for Responsive Politics. Available at: http://www.opensecrets.org. Accessed December 30, 2008.
Center for Science in the Public Interest, Press Release. *Conflicts of Interest on COX-2 Panel.* February 25, 2005.
Cray C, Drutman L. *The People's Business.* San Francisco: Berrett-Koehler Publishers, Inc.; 2004.
Democracy 21. Available at: http://www.democracy21.org/index.asp?Type=B_BASIC&SEC={BF5ECB7D-47F4-42A2-B73D-2655EA0A19AE}. Accessed November 9, 2008.

Elliot J. Notes of the Secret Debates of the Federal Convention of 1787, Taken by the Right Honorable Robert Yates, Chief Justice of the State of New York, and One of the Delegates from that State to the Said Convention. *Debates in the Federal Convention of 1787*, Published under the sanction of Congress, 1836.

Hedges C. Keynote Speech, Furman University, May 28, 2008.

International Dairy Foods Association v. Amestoy, 92 F.3d 67 (2nd Cir. 1996).

Keyssar A. *The Right to Vote: The Contested History of Democracy in the United States.* New York: Basic Books; 2000.

Korten D. *When Corporations Rule the World.* Connecticut: Kumarian Press, Inc., and San Francisco: Berrett-Koehler Publishers, Inc.; 1995.

Linzey T. Author Interview, Portland, Oregon, November 10, 2008.

Lundberg F. *The Myth of Democracy.* New York: Carol Publishing Group; 1989.

Madison J. *Notes of Debates in the Federal Convention of 1787 Reported by James Madison.* New York: W.W. Norton & Company, Inc.; 1987.

Morris JA. Speaking truth to power about campaign reform. In: Dean R, ed., *Defying Corporations, Defining Democracy: A Book of History & Strategies* (p. 192). New York: The Apex Press; 2001.

National Research Center for Women & Families. FDA Advisory Committees: Does Approval Mean Safety, 2006.

Project Vote. Available at: http://www.projectvote.org/index.php?id=14. Accessed November 6, 2008.

Sirota D. Interview with BuzzFlash. Available at: http://www.buzzflash.com/interviews/06/05/into6016.html. Accessed May 8, 2006.

Zinn H. *Voices of a People's History of the United States.* New York: Seven Stories Press; 2004.

13

Legal Strategies: You Are What They Say You Are Eating

Stephen Gardner and Katherine A. Campbell

Introduction

The Center for Science in the Public Interest (CSPI) has long sought to counter industry's powerful influence on public opinion and public policies, and to educate the public about industry's often-used misleading and deceptive marketing. Since 1971, CSPI has advocated for policies that are consistent with scientific evidence on public health issues including: nutrition and health, food safety, alcohol policy, and corporate influence on science and science-based public policy.

The Center for Science in the Public Interest 's Litigation Project uses state and federal courts to help correct corporate misbehavior. CSPI's legal actions have produced binding settlements resulting in more honest labeling and halting deceptive marketing. Litigation, or the threat of litigation, has spurred numerous companies to cleanup dishonest and unhealthy corporate practices—thus making the food available to us both safer and healthier. This chapter discusses the history and legal theories of the regulation of food marketing practices, both generally and with specific attention to CSPI's implementation of these theories.

Stephen Gardner had investments administered by a portfolio management company which itself purchased stock in some corporations described in this chapter, but divested the stocks upon realizing that they had been purchased.

Consumer Confusion—Lost in the Supermarket

Before discussing the current state of corporate marketing practices and government regulation of foods, it is appropriate to start with the person who is the target of advocates, companies, and the government alike—the consumer.

After all, it is for the consumer that consumer advocacy groups advocate. It is for the consumer that a consumer products companies produce. It is for the consumer that Congress congregates. And so on, through the whole feeding chain of interests that have been involved in these issues over the past decades.

Repeatedly, consumers express preferences for healthier foods. Consumer concerns with nutrition remain high. But consumers don't know what to eat. They are confused about watching their carbohydrate intake but still eating enough whole grains. They have heard they should eat a diet low in fat, but also heard that there are "good" fats to eat. They know that they should avoid sweets, but what about artificially sweetened food products? Nutrition science always seems to change: one day consumers hear coffee and chocolate are good for them, the next day consumers hear they should avoid them.

What Does the Consumer Want?

One problem with predicting actual consumer purchasing behavior based on polls of expressed needs and desires is that sometimes consumers give in to the natural tendency (familiar to priests, psychiatrists, and police) to admit to somewhat higher aspirations than they in fact have.[1] That is, consumers may indicate a preference for a low-sodium, nonfat hamburger in response to a mall-intercept pollster with a clipboard. But when subjected to a continuous onslaught of ads, commercials, and other marketing tools that urge the consumer to "have it your way," though the spirit is often willing, the flesh is weak. And there's too much flesh as a result.

A second problem with predicting consumer behavior with respect to diet and health is that there is a considerable gap between expressed consumer desires and actual consumer knowledge of the relative minutiae of nutrition. Thus, though most consumers report that health concerns have caused a major change in their diets[2] and that they use food labels in their search for healthier foods,[3] they are also lacking some of the most basic information necessary to make any significant change in their diet—such as the relationship between HDL and LDL cholesterol,[4] the saturated fat level of coconut oil,[5] and what a complex carbohydrate is.[6] (One suspects that many of the readers of this chapter—certainly many of whom are above the curve on nutritional issues—would hesitate to volunteer certain knowledge of these same bits of information if any sizable amount of money rested on it.)

Perhaps for this reason, consumers tend to express what would at first glance appear to be mutually exclusive desires. First, they want simple means of conveying information. Second, they want enough information to make an informed decision.[7]

Consumers indicate that their four primary sources of information regarding diet and health are (1) news stories, (2) health organizations, (3) physicians and other health professionals, and (4) food labels.[8] Except for labels (subject to manipulation by food companies), these various sources have never been seriously challenged as viable and trustworthy sources of information.

However, to the intense regret of all of us on the consumer side of the fence and the great joy of food marketers, consumers also report that they find informational statements by food companies—*advertising*—to be believable.[9] Presumably, if consumers believe a statement in an ad, they'll use it in their search for the truth.

The Point of Difference

If we could rely on the forthrightness of food marketers, we would probably be able to provide consumers exactly what they say they want—sufficient information that is simple to understand. However, we cannot.

Food marketers are not out to inform the public. Instead, they are out to sell a product. One primary way they sell their product over all others is by creating a point of difference.[10] This point of difference may well be created out of the whole cloth where no perceived difference had existed and where no meaningful difference does exist.[11]

Perhaps the best expression of the ethics of advertisers in this regard is by that grand old man of advertising, David Ogilvy, who bragged that "I could have positioned Dove as a detergent bar for men with dirty hands, but chose instead to position it as a toilet bar for women with dry skin. *This is still working 25 years later.*"[12] Actually, since Ogilvy said that in his 1983 book, *it is still working 50 years later*—on its web site, Dove says that "[e]veryday moisture is the key to beautiful skin. And who knows moisture better than Dove?"[13]

One method of creating a perceived point of difference is to add a smidgen of one or two healthy-sounding ingredients, say acai berry and ginseng, to an otherwise basic food product, say sugar-sweetened water, and sell the product as "Energy-Enhanced-Antioxidant-Immune-Boosting-Super-Berry-Powered Water!" Or add omega-3 to butter spread, and market it as a product that is "Smart." Or add flavanols to a food product otherwise known as a dessert, chocolate, and market it as a cholesterol reducer. Or, perhaps most brilliantly, add nothing at all and claim a point of difference: Jello-O pudding mix contains no added calcium, yet markets itself as a "good source of calcium." The pudding mix magically becomes a good source of calcium once the consumer adds in the milk that the product calls for. (Under this theory, an empty glass is an *excellent* source of calcium, if you add milk.)

Health Claims: What Happens When You Cross a Food Marketer with a Nutrition Scientist

Just over a century ago, the use of health claims to market and sell foods and dietary supplements was unregulated by the federal government. At that time, Congress believed regulation of food was a state issue. Then, in 1906, the Pure Food & Drugs Act (PFDA) was passed by U.S. Congress, and created the first systemic national food law. The PFDA defined "food" and "drugs," and centered on regulating "adulteration" and "misbranding." However, the law had little influence on the widespread use of health claims. Thus, although health claims were forbidden under PFDA, regulation was not enforced.

Then came the Federal Food, Drug & Cosmetic Act (FDCA) in 1938. The FDCA created a strong regulatory dichotomy between food and drugs. Under the FDCA, it was FDA policy that a food product that made any "health statement" resulted in the product's classification as an "unapproved drug," and permitted the FDA to seize the product. (It remains FDA policy that a food product that makes any health statement is classified as an unapproved drug and is subject to seizure. However, today there are myriad exemptions to this policy that are available to food products.) Strict enforcement of this policy forbade—largely successfully—bogus health claims for food for nearly 50 years.

Fast-forward three to four decades. Advances in medical science and concerns about chronic disease gained the public's attention. Press coverage of these issues increased interest in nutrition and the American diet. Food marketers saw potential in making nutrition-based health claims, and industry began to lobby for policy changes.

Meanwhile, U.S. Supreme Court rulings began expanding the rights of commercial speech for advertisers. Court rulings found First Amendment protection for commercial speech, if it concerned "lawful activity" and was not misleading.

In 1984, the Kellogg Company carefully crafted a print advertisement to challenge the FDA's policy that disallowed health claims for food. Kellogg's understated and mild campaign promoted its cereal, All-Bran, to be used to help prevent some forms of colon cancer.[14] The infamous ad ("At last, some news about cancer you can live with.") had the collaboration of the National Cancer Institute (NCI).[15] It was also thoroughly illegal.[16] The FDCA at the time strictly prohibited promotion of a food for prevention of disease without approval by the Secretary of Health and Human Services.[17] Which is precisely what Kellogg did, with the NCI as its perhaps unwitting accomplice.

The FDA took exception and began enforcement steps that would have stopped the claims made by Kellogg.[18] It would have done so, that is, had FDA had the chance to do its job. Instead, the deregulation mavens stepped in. At that time, officials at the Office of Management and Budget effectively muzzled the FDA and prevented it from enforcing the law.[19]

Further, the FTC allowed the advertisement, and the NCI (which was part of the same government agency—the Department of Health & Human Services—as the FDA) endorsed the claim on the ad. Thus, although use of health claims for foods remained forbidden, lax federal enforcement more or less equaled agency approval of their use.

The reaction of much of the marketing community and food industry to this deregulation was unhesitating and unequivocal. Once Pandora's cereal box had been opened a crack, all pandemonium then ensued. Companies of every ilk and repute began making a variety of disease-based claims, all without the scientific support—now largely discredited[20]—that Kellogg had compiled and without the cooperation and oversight of the NCI, or any other regulatory or nonprofit body that did not have a financial stake in the truthfulness and legality of the claims.[21]

The food industry took federal deregulation as a "Get Out of Jail Free" card and as an uncategorical imperative to go forth and profit by deception at the expense of consumers, who were left unprotected. The synchronous apex and nadir of these claims was probably oat bran beer. The very idea of promoting beer to Bubba as a way to fight cholesterol without having to do more than pull a ring-tab caused even some marketers to stop short. And consumer advocates stopped a lot shorter still.

In response, in 1987 the FDA proposed a policy that would have legitimated this tidal wave of health claims. But press coverage on advertising abuses, action against major food companies by state attorneys general, and congressional hearings questioning the FDA's authority to allow health claims, among other things, ensured failure of the policy. As a result of the complex and divided political, economic, and social issues at play here, the U.S. Congress passed the Nutrition Labeling & Education Act (NLEA) in 1990.

The NLEA amended the FDCA, and contained five major provisions: regulation of health and nutrient claims, mandated nutrition labeling, amended

ingredient declaration requirements, state power to enforce federal requirements, and federal preemption for nutritional labeling.[22] The NLEA was supposed to both *allow* health claims and *strictly enforce* health claim regulations.
In a nutshell: Congress cut a deal.

If one thinks the story ends with the passage of the NLEA, one is sadly
mistaken. The development of health claims regulation (and deregulation)
continued to evolve. Today, the extreme hands-off approach by federal authorities is the cause of much misleading corporate marketing. This is why some
health and nutrition advocates have turned to litigation.

Modern Federal Consumer Protection

Federal consumer protection has come full circle from 30 years ago.

1980s: Classic Deregulation

"Deregulation" was a byword of the Reagan Administration.[23] Conservative
ideologues within the government firmly believed in the principles of new
federalism—getting the federal government out of the business of regulating
the lives of Americans, and American business in particular, and leaving the
business of regulation up to the individual states, to act, as described by Justice
Brandeis, as "laboratories of democracy."[24] Each state was free to experiment
with differing manners and methods of governing, without interference from
the federal bureaucracy.[25]

So it went. The architect of President Reagan's transition team at the Office
of Management and Budget, dedicated to dismantling the federal system as
rapidly as possible, was James Miller, who was appointed chairman of the FTC
in 1981. The FTC under Chairman Miller was the antithesis of activist, fulfilling the role of deregulation with enforcement marked more by avoidance than
by observance.[26]

Cynics, unhappy with the prevailing winds at the White House during the
1980s, saw this shift from enforcement less as a true ideological shift than as
an intellectually supportable denial of protection to the average consumer in
favor of corporate America.[27]

Regardless whether this approach arose from altruism or opportunism,
the result of this free-for-all market was a call by consumer advocates and marketers alike for renewed federal activity. Unfortunately, this call fell on plugged
ears—there continued to be an enforcement vacuum at the federal level.[28]

1990s: Regulation Comes by Way of Enforcement Lawyers

Among the other forces of nature that abhor a vacuum are the state attorneys general. Before the 1980s, the attorneys general had focused their consumer protection efforts on problems in their own states, leaving most national consumer protection enforcement to their federal counterparts at the FDA and FTC. But with the advent of deregulation at the federal level came a rise in activity at the state level, which continues to this day.

The attorneys general had already come together to deal with deception in automotive repair,[29] in discount airline advertising,[30] and in rental car practices,[31] among other things. As they worked together, they learned that they could have a significant impact on the practices of major national companies that deceived the citizens of their states. Even if the federal agencies charged with consumer protection were out of commission, the state attorneys general were willing to pool their resources to protect their own citizens.[32]

Thus, several state attorneys general banded together to bring enforcement actions against a number of food marketers, including the makers of Campbell's soups, Sara Lee pastries, and Nabisco's Fleischmann's margarine, for a variety of health-related claims for foods that the attorneys general had concluded were deceptive in violation of state laws.[33] The state attorneys general had the authority—under the same consumer protection laws as private citizens (discussed in detail in section Consumer Protection Class Actions as a Reform Tool below)—to act to prevent deceptive acts within their states. In fact, in many instances there are remedies available to the attorneys general—including rulemaking,[34] penalties,[35] and the power to subpoena[36]—that are not available to private litigants.

Industry, which had reacted so positively to the new federalism when it meant no law enforcement at the federal level, began to raise all manner of objections to the several states that fulfilled the promise of the new federalism by enforcing their own consumer protection laws when necessary.[37] Claims of preemption, commerce clause problems, and First Amendment infringement began to be leveled against the states that chose to act against deceptive claims for foods.[38] They all proved fruitless.[39] The state attorneys general didn't go away. The cumulative effect of the rise in state activities was a renewed cry by marketers for the renascence of the FDA, the FTC and other federal agencies.[40]

Belatedly following on the heels of the state attorneys general, FDA and FTC activity increased in the late 1980s and through the 1990s.

The New Millennium: Deregulation Is Back

In the past decade, the FDA abandoned its longtime deference to state health officials and state food and drug enforcement in favor of an active program of intervention by its General Counsel office in private and public suits alike, urging that those suits are preempted by federal regulation (or the lack thereof).[41]

Federal regulatory efforts have been, in part, turned over to industry. For example, the Institute of Medicine of the National Academies proposed to turn federal regulatory efforts over to industry, to conclude that "[t]here is not enough evidence of food, beverage, and entertainment advertising's adverse impacts on children to support calling for a ban on all such advertising to kids." Instead of governmental action, the IOM favored letting food marketers police themselves: "Industry should develop and strictly adhere to marketing and advertising guidelines that minimize the risk of obesity in children and youth."[42]

Corporate voluntary codes, though seemingly a step in the right direction, do not adequately protect health. Often, the codes are weak, vaguely written, and do not provide a means of enforcement. For example, in alcohol advertising, industry has voluntary codes regarding advertising aimed at children that addresses advertisement placement, content, product placement, web site advertising, and marketing on college campuses. But the codes allow placement of alcohol ads during programs where half the audience is younger than 21 years. That standard results in many children viewing alcohol advertising.[43]

CSPI's Response to Corporate Malfeasance and Federal Deregulations

For decades, CSPI publicly criticized food companies for their deceptive marketing practices and sought to convince those companies to produce healthier foods, using a variety of approaches, including press releases, articles in CSPI's magazine Nutrition Action Healthletter, and sometimes direct contacts with the companies. While these efforts sometimes succeeded, often the companies would ignore CSPI's entreaties. CSPI then might turn to the FTC, or the FDA, or some other public enforcement agency, historically with mixed but sometimes positive results.

Come the new Millennium, the feds largely stopped enforcing federal laws prohibiting deceptive marketing practices, and did not actively push industry to provide healthier consumer food products in the interest of public health. CSPI decided to turn to the courts to stop deceptive labeling, fraudulent advertising, and the use of dangerous food additives, so it created its Litigation Project in 2004.

The rest of this chapter describes the legal construct that CSPI uses and illustrate the concept with specific results.

Consumer Protection Class Actions as a Reform Tool

The great bulk of lawsuits involving harmful or deceptive food and nutrition practices have been brought under state consumer protection laws (whether by CSPI, private lawyers, or public enforcers such as the state attorneys general).

These laws are often referred to as UDAP laws, shorthand for Unfair and Deceptive Acts and Practices laws. Use of UDAP laws to address marketplace predation is not new. The earliest large-scale attempt by states to regulate deceptive advertising came about almost a century ago, as the result of a 1911 model statute proposed by *Printer's Ink*, an advertising industry trade journal. Approximately 44 states adopted one version or another of the proposed statute.

For example, the California version of this model law first appeared in the California Penal Code in 1915[44] and in 1941 was transferred to the California Business and Professions Code. [45] Its scope is broad, in keeping with most other state UDAP laws:

> It is unlawful for any person, firm, corporation ... with intent
> directly or indirectly to dispose of real or personal property or to
> perform services, ... or to induce the public to enter into any obliga-
> tion relating thereto, to make or disseminate or cause to be made
> or disseminated before the public in this state, ... in any newspaper
> or other publication, or any advertising device, ... any statement,
> concerning such real or personal property or services, ... or concern-
> ing any circumstance or matter of fact connected with the proposed
> performance or disposition thereof, which is untrue or misleading,
> and which is known, or which by the exercise of reasonable care
> should be known, to be untrue or misleading ... .[46]

Starting in the 1960s, state legislators and politicians realized that an increasingly sophisticated marketplace was causing more and more problems for the "average" consumer. No longer did most purchasers go down to the "mom and pop" store to purchase what they needed, if in fact they ever did. Sales transactions became more and more impersonal, products were perceived as being less reliable than in "the good old days," and service was no longer what was being sold.

Three model UDAP laws were proposed as ways of equalizing the consumer's reduced position in the sales transaction.

The first of these, the Uniform Deceptive Trade Practice Act (UDTPA), was adopted in 1964 by the National Conference of Commissioners on Uniform State Laws. In its uniform version it is found at 7A U.L.A. 265 (West, Master Edition, 1985).[47] It lists 11 specifically defined deceptive trade practices, including trademark and trade name infringement; passing off goods as those of another; bait and switch; disparagement; misrepresentations of standards, origins, or quality of goods; misleading price comparisons; and a catchall provision which covers "conduct which similarly creates a likelihood of confusion or of misunderstanding." Although the UDTPA relieves a consumer from having to prove actual confusion, reliance, damage, or the intent to deceive, it does not provide for monetary recovery but only allows the plaintiff to obtain injunctive relief against future violations by the defendant. Some states that based their "consumer protection" statutes on the UDTPA therefore expanded its scope by adding provisions that give consumers the right to recover damages (sometimes setting forth a minimum damage amount), added to the list of defined deceptive practices reference to "unfair practices" as used in § 5 of the Federal Trade Commission Act, and provided for governmental enforcement.[48]

The second model act is the Uniform Consumer Sales Practices Act (UCSPA), which was adopted by the National Conference of Commissioners on Uniform State Laws in 1971. In its uniform version it is found at 7A U.L.A. 231 (West, Master Edition, 1985).[49] The stated purposes of the UCSPA were to provide sellers with more predictable standards for their conduct and to protect consumers against deceptive and unconscionable sales practices. The UCSPA was an attempt to modernize consumer sales practices, to require fairness in sales practices, to make state laws on consumer sales practice uniform, and to conform state requirements to FTC policies. The UCSPA prohibits unconscionable and deceptive sales practices. As with the UDTPA, it provides examples of 11 types of deceptive conduct, but these are not meant to be an exclusive listing of deceptive practices. There is some overlap with the 11 listed deceptive practices of the UDTPA.

The third model act is the Unfair Trade Practices and Consumer Protection Act (UTP-CPA). Starting in the mid-1960s the FTC began cooperating with state and local law enforcement officials in antitrust and consumer protection matters to a far larger degree than ever before. In 1971, the FTC issued a tentative draft Model Law for State Government, which came in the wake of its proposal that states adopt "Mini-FTC Acts."[50] The Model Act combines the basic language of section 5(a)(1) of the Federal Trade Commission Act[51] with the 11 specifically delineated deceptive practices of the UDTPA and some of the prohibited practices of the UCSPA, for a total of 19 "unfair methods of competition and unfair or deceptive acts or practices in the conduct of any trade or commerce" that are declared to be "unlawful."

Thus, although there are three separate model acts, the approach taken in each of them is similar, and thus most state UDAP laws allow both private and public protection of consumers.

Private protection is made possible by provisions in these UDAP laws that allow prevailing consumers to recover attorneys fees and costs.[52]

Food companies, and other UDAP defendants, usually raise defenses based on the First Amendment (commercial speech), the Commerce Clause of the Constitution, federal preemption, and the standing of the consumer to bring the lawsuit. Each of these defenses is the subject of numerous court opinions[53] and much scholarly writing.[54] Detailed discussion of these defenses is thus far beyond the scope of this paper.

False Claims Act

In addition to UDAP laws, there is another potential advocacy tool, the federal False Claims Act ("FCA").[55] Unlike virtually any other statute, the procedural mechanism for a FCA case involves three-party litigation—(1) the *qui tam* plaintiff, called the relator; (2) federal, state, or local government[56]; and (3) the defendant. This part of the chapter is a brief introduction to false claims, simply to describe the potential of this tool.

The *qui tam* plaintiff and the *qui tam* plaintiff's attorney are acting on behalf of two interests—that of the person filing the complaint and that of the United States: "A person may bring a civil action for a violation of section 3729 for the person and for the United States Government. The action shall be brought in the name of the Government."[57]

However, the interests of the relator and the government, as articulated by the United States Supreme Court, are not always harmonious:

> That a *qui tam* suit is brought by a private party "on behalf of the United States" ... does not alter the fact that a relator's interests and the Government's do not necessarily coincide. Moreover, as the statute specifies, *qui tam* actions are brought both "for the person and for the United States Government."[58]

Importantly, the *qui tam* plaintiff need not suffer any damage in order to bring the action.[59] The rationale of courts is that although the injury in fact is suffered by the United States, the FCA envisions "representational standing on the part of assignees" such "that the United States' injury in fact suffices to confer standing on" the relator.[60]

An FCA complaint cannot be based upon any information previously publicly disclosed or which was the subject of a government investigation.[61] The primary exception to the public disclosure bar is the "original source" rule. Even if there has been a public disclosure of the information on which the complaint is based, the "original source" of the information may still qualify to be a *qui tam* relator.

"Original source" means an individual who has direct and independent knowledge of the information on which the allegations are based and has voluntarily provided the information to the United States before filing an action under this part that is based on the information, and whose information provided the basis or catalyst for the investigation, hearing, audit, or report that led to the public disclosure.[62]

Corporations as well as individuals may be liable under the statute,[63] which imposes both joint and several liability[64] as well as conspiracy liability for acts taken in concert[65] under the FCA. Although local governments may be defendants, States may not be defendants.[66]

The penalties imposed under the FCA are severe. The statute provides for (1) mandatory payment of treble damages,[67] (2) government[68] and private counsel expenses, attorneys fees, and costs,[69] and (3) $5,000–$10,000 penalty per false claim.[70] If a defendant self-discloses to the government the fraudulent claims and cooperates with the investigation, liability under the statute is limited to double damages, expenses, attorneys fees, and costs, but no penalties.[71]

Claims filed under the FCA may be joined with other common law and statutory claims, such as unjust enrichment, breach of contract, and punitive damages.[72] The relator may also join in the same lawsuit individual claims for wrongful termination, retaliation or other employment-related claims. Under the FCA, there are specific whistleblower protections contained within the statute.[73]

The FCA grants the federal district court jurisdiction over supplemental claims arising under state law[74]:

A *qui tam* plaintiff, called a relator, has information about the submission of false or fraudulent claims to the government. The relator files a complaint under seal and serves a copy of the complaint on the United States.[75] Critically, the complaint is not served on the defendant to allow the government the time to investigate and determine whether or not it wants to intervene in the action. The complaint may not be served absent a court order.[76]

The complaint should be very detailed. The *qui tam* plaintiff and counsel can dictate the breadth and scope of the government's investigation only based upon the information they present. After the case is filed, government attorneys may effectively take over investigation of the case based upon information provided by the *qui tam* plaintiff. While the *qui tam* plaintiff and his or her attorney may focus government efforts in the government investigation, the degree of involvement remains dependent upon the type of information brought by the *qui tam* plaintiff and the credibility the *qui tam* plaintiff and his or her attorney can bring to the investigation. It is therefore critical that any *qui tam* plaintiff and his or her counsel thoroughly and competently investigate the case and present a complete factual basis of the laws that are alleged to have been breached, and the damages resulting.

A disclosure statement must accompany the complaint. It is not filed but is served directly on the government. The disclosure statement may contain several items, but typically contains at least the following three items: (1) the facts known to the relator's counsel based upon the prefiling investigation; (2) a summary of legal theories on which the claim is based; and (3) documentary evidence in the possession of the possession of the relator.[77] Evidence may include documents, correspondence, lists of potential witnesses; lists of documents to be subpoenaed, statement of relator, summary of liability, and a summary of damages.

Although the statute requires government to make its decision to intervene within 60 days after service of both the complaint and the disclosure statement,[78] the practice under the FCA is that the government often seeks multiple extensions[79] and may typically take as long as 1 or 2 years to decide whether to intervene in the action. However, the government must show "good cause" to obtain the extensions.[80]

If the government chooses to intervene, the U.S. Attorney may attempt to settle the action[81] or ask that the complaint be unsealed.[82] If the complaint is unsealed, it will be served on the defendant and the government will have primary responsibility for prosecuting the action.[83] The *qui tam* plaintiff, however, still has a statutory right to participate in the lawsuit, unless the government or defendant seeks to limit the *qui tam* plaintiff's involvement by court order.[84]

If the government declines to intervene, the *qui tam* plaintiff may continue the action on behalf of the government on his or her own,[85] while continuing to inform the government of the course of the litigation.[86] The government also retains its right to intervene at a later stage in the case.[87] Importantly, the government is not liable for any expenses, although if the United States does not intervene, the relator may be liable for defendants expenses where the court finds the "action was frivolous, vexatious, or brought primarily for purposes of harassment."[88]

The *qui tam* provisions of the FCA can be an invaluable tool for local governments to combat fraud and waste by government contractors. Because of the ability of private parties to bring *qui tam* actions under the statute, local government counsel need to develop expertise in litigating these cases. The rewards and benefits, both in money and deterrence, can be substantial.

Examples of Successful Use of UDAP Law in Food and Nutrition

The Center for Science in the Public Interest's Litigation Project has accomplished much during its short lifetime. The legal theory for its use of litigation as another form of public interest advocacy was based on the same UDAP laws already discussed.[89]

Examples of CSPI's use of consumer litigation advocacy are highlighted below.

Anheuser-Busch and Miller Brewing

In 2008, CSPI notified Anheuser-Busch and Miller Brewing Company of its intent to sue the companies over caffeinated alcoholic drinks such as Anheuser-Busch's Bud Extra and Tilt, and Miller's Sparks. The drinks, dubbed "alcospeed" by CSPI, have more alcohol than beer and contain stimulant additives that are not officially approved for use in alcoholic drinks, including caffeine, taurine, ginseng, or guarana.

No studies are available to support the safety of consuming those stimulants and alcohol together. On the contrary, new research does indicate that the young consumers of these type of drinks are more likely to binge drink, become injured, ride with an intoxicated driver, or be taken advantage of sexually than drinkers of conventional alcoholic drinks.[90] Therefore, drinking alcospeed is more dangerous than drinking alcohol alone.

The viral marketing campaigns[91] behind the drinks are clearly designed to appeal to young, and often underage, drinkers. For example, MillerCoors' marketing plan for Sparks is deliberately untraditional. It uses a chaotic, interactive website[92] that offers a local store and venue locator for the drink. It emphasizes the stimulant effect of Sparks, starting with the name "Sparks," which conveys the sense of an electric surge of energy, and continuing on the can itself, which resembles a battery (to deliver an electric charge).

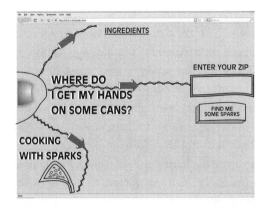

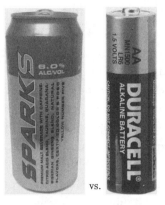

vs.

MillerCoors employed Street Attack, a firm specializing in so-called gue-rilla marketing, which uses "cultural curators" who "work with Street Attack account teams to continually build new networks, gain sponsorship oppor-tunities, open new bar accounts and create [word-of-mouth] buzz for Sparks. Target scenes included: hipster, indie, DJ, rock, art, graffiti, etc."[93]Last, and perhaps the most insidious form of viral marketing it uses, MillerCoors gives away Sparks for free at "house parties, concert backstage scenes, recording studios and art events."[94] Private gatherings do not have the same level of licensing requirements, strict regulations, or other safety nets that regulate alcohol—especially its consumption by minors—in public establishments.

Miller rejected CSPI's offer to attempt settlement without a lawsuit. Unlike MillerCoors, Anheuser-Busch promptly agreed to talk and CSPI was able to reach a settlement without needing to file suit.[95] As part of the settle-ment with CSPI, Anheuser-Busch removed the caffeine, guarana, and gin-seng from its alcoholic beverages Tilt and Bud Extra. The company, which also settled with 11 state attorneys general, agreed to remove the Tilt and Bud Extra web sites until those drinks are reformulated without the stimu-lants, and the company will urge competitors to cease production of their caffeinated alcoholic drinks.

Because Miller refused to do the same, CSPI filed suit in DC Superior Court in 2008. Following this suit and in large part because of an inves-tigation by state attorneys general, Miller agreed to essentially the same changes as Anheuser-Busch had cooperatively agreed to make months previous.[96]

Thus, the two major sellers of alcospeed have been forced out of that business.

Kellogg

In a landmark legal settlement with CSPI, the Campaign for a Commercial-Free Childhood, and two Massachusetts parents, the Kellogg Company agreed to adopt nutrition standards for the foods it advertises to young children. Foods advertised on children's media—such as Nickelodeon and other TV, radio, print, and third-party web sites that have an audience of 50% or more children under age 12—must meet Kellogg's new nutrition standards.[97] Also, Kellogg will not use licensed characters, such as SpongeBob, in advertising and on packages unless those foods meet the nutrition standards. For all products, Kellogg agreed to stop sponsoring product placements in children's media and to stop advertising in preschools and elementary schools.

School Soft Drinks

The Center for Science in the Public Interest's negotiations with the major soft drink companies to get soft drinks out of public schools contributed to an agreement announced through the Clinton Foundation and the American Heart Association. Coca-Cola, PepsiCo, and Cadbury Schweppes agreed to phaseout sugary soft drinks from schools.[98]

Starbucks

After CSPI publicized the possibility of a lawsuit against Starbucks for the presence of trans fat in numerous pastry products, Starbucks met with CSPI in July 2006. This meeting may have expedited Starbucks' January 2, 2007 announcement that it was immediately eliminating trans fat in half of its U.S. stores (with the other half changing by the end of 2007).

KFC

The primary purpose of this lawsuit was to force KFC to stop using oils rich in trans fat for frying and other purposes, or at least make the chain warn customers of the risks of partially hydrogenated oil. Several months after the lawsuit was filed, KFC announced that it would switch to a healthier cooking oil for most of its products. Presumably, the lawsuit accelerated KFC's action. CSPI dropped out of the lawsuit, which was filed jointly by a Washington law firm, as soon as KFC made its announcement.[99]

Sara Lee

In 2007, CSPI notified Sara Lee of its intent to sue based on misleading claims on labels for the company's "Soft & Smooth Made With Whole Grain White Bread." The label and advertising for the product led customers to believe that the product was mostly—or entirely—made of whole grains. Unfortunately this is not true. The product is mostly made with refined grains, and is only 30% whole grain.

As part of a settlement agreement with CSPI, Sara Lee will make it clear the product contains only 30% whole grains rather than claiming the product is nutritionally equivalent to 100% whole wheat bread. The new labels will also say that two slices of bread contain only 10 grams of whole grains, and that the government recommends consuming 48 grams of whole grains per day.[100]

Splenda

Splenda is an artificial sweetener, but its makers (McNeil-PPC, Inc. and McNeil Nutritionals, LLC) promote Splenda in a way that CSPI determined misleads consumers into believing that Splenda is a simply natural form of sugar without the calories: "Made from Sugar, Tastes Like Sugar." CSPI's consumer research surveys showed that consumers think that Splenda as "natural" or "not an artificial product." In truth, Splenda is a synthetic chemical that contains chlorine and is not natural. The Sugar Association[101] sued McNeil on behalf of its members, to stop this deceptive practice. McNeil moved to dismiss the suit, claiming in part that the Sugar Association had waited too long to sue. CSPI filed an *amicus curiae* ("friend of the court") brief, advising the court that it is in the public's interest to stop fraudulent and misleading marketing at any point—even four years after the start of the deceptive Splenda campaign. The court agreed with CSPI's position, and denied the motion to dismiss. In 2008, the Sugar Association and McNeil settled the lawsuit, the terms of which are sealed.

Quaker Oats

The Center for Science in the Public Interest contacted Quaker about label and ad claims that significantly exaggerated the minimal effect oatmeal might have on lowering cholesterol. The company agreed to modify its claims. However, as part of its monitoring of settlements, CSPI discovered that Quaker had not in fact changed all packaging and advertising as it had promised, so negotiations with Quaker have resumed. CSPI also previously negotiated with Quaker to revise labels for several varieties of instant oatmeal and grits so that consumers would know that the products did not contain any real fruit, real butter, or real meats (ham, bacon), as the labels imply.[102]

Capri Sun

The Center for Science in the Public Interest met with Kraft officials to obtain their agreement to stop calling Capri Sun drinks "natural" because they are sweetened with the very unnatural high-fructose corn syrup (HFCS). Kraft initially refused but after CSPI filed suit against Kraft,[103] the company announced that it was in the process of getting rid of the claim.

Cadbury Schweppes

The Center for Science in the Public Interest had also been in talks with Cadbury over its use of "100% Natural" to describe 7UP, also sweetened with HFCS. Within days of the suit against Kraft for Capri Sun, Cadbury agreed to drop the "100% Natural" claim, and CSPI dropped a planned lawsuit against the company. Shortly after that, Cadbury agreed that it would remove "100% Natural" from HFCS-sweetened Snapple drinks as well.[104]

Frito-Lay Lights

After a petition by Procter & Gamble and Frito-Lay, the FDA reversed a prior decision and allowed the companies to omit the warning on packages of foods containing the fake fat olestra, which causes mild to severe diarrhea and abdominal cramps in some consumers. Frito-Lay then removed all references to olestra, except in the ingredients statement, to make it less likely that consumers would not know what they were buying. Sales of the products increased significantly, as did the number of adverse reaction reports filed on CSPI's Web site. CSPI negotiated an agreement with Frito-Lay to change the labels of its chips to make the presence of olestra clearer.[105]

Fat Free Pringles

As with Frito-Lay, CSPI negotiated with Procter & Gamble to change the labels of Fat Free Pringles (now Pringles Lights) to make the presence of olestra clearer.

Betty Crocker

After CSPI met with General Mills about their Super Moist Carrot Cake Mix, which has only a tiny amount of dehydrated carrots, General Mills put a front label notice on the package to let consumers know that the product contains only carrot-flavored bits.

Aunt Jemima Frozen Blueberry Waffles

After CSPI contacted it, Pinnacle Foods agreed to revise labels to make it clear that there was no actual fruit in the waffles and that the so-called blueberries were artificial bits.[106]

Tropicana Peach Papaya

At the request of a private attorney, CSPI joined in a lawsuit against PepsiCo based on the fact that Tropicana Peach Papaya juice drink (1) contains no peach, (2) contains no papaya, and (3) is not a juice. Shortly after CSPI joined the litigation, PepsiCo agreed to modify its labels for Tropicana Peach Papaya, Tropicana Strawberry Melon, and Tropicana Twisters (even though the last two were not included in the lawsuit) to make it clear to consumers that these are artificially flavored drinks with very little actual juice (and pear juice at that). [107]

Conclusion

Although this chapter just scratches the surface of public interest litigation—whether by private lawyers, public lawyers, or (in the case of the False Claims Act) a true public–private partnership of lawyers—it demonstrates the potential for advancing the interests of consumers, and reining in the worse impulses of major marketers. Lawsuits should always be the last choice, but when the administrative agencies and Congress fail to do the job, there's only one branch of government left—the judicial branch.

NOTES

1 Robert B. Settle and Pamela L. Alreck, *Why They Buy: American Consumers Inside and Out*, 34–35 (1989).
2 CFSAN Study at 22.
3 CFSAN Study at 8.
4 CFSAN Study at 21.

5 CFSAN Study at 20–21.

6 CFSAN Study at 21.

7 Levy, Alan S. and others, *More Effective Nutrition Label Formats Are Not Necessarily Preferred*, 92 J. Amer. Dietetic Assn. 1230, 1234 (1992).

8 CFSAN Study at 7.

9 CFSAN Study at 19.

10 Theodore Levitt, The Marketing Imagination 85 *et seq.* (Expanded Ed. 1986).

11 *See, e.g.,* Theodore Levitt, The Marketing Imagination 86 (Expanded Ed. 1986).

12 David Ogilvy, Ogilvy on Advertising 12 (1983) [emphasis added].

13 http://www.dove.us/#/Products/BarSoapBodyWash/BB_White.aspx/ (last visited September 25, 2008).

14 S. House Comm. on Governmental Relations, Disease-Specific Health Claims on Food Labels: An Unhealthy Idea, H.R. Rep. No. 561, 100th Cong., 2d Sess. 2–3 (1988). This report, issued under the chairmanship of the late Congressman Ted Weiss of New York, provides an excellent summary of the activities and inactivities of the various federal players during this period.

15 It is likely that it was Kellogg's careful adherence to many criteria advanced by health professionals, consumer advocates, and regulatory officials that made its advertising campaign both informative and effective, although unfortunately unique in this regard. Bruce Silverglade, *A Comment on Public Policy Issues in Health Claims for Foods*, 10 J. Public Policy & Marketing 54, 55 (1991).

16 U.S. House Comm. on Governmental Relations, Disease-Specific Health Claims on Food Labels: An Unhealthy Idea, H.R. Rep. No. 561, 100th Cong., 2d Sess. 2–3 (1988). *See also* Bruce Silverglade, *Preemption—The Consumer Viewpoint*, 45 Food Drug Cosm. L.J. 143, 146 (1990). This article contains an excellent overview of the causes and effects of the mania for health claims, written from the perspective of the CSPI's director of legal affairs.

17 Under then-existing 21 U.S.C. § 321(g)(B) any "article[] intended for use in the diagnosis, cure, mitigation, treatment, or prevention of disease in man" is a "new drug." 21 U.S.C. § 355 prohibited the introduction of "new drugs" into commerce without prior approval. 21 U.S.C. §§ 321(f, p), 343 and 355. *See also* U.S. House Comm. on Governmental Relations, Disease-Specific Health Claims on Food Labels: An Unhealthy Idea, H.R. Rep. No. 561, 100th Cong., 2d Sess. at 6–11.

18 U.S. House Comm. on Governmental Relations, Disease-Specific Health Claims on Food Labels: An Unhealthy Idea, H.R. Rep. No. 561, 100th Cong., 2d Sess. 2–3 (1988).

19 U.S. House Comm. on Governmental Relations, Disease-Specific Health Claims on Food Labels: An Unhealthy Idea, H.R. Rep. No. 561, 100th Cong., 2d Sess. at 22–26.

20 *See, e.g.,* National Cancer Institute, U.S. National Institutes of Health, "The Polyp Prevention Trial and the Wheat Bran Fiber Study: Questions and Answers," available at www.cancer.gov/cancertopics/factsheet/polyp-prevention-fiber-qa (last accessed June 29, 2009); *also see* www.cancer.org/docroot/PED/content/PED_3_2X_Diet_and_Activity_Factors_That_Affect_Risks.asp (last accessed June 29, 2009).

21 Many nutritionists now believe that the link between dietary fiber and cancer prevention is less certain than was thought to be the case in the mid-1980s. *See, e.g.,* Fuchs, C.S., Dietary Fiber and the Risk of Colorectal Cancer and Adenoma in Women, New England J. Med. 340:169–176 (1999). This illustrates why leaving it up to food marketers to cure disease is an idea whose time has come and gone.

22 Pub.L. 101–535, § 1(a), Nov. 8, 1990, 104 Stat. 2353; codified at 21 U.S.C. 301 *et seq.*; see also www.fda.gov/ora/inspect_ref/igs/nleatxt.html.

23 *See* Exec. Order No. 12,612, 52 Fed. Reg. 41,685 (1987).

24 *New State Ice Co. v. Liebmann,* 285 U.S. 262, 311 (1932) (Brandeis, J., dissenting).

25 Exec. Order No. 12,612, 52 Fed. Reg. 41,685 (1987).

26 *Report of the American Bar Association Section of Antitrust Law Special Committee to Study the Role of the Federal Trade Commission,* 56 Antitrust & Trade Reg. Rep. (BNA) No. 1410, at S-11 to S-12 (Apr. 6, 1989).

27 Burros, *Eating Well,* N.Y. Times, Feb. 27, 1991, at C3, col. 1.

28 One consumer advocate commented that the problem was that the FDA and FTC were "understaffed, underfunded, and under Reagan."

29 *Big Suits. Texas v. AAMCO,* Texas Lawyer, Mar. 2, 1987, at 12, col. 1.

30 National Association of Attorneys General, *Report and Recommendations of NAAG Task Force on Air Travel Industry: Guidelines for Air Travel Advertising,* 53 Antitrust & Trade Reg. Rep. (BNA) No. 1345 (special supp.) (Dec. 17, 1987). This particular state enforcement effort came for naught when the United States Supreme Court held that states were preempted from enforcing state laws against deceptive airline advertising. *Morales v. Trans World Airlines, Inc.,* 112 S.Ct. 2031 (1992).

31 National Association of Attorneys General, *Final Report and Recommendations of the Task Force on Car Rental Advertising and Practices,* 56 Antitrust & Trade Reg. Rep. (BNA) No. 1407 (special supp.) (Mar. 16, 1989).

32 *Report of the American Bar Association Section of Antitrust Law Special Committee to Study the Role of the Federal Trade Commission,* 56 Antitrust & Trade Reg. Rep. (BNA) No. 1410, at S-12 (Apr. 6, 1989).

33 Sugarman, *The New Chow Hounds. States Join Forces to Monitor Product Claims,* Wash. Post, Sept. 21, 1988, at El, col. 3; Burros, *Eating Well,* N.Y. Times, Feb. 27, 1991, at C3, col. 1.

34 E.g., Maryland Com. Code Ann., § 13–205(a); Maine Rev. Stat. Ann. title 5, § 207(2).

35 E.g., California Business and Professions Code, §§ 17206 and 17536 (the court shall assess a "civil penalty not to exceed two thousand five hundred dollars ($2,500) for each violation"). A standard sales presentation that is repeated to 1000 different individuals may result 1000 separate penalties. People v. Superior Court (Jayhill) (1973) 9 Cal.3d 283. And penalties are not limited to the corporate entity, but corporate officers and those responsible for the institution of the deceptive plan or advertising are also liable for civil penalties. See, e.g., United States v. Park 421 U.S. 658, 672; Consumers Home Equipment Co. v. FTC, 164 F.2d 972 (6th Cir. 1947).

36 Attorney general subpoenas are usually called Civil Investigative Demands. See, e.g., Md. Com. Law Code Ann., § 13–405; New York Exec. Law, § 63(12); and Texas Bus. & Comm. Code, §§ 17.60 and 17.61.

37 Probably the finest example of these arguments can be found in an instance of the FTC carrying the industry's water. John E. Calfee and Janis K. Pappalardo, *How Should Health Claims for Foods Be Regulated? An Economic Perspective*, Bureau of Economics, Federal Trade Commission (1989). As an artifact of a failed regulatory approach, this piece is must reading. One way for those opposed to consumer protection efforts in the Eighties to advance an intellectual justification for their inactivity was to use a cost-benefit analysis. Because they found any inconvenience to industry a major cost and found no benefit to a deception-free marketplace, the cost-benefit battles were over before they began, as far as this breed of economists was concerned. Calfee and Pappalardo's attempt to quantify that which is essentially metaphysical reached its charmingly nutty peak when they put forth the proposition that the best justification for FDA failing to act on illegal health claims was derived from the formula: $EV = PtBt - (l-Pt)Cf$, where EV is the expected value of allowing a health claim, Pt is the probability that the claim will turn out to be true, Bt is the estimated net benefit of allowing the claim if it turns out to be true, and Cf is the estimated net cost of allowing the claim if it turns out to be false. *Id.*, at 39–44. Got it?

38 For good discussions of the ill effects of preemption, and the lack of legal underpinnings for it, *see* Charles P. Mitchell, *State Regulation and Federal Preemption of Food Labeling*, 45 Food Drug Cosm. L. J. 123 (1990); and Richard L. Cleland, *The Regulation of Food Labeling: An Effective, Uniform National Standard Without More Preemption*, in James E. Tillotson (Ed.), America's Foods: Health Messages and Claims: Scientific, Regulatory, and Legal Issues (1993).

39 *See, e.g., Kellogg Co. v. Mattox*, 763 F. Supp. 1369 (N.D. Tex. 1991), *aff'd* 5th Cir. 1991. Kellogg sued Texas Attorney General Jim Mattox claiming several constitutional grounds—including the Commerce Clause and the 1st Amendment—for its right to violate state food labeling laws. The court denied Kellogg's motion for preliminary injunction, in a strongly worded opinion.

40 *FTC's Welcome Return*, Advertising Age, Feb. 6, 1989, at 16, col. 1; Saddler, *FTC, Under Industry Pressure, Shows New Life in Backing Deceptive Ad-Laws*, Wall St. J., Apr. 17. 1989. at B4. col.

41 *E.g.*, seattletimes.nwsource.com/html/nationworld/2001925357_fda11.html (accessed September 28, 2005).

42 Kaplan, J.P., Preventing Childhood Obesity: Health in the Balance (2005), summary available at www.iom.edu/Object.File/Master/25/858/0.pdf.

43 Margo Wootan, *Pestering Parents: How Food Companies Market Obesity to Children*, Part III, available at www.cspinet.org/pesteringparents (Nov. 2003); Federal Trade Commission, *Self-Regulation in the Alcohol Industry: A Review of Industry Efforts to Avoid Promoting Alcohol to Underage Consumers*, (Washington, D.C.: FTC, 1999).

44 Cal.Penal Code § 654a (repealed).

45 Cal. Bus. and Prof. Code § 17500.

46 Cal. Bus. and Prof. Code § 17500.

47 States that have used all or parts of the UDTPA include: Colorado (C.R.S., §§ 6-1-101 to 6-1-115), Delaware (6 Del.C., §§ 2531 to 2537), Georgia (O.C.G.A., §§ 10-1-370 to 10-1-375), Hawaii (HRS, §§481a-1 to 481a-5), Illinois (I.R.S., ch. 121 1/2, §§ 311 to 317), Maine (10 M.R.S.A., §§ 1211 to 1216), Minnesota (M.S.A., §§ 325D.43 to 325D.48), Nebraska (R.R.S. 1943, §§ 87–301 to 87–306), New Mexico (NMSA 1978, §§ 57–12-1 to 57–12-16), Ohio (R.C., §§ 4165.01 to 4165.04), Oklahoma (78 Okl. S.A., §§ 51 to 55), and Oregon (ORS 646.605 to 646.656).

48 E.g., Tex. Bus. and Com. Code, §§ 17.46(c)(1) & 17.47 ; Colo.Rev.Stat. § 6-1-103; Ore. Rev. Stat. § 646.632.

49 States that have used major portions of the UCSPA include: Kansas (K.S.A., §§ 50–623 to 50–643; called the "Kansas Consumer Protection Act"), Ohio (R.C., §§ 1345.01 to 1345.13) and Utah (U.C.A. 1953, 13–11-1 to 13–11-23).

50 Prior to its 1971 draft, the FTC in cooperation with the Council of State Governments had in 1967 proposed an *Unfair Trade Practices and Consumer Protection Law (UTP-CPL)*. The 1971 draft reincorporated many of the same proposals. The major differences were that the 1971 FTC proposal permits a state attorney general to obtain restitution for injured consumers and it provides for private causes of action by consumers for violations of the act. The UTP-CPL provides for neither of these remedies.

51 "Unfair methods of competition in commerce, and unfair or deceptive acts or practices in or affecting commerce, are declared unlawful." 15 U.S.C. § 45.

52 *See, e.g.,* Cal. Civil Code, §1780; Tex. Bus. & Com. Code, § 1750; and *Chrysler v. Maiocco*, 522 A.2d 1207 (Conn. 1988), (state lemon law arbitrator has power to award attorneys fees to consumer). The statutes, however, vary in the requirement of awarding attorneys fees in that some of them make it mandatory, e.g., Mass. Gen. Law Ann. c. 93A, § 9 (4) and Tex. Bus. & Com. Codes, § 17.50) while others make it discretionary, e.g., Md. Com. Law Code Ann., § 13–408(b). Most of the state unfair trade practices acts allow private citizens to obtain injunctions to halt violations of the act. Some of the acts require that the consumer suffer actual damages before bringing an action, whereas others allow actions under the theory of "private attorney general" where consumers are merely attempting to obtain injunctive relief to halt the continuation of the illegal conduct. Some state consumer statutes allow for class actions to be brought under them, e.g., Cal. Civil Code, §1781. Approximately 20 states provide for double or treble damages, and some of the statutes provide that the prevailing consumer will recover either the actual damages or a minimum damage award, whichever is greater. *See, e.g.,* Tex. Bus. & Com. Code, § 17.50(b)(1) and *Taylor v. Volvo North America Corp.*, 421 S.E.2d 617 (N.C.App. 1992).

53 E.g., *Nike v. Kasky*, 27 Cal.4th 939 (2002) (commercial speech); *U.S. v. Lopez*, 514 U.S. 549 (1995) (Commerce Clause); *Hunt v. Washington State Apple Advertising Comm'n*, 432 U.S. 333 (1977) (Commerce Clause);Altria v. Good, 555 U.S. __, 2008 WL 5204477 (2008) (preemption); *Cipollone v. Liggett Group, Inc.*, 505 U.S.

504 (1992) (preemption); *Pelman v. McDonald's Corp.*, 237 F.Supp.2d 512 (S.D.N.Y. 2003) (preemption); *Williams v. Purdue Pharma Co.*, 297 F.Supp.2d 171 (D. DC 2003) (standing); *Stop Youth Addiction, Inc. v. Lucky Stores, Inc.*, 17 Cal.4th 553 (Cal. 1998) (standing).

54 E.g., D. Vladeck, Lessons from a Story Untold: Nike v. Kasky Reconsidered, 54 Case W. Res. L. Rev. 1049 (2004) (commercial speech); C. Fischette, A New Architecture of Commercial Speech Law, 31 Harv. J.L. & Pub. Pol'y 663 (2008); D. Wilson, The Fate of the Dormant Foreign Commerce Clause after Garamendi and Crosby, 107 Colum. L. Rev. 746 (2007); A. Zieve, Rebutting the Implied-Preemption Defense, 39 Trial 46 (2003); S. Karas, The Role of Fluid Recovery in Consumer Protection Litigation: Kraus v. Trinity Management Services, 90 Cal. L. Rev. 959 (2002) (standing).

55 31 U.S.C. § 3729 to 33. (Claims Against the United States Government).

56 In practice, the federal and state governments often coordinate investigative efforts in cases which involve both federal and state funds.

57 See 31 U.S.C. § 3730(b).

58 *See Hughes Aircraft Co. v. United States ex.rel. Schumer*, 520 U.S. 939, 949 n.5, 117 S.Ct. 1871, 1876 n.5, 138 L.Ed. 2d 135, 145 n.5 (1997).

59 Helmer, Lugbill & Neff, False Claims Act: Whistleblower Litigation (Second Edition 1999) § 4–3 at 128 to 148.

60 Vermont Agency of Natural Resources v. U.S. ex rel. Stevens, 529 U.S. 765, 774, 120 S.Ct. 1858, 1863, 146 L.Ed.2 836 (2000).

61 See 31 U.S.C. § 3730(e).

62 See 31 U.S.C. § 3730(e)(4)(b).

63 Boese, Civil False Claims and *Qui tam* Actions § 2.06 (2001–2 Supplement).

64 Boese, Civil False Claims and *Qui tam* Actions § 2.08 at 2–206 to 2–207 (2001–2 Supplement).

65 See 31 U.S.C. § 3729(a)(3).

66 *Cook County, Ill. v. U.S. ex rel. Chandler*, 538 U.S. 119 (2003) (counties are defendants); *Vermont Agency of Natural Resources v. U.S. ex rel. Stevens*, 529 U.S. 765, 120 S.Ct. 1858, 146 L.Ed.2d 836 (2000) (states are not defendants).

67 See 31 U.S.C. § 3729(a).

68 31 U.S.C. § 3729(a)("A person violating this subsection shall also be liable to the United States Government for the costs of a civil action brought to recover any such penalty or damages.")

69 See 31 U.S.C. § 3730(d).

70 See 31 U.S.C. § 3729(a).

71 See 31 U.S.C. § 3729(a).

72 See 31 U.S.C. § 3730(c)(2)(D)(5).

73 31 U.S.C. § 3730(h).

74 31 U.S.C. § 3732(b).

75 See 31 U.S.C. § 3730.

76 See 31 U.S.C. § 3730.

77 See generally Helmer, Lugbill & Neff, False Claims Act: Whistleblower Litigation (Second Edition 1999) § 7–9 at 272–74 and Boese, Civil False Claims and *Qui tam* Actions § 4.04[A] at 4–118.7 to 11.9 (2001–2 Supplement).

78 See 31 U.S.C. § 3730.

79 See 31 U.S.C. § 3730(b)(3).

80 31 U.S.C. § 3730.

81 One method of attempting to settle the case is to request a "partial unsealing" of the complaint for review by the defendant, in order to attempt a resolution of the case. If the case does not settle, then the county attorney may request a full unsealing and then decide whether or not to intervene.

82 See 31 U.S.C. § 3730(b)(4).

83 See 31 U.S.C. § 3730(c).

84 See 31 U.S.C. § 3730(c)(2).

85 See 31 U.S.C. § 3730(b)(4).

86 See 31 U.S.C. § 3730(c)(3).

87 See 31 U.S.C. § 3730(c)(3).

88 See 31 U.S.C. § 3730(d)(4).

89 State UDAP laws that CSPI has invoked include Mass. G.L. c. 93A, Tex. Bus. & Commerce Code § 17.41 *et seq.*, DC Code § 28–3905 *et seq.*, N.J. Stat. Ann. 56:8–1 *et seq.*, and Cal. Bus. & Prof. Code § 17200.

90 Mary Claire O'Brien, MD, et al., *Caffeinated Cocktails: Energy Drink Consumption, High-risk Drinking, and Alcohol-related Consequences among College Students*, 15 Acad. Emergency Med. 1, 4 (2008).

91 "Viral marketing" describes deliberate marketing efforts that bypass traditional marketing channels such as television or print advertising. It is dependent on individuals passing along information about a product, whether in person, online, or otherwise. See, e.g., J. Phelps et al., Viral Marketing or Electronic Word-of-Mouth Advertising: Examining Consumer Responses and Motivations to Pass Along Email, J. Advertising Research , Volume 44, Issue 04, pp 333–348 (December 2004).

92 www.sparks.com. This website has been pulled, as part of Miller's resolution of the various claims against it.

93 Street Attack, http://streetattack.com/work.php (last visited August 13, 2008; subsequently revised).

94 Tom Daykin, *Miller's Marketing Goes Under the Radar*, The Milwaukee Journal Sentinel, Dec. 14, 2007, *available at* http://www.jsonline.com/story/index.aspx?id=696926.

95 http://cspinet.org/new/200806261.html.

96 http://cspinet.org/new/200812182.html.

97 http://www.cspinet.org/new/200706141.html. These standards do not prohibit all but the most healthy of foods; instead, they prevent marketing junk foods to kids.

98 http://www.cspinet.org/new/200605031.html.

99 http://www.cspinet.org/new/200610301.html.

100 http://cspinet.org/new/200807212.html.

101 The Sugar Association is the trade group for sugar companies. www.sugar.org.

102 http:// cspinet.org/new/200704171.html.

103 http://cspinet.org/new/200701081.html.

104 http://cspinet.org/new/200701121.html.

105 http://www.cspinet.org/new/200606011.html.

106 http://www.cspinet.org/new/200508111.html.

107 http://www.cspinet.org/new/200508112.html.

14

Anticorporate Social Movements: A Global Phenomenon

Thomas E. Mertes

Late in 1773 the colonies of New York, Pennsylvania, and South Carolina were the scene of local direct actions against the British monopolistic East India Company. Colonists refused to allow East Indian tea to be unloaded. It would have been cheaper than tea smuggled through Holland and other places. They denounced the imposition of an import duty (taxation without representation) and because the tea was shipped by a monopoly and intended to wipe out local merchants.[1] In Boston, the famous Tea Party dumped the company tea into the harbor. In response, the British government decided that the Bostonians and the citizens of Massachusetts would have to be taught a lesson. The subsequent Coercive Acts further escalated tensions between the colonies and London adding momentum toward the U.S. revolution 3 years later. The tension between citizen activists, states, and corporations continue to this day though the balance of forces and contexts have changed dramatically.

Much as the colonial critics of the British imperial system took many years to coalesce, our latter-day democrats have also reached a critical mass. Since the late 1990s, a "movement of movements" has become a powerful force in opposition to neoliberal economic globalization. In large part, nongovernmental organizations (NGOs), social movements, and activists critique the vast increase in corporate power that has been part and parcel of the present form

of economic globalization. The movements have been labeled as "antiglobalization," usually by detractors, but are also characterized as "anticorporate,"
"alter-globalization," a "network of networks," "global justice movement," and
a number of other names reflecting the changing and diverse nature of the
phenomenon. Despite the morphing aspects of the movements, it is clear they
have had and will continue to have resonance related to economic globalization. In a newspaper content analysis of over a thousand protests, it was found
that from January 1999 to June 2004: eight governments were overthrown in
part by protests; seventy "difficulties or crisis" were created for political leaders; seventy talks were held between political leaders and protesters; nineteen
leaders acknowledged protesters issues; thirty liberalization and/or austerity
programs were diluted; twenty-four World Bank/International Monetary Fund
projects were eliminated, stalled or revamped; twenty meetings (i.e., World
Trade Organization's [WTO] Seattle and Cancún, G8 summits, etc.) were disrupted, altogether 198 events with a "discernible result" (Podobnik, 2005: 67).
Another estimate has the movement consisting of between one and two million local organizations "working towards ecological sustainability and social
justice [that includes economic justice] .... the largest social movement in all
of history" (Hawken, 2007: 2–4).

The purpose of this chapter is to explore the rise of social movements and
NGOs worldwide to stop and roll-back corporate power that has been advanced
by neoliberal policies. Since the late 1970s, these toxic policies have made the
lives of a huge percentage of the earth's population more difficult. The chapter
will focus on the main targets of these movements, international financial institutions (IFIs) that have pried open economies for corporate plunder, thereby
creating solidarities for international struggle because national governments
have failed to protect and aid all of their citizens. It will outline the rise of neoliberal ideology and how it became the primary blueprint for IFIs and nation
states to reconstruct economies more favorably for corporations. We then turn
to what some of the effects of these policies have been on local populations
and how they have formed movements and organizations to fight back. More
importantly, the chapter also points to alternatives that exist beyond the current
unsustainable balance of forces. The new social movements have also increased
various forms of democracy outside of the old political system in an effort to
build new platforms for popular participation in policy formation and practice.
The chapter concludes with some reflections on successful organizing and the
way forward for social movements and NGOs at this critical conjuncture.

Charles Tilly describes a social movement as "a sustained, organized
public effort making claims on target authorities" that deploys various forms
of political action (demonstrations, petition-drives, etc.) and demonstrates

solidarity (Tilly, 2004: 3–4). Within this definition, a movement of movements is clearly discernible though critics have argued that it is not sustained because it has no central governing body. The World Social Forum (WSF) is an ongoing forum that gives continuity to the movements though it does not organize actions nor make proclamations in the name of movements.[2] The above-mentioned protests were not discrete; actions only at the national level but more to the point transnational aimed at nation states, IFIs, and corporations. They have a transnational character because of their multinational composition often with the same agenda. Furthermore, they coordinate actions through networks with specific targets and goals.

At the local level social movements have their most powerful solidarities but as the power of corporations and IFIs has outpaced nation states, local and national movements have constructed solidarities (networks) by extending their frame of analysis and by calling for another world. This "scale shift" is evident at Seattle in 1999 when the WTO ministerial ground to halt, in part, because protesters from Europe, United States, South America, and Africa heeded a call from the People's Global Action and other networks to shut down the ministerial.[3] This event was one of a growing number of transnational actions against IFIs and corporations. Opposition to IFIs by social movements and radical NGOs is rooted in a critique of corporations that can no longer be held accountable by states. They are thus "anticorporate." For example, at the first WSF in 2001 José Bové of the Europe's Confédération Paysanne and João Pedro Stedile of Brazil Landless Workers Movement (MST) led 1,300 protesters who up-rooted acres of Monsanto's genetically modified soybeans. Bové commented afterward that, "What we did at the Monsanto farm should have been the job of the police. [They] are trying to scare Brazilian farmers [by arresting me for the action] (Smith 2001)."

The WSF is one of the most critical convergences of the anticorporate movements. The original WSF at Porto Alegre was an alternative to the World Economic Forum at Davos. It kicked off with a teledebate between two very different gatherings. Thus, some of the richest CEOs and IFI lieutenants from one of the world's most exclusive resorts contended with alter-globalization activists and thinkers from Porto Alegre, an industrial city with a participatory budget.[4] The event marked another step forward for the critique of corporate domination as the activists made a compelling case. The first WSF saw an estimated 12–15,000 participants, primarily from the Global South and Europe. It expanded quickly at the next few gatherings, doubling in both 2002 and 2003; the 2004 WSF at Mumbai attracted 75,000 participants. By 2005 the WSF hosted 155,000 activists again in Porto Alegre.

The WSF is an "open space" for discussions and debates among social movement activists, academics, NGOs, and politicians. It is organized along various themes chosen by that year's organizing committee. The themes are addressed and debated in large lectures, panel discussions, workshops, youth encampments, marches, cultural events, and many other forms of social engagement. The WSF as a body does not organize actions, pass legislation, issue statements nor support political parties though activists are encouraged to do so at the forum. However, it is a "space for reflection and for organization of all those who counter neo-liberal policies and are constructing alternatives to prioritize human development and overcome market domination" (Leite, 2005: 80). Moreover, the WSF has spin-offs recognizing the importance of local organizing and actions. These local forums can be continental, a city or even a particular theme. Thus, as the U.S. reinvasion of Iraq loomed large, activists throughout the world began to focus intently on stopping yet another aggressive action by the world's hegemon. In European elections and polls, one point unified most Europeans and that was rejection of the impending war on Iraq. The European Social Forum (ESF) at Florence galvanized this sentiment into an antiwar march. Planners expected 200,000 but by 9 November 2002 over 500,000 activists marched. The activists at the WSF and the ESF did the early planning for perhaps the largest call for peace in world history. The worldwide marches and demonstrations on 15 February 2003 against the possible invasion of Iraq marked a renewed and reinvigorated mobilization with global justice advocates at the forefront (Leite, 2005: 18). Estimates of the turnout range from six to ten million people in most of the world's major cities (Hawken, 2007: 24).

The forum remains a powerful source for building solidarity, sharing tactics and information as well as critiques of TNCs, IFIs and governmental policies. The WSF international organizing committee decided that instead of a forum in 2008, a "day of action" should be promoted wherever local activists chose. It hopes that local actions could speak loudly to global problems and alternatives. The WSF 2008 website collected reports on these local actions at http://www.wsf2008.net/.

Of course, the WSF has critics and detractors. Many activists argue that it is "star-driven" and too influenced by NGOs. Politicians have become regular participants pressing their policies and parties blurring the original intent of the forum to stay beyond partisanship. Moreover, it is difficult for poor and disenfranchised to attend. And yet, the WSF claims to represent them. Many movement spokespersons and small NGOs have decided that their resources and time are better deployed locally. Finally, some activists and critics argue that the forum is too much talk and a distraction from organizing effective actions, challenging corporations, building coalitions, and strategizing for the long term.

The Battle of Seattle and WSF just scratch the surface of actions that Sidney Tarrow characterizes as "event coalitions" but these coalitions can foster "enduring coalitions." In longer campaigns, activists who cut their teeth in events often become more committed to causes and fellow activists. Moreover, events can also create opportunities for extending solidarities and bringing in other organizations. In Seattle the brutality of the police and military against protestors expanded the focus from WTO to global justice thereby incorporating civil rights organizations. Finally, event coalitions can and do morph into "institutions" though most of the activists prefer decentralized and creative actions especially ones that focus on a single corporation or problem. The WSF, the Zapatistas, the People's Global Action, and host of other radical organizations do consistently challenge corporate-driven globalization and toward alternative economic, social, and political models (Tarrow, 2005: 169–171).

Besides event coalitions, social movements and NGOs also engage in direct action in a wide variety of responses not only to IFIs but also to corporations specifically. Researching and creating well-formed opinions are often the first steps in both critiquing corporate practice but also in formulating alternatives. While self-publishing and other forms of presentations are utilized, transmitting critiques of corporations are more difficult because most social movements lack money and easy access to the mainstream media. Moreover, corrupt corporate behavior is so rampant that it is more often considered as business as usual than as news. Like the Boston Tea Party, sometimes a ruckus needs to be raised to get public attention and increase pressure on corporations and IFIs to change destructive policies. This might take the form of a protest in front of or at stockholder meetings, a march, hanging a banner from corporate headquarters, hunger strikes, press conferences, other consciousness-raising pranks, and the like. These are often only annual or semiannual events but more enduring campaigns can include boycotts, legislative testimony and lobbying, legal action, and occupation of production sites (factories and farms) or company buildings and empty urban spaces (i.e., squatting and reconnecting services from electricity to water). More widely, activists often try to build and live through alternatives to the corporate-dominated economy with independent media centers, guerilla gardening and growing organic crops, shopping at farmers markets and buying locally whenever possible, creating social centers and community groups, and bartering goods and services. This list is, of course, very partial but points to the many arrows in the quiver of anticorporatists.

Becoming Fundamentalist

To understand the rising tide against greater depredations of corporations and the apparently receding power of states, let us turn briefly to the historical trajectory of the movements. In large part, anticorporate activists grew in numbers in response to economic turmoil created by dislocations in the world economy as well as the weakening of labor unions, formerly a counter-balance of sorts. The economic restructuring did not occur as a matter of happenstance but rather because of the stagflation of the 1970s in the developed world and the looming debt crisis in the developing world. These conditions motivated corporate elites and government officials to experiment with new models of capitalism. The agenda with the most traction was inspired by economists like Ludwig von Mises and Frederic von Hayek but also popularized by Milton Friedman and some of his colleagues at the University of Chicago. They argued that states inhibited businesses from fully utilizing market signals to make investments and profits. Thus, the most efficient allocation of resources was not being achieved because the "invisible hand of the market" was tethered by states (Harvey, 2005: 19–24).

The ideas of Hayek and Friedman paralleled much of corporate thought in the 1970s and led to a political offensive to capture the U.S. government. A new dispensation did not arise organically rather it was the result of luck, hard work, hard cash, and hard bargaining. In the 1970s the Business Roundtable, National Association of Manufactures, and the Chamber of Commerce shifted their fields of operation from New York to Washington DC. Along side this shift came an outpouring of funds from free market foundations into think tank start-ups like the Heritage Foundation, Manhattan Institute, and the Cato Institute. Older brothers like the American Enterprise Institute saw fundraising explode and the Hoover Institute sprang again to life (Faux, 2006: 80–84). Their univocal demands were for the dismantling of the Keynesian state in the United States (and the First World by extension) and eviscerating the developmental state in the Third World. In place of governments, they sought ever-increasing autonomy for corporations.

Though neoliberal policies began to be implemented in the United States with Carter's deregulation and a Federal Reserve interest rate hike in 1979, Reagan, following in the footsteps of Margaret Thatcher, pushed these ideas further as think tankers entered his administration. Thatcher privatized much of public sector industry including water companies, railroads, automobile, steel, telecommunications, coal, and electricity. In part, breaking unions and offering hidden subsidies for corporate takeovers or undervaluations of state properties to guarantee quick sales (Harvey, 2005: 59–63). Reagan attacked the power of labor early in his administration by crushing the Professional Air Traffic Controllers Organization strike in 1981 signaling to corporations that the administration would be very flexible in allowing corporations to set lower wages. The turn to even more corporate friendly policies also included very probusiness appointments to the National Labor Relations Board as well as other key agencies like Environmental Protection Agency (EPA) and the Interior Department. Moreover, he cut the funding of regulatory agencies like the EPA (22%), Occupational Safety and Health Administration, and Equal Employment Opportunity Commission. His tax cuts strongly favored the highest income brackets and corporations (Baker, 2007: 65–81).

The rising power of the new conservatives could also be seen in the antagonistic positions of the U.S. government toward the UN. The United States sought to undermine the UN Conference on Trade and Development (UNCTAD) from the mid-1970s onward because it was a powerful forum for the Third World to critique First World policies and resist imposition of Northern ideas especially in trade talks. The United States also successfully neutralized the UN Center on Transnational Corporations. It had been an effective tool for tracking and publicizing the activities of transnational corporations (TNCs) in the Third World (Bello, 2001: 16–17).

Reagan era fiscal deficits coupled with the high-interest rates had a terrible effect on world capital markets. High-interest rates caused countries that had to borrow to keep up with old debts to pay an even higher interest rates. Thus, United States borrowing on international markets crowded out other debtors. Commercial bankers and countries with current account surpluses lent to the United States rather than countries that had very deepening debt problems. If countries began defaulting on their loans it would have severely undermined U.S. commercial banks, some foreign banks and the international finance system as a whole. Since no commercial banks would loan, the International Monetary Fund (IMF) and, then, the World Bank were called upon to help bridge the growing debt crisis in the Third World. As lenders of last resort, they had a great deal of leverage to impose conditions with each new loan (Freiden, 2006: 372–375).

Sapped into Action

The World Bank and the IMF were market oriented from their very origins but had altered their policies in keeping with their national directorships and, especially as a reflection of U.S. policy (Woods, 2006: 39–64). Thus, by the late seventies and early eighties they turned toward more rigid conditions on loans. The Reagan administration saw to it that the managers of these institutions had the same blueprint for loan concessions that were intended to free the "competitive spirits" of capital so that it could allocate the factors of production to produce maximum efficiency, at least in theory (Bello, 1994: 18–31).[5] The blueprint for conditionalities or structural adjustment programs (SAPs) set the conditions for TNCs to be able to exploit local markets without the interference of governments because they relinquished their controls as their terms make clear. The conditionalities included

1. Fiscal austerity and discipline through significant cuts in state spending, especially reducing subsidies for agriculture, energy, food, health care, and education. It was argued that public spending and state institutions crowded out the private sector, that is, corporations.

2. Revocation of capital controls so that money could easily flow in and out of nations determined by their comparative advantages. Corporations could invest, export the profits, and exit more easily as a result.

3. Flexible labor markets—this was a linguistic cover for cutting wages and destroying unions. Companies could pay lower wages and threaten workers with moves to lower income countries to discipline them.

4. Elimination of tariff barriers so that cheap goods from the Global North could enter domestic markets, undermines "uncompetitive producers," and requires domestic producers to compete internationally.

5. Lastly and most importantly, privatizations. Selling-off state owned enterprises and resources, often at fire-sale prices, both to make them more efficient but also to use the proceeds to pay back IMF and World Bank loans as well as debts to commercial banks from the Global North.

SAPs could not be imposed uniformly but on a country-by-country basis because of resistance from governments and because they had different effects given national histories, endowments, commodity prices, and the like.

SAPs are one of the primary levers that opened economies to neoliberal globalization. While it can be argued that these structural changes have brought some aggregate growth to some societies, it is certain that the benefits have not trickled down to all citizens (Weisbrot et al., 2006). This is one of the primary reasons that struggles have increased significantly and shifted to the international level. The UN has described grimly some of the effects:

The major disadvantage [of neoliberal globalization] is the wholesale *loss of formal-sector job opportunities* in both the public sector and the private import-substitution industries, so that informal-sector jobs, with no security and often with subsistence wages, are all that is left. As well, *inequality* increases as the part of urban society able to access global opportunities increases its income. This means that the prime resources of the city are increasingly appropriated by the affluent. And globalization is *inflationary* as the new rich are able to pay much more for a range of key goods, especially land. This is exacerbated by removal of price fixing on subsistence goods, and increased utility charges through privatization and the removal of cross-subsidy. The poor are *marginalized* in the worst parts of the city—the slums. The ability of national governments to act on their behalf is curtailed, while local governments in poor areas have no tax base with which to assist. In addition, *social cohesion* is damaged through a bewildering array of new ideas, images and international norms, and through the general precariousness of existence, all of which undermine the traditional bases of authority. (United Nations, 2003: 52)

Neoliberal SAPs contribute to poverty and lower health-care provision in very specific ways. Trade and financial liberalization caused declines in national manufacturing in many states. Domestic petty producers often cannot compete with large TNCs who can sell their products for lower prices. A multi-country study found that SAPs trade policy (see also below WTO) bankrupted much of traditional manufacturing and thus, "the benefits of export growth have gone primarily to TNCs at the expense of domestic producers. ... Overall, real wage rates have tended to decline, income inequality has increased, and job insecurity and informalization have become more pervasive" (SAPRIN, 2004: 70).[6]

With fewer jobs and paychecks, poverty increased dramatically and fueled further the rise of slums and all of the problems associated with them: lack of sanitary conditions, little electricity, degraded water sources, and crime. In 2007 the world's population became more urban than rural for the first time in world history. There may well be as many as 924 million people living in slums of which well over 90% are in low- or middle-income countries (United Nations, 2005: 11). The UN concluded that

Almost half of the urban population in Africa, Asia, and Latin America is suffering from one or more of the main diseases associated with inadequate water and sanitation provision, including diarrheal diseases and worm infections. High levels of overcrowding also make poor urban residents vulnerable to contracting communicable diseases, such as tuberculosis, acute respiratory infections, and meningitis, the spread of which is often facilitated by low resistance among the population due to malnutrition. Vaccine-preventable childhood diseases (measles, diphtheria, whooping cough) also spread more rapidly in overcrowded urban areas, where the number of nonimmunized people is high. Inadequate provision for drainage can increase the risk of malaria, as its mosquito vector breeds in swamps and ditches. Inadequate provision for sanitation often increases the risk of urban dengue and yellow fever, as the vector breeds in latrines, soakaway pits, and septic tanks. (United Nations, 2005: 11)

While conditions are dire, attempts to address fundamental problems have increased for slum dwellers and squatters. One example is the South African Anti-Privatization Forum (APF). It is a network of community organizations and citizens whose main campaigns are directed at gaining access to water and electricity, and fighting against evictions. "We set up APF with very simple terms of reference: 'We are not here to debate privatization, or find some 'Third Way' to finesse it. Everyone here has decided that privatization is bad, and wants to do something to fight it'" (Ngwane, 2004: 126). Likewise, the Shack/Slum Dwellers International is a network of local and regional NGOs that had its origins in as far back as 1987 when the South African Homeless Peoples Federation was established. After 10 years, it was joined by the Asian Coalition for Housing Rights, an Indian NGO (Society for the Promotion of Area Resource Centers) and two social movements (National Slum Dwellers Federation and Mahila Milan) as well as a number of South American movements. The various movements and organizations vary in ideological orientation and some work closely with the World Bank. They primarily agitate and organize to secure tenure on lands, adequate and durable housing, and access to urban infrastructure, notably to electricity, transport, sanitation, and allied services. Many of these services had been publicly run but are now managed for profit. The move from the local to global exemplified by increasingly international linkages will be taken up below.

On the rural front, SAP-imposed agricultural and mining reforms have reduced the income of poor farmers and small communities. Food insecurity especially in the countryside has risen as households have less capital to purchase necessities and reinvest in their farms. Bad harvests and smaller plots of land put many farmers in an evermore tenuous position so that they have been forced into putting more or all of their land into producing for the market and not in the subsistence-first tradition. In other words, they devote all of their land to producing one crop such as cotton, coffee, or tobacco. Austerity measures cut subsidies for machinery, fuel, water, and credit that the World Bank had promoted in the 1950s and 1960s to encourage capital intensive agriculture as part of the "Green Revolution." Commodity boards that helped to stabilize prices and state-sponsored extension programs also came under the cost-cutting axe. As a result, many farms have gone into debt and have been foreclosed leading to a rise in farmer suicides (Patel, 2008: 21–43).

At first, farmers organized at the national level to oppose the new economic regime but increasingly they agitated for reform at the transnational level because of the lack of results from their individual governments. Though there were regional organizations in the early 1990s, formation of Via Campesina in 1993 was the beginning of an enduring and powerful network of farm and peasant organizations. It became a visible international actor 2 years later at the Global Assembly on Food Security and grew significantly as a result of the inclusion of agriculture in General Agreement on Trade and Tariffs (GATT) talks and the formation of the WTO (Edelman, 2003: 190–205). Today, its member organizations represent at least 150 million people. It is probably the most powerful network in the alter-globalization movements. It is also clearly anticorporate:

> The monopoly of certain multinational corporations in each one of the links in the chain of food production, from seeds to fertilizers to marketing and distribution of what we eat, is something that was not dealt with during this [UN Food and Agriculture, 2008] summit. However, despite the [present food] crisis, the principle seed companies, Monsanto, DuPont and Syngenta, have realized a growing increase in profits as have the principle chemical fertilizer corporations. The largest food processing companies such as Nestle and Unilever have also announced an increase in benefits, though less large that those who control the first rungs in the food system ladder. In the same way the large distributors of food such as Wal-Mart, Tesco and Carrefour have confirmed that their profits continue to rise. . . .
>
> A resolution of the crisis situation implies putting an end to the current agricultural model and food system which puts the interests of the large TNCs ahead of the food needs of millions of people. It is necessary to deal with the structural causes; the neoliberal policies that have been systematically applied in the last 30 years, promoted by the WB, the IMF, and the WTO, with the United States and the

European Union in front. Some policies have meant an economic liberalization on a global scale, the unrestrained opening of markets, and the privatization of lands dedicated to local supply and a conversion of that land to export monocultures, which have all led us to the grave situation of food insecurity at the present time. (Vivas, 2008)

Agrarian skeptics of the present corporate-dominated food system are not limited to the Global South (formerly known as the Third World and or the developing world). In Europe, for example, the Confédération Paysanne has blazed a path for noncorporate farm movements and was instrumental in the founding of Via Campesina. Even in the United States, forums like the Agribusiness Accountability Initiative and National Family Farm Coalition oppose the corporate-driven food system. Another important point that links farmers and peasants, North and South, is they also have alternatives to industrial farming including land reform, organically grown and locally sold produce, collectively owned seed banks, cooperatives and, above all, strongly endorse food sovereignty.

While austerity programs have affected agriculture, they have, along with privatizations, also led to higher job insecurity for government workers, lower wages for workers in most sectors, less benefits, fewer rights, and diminished bargaining power. In the 1980s Africa agreed to 156 IMF and 52 World Bank structural adjustment loans. One result was the shrinkage of support for social services across much of Africa. For example, in accordance with SAP austerity measures the Democratic Republic of Congo (formerly Zaire), slashed the civil service from 429,000 to 289,000 from 1980 to 1985 of which 80,000 had been health and education workers. Ghana employed 1,782 doctors in 1985 but only 965 7 years later (United Nations, 2003: 46).

SAPs have substituted public provision of health services for user fees expanding the percentage of the population that relies on home care and self-medication instead of hospitals and clinics. Women have been particularly affected. Increasingly, the ill and the injured have reduced hospital time and/or cannot finish their prescribed treatment because they cannot afford the medication. More people now wait to see trained medical professionals only when their illnesses are at an advanced stage, causing many more deaths from curable diseases and often creating community health hazards from contagious but treatable diseases such as tuberculosis, bronchitis, and pneumonia (SAPRIN, 2004: 46).

In the Philippines, for example, structural adjustment cuts and a drive for profits in the health-care sector have created a two-tier system. Yet even in the public tier user fees are charged and getting signed on is difficult. Without the means to pay fees, many of the poor forgo treatment. As a result of adjustment, health institutions have put in place "stricter screening of indigent patients; imposing a ceiling on the amount of assistance for indigent or charity patients; requiring a deposit from indigent patients before treatment is administered; and requiring all types of patients to buy all the medical supplies needed for their treatment or operation, such as cotton, bandages, sutures, plaster, intravenous fluids, syringes and needles" (SAPRIN, 2004: 189). Even health-care workers suffer because they are experiencing labor speedups with heavier caseloads but less economic incentives including hazard pay, solely to increase productivity and profit.[7]

One group that has organized to provide health care and training in poor Filipino communities is Likhaan, a nation-wide women's advocacy and health-care NGO. It is also a community organizer and agitates for women's rights. Its co-founder explained that health care should not be privatized:

> [Likhaan is] one in the belief that health is a basic right that cannot be made to follow the logic of profit. There is a difference between being efficient in our use of resources and the criminal assault that has resulted from such "reform measures" like user fees, health sector reform and privatization that purportedly increase cost-efficiency and self-sufficiency. Like [Inter Pares] we believe in the standard of accessible, appropriate and competent health care for all. The multinational corporations, the IMF-WB, and our own governments attempt to convince us that this is impossible and should not be the gold standard. They are wrong. Their attempts to find a better system have failed. ... The truth of the matter is, unbridled capitalism, the kind increasingly pushed by neoliberal globalization is contradictory to the kind of health care necessary to ensure human dignity. (Estrada-Claudio, 2006)[8]

Privatizations and smaller budgets have cut the ability of states to provide vital services to the poor, insuring continued poverty. SAPs did not produce the projected growth and, has, thus, made it much more difficult for loans to be paid back. Africa pays three dollars in debt for every dollar it receives in aid. Uganda uses 80% of its export earnings to service debt, funds not spent for the greater good of Ugandans (United Nations, 2003: 46). These dire effects are what have galvanized so many citizens to unite at the local, regional, national, and international level to repeat the refrain of the Zapatistas against neoliberalism, "Ya Basta" or "enough is enough" to "privatizing profits and socializing risk." Debt is one of the central animating frames of the movement of movements. The problems of debt in the Global South led to the formation of a number of networks in Europe, Asia, and North America. It was not until the 1990s that they became a network of networks.

Two networks stand out because of their activism on debt, 50 Years is Enough and Jubilee 2000 (J2000). In 1994 50 Years brought together a number of North American NGOs and their activists who were determined that WB and IMF take "far-reaching changes in the lending policies, internal processes and structure." They are currently about 200 U.S. grassroots organizations are informed by its network of over 185 organizations in 65 countries who correspond and coordinate mass actions, policy goals, and share information. Launched in 1997, J2000 grew out of a coalition of NGOs and religious groups who had been pressuring the IMF and World Bank to reduce or "forgive" loans to some of the poorest countries. In part their campaigning had already yielded some policy change by IFIs with the 1996 Heavily Indebted Poor Countries initiative. While it was considered an ideological step forward, it was not significant enough to ease pressure on the institutions, especially because IFIs still put conditions on countries for their participation. J2000 was important in organizing for the Seattle WTO meeting. One scholar argues that if the movement of movements was born at this meeting, "J2000 network could rightfully be named its *comadre*—godmother and midwife" (Reitan, 2007: 83).

One important coalition that grew out of J2000 was Jubilee South (1999). It feared that many of the Northern groups in the coalition would too readily concede to the IMF/WB repackaging of policy in HIPC. Jubilee South is a network of Southern activists from 85 antidebt groups from 40 countries that have been particularly effective because they provide first-hand experiences of what debt is doing to their societies. Moreover, they have a much more comprehensive agenda that includes the zeroing of debt obligations, reversal of SAPs, sustainable development, and economic democracy. At its founding Jubilee South made clear their position, "Debt is essentially an ideological and political instrument for the exploitation and control of our peoples, resources, and countries by those corporations, countries, and institutions that concentrate wealth and power in the global capitalist system" (Jubilee South, 1999).

WTO and Democracy

Created in 1948, the GATT has had eight rounds before it was transformed into the WTO. Up to the seventh round in Tokyo (1973–1979), the GATT attempted to manage trade primarily in manufactured goods. But Washington's market-driven ideology and the emergence of TNCs put more pressure on transforming the parameters of debates on trade. In particular, TNCs and Washington advocated more market access for raw materials, consumer goods, and the ability to tap into "liberalized" labor markets. Its establishment opened a whole new range of debates that promoted liberalization, privatization, and deregulation. The Uruguay Round (1986–1994) opened even further the negotiations for a new trade regime that gave birth to an organization that unlike the GATT had much stronger coercive mechanisms that could be imposed for the rules set in place by the ministerial rounds. Corporations now had the benefit of having, basically, the same set of rules in all member states. Like the IMF, World Bank, and North American Free Trade Agreement, the WTO lacks transparency both in decision making as well as administration, especially dispute resolution (Jawara & Kwa, 2003: 293–301; Wallach, 2000: 773–778). Barlow and Clarke caution that national laws and regulations are contravened by WTO rulings because

> The losing country has three choices: change its law to conform to the WTO ruling; face harsh, permanent economic sanctions; or pay permanent compensation to the winning country. Because their only task is to judge whether or not a country's policy is a "barrier to trade," the panels do not have to consider other factors such as public health, economic justice or democratic sovereignty. ... Unlike the GATT, which was effectively a business contract between nations, the WTO has a "legal personality" and the power to enforce its rulings. It has an international status equivalent to the United Nations, but unlike the UN, it carries the powers and tools of a global government. WTO rulings are so powerful, they take precedence over Multilateral Environment Agreements (MEAs) such as the Convention on Biological Diversity; human rights agreements like the UN's Universal Declaration of Human Rights; and international labor codes, such as those of the International Labour Organization (ILO). WTO rulings also apply to laws at every level of domestic governance—federal, provincial, state and municipal. (Barlow & Clarke, 2003)

The WTO is thus, considered the youngest member of the "Unholy Trinity" and has become the primary focus of anticorporate/alter-globalization movement opposition. João Pedro Stedile, a spokesperson for the MST,[9] declared that "We are against the WTO, and against the monopolization of world agricultural trade by multinational corporations" (Stedile, 2004: 43). The WTO is the focus of some of the greatest turn-outs by event coalitions. Seattle became a pivotal moment in the exercise of opposition both within and outside of ministerials in 1999. Not unexpectedly, most of the trade rounds have since failed whether they were held at distant authoritarian outposts (Doha) or fenced in militarized cities (Cancún). Ironically, while the IFIs attempt to seize evermore power from governments, more democratic actions sprout up in opposition.

The WTO has been under particularly strong criticism from alter-globalization groups over Trade-related Agreements on Intellectual Property Rights (TRIPS) because they have protected corporate patents of the Global North TNCs at the expense of the health of the Global South. Antiretrovirals used in treating human immunovirus-acquired immunodeficiency syndrome (HIV-AIDS) have been a bone of contention given the extent of its spread in Africa as well as the rest of the developing world and the high level of poverty combined with little or no governmental provision. In 2007 over a quarter of a million people petitioned Novartis to halt a suit against the Indian government for its protection of a leukemia drug patent. They argued that if the patent was overturned then pharmaceutical companies would have an even freer hand to enforce the patents on current and future drugs. Dr. Unni Karunakara, medical director of Medecins Sans Frontieres Campaign for Access to Essential Medicines argued that, "Novartis is trying to shut down the pharmacy of the developing world. Indian drugs account for at least a quarter of all medicines we buy, and form the backbone of our AIDS programs, in which 80,000 people in over 30 countries receive treatment. Over 80% of the medicines we use to treat people living with HIV/AIDS come from India. We cannot stand by and let Novartis turn off the tap." In India, many groups and organizations lobbied forcefully for protections against international patent laws that would affect the price of drugs including the People's Health Movement because they wanted to "put people's health before patents and profits. But now, Novartis is trying to force a change in our patent law, which could deprive people suffering from life-threatening diseases and conditions." Novartis argued that incremental patents "ensure incentives are in place that stimulate long-term research and development efforts critical for medical progress" (Médecins Sans Frontières, 2007a). The corporation argued that the WTO has chastised the Indian government for not "taking steps to align its national standards with international requirements" (Novartis, 2007).[10]

Novartis's criticism of the world's largest democracy is symptomatic of corporate ideology flying in face of social realities. In contrast, Jackie Smith argues that alter-globalization movements and NGOs are actually "democratic globalizers" (Smith, 2007). Citizens can no longer rely on their government to protect them from the whims of the global economy and TNCs. In numerous cases they have taken down these governments. Bolivia, Argentina, and

Ecuador are just three examples of people rejecting governments that had forfeited powers to international forces.[11] Moreover, citizens have put increasing pressure on their own governments to resist further concessions at trade rounds. The Doha Round of the WTO trade talks is for all practical purposes dead in the water especially as the price of food has spiked. Food riots have broken out in numerous nations so further concessions on agriculture, a central plank in the round, are unlikely to go forward (BBC, 2008).

The WTO also acts as a powerful target that helps to build solidarities across the Global North and South because it is so clearly a front for corporations. Corporations are by their very nature antidemocratic, even the most horizontally organized companies. Thus, citizens are demanding more accountability from corporations and by extension some voice in the decisions taken by IFIs. Conditionalities made by the WB and IMF are rarely formulated in the countries they effect. In large part, the outcomes of trade agreements and conditionalities limit the influence of governments and by extension their citizens. Policymakers do represent their nations in the negotiation process but they are usually in an unenviable position to debate. Many of these representatives are themselves from business backgrounds or from wealthy families and thus stand to gain by implementing the policies insisted upon by World Bank and IMF economists. Furthermore, many of the state representatives have been trained in United States and European universities that are dominated by neoclassical economic orthodoxy.

Though they are separate and distinct institutions, the Bretton-Woods institutions are mutually reinforcing with the U.S. Treasury strongly influencing their decision making (Stiglitz, 2002: 15–22, 80). U.S. trained and inspired academics and critics currently dominate WB, WTO, and IMF bureaucracies; "One unmistakable factor that contributed to this homogenizing [of the WB] and that grew stronger over time was economics ... the Bank's hallmark scholarly discipline ... To a large degree, however, [the staff] were the product of the graduate economics departments of English-speaking, but especially America, universities" (Buira, 2003: 4–5; Kapur et al., 1997: 4). This training gives the United States a greater degree of influence beyond formal procedures and by the same token less power for smaller nations and different ideas. Norms determine the terms of debate to a focus on resource allocation and market performance rather than what best serves each nation or community in a wider sense.

Often the economics profession fails to consider that some economic policies and socio-political power favor some individuals, most often capitalists, and corporations at the expense of others like workers and peasants. From another perspective, TNCs have grown tremendously in terms of political sway as a result of the neoliberal policies and have themselves grown in size through mergers and acquisitions. Some corporations are so big that governments will not allow them to fail. In fact, of the top 100 wealthiest economic units less than 50% are nation states and majority are TNCs (Rosenkrands, 2004: 61). Thus, Global North TNCs are competitively more advantaged than local business in filling voids created by the recession of state power. The result is that inequality within nations has risen significantly since the late 1970s as well as between nations, in particular those nations that have had SAPs or have followed the economic recipes of Reagan and Thatcher. Inequality significantly limits the ability of lower- and middle-income people to have a powerful impact on policy making. In the United States both the major political parties are beholden to corporations for fundraising and the authorship of legislation. Corporations influence the WTO more than citizens so its veneer of democracy is dubious at best. For example, while thousands gathered outside the Cancún ministerial to say Ya Basta, on the inside over 250 corporate lobbyists were accredited to offer their input and pressure on policy negotiations (Friends of the Earth International, 2003). Finally, democracy promotion under the ideological hegemony of neoliberalism is subsumed into voting occasionally and being able to purchase a wide array of consumer products at cheap prices. In practice, it destroys economic democracy.

Organizing

Movements are by nature coalitions, often, of diverse groups of people. There is no single model for building coalitions and movements but the study of successful movements has burgeoned in the last two decades so that some solid generalizations can be asserted. Most of the movements that have been noted so far are community based rather than agency based (state or NGO organized). Initially, they were organized around a local or regional issue. This is often called "globalization from the bottom up." In its initial phases, problems in social relations rise to a level that inspires change. Often particular groups hold common religions, political views, class orientation, ethnicity, or gender that is more affected than other groups in society. As a result, they begin to consider, internally, both critiques and alternatives to the status quo. Thus, movement building "becomes a social process as people discover that others are having similar experiences, identifying the same problems, asking the same questions, and being tempted to make the same rejections." The potential for collective action is reinforced and gains momentum (Brecher et al., 2000:19–31).

One of the most important aspects of building any movement is the choice of frame. How is the issue constructed and what is to be achieved? Critically, the frame is often adjusted as movements grow and as critiques from below diffuse upward or if the leadership can offer a better vision. Organizers emphasize that goals and objectives have to have credibility for grassroots solidarity. A legitimized frame draws in a critical mass of participants with enough intensity and intentionality to sustain activities long enough to gain credibility so that it could develop further linkages and/or deepen its roots in the community. One of the singular aspects of the current movements is their emphasis on respecting each other's identities whether it is race, gender, sexuality, class, or place of origin. As a consequence, one of the most perceptive analysts of the alter-globalization movement suggests casting a wide net:

> The promise of anti-corporatism is its ability to develop a diverse and unified constituency mutually threatened by the corporate hijacking of economy and politics. Many possibilities for alliance have yet to be explored. It seems that we should be careful not to jump to conclusions about social movements' goals, particularly when apparent enemies (like religious and other nationalists) are being demonized by neoliberal elites. Obviously, people interested in "globalization from below" must work as hard within national borders as across them, and also across generations, class and ideology within nations. (Starr, 2000: 164–165)

Tilly outlines the legitimization of movements as WUNC: worthiness, unity, numbers, and commitment. In other words, movements should have all of the following aspects: socially acceptable tactics, similar costuming and/or marching in ranks, petitions and/or critical mass, and sacrifice in the face of opposition and/or bad environments (Tilly, 2004: 4–5).

In the first phases community-based movements are "relational" (face-to-face). Community-based coalitions have difficult challenges because they often lack funding that would allow for the development of an organization that can provide the capacity for a long-term struggle, cultivate wider linkages, and keep activists engaged through newsletters, regular meetings and actions. An additional element in the legitimization process is in the area of action. Developing a track record for change, albeit political, economic, or social, is important because it gives members a sense of accomplishment, it increases the power of the organization, and it attracts attention and support to the cause (Wolff, 2001).

One example of movement building can be seen in the Association for the Tobin Tax to Assist the Citizen (ATTAC). It was created from a proposal floated in the December 1997 edition of *Le Monde Diplomatique* by Ignacio Ramonet. It met with such overwhelming response that Bernard Cassen, an editor of the journal, organized a meeting of trade unions, social movements, journals, and NGOs who had expressed support. By October 1998 a "national get together" occurred and ATTAC was officially founded two months later. It called for a tiny tax on international currency transactions (Tobin Tax, .01%), the proceeds to be used for poverty relief especially in the Global South, sustainable development and food security. The frame of the movement was a critique of financial globalization that undermined democracy. Its goal is to reassert democratic control of economies in place of "purely speculative logic that expresses nothing more than the interests of multinational corporations and financial markets" (ATTAC, 1998; Cassen, 2004: 152–156). Because of the great outpouring of support, the intensity for organizational lift off had been achieved. Moreover, community-level (relational) chapters were formed who were given wide latitude for developing their own critiques and goals. Therefore, ATTAC was not merely a movement for a tax but rather for regulating multinational corporations and addressing problems associated with neoliberal globalization. Within 2 years ATTACs were formed in most of the rest of Europe and by 2004, 38 countries worldwide. They have been important in mobilizing actions against the IMF, WB, WTO, and G8 summits and the formation of the World and ESFs. Even more to the point, they are an important channel for communication and education. ATTAC was perhaps the most important educators for the French "No" vote on the 2005 European Constitution (*Le Temps*, 2005). It has also achieved WUNC. It should be noted that ATTAC was created because the moment was propitious. It came in the wake of the 1997 Asian Currency crisis and as many European states were becoming more and more neoliberal.

ATTAC did reflect the trend of community-based and nationally based movements becoming part of international coalitions in the late 1990s. This transformation has recently been documented in a number of works. Ruth Reitan building on the pioneering work of Sidney Tarrow has developed the most compelling and detailed analysis of the rise of a "network of networks" (see also Juris, 2008). She concludes that framing goals widely can create the ground on which international solidarities can be built. This is especially the case where activists have experienced similar processes that create a shared identity. This is a shift in scale from local to global. From her case studies she has determined that "identity-based solidarity is increasingly foundational to transnational activism. But in addition, this type of solidarity is facilitated, sometimes greatly, by relationships of reciprocity with those with whom activists empathize and perceive some connection among struggles" (Reitan, 2007:

54). A weaker form of solidarity is one based on altruism or substitutionism. This is a common form of solidarity of Northern NGOs and activists in global networks whereby they "stand in" for movements in the South. It can take many forms from life-style changes to demonstrations in front of corporate headquarters, boycotts, petitions, lobbying, and so on. This form of solidarity is treated with much more skepticism.

Another important finding in the development of networks is the importance of brokering. For example, Cassen was critical in the formation of ATTAC because he brought together otherwise disparate and even perhaps antagonistic groups and organizations. It was predicated on the trust that they had in Cassen. Once ATTAC had made discernable headway in meetings and actions the trust could and did deepen. Brokering has the potential for multiplication because once trust is established between groups then they can bring in their own coalitions building more capacity and power.

Anticorporate coalitions also face a number of problems that have made enduring campaigns difficult. Casting a frame too widely can cause the coalition to fall apart when the goals of part of the coalition seem to have been met. In part, the split between the Jubilees mentioned above reflects this tension. The eradication of poverty and elimination of debt was agreed upon but when IMF-WB launched the HIPC initiative and, later, with the UN Millenium Development Goals, many of the Jubilee 2000 groups especially in the North thought that it was substantial progress without accepting the more radical program of many in the South. Similarly, coalitions or some of their NGOs also face cooptation by corporations and IFIs who use carrots and sticks to drive a wedge through a movement. Often a corporation will offer to reform some part of their operations and ask a more conservative NGO to monitor an activity and, thus, gain leverage over the NGO alienating former coalition partners. For example, the Environmental Defense Fund (EDF) has been partnering with corporations to create the trade in carbon emissions, something that most environmental groups find repugnant (Birchall, 2008). It has even partnered with Wal-Mart to reduce their use of plastic and "greenwash" other company activities. Moreover, some NGOs are more interested in their corporate sponsors than in representing a social sector. Thus, during the negotiations at World Health Organization (WHO) in 2004 over the Global Strategy on Diet, Physical Activity and Health, Infact (now known as the Corporate Accountability International) called on the WHO to distinguish between public interest NGOs and those linked to business interests such as Kraft and other TNCs (Infact, 2004).

The World Bank has been particularly effective at pushing "public-private partnerships" that have the same detrimental outcomes for NGOs (Oppenheim

& MacGregor, 2004). Public-private partnerships can take a number of forms but generally they link a corporation with a government agency or an NGO to provide a service or build infrastructure. Yet, the same logic of corporations applies: cost cutting, skepticism of unions, and profit-maximization including cutting off services to those least able to pay. If there is no profit, the corporation exits and sometimes is paid a fee in lieu of profit. On the other hand, NGOs that receive grants from the World Bank where the state had previously provided a service imprint a neoliberal ideology into their work. Rather than providing a service to a citizen, the individual is transformed into a client reinforcing the logic of the market. Lastly, public-private partnerships also often subordinate NGOs in their power relationship with providers of funds (Miraftab, 2004: 89–101).

Likewise, coalition pitfalls also include a strong tension between NGOs and social movements. Many activists in social movements see many NGOs as shock-absorbers for IFIs and TNCs. They also find it distasteful that some NGOs claim to be speaking for the masses when they are actually hierarchical organizations that only have little knowledge of conditions and challenges on the ground. In addition, many of the event coalitions are composed of a very wide ideological spectrum that on other issues diverge considerable. For example, many Northern labor unions might favor protectionism but that might translate into more joblessness for workers elsewhere. Another example is the divide between environmentalists and workers in some industries. In the timber industry in the 1980s and 1990s, lumber men fought greens who sought an end to clear-cutting and harvesting old growth trees especially redwoods.[12] This was just one point of contention between labor and environmentalists similar ones exist in many of the other extractive industries, the auto industry, and industries that have considerable pollution problems.

Another possible obstacle for enduring coalitions is the role of leadership and the loss of legitimacy. Leaders have to walk a narrow path between listening to their base and arriving on course to proceed. Infighting in the leadership can spill over into the ranks causing factions to develop. One of the most potent criticism of the World Social Forum is that it seems to have a handful of "stars" that do not necessarily reflect the ideas and struggles of local social movements. Moreover, since the WSF does not organize or campaign, the leaders aren't actually moving the ranks to action. Once leadership is put in question, coalitions, campaigns, and social movements can lose their legitimacy and capacity building moves in reverse. Legitimacy can also be lost because campaigns don't demonstrate the ability to achieve their goals. In addition, not gathering good information or creating false critiques can undermined arguments and delegitimize campaigns. For example, many environmentalists and

NGOs who fought for indigenous rights also argued for returning forests, wet-lands, and other terrain back to its pristine condition, that is, without humans. Obviously, indigenous peoples took offense to this critique diminishing soli-darity between the groups though many of Northerners became more edu-cated and rethought their positions.

A final obstacle for coalitions and social movements lies outside of their control. They are often the subject of police and corporate surveillance and espionage. The use of information gathered can be used to preempt or break up actions, arrest and imprisonment of leaders, physical abuse, and even mur-der. Corporations usually have more capacity to fight back on a number of fronts. They can afford valuable lawyers who can keep litigation of a single case in the courts for years. In response to these deep pockets, activists have their own legal allies like Community Environmental Legal Defense Fund, EDF, Natural Resources Defense Council, Public Citizen, and the American Civil Liberties Union. Corporations have much better access to the media with pub-lic relations departments and deep pockets for advertising. They often have the sympathetic ear of local and state authorities as well as legislators and execu-tives. It is more difficult to make change happen because corporations and states are inherently conservative, preferring the status quo to another possible world. Events can also conspire to destroy campaigns and movements or, at least, disrupt them significantly. Many analysts of the movements critical of TNCs point to the crime of 9/11 as sapping momentum and directing attention toward terrorism and war. Some officials and pundits cynically used it to paint activists as allies or fellow travelers of Al Qaeda (Zoellick, 2001). On a more optimistic front, sometimes campaigns are successful in their goals and their *raison d'etre* is lost. If we could only always be so lucky!

Conclusion—Where We Need to Go

We now live in a time where the economy has nosedived and people are very anxious about the state of their world. The financial system has proven that it cannot regulate itself[13] nor have the prescriptions of neoliberalism produced their promised results, at least for the vast majority of the planet (Stiglitz, 2008). Critiques and alternatives that would have once fallen on deaf ears are now being sought after desperately. This is a great moment for debates, dialogues, organizing and advocating for structural change. It would take several heavy tomes to consider what is to be done and what the possible results might be.[14] One strong point of agreement among activists is that more decision-making power must be devolved to communities where more democratic decisions can be taken. One-size fits all models do not seem to work well whether it is state-centered communism or neoliberal capitalism.

I think that it is important to first suggest some ways to avert some of the pitfalls of organizing mentioned above. First, avoid any entanglements with corporations, however, progressive their intentions appear to be. In particular, do not rely on funding from corporations or on a small number of donors. This will insure independent decision making and action. Beware of "win-win" situations and decisions. NGOs and movements are also criticized for being too chaotic. The most successful campaigns have a strong central critique or alternative. They often target a single corporation. Most corporate sectors are oligopolistic so if one of the major competitors can be driven to change a harmful practice then competitors often reform in fear of becoming the next target of negative publicity or potential increased regulation. Another criticism is that key personalities control their organizations and lose touch with the people they are representing. Thus, the experiences, ideas, and desires of the base should drive the organization. A third concern is that too many of the coalitions are based on affinities and not strong in solidarity. Official and actual support of other struggles builds the strength of networks. Many environmentalists now realize that they have to stand with minorities in their fight for social justice, if they expect to get support from civil rights activists in their struggles.

On the flip side of the organizational coin, organize and act locally. This is where grass roots action is more effective because the lay of the land is most familiar. Movements or organizations structured horizontally have a greater capacity for positive feedback loops as well as keeping the base engaged and empowered. To cast a broad net, frame issues in public statements, and actions without ideologically loaded language. It will have the most impact. Anticorporate struggles in health-care sector have the potential for strong coalitions. For example, Big Pharma has generated a host of critiques from movements already in place such as: environmental destruction (pesticides and fertilizers), harmful animal testing, genetically modified seeds, patenting of life forms, construction and imposition of the codex alimentarius, and the increasing privatization of health care. The potential for cooperation among these groups is strong. The campaign against Novartis mentioned above led to the corporation dropping the case after receiving a petition of over 420,000 signatories gathered by a coalition of NGOs and social movements (Médecins Sans Frontières, 2007b).

Humbly, I also suggest some alternatives that I believe are worthy of debate. A first critical step is redefining what should be the areas where corporations will be allowed to determine the allocation and production of resources. This would require setting out clearly what should be part of the "commons" or areas where the interest of society or community as a whole is paramount. The International Forum on Globalization argues that there are three categories that make up the commons and cannot be allowed to be privatized:

> The first category includes the water, land, air, forests, and fisheries on which everyone's life depends. The second includes the culture and knowledge that are collective creations of our species. Finally, more modern common resources are those public services that governments perform on behalf of all people to address such basic needs as public health, education, public safety, and social security, among others. (International Forum on Globalization, 2002: 63–64)

These commons have to be treated as the inheritance of future generations and must be decommodified. In the United States we have seen that health provision is being denied to millions because they cannot afford private insurance. Instead they are only being treated when their injuries and diseases turn catastrophic. Decisions about the health of our families and communities should not be left in the hands of accountants, actuaries, and entrepreneurs. The present economic troubles portend even greater numbers of uninsured. A national health-care system can and should be constructed in this new light.

Second, corporations must be much more highly regulated and executives must be held personally responsible for the actions of their corporations whether they were directly responsible or not for transgressing the law. This would certainly reduce problems of moral hazard. Third, we must fight the ideology of consumption as the primary framework for identity in the United States that will require a much greater emphasis on the community and downplaying the supremacy of the individual. On the international front, Walden Bello has suggested that to "deglobalize" economically we must radical alter the nature of IFIs and the range of action of corporations. Bello takes aim at the WTO suggesting that it not be allowed to move forward with its agenda and if possible roll-back some of its worst aspects in collaboration with advocates from the Global South. He also argues for defunding the IMF and restructuring it into a research organization devoted solely to tracing capital flows and exchange rate fluctuations. As for the World Bank, its power to make loans should be given to regional and local institutions where people most affected can participate through grants especially for poverty and food relief as well as health-care provision. He wants to increase the power of the International Labor Organization to protect workers rights around the world as well as strengthening UN, especially UNCTAD (Bello, 2002: 112–118).

Globalization has a number of very positive aspects. The circulation of people, technology, and knowledge has sped up immensely. It has led to a much greater awareness and appreciation of different cultures but also the interdependence of humankind on one another. Curative plants have been discovered, farming techniques improved, new sources of sustainable energy developed, better prevention and treatment of diseases, healthier diets, and solidarities in opposition to war. These advances are too precious to be left to the rule and ruination by corporations. This scheme of neoliberal disorder is too dangerous for us to permit the experiment upon us to continue.

NOTES

1 As "A Citizen" noted at the time, "Whether the duty of tea is taken off or not, the East India Company's scheme has too dangerous aspect, for us to permit an experiment to be made of it among us; whether we consider it as it may create a monopoly; or, as it may introduce a monster, too powerful for us to control, or contend with, and too rapacious and destructive, to be trusted, or even seen without horror, that may be able to devour every branch of our commerce, drain us of all our property and substance, and wantonly leave us to perish by thousands, for want of the necessaries of life, as they did the poor unsuspecting Indians . . ." *New York Journal*, November 4, 1773.

2 The Porto Alegre Manifesto coming out of the 2005 WSF was an attempt to give coherence to the main arguments and alternatives of the movements. The manifesto has not become a mission statement but the ideas in it reflect a broad consensus across a wide spectrum of the network of movements (Group of 19 2005).

3 As protesters were beaten and tear-gassed in Seattle, opposition to the WTO was on the streets of London, Paris, Hong Kong, Ankara, New Delphi, Brisbane, Buenos Aires, and Mexico City. Movements represented at Seattle included labor, environmental, indigenous, feminist, and anti-imperialist.

4 A participatory budget is one in which citizens have a much larger influence on decisions, that is, the budget is submitted to local counsels and communities who are given specific powers to insert and veto parts of the budget as well as set priorities.

5 In 1981, President Reagan spoke to the World Affairs Council. He asserted that, "Free people build free markets that ignite dynamic development for everyone; and that's the key but that's not all." He went on to note that cooperation is important and there is *even* a role for government (Reagan 1981: 1–2).

6 SAPRIN is The Structural Adjustment Participatory Review International Network. It conducted a long-term multicountry (both low- and middle-income nations) study of the effects of SAPs with the assistance of the World Bank who later refused consultation with the network when it was clear that the conclusions

would prove decisively that neoliberal proscriptions were hurting the poor in the countries studied.

7 SAPs have increased the number of immigrants from the Global South to the North finding work in the health-care industries. While it has probably lowered costs, it has also led to immigrants hiring poorer women to take care of their families in their country of origin (Misra et al., 2006: 317–332).

8 Inter Pares is a Canadian social justice organization.

9 The MST is the largest social movement in Latin American and a member of Via Campesina.

10 A Novartis press response conceded that its profits in 2006 were $7.2 billion of which approximately $5.4 billion was invested in research and development (Novartis, 2007). Yet, the budgets of big pharmaceutical companies are dominated much more with advertising and administration than in research (Angell, 2004).

11 In 1999 the Bolivian's President Hugo Banzer (former dictator) imposed World Bank proscriptions to privatize the economy including water provision. A local analyst from the Democracy Center joked that the "Bank water officials believe in privatization the way other people believe in Jesus, Mohammad, Moses or the Buddha." In Cochabamba the sole bid for its water works was a subsidiary of Bechtel who promptly raised rates by 35% sparking massive protests organized by the La Coordinara (Coalition in Defense of Water and Life) that led to a violent repression of the strikes by the military. As an international outcry spread, Bechtel fled Bolivia only to sue it for $25 million at a closed trial under the auspices of the World Bank (Schultz, 2003).

12 Deregulation and other financial policies helped the junk bond market explode leading to the mergers and acquisitions wave in the 1980s. Pacific Lumber was one of the companies acquired with junk bonds. To strip the company of its assets to pay for the acquisition, Charles Hurwitz tried to speed up the harvesting of trees and mow down Redwood groves in California. This led to a strong direct action campaign that pitted timber men against environmentalists. Workers in the timber industry had been hit with hard times including deskilling and wage cuts as the production process was significantly industrialized. They saw greens as a direct threat to their jobs.

13 The Chief Economist of IMF warns, "The global economy is facing its worst crisis in 60 years" (Blanchard, 2008: 8).

14 I am largely in agreement with the authors of the *Porto Alegre Manifesto* that lays out a *general* agenda for the alter-globalization movement (Group of 19 2005).

REFERENCES

Angell M. *The Truth about Drug Companies: How They Deceive US and What to Do About It.* New York: Random House; 2004.

ATTAC. *Platform of the International Movement ATTAC.* Available at: http://www. attac.org/spip.php?article2. Published December 11–12, 1998. Accessed October 5, 2008.

Baker D. *The United States Since 1980*. Cambridge: Cambridge University Press; 2007.

Barlow M., Clarke T. *Making the Links: A People's Guide to the WTO and the FTAA*. Ottawa: Council of the Canadians; 2003.

BBC. *Dismay at Collapse of Trade Talks*. Available at: http://news.bbc.co.uk/2/hi/ business/7532302.stm. Published July 30, 2008. Accessed December 7, 2008.

Bello W. *Dark Victory: The United States and Global Poverty*. Oakland: Food First; 1994.

Bello W. *The Future in the Balance*. Oakland: Food First; 2001.

Bello W. *Deglobalization: Ideas for a New World Economy*. London: Zed Books; 2002.

Birchall J. Wal-Mart joins logging initiative. *Financial Times*. July 15, 2008.

Blanchard O. Cracks in the system: repairing the damaged global economy. *Finance and Development* 45:#4 (December 2008).

Brecher J, Costello T, Smith B. *Globalization from Below: The Power of Solidarity*. Cambridge, MA: South End Press; 2000.

Buira A. Introduction. In Buira A, ed., *Challenges to the World Bank and IMF: Developing Country Perspectives* (pp. 1–12). London: Anthem Press; 2003.

Cassen B. Inventing ATTAC. In: Mertes T, ed. *A Movement of Movements: Is Another World Really Possible* (pp. 152–174). London: Verso; 2004.

Edelman M. Transnational peasant and farmer movements and networks. In: Anheier H, Glasius M, Kaldor M, eds. *Global Civil Society 2003* (pp. 185–220). London: Oxford University Press; 2003.

Estrada-Claudio S. *Lessons from the Philippines: Public Health, Privatization, and Women's Activism*. at Inter Pares Annual General Meeting on Democracy, Health and Justice: Health Care in the Public Interest, Ottawa, April 24, 2006.

Faux J. *The Global Class War: How America's Bipartisan Elite Lost Our Future—and What It Will Take to Win It Bank*. New York: Wiley & Sons; 2006.

Freiden, J. *Global Capitalism: Its Fall and Rise in the Twentieth Century*. New York: W.W. Norton; 2006.

Friends of the Earth International. "Business Rules: Who Pays The Price? How Corporate Influence in the WTO Impacts People and the Environment." Issue #103 Amsterdam: Corporate Europe Observatory.

Group of 19. "Porto Alegre Manifesto." Available at: http://www.openspaceforum.net/ twiki/tiki-read_article.php?articleId=276. Published January 2005. Accessed July 15, 2008.

Harvey D. *A Brief History of Neoliberalism*. New York: Oxford University Press; 2005.

Hawken P. *Blessed Unrest: How the Largest Social Movement in History is Restoring Grace, Justice and Beauty to the World*. New York: Penguin Books; 2007.

Infact. NGOs Decry Industry-Driven Policymaking. Available at: www.ibfan. org/english/pdfs/press22jan04.pdf. Published January 22, 2004. Accessed November 15, 2008.

International Forum on Globalization. *Alternatives to Economic Globalization*. San Francisco: Berrett-Koehler Publishers; 2002.

Jawara F, Kwa A. *Behind the Scenes at the WTO: The Real World of International Trade Negotiations*. London: Zed Books; 2003.

Jubilee South. Founding Assembly. Available at: http://www.jubileesouth.org/index. php?option=com_content&task=blogcategory&id=61&Itemid=56. Published November 21, 1999. Accessed August 15, 2008.

Juris J. *Networking Futures: The Movements Against Corporate Globalization*. Durham: Duke University Press; 2008.

Kapur D, Lewis JP, Webb RC. *The World Bank: Its First Half Century*. Washington DC: Brookings Press; 1997.

Le Temps. Attac, enquête sur le fer de lance du non français June 3, 2005. Accessed December 12, 2008.

Leite JC. *The World Social Forum: Strategies of Resistance*. Chicago: Haymarket Books; 2005.

Médecins Sans Frontières Press Release. "Quarter of a Million People Urge Novartis To Drop Case Against India. Company Would Effectively be Shutting Down the 'Pharmacy of the Developing World.'" New Delhi/Geneva; January 29, 2007a. Accessed July 11, 2008.

Médecins Sans Frontières Press Release. "After Indian court ruling, MSF hands over petition with 420,000 signatures to Novartis." Basel; August 8, 2007b. Accessed November 14, 2008.

Miraftab F. Public-private partnerships: the Trojan horse of neoliberal development. *J Plan Educ Res*. 2004;24(1):89–101.

Misra J, Woodring J, Merz S. The globalization of care work: neoliberal economic restructuring and migration policy. *Globalizations*. September 2006;3:3.

Ngwane T. Sparks in the townships. In Mertes, ed. *A Movement of Movements* (pp. 111–134). London: Verso; 2004.

Novartis Press Release. Novartis concerned Indian court ruling will discourage investments in innovation needed to bring better medicines to patients. Available at: http://www.drugs.com/news/novartis_concerned_indian_court_ruling_discourage_investments_innovation_needed_bring_better-6653.html. Published June 8, 2007. Accessed July 11, 2008.

Oppenheim J, MacGregor T. *Democracy and Public-Private Partnerships*. International Labor Organization Working Paper 213. Geneva: International Labor Office; 2004.

Patel R. *Stuffed and Starved: The Hidden Battle for the World Food System*. Brooklyn: Melville House; 2008.

Podobnik B. Cycles and trends in the globalization protest movement. In Podobnik, Reifer T, eds. *Transforming Globalization. Challenges and Opportunities in the Post 9/11 Era* (pp. 51–68). Boston: Brill Academic Publishers; 2005.

Reagan R. Cooperative Strategy for Global Growth. Current Policy #328 (October 15, 1981).

Reitan R. *Global Activism*. New York: Routledge; 2007.

Rosenkrands J. Politicizing *homo economicus*: analysis of anti-corporate websites. In van de Donk W, Loader B, Nixon P, Rucht D, eds. *Cyperprotest: New Media, Citizens and Social Movements* (pp. 57–76). New York: Routledge; 2004.

Schultz J. Bolivia: The Water Wars Widen. *NACLA Report on the Americas.* January/ February 2003;36:3.

Smith J. *Social Movements for Global Democracy.* Baltimore: Johns Hopkins University Press; 2007.

Smith T. French economic activist arrested in Brazil: man ordered to leave country after protest at US business plant. *The Independent,* January 30, 2001.

Starr A. *Naming the Enemy: Anti-corporate Movements Confront Globalization.* New York: Zed Books; 2000.

Stedile JP. Brazil's landless battalions. In Mertes, ed. *A Movement of Movements* (pp. 17–48). London: Verso; 2004.

Stiglitz J. *Globalization and Its Discontents.* London: Allen Lane; 2002.

Stiglitz J. The end of neoliberalism? *Project Syndicate.* Available at: http://www. project-syndicate.org/commentary/stiglitz101. Published July 8, 2008. Accessed December 10, 2008.

Structural Adjustment Participatory Review International Network (SAPRIN). *Structural Adjustment: The SAPRI Report.* London: Zed Books; 2004.

Tarrow S. *The New Transnational Activism.* Cambridge: Cambridge University Press; 2005.

Tilly C. *Social Movements 1768–2004.* Boulder: Paradigm Press; 2004.

United Nations Human Settlements Programme. *The Challenge of Slums: Global Report on Human Settlements.* London: Earthscan; 2003.

United Nations Millennium Project. *A Home in the City Task Force on Improving the Lives of Slum Dwellers.* New York: United Nations; 2005.

Vivas E. FAO: More Free Trade, More Hunger. Via Campesina. Available at: http:// www.viacampesina.org/main_en/index.php?option=com_content&task=view&id =563&Itemid=1. Published June 17, 2008. Accessed July 22, 2008.

Wallach L. Transparency in WTO dispute resolution. *Law Policy Int Business.* 2000;31:3.

Weisbrot M, Baker D, Rosnick D. Scorecard on development: 25 years of diminished progress. *Int J Health Serv.* 2006;36:2.

Wolff T. A practitioner's guide to successful coalitions. *Am J Community Psychol.* 2001;29:2.

Woods N. *The Globalizers, The IMF, World Bank and Their Borrowers.* Ithaca: Cornell University Press; 2006.

Zoellick R. *American Trade Leadership: What is at Stake?* Washington DC: Institute for International Economics; September 24, 2001.

15

Labor Movement Strategies to Address Corporate Globalization

Jane Lethbridge

In Algeria, on the 14th July 2008, 35 contract teachers went on hunger strike, to protest against the increasing casualisation of the teaching sector. According to the trade union "Syndicat National Autonome du Personnel de l'Administration" (SNAPAPr) there has been no direct recruitment since 1995 and contract or "casual" teachers will soon outnumber permanent teachers. Some teachers have been in this position for 14 years. They were also protesting against the non-payment of salaries. In some cases the teachers were owed more than three years back pay. (PSI News July, 2008)

This is just one example of the actions that workers have taken to protest against increasing employment and income insecurity. Policies of liberalization, deregulation, privatization, and structural adjustment have led to workers becoming more insecure in their work, through lack of employment rights, benefits, and poor wages. Even though the position of labor has worsened in many countries, levels of unionization have also declined.

The key role of neoliberalism and its related policies has been to support the expansion of multinational and transnational companies. This has been achieved through the privatization of public services, which results in multinational companies expanding ownership of previously publicly owned enterprises. Deregulation of national markets has resulted in the opening of new markets to multinational companies. This chapter discusses five main approaches that labor has taken to fighting for the rights of workers in the face of multinational and transnational company expansion.

A survey by the International Labour Office (ILO) (2001)—Public Services International (PSI) (2006) found that trade unions have responded to attacks on labor rights with a diversity of responses, although with some common approaches. Some of the traditional forms of protest, for example, strikes and demonstrations, are still widely used, but there are also newer activities that show that protests are taking on different forms throughout the world (Lethbridge, 2006).

Trade union responses often start with information gathering and training. Collaboration with nongovernmental organizations and other community organizations has become more widely used in the past two decades. The development of networks with trade unions around the world have expanded and international support is often a key part of a campaign. There are regional differences in the extent to which negotiations with government and lobbying for involvement in reforms have been the prime focus of campaigns. In high-income countries, trade unions have increased the resources for recruitment of new members and improved member benefits. Trade unions often use campaigns for equal pay and workers' health as a focus for campaigning against neoliberal policies.

A classification of how labor has engaged with multinational companies provides a framework for examining different struggles and evaluating the effectiveness of each approach. These five categories of union organizing can be presented as parts of a continuum. They draw from different political philosophies about the position of labor and workers rights. A Marxist perspective on labor and workers rights, places labor at the center of the production process. How to expand the control that labor has of the means of production is a vision that should not be forgotten. The following five approaches represent different goals for trade unions.

1. *Multinational collective bargaining—the starting point for trade unions*
   Multinational collective bargaining was an initial response of trade unions to the expansion of multinational companies in the 1960s onward. It represented an attempt to adapt a national approach to an international context.

2. *Labor codes and codes of conduct*
   The development of labor codes and codes of conduct represented another approach to working within the existing arrangements, by nongovernmental organizations and trade unions. It also reflected the failure of international organizations and national governments to implement existing international labor standards and the weakness of labor at all levels.

3. *European/global workers councils and social dialogue*
   The creation of workers councils and social dialogue has its origins
   in a more social democratic or reformist approach to the position of
   labor, where management and labor are considered equal partners.

4. *New labor internationalism and coalitions/community organizing*
   Although trade unions have not abandoned the first three approaches,
   there has been a growing awareness that there is a need for different
   strategies to safeguard the interests of labor. Some trade unions
   at local, national, and international levels have started to develop
   coalitions with local communities, also fighting against the effects of
   corporate globalization. This approach has also been supported by the
   World Social Forum and related regional meetings.

5. *Organizing marginalized workers—new forms of transnational labor
   solidarity*
   The development of new forms of labor solidarity is a response to
   the extensive reach of neoliberal policies. Social justice and income
   inequality are the defining goals, with more emphasis on bringing
   workplace and community struggles together.

Multinational Collective Bargaining—The Starting Point for Trade Unions

> There is no respect for freedom of organisation and industrial action.
> Male and female workers who promote the trade union movement
> are dismissed, and there are "black lists" of those who have been
> union leaders in other bonded assembly plants. (Torres, 2008)

The reactions of trade unions to the growth of multinational companies and
the implications of these changes for collective bargaining need to be seen
as part of a wider process of trade union internationalism. Recent challenges
to corporate power by workers have to be seen in the context of a longer history of labor struggles that started in the 19th century. By the early 20th century, growing national union movements were linked to labor, cooperative,
and socialist internationalisms, which often took separate paths (Waterman &
Timms, 2004–05)

Organizations that linked trade unions were often determined by politics
or regional groupings. The World Federation of Trade Unions (WFTU) linked
trade unions in communist states until 1989. The International Federation
of Free Trade Unions, formed as a counter balance to the WFTU in 1949 has
become the International Trade Union Confederation. It has worked to develop

a mechanism of social regulation into emerging global governance structures. Regional trade union movements were set up in Africa, the Middle East, and Europe (Ghigliani, 2005).

Global Union Federations

The creation of International Trade Secretariats (ITS), which affiliated national unions from specific sectors, was another form of international labor solidarity (Ghigliani, 2005). However, although they starting to fight for an 8-hour day and union rights, the struggle soon focused on social reform at national level (Hyman, 2002). The ITS were effectively interrelationships of national trade unions. From the 1960s, the ITS made attempts to challenge international capital or multinational companies through the development of "networking, information gathering and provision" Ramsay (1997).

Cooke (2005) argues that trade unions have not changed their collective bargaining structures from national to global levels (Cooke, 2005). Although national trade unions have taken part in ITS and other global groupings, their activities have been mainly information sharing, consultation, and some support for national struggles. They have also pursued wider political and social aims for improved working conditions and protecting rights to freedom of association and collective bargaining (Cooke, 2005).

In 2002, the ITS became the Global Union Federations (GUFs). They continue to play a role in negotiations with sectors, which can be seen as a form of "bottom-up" internationalism. There are now 10 GUFs, which cover the sectors mentioned in Table 15.1.

The Union International Network (UNI) was created through a merger of several ITS that brought 1,000 service industry unions together. It was set up specifically to promote transnational negotiations between multinational companies and trade unions (Cooke, 2005). UNI provides an example of an increasingly coordinated international trade union action for collective bargaining.

International Framework Agreements

International Framework Agreements (IFAs) are the most significant recent development in multinational collective bargaining. Hammer (2005) defines the minimum provisions of an IFA. It must be a global agreement between a multinational company and a global union federation. It has to make a multinational company exert influence over its suppliers. Trade unions have to be involved in the implementation and monitoring and have a right to bring complaints (Hammer, 2005; Nilsson, 2002). GUFs are recognized as legitimate

TABLE 15.1. Sectors Covered by Global Union Federations.

• Chemical energy, mine, and general workers	• Textile Garment and leather workers	• Public Services International—public services
• Building and wood workers	• Transport workers	• Union Network International (UNI) services
• Metal workers	• Food, Agriculture, Hotel, Restaurant, Catering, Tobacco, and Allied Workers (IUF)	• Education

bargaining partners. The agreements include labor standards that are part of the ILO Declaration on Fundamental Principles and Rights at Work and ILO Conventions 29, 87, 98, 100, 105, 111, 138, and 182, which cover freedom of association and protection of right to organize, the right to organize and take part in collective bargaining, and minimum age of forced labor discrimination.

Hammer (2005) analyzed IFAs up until 2005 and found that there are differences between IFAs. Some established basic labor rights, whereas others set out details for bargaining procedures. It can be argued that rights set out the conditions for bargaining so that the two types are not mutually exclusive. More generally, IFAs tend to deal with bargaining issues as well as key ILO core conventions (Hammer, 2005). About 75% of IFAs cover health and safety working conditions and focus on trade union rights.

Global Union Federations have played an important role in developing IFAs, although some IFAs do not include a GUF as a signatory. The success of IFAs often depend on local unions being involved in implementation and monitoring. Another significant characteristic of an IFA is that it exerts influence on all stages in the supply chain, including suppliers used by a multinational company. Interestingly, by 2005, no IFAs had been signed with North American multinational companies.

Stevis (2008) argues that the adoption of IFAs by global union federations was a result of the failure to obtain a labor rights clause in the WTO and a move toward global social dialogue and global industrial relations. Forty-seven of the 59 IFAs in existence have been signed since 2002. More southern unions in Latin America, South Africa, and Asia support IFAs.

A less positive development is that some multinational companies have started to develop partnerships with other corporate stakeholders to define corporate responsibility (Egels-Zandon & Wahlqvist, 2007). These partnerships leave out the trade unions/nongovernmental organizations and are a response by companies to the sometimes problematic dynamics between trade unions and nongovernmental organizations, which they consider increase the complexity of the partnerships. This can be interpreted as a sign that companies have failed to recognize the value of involving a range of stakeholders.

Riisgaard (2005) examined the process of drawing up an IFA between Chiquita, a banana company and COLSIBA, a transatlantic network of organizations, which included 42 unions with 45,000 workers. COLSIBA was set up in 1993, and it was the first time that banana workers has cooperated internationally. This enabled them to gather information and coordinate strategies about the companies. In 1998, there was a campaign that coordinated international actions in the Americas and Europe and successfully put pressure on Chiquita. In 2001, Chiquita and COLSIBA signed a framework agreement, which includes giving each worker the right to be the member of a trade union and to have access to collective bargaining (Riisgaard, 2005).

However, Riisgaard (2005) also shows that due to lack of experience, the union did not use the framework as effectively as it might have done. Dissemination of the agreement to workers varied from country to country. In Honduras, there were higher levels of awareness, perhaps because it had led the process of setting up COLSIBA. Managers felt the agreement was being adhered to, but workers reported violations. One of the major problems was that although Chiquita-owned plantations reported improved conditions, those on supplier plantations had not improved. Pressure on supplier plantations could also lead to loss of jobs if Chiquita terminated contracts. The review committee only functioned in a limited way. COLSIBA members had not always prepared for meetings partly through lack of experience but also due to political differences, which weakened interunion collaboration.

The development of IFAs by unions, as in the case of Chiquita, shows that the strategies of trade unions are changing. From blocking capital's access to labor, unions are now controlling access to the retail market, consumers, and investors, although they have to be shaped to the specific industry (Bergene, 2007). This has also involved working more closely with nongovernment organizations (Riisgaard, 2005).

Increasingly, global framework agreements (GFAs) are negotiated between management and labor to define basic labor standards as well as conditions for collective bargaining. This represents an important development in multinational collective bargaining but IFAs require careful implementation if they are to be successful in safeguarding workers rights. Capacity building for trade unions is required.

Labor Codes and Codes of Conduct

> "Workers labor from sunrise to sunset. They never see day light,"
> says Ojeda, a maquiladora worker for 20 years. "They are sometimes
> exposed to toxic chemicals, and in one case workers were given
> 'vitamins' which turned out to be amphetamines. They rarely see
> their families." Sexual harassment of women employees, who are the
> majority of maquiladora workers, is common and not prohibited by
> Mexican law. (Sorriano, 1999)

In 1919, the ILO was set up as an interstate organization with national governments holding 50% of voting rights and trade unions and employers 25% each.
One of the main roles of the ILO has been to develop labor conventions and
standards. One *hundred* and *seventy-six* labor conventions have been drawn up
since the foundation of the ILO and there are 174 member states. The major
conventions cover freedom of association and protection of right to organize
convention 1948 (no. 87); the right to organize and collective bargaining convention 1949 (no. 98) and labor inspection (Pearson & Sayfang, 2001).

The power of the ILO to make national governments implement these
standards is limited. ILO conventions are not fully ratified and, in the past 20
years, with increased labor deregulation, there has been a decline in the ratification of conventions by national governments, especially the new conventions
for occupational health and safety, health services, and training (Standing,
1999). The lack of enforcement of ILO conventions has shown the limitations
of statutory code of conduct and labor standards coupled with the reluctance of
national governments to play an active role in safeguarding labor rights. This
is reflected in the varying levels of commitment that national governments
have shown to actually implementing conventions (Waterman & Timms,
2004–05).

The example of health and safety shows the limits of ILO influence.
Although ILO plays a central role in providing recommendations and guidance
for national occupational safety and health (OSH) policies, it does not have the
power to make countries ratify its own conventions. The ILO publishes instruments, which outline varying levels of obligations for member countries, but
ILO members still have to ratify each instrument before implementation takes
place. Ratification does not guarantee implementation. The recommendations
are for national governments to implement and use in an advisory capacity.

Although labor standards and codes have emerged as one of the main
vehicles for addressing labor rights there has been a move away from statutory
codes to voluntary codes because of the reluctance of national governments

to implement statutory rights. As a response to the limitations of statutory codes, a series of voluntary codes of conduct have been developed between specific firms, groups of firms or firms in a certain sector, and to certain groups of workers (Pearson & Seyfang, 2001). Voluntary codes can be defined as "Voluntary measures taken by a private firm to impact upon some aspect of their labour conditions and workforce" (Pearson & Seyfang, 2001).

One of the first voluntary agreements was drawn up by the ILO in 1977, It was entitled the "*Tripartite Declaration of Principles Concerning Multinational Enterprises and Social Policy,*" which aims to make multinational companies contribute to economic and social progress (Pearson & Sayfang, 2001). It provides guidelines for governments, and employers' and workers' organizations in areas such as employment, training, and industrial relations (ILO, 2001). The principles are not legally binding, although governments have agreed to them. Attempts to agree on a United Nations code for multinational companies failed in the 1960s (Vannieuwenhuyse, 2003). However, a UN Global Compact was launched in 2006, which aims to bring together the United Nationals and multinational companies in a form of global public–private partnership. This is a significant step in seeing multinational companies as subjects of international law (Deva, 2006). However, the commitment by the various companies is uneven, drawing in companies, which have made significant efforts to improve working standards with those whose practice remains questionable (Deva, 2006).

An increasing number of companies are introducing voluntary codes of conduct. There are a wide range of different types of codes of conduct. The wording of many voluntary codes is often vague and does not refer to specific ILO standards. Not all voluntary codes of conduct have been drawn up with trade union involvement. Making voluntary codes apply to the multinational company but not to the suppliers used by the company results in a weakening of the impact of the code.

The Ethical Trade Initiative (ETI) is one example of a voluntary code of conduct. It was set up and promoted by the UK Department for International Development. Members include 17 companies, 18 nongovernmental organization, and 4 domestic and international trade union federations. There are pilot projects in China, Zimbabwe, and South Africa. The ETI core code is based on ILO core labor standards but its effectiveness has been limited by problems of implementation, monitoring, adaptability, and accountability (Pearson & Seyfang, 2001).

By using the threat of consumer boycotts, NGOs have campaigned to force multinational companies to consider working conditions. International social standards (SA8000) have been used to promote socially responsible business behavior (Riisgaard, 2005) but corporate social responsibility is seen as a process whereby consumers, investors, and NGOs exert pressures on companies. Nongovernmental organizations involvement in labor standards has been criticized for not recognizing the rights of workers to organize and negotiate with management (ILO, 1998). A recent survey found that only 15% of codes included the right to freedom of association and collective bargaining (Riisgaard, 2005).

Some examples of voluntary codes of conduct that include trade unions, either as initiators or as partners are as follows:

- ICFTU Code on Labour Practices (model code);
- Central American Network of Women in Solidarity with Maquila Workers (Voluntary code);
- Clean Clothes Campaign and International trade unions and FTCG (Dutch);
- Clean Clothes Campaign, NOVIB and trade unions (voluntary and label);
- EURATEX—ETUC—European employers association and ETUF-TCL—textiles trade union voluntary and label;
- Hong Kong based Coalition of Workers for the Safe Production of Toys and NGOs.

(*Source*: Pearson & Sayfang, 2001)

Codes which have originated in workers organization are more likely to include payment of nonwage benefits, health and safety issues, reproductive rights, provision of information on standards, and banning physical abuse (Jenkins, 2001; Pearson & Sayfang, 2001). Voluntary codes do not include all ILO standards. Age of workers was one of the most common issues.

LaCroix (1998) provides an account of how the Network of Central American Women in Solidarity with Women Maquila Workers, set up to improve working conditions, persuaded the Nicaraguan Minister of Labor to formalize a Code of Ethics, developed by Network members in consultation with the workers. The Network had persuaded each maquila factory owner in Nicaragua to endorse the Code, which includes such basic guarantees as a safe working environment, the right for pregnant women to retain their jobs, and payment for overtime work (LaCroix, 1998). The approach that the Network took is also significant. Many women in the Network felt that the labor movement was too confrontational, and they were afraid of losing their jobs in working environments that were hostile to labor. As a result, a different approach was chosen; working with women in their communities on issues such as health education and labor rights. Research established baseline survey information and other information about working conditions. This was used to inform the development of resources and a public awareness campaign (LaCroix, 1998).

Corporate codes of conduct are often weak and do not provide adequate protection for the rights of workers (Ferus-Comelo, 2008). They rarely go further than local labor legislation, even when international standards are significantly higher. The actual process of enforcement is often not clearly set out and when violations occur, are difficult. These shortcomings have generated a corporate monitoring industry that monitors codes of conduct but without adhering to government legislation and union representation. These have been called "labor campaigns without labor" (Ferus-Comelo, 2008). Examples of companies involved in these private monitoring activities include PriceWaterhouseCoopers, a large multinational accountancy company, which has consistently provided a range of "professional services" for multinational companies and governments to facilitate and implement neoliberal policies.

Recent research on the effectiveness of voluntary labor codes, through the Ethical Trading Initiative, shows that codes of labor practice have a positive effect on the more "visible" code principles: health and safety, child labor, minimum wages, and documented employment benefits. Codes had little impact on the "less visible" principles: freedom of association, discrimination, and regular employment. Permanent and regular workers benefited most but migrant or casual workers were often not affected by the codes. Third party labor contractors were often beyond the reach of the codes (Barrientos and Smith, 2007).

There are several examples of unions taking a "bottom-up" approach to international organizing. Forus-Comelo provides examples of successful international organizing, for unions that were also involved in GUFs. The 1997 United Parcels Service (UPS)—Teamsters strike was supported by over 150 job action or demonstrations on UPS World Action Day.

During a labor dispute with the Ravenswood Aluminum Corporation (RAC), the United Steel Workers of America (USWA) met with local unions and politicians to convince them to fight against an international commodities trader, Marc Rich, who was a co-owner of RAC. Workers from two global union federations organized demonstrations in Eastern Europe, Latin America and the Caribbean. Together they successful stopped any further acquisitions by Marc Rich (Ferus-Comelo, 2008; Herod, 2001).

These two examples illustrate the power of labor in targeting areas of company expansion through strikes and demonstrations. The demonstrations by unions in Europe, as part of the UBS dispute, showed the company that borders do not limit trade union activities. Sophisticated media campaigns were also used by unions to show companies in an unfavourable light (Ferus-Comelo, 2008).

Changing Role of State

The introduction of voluntary codes of conduct also reveals a change in the role of the state, from setting standards to a facilitator of voluntary codes. This is part of the wider changing role of state from provider to facilitator and regulator. Governments are rarely involved in the development of voluntary codes and governments in many low-income countries often view voluntary codes as a form of protectionism (Pearson & Sayfang, 2001).

The relationship between global economy, domestic politics and institutions, and labor rights is explored by Mosley (2008). Mosley and Uno (2007) showed that there is a positive relationship between the level of democracy and recognition of labor rights. Domestic institutions can play a mediating role. Leftwing governments have often promoted sympathetic labor legislation. Collective rights are easier to support but, at the same time, wage flexibility and making dismissals easier can be part of economic strategies. The industrial structure of the workforce also influences levels of organization, with agricultural and service sectors having lower levels of organization than manufacturing and public services (Mosley, 2008).

In the 1990s, Costa Rica saw a shift from agricultural production, due to a decline in coffee production, to the services sector. Manufacturing also changed to a high technology production (Mosley, 2008). By 2005–06, there were 227 companies, mainly from the United States, in Export Production Zones with 36,000 workers. Between 2002 and 2005, the government budget for inspection increased by 25% and it compliance budget doubled. Costa Rica may be considered to have a weak record on collective labor rights but increasingly individual labor rights are being strengthened and wages increased, although these may only benefit workers in the Export Production Zones (Mosley, 2008).

European/Global Workers Councils and Social Dialogue

The establishment of Workers Councils and social dialogue arrangements are another approach that brings labor and multinational companies together. These are based on the recognition of partnership and collaboration between capital and labor. The European Commission has played an important role in providing legislation and guidance for the creation of European Works Councils (EWC) and Social Dialogue committees.

The EWC Directive (94/45/EC), initially adopted in 1994, aims to improve the right of workers to information and consultation in multinational companies. Companies, or groups of companies, are required to establish information and consultation agreements covering their entire European workforce, if they have:

- at least 1000 employees across the member states, *and*
- at least 150 employees in each of two or more distinct member states. (European Commission, 1994)

The content of these agreements is not specified and is up to the management and employee representatives to negotiate. There are minimum requirements, which include the requirement of annual reports to the EWC on the company's business prospects, and the right to be informed about exceptional circumstances affecting employees' interests, such as closure or collective redundancy.

There are several examples that show how a EWC has contributed to improving pay and conditions for workers, worldwide, in a multinational company. The EWC for the French multinational company, Suez, involved in water, waste, and energy services, has negotiated a 3-year profit-sharing agreement, which will provide for a system in which all workers, worldwide, will share in the results of the company. For 2007, €80 million has been placed in a fund. Due to legal, technical, and taxation issues, the results will be distributed in the form of free shares. The EWC and unions have demanded that a different way is found to distribute a share of the profits in 2008 and 2009. Discussions in the Suez EWC have also covered a range of other issues such as training and qualifications. Less satisfactory discussions cover issues such as inflation-linked pay increases, funding for social activities, and the improvement of trade union rights (EPSU, 2008).

Waddington (2006) outlines some of the shortcoming of EWCs in the engineering sector. There are variations between EWCs, which are influenced by the country of origin of the company, the sector, and the level of internationalization of the workforce. Some of the information and consultation practices also vary. Some of the issues identified cover the frequency of EWC meetings. There is only a requirement for a EWC to meet once a year. Some representatives question whether this is often enough to be able to operate. Links between the EWC representatives and the workers represented may be influenced by national structures of representation. Waddington (2006) found that the ways in which EWC representatives reported back to members was influenced strongly by the country they originate from. Anglo-Irish representatives circulate minutes, whilst representatives from Continental Europe report back via their Local Works Council (Waddington, 2006).

The European Trade Union Confederation (ETUC) and the European Federation of Public Services Unions (EPSU) have played an important role in supporting trade unions representatives in EWCs, through information exchange, commissioning research, and providing training. The EPSU has recently set up a EWC legal fund to help trade unions fight companies that do not adhere to an agreement (EPSU, 2008).

EWCs raise important questions for trade unions about how to operate at a European level, acknowledging local and national issues but also coordinating on issues that affect labor at a European level. This process is also influenced by the attitude of national trade unions to European integration (Bieler, 2008).

World Company Councils

There have also been attempts to establish world company councils in global multinational companies. A world company council is "a consortium of union representatives employed by the company in different location coordinated by global union federations" (Ferus-Comelo, 2008). World company councils aim to bring union representatives together every few years, develop union strategies and exchange information on the company's strategy, business models, financial situation, and investment plans. One of the difficulties in realizing these activities is that unions are fragmented both politically and physically. The costs of international meetings and language barriers and different trade union approaches make information exchange difficult (Ferus-Comelo, 2008).

Social Dialogue

Social dialogue is defined by the ILO as "all types of negotiations, consultations or exchange of information between or among governments/employers/unions (labor administrations, trade unions and employers' associations) to develop consensus on policy approaches and practical measures to ensure equitable social and economic development" (International Labour Organization, 2008). In the European Union (EU), social dialogue is seen as a way of promoting a new organization of work (European Union , 1993). The EU defines social dialogue as a bipartite arrangement between employers and trade union organizations and as a tripartite arrangement between social partners and public authorities. Social dialogue is presented as the way "social partners assist in the definition of European social standards, and play a vital role in the governance of the Union" (European Union, 1993).

Social dialogue in Europe has evolved in the past two decades. The introduction of bipartite social dialogue in 1985, was followed by the Protocol on Social Policy, annexed to the Maastricht Treaty (1993), which allowed agreements by social partners to be "given legal effect by a Council Decision and transposed into national legislation of Member States" (EU, 1993). These led to three agreements, which covered parental leave (1995), part-time work (1997), and fixed-term contracts (1999), formalized through Council directives.

In 1998, sectoral social dialogue committees were created (European Commission, 1998). The social partners of a sector have to apply jointly to the European Commission in order to set a sectoral social dialogue committee at European level. Both social partners have to satisfy a number of criteria that include: having an organizational structure at European level; recognition as part of Member States social partner structures; capacity to negotiate agreements and be representative of several member states; and adequate structures to ensure their effective participation in the work of committees.

Sectoral social dialogue committees have a maximum of 50 representatives of social partners, with an equal number of employers' and workers' representatives. They are chaired either by a representative of the social partner or by a representative from the European Commission. The European Commission provides the secretariat for each social dialogue committee as well as plays an active role in formalizing and administering each committee.

There is extensive debate about whether social dialogue is the most effective way for trade unions to fight for improved recognition of the needs of workers. Ikanova and Turner (2004) identified neoliberal policies within Europe as driving the creation of social dialogue structures in Western Europe. Nevertheless, they also argue that some of the tripartite arrangements in the countries of Eastern and Central Europe have contributed to easing some of the problems of the transition countries (Ikanova & Turner, 2004). Degryse (2000) recognizes that the agreements that have been achieved through sectoral dialogue committees have had some influence on working time, promotion of employment, vocational training, and health and safety but does not think that social dialogue can influence macroeconomic issues.

Curtin (1999) argues that social dialogue as a form of democracy depends on access to information and access to dialogue. In this discussion, the issue of what additional powers social partners need is set alongside the powers of the Commission in the social dialogue process. With some increased powers given to the partners, Degryse feels that the powers of the Commission have declined, moving from "endeavouring to develop the dialogue between management and labour" (Single Act) to "facilitate their dialogue" (Amsterdam Treaty).

As with European Works Councils, both the ETUC and the EPSU have helped to set up sectoral social dialogue committees, often playing an important leadership role. A recent example can be seen in the South East European gas sector. The trade unions and EUROGAS (for the employers/companies) have agreed to seek a constructive involvement in building a social dimension to the European Energy Community for South East Europe and to contribute to the development of the social dialogue with their expertise (EMCEF/ EUROGAS/EPSU, 2007).

Streek (1998) considers that European Works Councils and social dialogue, as well as the concept of subsidiarity set out in the Maastricht Treaty and the common currency, form a new set of "rules" that are part of the process of liberalization. He argues that although liberalization involves the elimination of many regulations, it also required new "rules" to organize decision-making process between players at national and European level. These new rules can also be seen as part of the internationalization of industrial relations.

In the European Union, there are well-developed structures and some institutional support for social dialogue. In other regions, although social dialogue is a rhetoric used by governments and international institutions, the reality is that social dialogue is being used to promote neoliberal economic policies, which require some communication between capital and labor.

New Labor Internationalism and Coalitions/Community Organizing

> In Turkey in 2007, dozens were injured in violent street battles on
> the 30th anniversary of the deaths of 37 people who were shot by an
> unknown gunman or trampled to death in May Day demonstrations
> in Taksim Square in 1977 (Reuters May 1, 2008)

Over the past two decades, trade unions have had to deal with falling membership, the rapid movement of capital and increasingly "precarious" employment, accompanied by a hostile environment toward organized labor. The search for new strategies that will strengthen trade unions has focused on the development of community alliances and an increased international perspective. These have informed new forms of trade union organization and activity.

Social Movement Unionism

"Social movement unionism" is characterized by unions taking action on issues, which effectively combine collective bargaining activities and collective action (Hyman, 1997; Moody, 1997; Schiavone, 2007). This may involve campaigns for housing, social services, health, education, and other basic public services. Union democracy is an important feature of "social movement unionism." Unions fight for power and organization in the workplace as well as reaching out to other unions at local, national, and global levels; community organizations, and other social movements (Hyman, 1997; Moody, 1997).

In South Africa, during the 1980s, the labor movement and civil society organizations worked together to promote the cause of democracy, bringing workplace and community struggles together. COSATU worked with the African National Congress (ANC) to mobilize for elections in the early 1990s (Hirschsohn, 2007). Since the ANC came to power, some of these relationships have become more complex. The continued alliance between COSATU and the Treatment Action Campaign (TAC) has shown how a partnership can continue to grow at different levels and in different contexts. Formed to support the campaign for improved treatments for people with HIV/AIDS, the alliance has continued to provide support for each other's campaigning on nonhealth and labor issues.

Greer (2006) looked at the experience of Hamburg, over a 10-year period, which covered the transformation of public hospitals into corporate institutions and subsequent privatization. External factors, such as the loss of power of the Social Democratic Party in the municipal government, forced the trade union to develop alliances with local community organizations (Greer, 2006). At the moment, there is no evidence to show that this strategy has been a success. There have been no noticeable improvements in collective bargaining and wages. The new private sector owner of the hospitals is running hospitals with a wage freeze (Greer, 2006).

For Germany, with a long history of trade union social dialogue with management, the change to "social movement unionism" is a fundamental one. There are indications that this process of bringing together unions with other stakeholder groups has continued to develop. On September 25, 2008, in Berlin, 130,000 people protested against the declining working conditions in German hospitals. For the first time ever, trade unions, civil servants' organizations, doctors' professional associations, municipalities, and employers demonstrated together in order to tell the conservative German government: "STOP saving our hospitals to death!" The federal government has refused to allocate more than €3 billion when at least €7 billion is needed to maintain the health care system (PSI News September/October, 2008).

To maintain partnerships with community organizations, the trade unions requires different ways of working and dividing power and can even mean giving up power. Reiss (2005) found that there was a culture gap between unions and community groups in New York. The process of developing consensus in a diverse movement was slow, especially in a difficult social, political, and economic context.

Wills (2001a) identifies some of the barriers that trade unions have found in working with community organizations in the United Kingdom on social justice issues, particularly the need to identify economic issues that they can work on collaboratively with other groups, as well as reorganizing themselves if they are to develop successful alliances with political and community groups. The recent experience of TELCO, in East London, indicates that some of these issues are being addressed. It also requires a balance between workplace interests and wider political struggles, which can often become obscured.

Novelli (2004) provides an interesting study of how a regional trade union transformed itself into a social movement union that operated, at many levels, from local to global. SINTRAEMCALI, a Colombian trade union, recognized that it was no longer effective in defending public services under threat from neoliberal policies. Novelli attributes the subsequent success of the union in generating local, national, and international support as due to "strategic learning," which emerged as a response to changing conditions. This involved action on alternative economic plans, publicity to counter the effects of the mainstream media, the development of a union–community alliance and human rights campaigns. The use of research, education, and learning to produce alternative globalizations was crucial to the success of the campaign.

Networks and networking can facilitate ways in which workers can articulate their needs (Waterman, 2001). One of the major criticisms of "social movement unionism" is the lack of systems of "representativity" of community groups or nongovernmental organizations. Waterman asserts that to criticize them for lack of "democracy" or "representativity" is to misunderstand the nature of the new radical-democratic movements (Waterman, 2001).

Webster and Lambert (2003) provide an account of some of the practical issues of drawing different national trade unions together through an analysis of a southern based trade union network, "Southern Initiative on Globalisation and Trade Union Rights" (SIGTUR). It is a network organization based on democratic trade unions in the South. SIGTUR operates in "cyberspace campaigning and organization." There is no hierarchy, structure, or control (Webster & Lambert, 2003). They identified several challenges facing the new labor internationalism. There are resource implications if conferences are to be run in home languages. Decision making at meetings can be difficult because of different degrees of union autonomy of SIGTUR members and different levels of capacity. There are gender imbalances within conferences, where the majority of members are men but some delegations are all women.

The development of trade union–community alliances has been evolving over several decades at local and global levels. The World Social Forum and regional social *fora* have contributed to bringing trade unions, civil society groups, and social justice networks together. These have helped to strengthen links and provide the basis for future campaigning (Bieler & Morton, 2004).

Organizing Marginalized Workers—New Forms of Transnational Labor Solidarity

> Guangdong Province, in the south-eastern part of China, has long been a symbol of China's economic strength and many electronics factories are located there. ... However, young women behind the growth are paying a very high cost. .... Working 10–12 hour shifts in a standing position for six or seven days a week negatively affects the health of the workers. Wage reductions for falling asleep or making minor mistakes ... are common, even though they are obvious consequences of the working conditions offered by the employer (Chan et al., 2008).

Some of the *labor* responses to neoliberalism, trade agreements, and privatization have highlighted the divisions between organized and unorganized labor. One of the results of privatization and deregulation is the growth of contracting out of services, so that suppliers of services may be diverse and not linked directly to a multinational company. Workers in these supplier companies are often poorly paid with few labor rights and are often nonunionized. In this section, the focus will be on approaches to organizing workers involved in contracted-out services. It will also show that gender issues within labor organizing are becoming more widely recognized because many of these workers are women.

Challenging the effects of liberalization has to continue after policies have been implemented. Two of the major results of neoliberal policies has been the rise of "precarious" work and flexibilization, often creating a "two-tier" workforce, where some workers have rights and others have none. The fight for a "Living Wage," a campaign that was initiated in the United States, has spread throughout the world. The "Justice for Janitors" campaign in the United States and the TELCO "Living Wage" campaign in the United Kingdom is discussed in the following section.

Justice for Janitors

In the United States, the Service Employees International Union (SEIU) started the "Living Wage" campaign in 1985. Subsequent campaigns have contributed to raising the public profile of SEIU (Chun, 2008). One example of a "Living Wage" campaign is the one that was fought in the University of Miami, where conflicts over low wages and poor benefits for janitors started in 2001, when academic staff and other workers were given wages increases. In 2006, a 9-week strike was crucial to winning improved terms and conditions for janitors. SEIU provided resources, support, and training for several key groups that took on a leadership role in the dispute. Students, who were linked to the United Students against Sweatshops, were trained by SEIU. The national Interfaith Worker Justice organization was involved. Faculty staff held off-campus classes during the strike (Albright, 2008).

Toward the end of the strike, workers took a stronger position by starting a hunger strike, supported by a range of nonviolent actions. They achieved an increase in hourly rate, a week-paid holiday with three personal days, and three statutory holidays. As well as these specific material benefits, the campaign also created stronger bonds between different groups, students, faith groups, faculty, and local communities. It has also created an "ethical discourse" among the communities in Miami as well as demonstrating the value of trade union organizing (Albright, 2008).

TELCO

Set up in 1997, as a coalition of 37 local community organizations and local trade union branches in East London, UK, The East London Communities Organisations (TELCO) aims to bring these diverse communities into an effective alliance to:

> Press power-holders, in the public private sectors, to act for the
> benefit of families and communities in East London. TELCO trains
> leaders from its member organisations to be skilled and capable
> citizens, who can act collectively for the common good and take their
> case wherever it needs to be heard. (TELCO, 2003)

In 2001, TELCO published "Mapping low pay in East London" which highlighted the gap between minimum and living wages and poor working conditions. In May 2002, TELCO bought shares in HSBC, a major bank in the financial center, Canary Wharf, which paid its cleaners poor wages. At the HSBC AGM, TELCO raised concerns about how the bank contracted out its cleaning services. After many demonstrations and strikes, effective publicity and the development of widespread support for the "Living Wage" campaign, both Barclays Bank and HSBC agreed to new terms and conditions for their contract cleaners in Canary Wharf in 2004. In the same year, the T&G union started to employ two full time organizers based in Canary Wharf (Queen Mary College, Department of Geography, 2008).

Another TELCO campaign led to improved pay and conditions, for catering and cleaning services, in local hospitals. This campaign was successful in establishing a coalition between users and workers. It used arguments about reducing health inequalities, which were part of central government policy, to provide a rationale for the campaign. In the United Kingdom, there has been a growing awareness of the role that the public sector play as major employers, in disadvantaged areas (Lethbridge, 2009)

The work of TELCO is informed by research into working conditions, within the East End of London (Wills, 2001b). TELCO also provides an important training role for members of the coalition. This means that any campaign supported by TELCO, uses research and training to inform strategies and action and prepare activists, within the campaign. This recognizes that effective campaigning needs people with different skills, who are prepared to adopt multiple approaches to campaigning (Lethbridge, 2009).

Both the "Justice for Janitors" Miami campaign and the East London TELCO "Living Wage" campaign drew in many local community groups as well as faith communities with trade unions. These alliances have been powerful in providing support and introducing "ethical discourses" into institutions.

Rural Women Workers

In other regions, the organization of marginalized workers has often built on existing social movements. In Brazil, during the 1980s, the Workers' Party started to mobilize workers on the basis of their involvement in local community and neighborhood organizations and well as workplaces. This introduced a form of "new unionism."

The rural women workers' movement in Southern Brazil provides an example of how landless and smallholder women started to organize as "working class women" after their initial experiences of working as a part of wider rural worker movements. In the late 1980s, they campaigned to "secure the constitutional rights of rural women workers" (Stephen, 1997) as part of the process of rewriting the Constitution, which was taking place in Brazil at the time. Many women felt that their specific gender concerns were not taken seriously by wider campaigns. Organizing initially as the organization of country women, the rural women workers' movement in Southern Brazil campaigned for equal working conditions and benefits for rural women as well as reproductive health rights, domestic violence, and representation of women in the political system (Stephen, 1997).

Conclusion

Each of the five approaches to labor organizing, outlined in this chapter, have strengths and weaknesses, which are set out as follows:

1. *Multinational collective bargaining—the starting point for trade unions*
   Multinational collective bargaining was an important attempt to engage with multinational companies but was sometimes undermined by the perspectives of trade unions, which remained national in focus. National trade unions need to develop coherent transnational strategies by sector.

2. *Labor codes and codes of conduct*
   Voluntary codes of conduct were a response to some of the failures of governments and international agencies to implement labor standards. However, they would be more effective if governments played a more active role in implementation. It is also becoming clear that codes of conduct must cover all stages in the supply chain.

3. *European/global workers councils and social dialogue*
   Workers councils are structures, within multinational companies, that enable workers and management to discuss issues of concern. The shortcomings of these arrangements are that they are often under-resourced and meetings are only annual events. The evolution of social dialogue between labor and employers in different sectors in Europe, has led to some significant agreements on issues, such as part-time working. More negatively, social dialogue can be used as a "veneer" when more fundamental issues of labor-management relations or the implementation of neoliberal policies are not addressed.

4. *New labor internationalism and coalitions/community organizing*

The development of union–community coalitions draws in a wider range of groups into labor struggles but understanding different organizational cultures and ways of organizing takes a long time. The main issue for the future is how to maintain and sustain long-term coalitions.

5. *Organising marginalised workers—new forms of transnational labor solidarity*

   Specific initiatives to organize marginalized workers may pose some challenges for existing trade unions but workers in both informal and formal sectors need to work together. As with the development of union–community coalitions, this approach widens the cope of labor constituencies. In future, the momentum will need to be maintained and may require fundamental changes in the ways in which trade unions operate.

Issues for the Future

Labor, workers, and trade union responses to globalization raise issues of how place, space, and scale influence campaigns (Herod, 1997). How workers organize, at different levels, has a direct influence on workers' solidarity across space (Ghigliani, 2005). There is increasing recognition of the interdependence of workers through processes, institutions and relationships, operating at local, national, and global levels (Castree, 2007). International support has often proved essential for a campaign that started as a local campaign. This shows that workers recognize the need to support similar struggles elsewhere in the world. This is not always an easy process and effective ways of working internationally are still being refined. The importance of research and information sharing has started to emerge as crucial in campaigns that cover local, national, and global issues.

There is a growing recognition of the influence of workers on global labor markets, as shown in the recent living wage campaigns. These campaigns are also changing trade unions, which in the past have focused on specific organized groups of workers, sometimes ignoring unorganized workers. Trade unions now recognize that one way of reversing declining membership, is to start to organize disparate unorganized groups. This will require different strategies and will be strengthened by involving local communities and working on wider campaigns outside the workplace.

The needs of women workers are being recognized more widely. One of the results of working on workplace and community issues together, is that work is placed in the context of people's lives. Neoliberalism and privatization have affected all aspects of people's lives and these also need to be challenged.

Within the past 2 years I have not received gifts, grant funds, payments as a consultant, representative, writer or other services to a corporation, nor served on a corporate board, corporate advisory group, corporation sponsored institute or foundation, nor have I held financial interest in a corporation or industry about which I have written.

REFERENCES

Albright J. Contesting rationality, leadership and collective struggle: The 2006 Justice for Janitors campaign and the University of Miami. *Labor Studies Journal.* 2008;33:63–81.

Barriento S. and Smoth S. Do workers benefit from ethical trade? Assessing codes of labour practice in Global Production System. *Third World Quarterly.* 2007 28;4:713–729.

Bergene AC. Trade unions walking the tightrope in defending workers' interest Wielding a weapon too strong? *Labor Studies Journal.* 2007;32(2):142–166.

Bieler A. Labour the struggle for the future European model of capitalism: British and Swedish trade unions and their position on EMU and European cooperation. *BJPIR.* 2008;10:84–104.

Bieler A, Morton A. Another Europe is Possible? Labour and social movements at the European Social Forum. *Globalizations.* 2004;1–2:303–325.

Castree N. Labour geography: a work in progress. *Int J Urban Reg Res.* 2007;31(4):853–862.

Chan J, de Haan E, Nordbrand S, Torstensson A. *Silenced to Deliver: Mobile Phone Manufacturing in China and the Philippines.* SOMO & SwedWatch; 2008.

Chun JJ. The limits of labor exclusion: redefining the politics of split labour markets under globalization. *Crit Sociol.* 2008;34(3):433–452.

Cooke W. Exercising power in a prisoner's dilemma: transnational collective bargaining in an era of corporate globalization. *Industrial Relations Journal.* 2005;36A:283–302.

Curtin DM. Transparency and political participation in EU governance: a role for civil society? *Cultural Values.* 1999;3(4):445–471.

Degryse C. European social dialogue: a mixed picture *DWP* 2000.01.02. European Trades Union Institute; 2000.

Deva S. Global compact: a critique of the UN's public –private partnership for promoting corporate citizenship. *SJILC.* 2006;34:107–151.

Egels-Zandon N, Wahlqvist E. Post-partnership strategies for defining corporate responsibility: the Business Social Compliance Initiative. *J Bus Ethics.* 2007;70(2):175–189.

EMCEF/EUROGAS/EPSU. *Joint statement of the European social partners in the European gas industry on the Memorandum of Understanding on social aspects of the Energy Community for South East Europe.* Available at: http://www.

energy-community.org/pls/portal/docs/54176.PDF. Published 2007. Accessed December 17, 2008.

EPSU. Profit sharing, equality and diversity, employment and qualifications on Suez EWC agenda. Availbale at: http://www.epsu.org/a/3050. Published 2007. Accessed December 17, 2008.

EPSU. Suez EWC expresses its opinion on the merger with Gaz de France. Availbale at: http://www.epsu.org/a/3460. Published 2008. Accessed December 17, 2008.

European Commission Council Directive 94/45/EC of 22 September 1994 on the establishment of a European Works Council or a procedure in Community-scale undertakings and Community-scale groups of undertakings for the purposes of informing and consulting employees. Available at: http://europa.eu.int/comm/ employment_social/soc-dial/labour/directive9445/9445euen.htm. Published 1994. Accessed December 17, 2008.

European Commission Directive 94/45/EC. Available at: http://eur-lex.europa.eu/ LexUriServ/LexUriServ.do?uri=CELEX:31994L0045:EN:HTML. Published 1994. Accessed December 17, 2008.

European Commission. Commission Decision of 20 May 1998 on the establishment of Sectoral Dialogue Committees promoting the Dialogue between the social partners at European level (notified under document number C(1998) 2334) (Text with EEA relevance) (98/500/EC). *Official Journal of the European Communities.* 1998. Available at: http://eur- lex.europa.eu/LexUriServ/ LexUriServ.do?uri=OJ:L:1998:225:0027:0028:EN:PDF. Accessed May 2009.

European Union. Articles 3&4 Maastricht Treaty, 1993 Protocol on Social Policy (annexed to the Maastricht Treaty, 1993); 1993.

Ferus-Comelo A. Mission impossible?: raising labor standards in the ICT sector. *Labor Studies Journal.* 2008;33:141–162.

Ghigliani P. New Labour internationalism. *Economic and Industrial Democracy.* 2005;26(3):359–382.

Gill L. 'Right there with you': Coca-Cola, labor restructuring and political violence in Colombia. *Crit Anthropol.* 2007;27:235–260.

Greer I. *Social Movement Unionism and the Breakdown of the Neo-Corporatist Relations: The Case of Hamburg's Hospitals.* Worldwide Universities Network Paper presented 1 June 2006 Available at: http://www.wun.ac.uk/rcc/pdfs/econference/ papers/Ian%20Greer.pdf. Published 2006. Accessed December 18, 2008.

Hammer N. International Framework Agreements: global industrial relations between rights and bargaining. *Transfer.* 2005;11(4):511–530.

Herod A. From a geography of labor to a labor geography: labor's spatial fix and the geography of capitalism. *Antipode.* 1997;29(1):1–31.

Herod A. Labor internationalism and the contradictions of globalization: or, why the local is sometimes still important in a global economy. In: Waterman P, Wills J, eds. *Place, Space and the New Labor Internationalism* (pp. 103–122). London: Blackwell; 2008.

Hirschsohn P. Union democracy and shopfloor mobilization: Social movement unionism in South African Auto and Clothing Plants. *Economic and Industrial Democracy.* 2007;28(1):6–48.

Hyman R. Trade unions and interest representation in the context of globalization. *Transfer.* 1997;3(3):3515–3533.

Hyman R. *The International Labour Movement on the Threshold of Two Centuries Agitation, Organisation, Bureaucracy, Diplomacy.* Available from Arbetarrörelsens arkiv och bibliotek, Stockholm, 2002 http://www.arbark.se/pdf_wrd/Hyman_int.pdf. Accessed May 2009.

Ikanova E, Turner L. Building the New Europe: Western and eastern roads to social partnership. *Industrial Relations Journal.* 2004;35(1):76–92.

International Labour Organisation (ILO). Overview of global developments and Office Activities concerning codes of conduct, social labelling and other private sector initiatives addressing labour issues Working party on the social dimensions of the liberalization of international trade International Labor Organization LO Governing Body 273rd session. Geneva: ILO; 1998.

International Labour Organization (ILO). *Tripartite Declaration of Principles Concerning Multinational Enterprises and Social Policy.* Geneva: International Labour Organization; 2001.

International Labour Organization (ILO). What is social dialogue. Available at: www.ilo.org/public/english/dialogue. Accessed December 17, 2008.

Jenkins R. *Corporate Codes of Conduct Self-Regulation in a Global Economy.* Technology, Business and Society Programme Paper Number 2 April 2001 Geneva: United Nations Research Institute for Social Development; 2001.

LaCroix P. Improving Workplace Conditions in the 'Maquilas' of Central America. *IDRC Bulletin.* May 29, 1998. Available at: http://www.idrc.ca/en/ev-5539–201-1-DO_TOPIC.html. Accessed December 17, 2008.

Lethbridge J. Hidden Dimensions of Liberalisation and Privatisation: The Impact on Public Sector Workers. Unpublished 2006.

Lethbridge J. Trade unions, civil society organisations and health reforms. *Capital and Class.* 2009. Issue 98:101–130.

Moody K. *Workers in a Lean World.* London: Verso; 1997.

Mosley L. Workers' rights in open economies: global production and domestic institutions in the developing world. *Comp Polit Stud.* 2008;41:674–714.

Mosley L, Uno S. Racing to bottom or climbing to the top? Economic globalization and collective labour rights. *Comp Polit Stud.* 2007;40(8):928–948.

Nilsson J. A Tool for Achieving Workers' Rights' Metal World 4. 2002.

Novelli M. Globalisations, social movement unionism and new internationalisms: The role of strategic learning in the transformation of the Municipal Workers Union of EMCALI. *Globalisation, Societies and Education.* 2004;2(2):161–190.

Pearson R, Seyfang G. New hope or false dawn?: voluntary codes of conduct, labour regulation and social policy in a globalising world. *GSP.* 2001;1:49–78.

PSI News. July, September, October. Available at: www.psi-world.org. Accessed December 17, 2008.

Queen Mary College, Department of Geography Living Wage campaign. Available at: http://www.geog.qmul.ac.uk/livingwage/chronology.html. Accessed December 17, 2008.

Ramsay H. Solidarity at last? International trade unionism approaching the millennium. *Economic and Industrial Democracy.* 1997;18(4):503–537.

Reiss J. Social movement unionism and progressive public policies in New York City. *Just Labour*. 2005;5:36–48.

Reuters Turkish Police breakup Istanbul May Day protests. Thursday May 1, 2008. Available at: http://in.reuters.com/article/worldNews/idININdia-33341220080501 Accessed November 29, 2009

Riisgaard L. International Framework Agreements: a new model for securing workers' rights? *Industrial Relations*. 2005;44(4):707–737.

Schiavone M. Moody's account of social movement unionism: an analysis. *Critical Sociology*. 2007;33:279–309.

Sorriano J. Globalization and the maquildoras November 24, 1999. Available at: http://www.motherjones.com/news/special_reports/wto/soriano1.html. Published 1999. Accessed December 17, 2008.

Standing G. *Global Labour Flexibility: Seeking Redistributive Justice*. Basingstoke: Macmillan; 1999.

Stephen L. *Women and Social Movements in Latin America Power from Below*. London: Latin America Bureau; 1997.

Stevis D. 'International Framework Agreements between unions and multinationals: Corporate social responsibility or social regulation' Paper presented at the 2008 Convention of the International Studies Association. San Francisco March 26–30, 2008.

Streek W. The Internationalisation of industrial relations in Europe: Prospects and problems. *Working Paper Series in European Studies* 1(1) European Studies Program International Institute University of Wisconsin-Madison, Wisconsin; 1998.

TELCO. *Funding the Poorest in the NHS: The Case for East London*. London: TELCO; 2003.

Torres B. Honduras: Analysis of the impact of the Collective of Honduran Women (CODEMUH) on workers' rights and occupational health, 2002 to 2005 in *From Poverty to Power: How Active Citizens and Effective States Can Change the World*. Oxfam International; 2008.

Vannieuwenhuyse F. *The ILO Tripartite Declaration of Principles concerning Multinational Enterprises and Social Policy and The OECD Guidelines for Multinational Enterprises* Presentation to the International Training Centre of the ILO, Turin, Italy; 2003. *training.itcilo.it/actrav/courses/2003/A4–00243_web/ resource/fons/ILODeclarationOECDguidelines.ppt. Accessed December 17, 2008.*

Waddington J. The performance of European Works Councils in engineering: Perspectives of the employee representatives. *Industrial Relations*. 2006;45(4):681–708.

Waterman P. Trade union internationalism in the Age of Seattle. *Antipode*. 2001;312–336.

Waterman P, Timms J. Trade union internationalism and global civil society in the making Chapter 8 of Helmut Anheier, Marlies Glasius and Mary Kaldor. (eds.) *Global Civil Society*. 2004–05;175–202.

Webster E, Lambert R. What is new in the new labour internationalism: A southern perspective. *RAU Sociology Seminar Series.* (First Term) March 7, 2003;1–36.

Wills J. Community unionism and trade union renewal in the UK: Moving beyond the fragments at last? *Trans Inst Br Geogr.* 2001a;26:465–483.

Wills J. *Mapping low pay in East London* September 2001, written for TELCO's Living Wage campaign UNISON, Queen Mary College, London; 2001b.

16

Campaigns to Change Health-Damaging Corporate Practices

Nicholas Freudenberg

Introduction

In the 20th century, corporations became the dominant institution in the global economy and corporate business and political decisions became an increasingly important influence on all aspects of life, including health. The growing power of corporations to shape patterns of health and disease has forced the public health community to consider how best to change corporate practices and policies that harm health and to encourage those that promote well-being. In this chapter, I consider the role of public health campaigns in altering corporate activities that affect health. My goals are to define and describe such campaigns, analyze factors associated with success and failure, assess their potential and limitations for improving population health, and examine the linkages between public health campaigns and social movements. To illustrate the dynamics of such campaigns, I present three case histories of efforts to change corporate practices. Finally, I suggest how public health professionals, advocates, and researchers can contribute to campaigns to modify health-related corporate practices.

Case History 1 Coalition against Uptown Cigarettes

In 1990, RJ Reynolds Company announced its intention to test market in Philadelphia a new brand of cigarettes called Uptown designed to appeal to African Americans. In response, the Coalition against Uptown Cigarettes organized to stop Reynolds. The campaign included African American church groups, local and national health leaders, civil rights groups, elected officials and others. One of the group's leaders, Charyn Sutton, explained their strategy:

> The Coalition against Uptown Cigarettes decided to focus their outreach efforts primarily to Black smokers. The goal was to derail the test market by getting smokers to refuse even to sample the new cigarette during the proposed six-month test market period. To do this the Coalition crafted messages that targeted Reynolds Tobacco as the enemy rather than focusing their attacks on smokers or on other Blacks who stood to benefit financially from the product, such as Black-owned media and neighborhood grocery stores. The aim of the Uptown Coalition was to form a partnership among Black smokers and nonsmokers around the issues of youth access to flashy new product. (Robinson & Sutton, 1994).

Faced with growing media coverage and national opposition, RJ Reynolds decided to halt the test before any cigarettes hit the shelves. The Uptown cigarette campaign was uniquely successful in that it used primarily local grassroots strategies to stop the marketing of Uptown cigarettes before the cigarettes and accompanying promotional products could be distributed to retailers. Moreover, by creating a campaign that was rooted in Philadelphia's African American neighborhoods and framing the issues as one of community choice, the campaign was able to appeal to a board cross-section of the community. As Sutton explained

> The Uptown struggle was one of taking back the issue of choice and redefining it in a larger community context, rather than an individual context. Excessive tobacco advertising in African American communities pushes tobacco products in a way that takes away choice. The Coalition believed that African Americans were exercising their right of free choice—by rejecting Uptown. (Robinson & Sutton, 1994)

In the following decade, several other African American communities picked up on Philadelphia's example and took action against racially targeted tobacco marketing. In 1999, veterans of the Uptown campaign joined other activists to create the National African American Tobacco Prevention Network, a national organization that supports grassroots advocacy for tobacco control.

Public Health Campaigns to Change Corporate Practices

Public health advocates and corporate reformers have used many strategies to modify corporate practices. These include legislation, regulation, litigation, shareholder resolutions, community mobilization, boycotts, strikes, and other strategies, some of which are described in other chapters in this volume. In this chapter, the focus is on *public health campaigns,* defined as advocacy initiatives in which one or more organizations launch targeted activities designed to achieve explicit changes in corporate or industry practices perceived to influence health. These campaigns can be of variable duration and intensity; target a specific corporation (e.g., Nestlé), industry (e.g., tobacco), or product [e.g., trans fat or Sports Utility Vehicles (SUV)]; and operate at the local (e.g., campaign to Stop Uptown Cigarettes), national (e.g., campaigns to ban junk food advertising to children), or global levels (e.g., campaign to stop Nestlé from promoting infant formula over breast feeding).

Public health campaigns seek to change corporate practices directly, using strategies such as boycotts, shareholder resolutions or media advocacy, or indirectly by passing new legislation, convincing government to enforce regulations, or winning lawsuits that require companies to pay damages and/or modify their practices.

While public health campaigns to change corporate practices are often supported by and contribute to social movements, broader and more ongoing popular mobilizations (Lofland, 1996), the definition used here distinguishes between the more time and objective limited campaigns and broader social movements. In addition, this definition of public health campaigns encompass broader goals and a wider repertoire of strategies and tactics than electoral or legislative campaigns, which seek to pass or defeat a referendum, law, or elect or reject a candidate, sometimes for reasons related to health (Oliver, 2006). Some public health researchers have also used the term campaign to describe media or social marketing effort to change health-related behaviors or attitudes (Randolph & Viswanath, 2004; Grier & Bryant, 2005; Noar, 2006). Although these efforts may share certain characteristics with campaigns to change corporate practices, our focus here is on campaigns that seek to bring about institutional or policy change, rather than individual change.

Finally, campaigns to modify corporate practices extend beyond health to include, for example, efforts to improve pay and working conditions for sweatshop workers, to limit executive compensation, to prevent companies from shutting down facilities without prior notice, or to limit rain forest destruction (Manheim, 2002; Cray, 2007). While some of these corporate campaigns touch on health, the focus here is on campaigns with the explicit goal of improving population health.

Characteristics of Campaigns to Change Corporate Health
Practices

The goal of studying public health campaigns is to identify the characteristics of effective efforts so as to provide an evidence base to inform policy and practice that can promote health. Prior research on community mobilization for health and public health advocacy suggests several key variables of interest (Freudenberg et al., 2009; Minkler et al., 2008; Minkler & Wallerstein, 2008) These include campaign goals and objectives; the target of change; the response of the target; the campaign's organizational structure and participants; the political, social, and economic context; the strategies and tactics; and the intensity and duration of campaign activities. Previous research shows considerable variability on these characteristics, suggesting that analyses of the associations between these traits and campaign outcomes may yield insights that can improve their effectiveness in protecting health.

Campaign Goals and Objectives

Public health campaigns seek to alter corporate business practices such as advertising, employment, pricing, production processes, product design, and retail distribution. They also seek to bring about political changes such as restrictions on lobbying, campaign contributions and public relations, and they work to educate and mobilize the public at large or specific constituencies to play a more active role in protecting health against corporate harm. For example, public health campaigns have sought to improve fuel efficiency and safety standards for SUVs, impose taxes on alcohol, tobacco and soda, require infant formula and gun manufacturers to better monitor retail distribution of their products, prevent soda companies from signing exclusive "pouring rights" contacts with school districts, and restrict secrecy requirements attached to corporate funding of scientific research.

Campaign Target

Campaigns can target a specific corporation, product or practice, or an industry as a whole. The Stop Uptown Cigarettes campaign prevented a new product, the Black-oriented Uptown cigarette, from being introduced. Similarly, in Seattle, a coalition of parents and food advocates forced the Seattle school board to cancel an exclusive "pouring rights" contract with Coca-Cola thus removing the one brand of soda the school had authorized selling (Ervin, 2002). In these two cases, campaigns removed a single product of a single company from a defined space, a victory that was both "real" in that it reduced access to an unhealthy product but also symbolic since Coke and other sodas were still available in Seattle and other brands of Black-targeted cigarettes were still sold in Philadelphia.

Campaigns can also target an entire class of products, as shown in Case History 2 on trans fats. In addition, gun control advocates have sought to limit production and sales of Saturday night specials, cheap handguns readily available to the impulsive shooter (Wallack, 1999), and the national environmental organization Sierra Club organized a campaign against SUVs because of their high levels of pollution and their contribution to automobile injuries and deaths (Sierra Club, 2002). By targeting an entire class of products rather than a single brand, it may be possible to have a wider public health impact (Borra et al., 2007).

Campaigns can also take on an entire industry. The tobacco control movement has targeted practices of the tobacco industry as a whole, including their advertising to young people, their obfuscation of scientific evidence showing tobacco's harm, and their introduction of additives to make their products more addictive (e.g., nicotine) or more attractive (e.g., menthol) to vulnerable populations (Schroeder, 2004; Brandt, 2007). Tobacco control advocates continue to debate whether their ultimate goal should be to eliminate or reform the tobacco industry (Pertschuk, 2001).

Public health campaigns can set either negative or positive goals or some of each. Food advocates, for example, may urge supermarket chains to make healthy products like fresh fruits and vegetables more available by lower pricing, more advertising and allocation of more or better supermarket shelf space, or they may work to make unhealthy food less available by contesting deceptive health claims, limiting shelf space for junk food, or taxing products like sweetened soda (Kristal et al., 1997; Sustainable Development Commission, 2008). Positive goals may help to activate constituencies motivated by a vision of a healthier world whereas negative goals can help to unite groups facing a common enemy. Both approaches can be useful campaign organizing tools.

Case History 2 Campaigns to Eliminate Trans Fats from American Diet

In 1994, the Center for Science in the Public Interest (CSPI) petitioned the Food and Drug Administration (FDA) to require that food manufacturers label the *trans* fatty acid (*trans* fat) content of their food products (FDA, 2003). The petition was based on new research that showed that replacing *trans* fat with healthier oils could prevent between 30,000 and 100,000 premature deaths from cardiovascular disease in the United States each year. Artificial *trans* fats are used to enhance the crispness, stability, and flavor of many processed foods. By the late 1990s, 40% of US supermarket products contained *trans* fats. In 1999, five years after the CSPI petition, the FDA proposed to include the *trans* fat content of food on the standard food label, claiming that the change would yield significant health and economic benefits (FDA, 2003).

In May 2003, Ban *Trans* Fat, a California-based nonprofit advocacy group, filed a lawsuit against Kraft Foods North America, Inc. seeking an injunction against the sale and marketing of Oreo cookies to children in California (Severson, 2003). One of the legal bases for the lawsuit was that the cookies contain *trans* fat which is not shown on the Nutrition Facts panel on the packaging. The lawsuit relied on a provision in California law that deems companies accountable for unknown dangers of substances they add to their products (Burros, 2003). One effect of the lawsuit was to educate people about the risks of *trans* fat. A few weeks later, Kraft announced it would stop marketing certain products in schools and develop a *trans* fat free Oreo. As a result, Ban *Trans* Fat voluntarily dismissed the lawsuit, claiming they had won their demands (Severson, 2003). The group also filed a lawsuit against McDonald's for its failure to live up to its 2002 promise to reduce *trans* fat.

Meanwhile, CSPI launched a major grassroots campaign to encourage food manufacturers to reformulate their products. Twenty-eight nationally prominent scientists sent a letter to FDA in support of CSPI's call for a ban on *trans* fat. CSPI also called on restaurants to disclose to their customer the *trans* fat contents of their food (Jacobson, 2004) and ran a full-page ad in the *New York Times* calling on McDonalds to live up to its previous pledge.

In early 2005, Ban *Trans* Fat and McDonalds reached a settlement in the *trans* fat lawsuit that required Big Mac to inform the public about its *trans* fat policies and to donate $7 million to the American Heart Association for public education regarding *trans* fat (Garofoli, 2005).

In 2007, New York City modified its health code to ban the use of *trans* fat in all food service establishments. By 2008, the American Medical Association had endorsed a ban on *trans* fat, the amount of *trans* fat in the American diet had declined almost 50% since 2005 and bans on *trans* fats in restaurants had been passed in cities and states with 20% of the U.S. population (CSPI, 2008).

Level of Action

Campaigns operate at the institutional, local, national, or global levels. For example, parents mobilize to force their children's school to remove unhealthy food from school vending machines. A local campaign seeks to force gun manufactures to compensate a municipality for the cost of gun injuries attributed to their inadequate oversight of retail distribution of their products. National campaigns like the Million Mom March for regulation of the gun industry (Wallack et al., 2004) or the Prescription Project's campaigns to ban gifts to physicians (Rothman & Chimonas, 2008) use both legislative and media strategies to alter the practices of these industries.

Global campaigns cross national boundaries and often involve global organizations. South Africa's Treatment Action Campaign, profiled below, partnered with Doctors without Borders, Health Gap and Act Up as well as the governments of South Africa, India, and Brazil, to force the pharmaceutical company Glaxo to lower the price of antiretroviral medications for HIV infection (Powers, 2003). In 1977, activists launched an international boycott of Nestlé's products to protest their promotion of infant formula. This campaign brought together health professionals and advocates first in the United States and Europe and then from around the world. In 1981, the World Health Assembly passed a new international code on the marketing of breast milk substitutes and in 1984, Nestlé agreed to follow this code (Nestle, 2002). At present, the International Baby Food Action Network, which consists of more than 200 groups in more than 100 countries, continues to monitor infant formula companies' compliance with these guidelines (Baby Milk Action, n. d.). Given the tendency of many manufacturers to export risky products to developing markets when oversight increases in the developed world, global campaigns can help to prevent public health successes in wealthier nations from turning into health threats to poorer countries.

Organizational Structure and Allies

Campaigns also differ in their organizational structure and their partnerships with allies. In some cases, a single independent organization sponsors or leads a campaign. The national organization Center for Science in the Public Interest has served as the catalyst for dozens of campaigns designed to modify the practices of the food and beverage, pharmaceutical, and other industries. With a small staff, decades of experience in Washington politics and the ability to form partnerships with local and other national organizations, CSPI is one of a handful of groups that have the capacity to sustain national campaigns over an extended time. Other such groups include the Union of Concerned Scientists, the Sierra Club, the Brady Center to Prevent Gun Violence and the Marin Institute, a California-based organization that monitors the alcohol industry. These groups often have ready access to scientific expertise, strong links to other national advocacy organizations, and an insider's knowledge of corporate resistance to policy change. On the other hand, their national focus may reduce their capacity mobilize grassroots constituencies or sustain the community mobilization needed to achieve more than token victories.

In other cases, an organization is formed for the specific purpose of carrying out a campaign and may disappear once the campaign is over. The Stop Uptown Cigarettes Coalition and the Million Mom March (Wallack et al., 2004) are examples of such transient campaign sponsors. One advantage of this approach is that it is less expensive and does not require the ongoing commitment to maintain an organization. On the other hand, this short lifespan may make it difficult for the organization to monitor and sustain victories.

Finally, some grassroots social change organizations may choose to launch public health campaigns as one part of a broader portfolio of activities. The South African Treatment Action Campaign, for example, provides direct services to people with HIV, challenges government AIDS policies, and campaigns to change pharmaceutical industry practices. A church in Harlem, New York, played a lead role in mobilizing the community to paint over alcohol and tobacco billboards, viewing this action as one more way to protect their young people from harm (Navarro, 1990).

Campaigns choose to partner with a wide variety of organizations, including government agencies, public officials, university researchers, civic or civil rights groups, health professionals, neighborhood associations, and others. These partners bring unique assets – and limitations – to the campaign, as illustrated in the three case histories in this chapter. In some cases, public health campaigns choose to work in partnership with, rather than oppose, a company or industry. For example, the Sierra Club for a time worked with Ford Motor Company to build and promote a more energy efficient SUV, the Mercury Mariner (Sierra Club, 2005), and through the Alliance for a Healthier Generation, the William Jefferson Clinton Foundation partners with 11 major food companies to reduce the amount of unhealthy food in schools and reformulate high calorie low nutrient products marketed to children (Clinton, 2008). Some activists assert these partnerships compromise the campaign's health goals and inevitably lead to problematic concessions (Simon, 2006), while others suggest that coalitions should carefully define their goals and bottom line *before* entering any discussions with industry representatives (Dorfman et al., 2005a).

Context

Evidence suggests that the social context in which advocates and industry compete for the dominant interpretation of corporate practices is a critical component to the success or failure of campaigns to change corporate practices. For example, a comparison of the campaigns to change the practices of tobacco corporations and gun manufacturers illustrates the importance of national and local popular opinion, elected officials' willingness to act on the issue, and the role of mainstream news media in influencing the more favorable outcomes for activists in tobacco control as compared to gun control (Nathanson, 1999). In some cases, the cumulative successes of previous campaigns may create a more favorable climate for advocates, as in the case of efforts to change food industry practices in the current decade, and the campaign to restrict advertising of tobacco, which built on the 1998 Master Settlement Agreement.

In other cases, the shifting social and political climate during the course of campaigns suggests the importance of context. For example, when the Seattle-based campaign to remove Coca-Cola from the public schools was launched in 1996, the school district was facing a budget crisis and many board members felt the financial opportunities presented by the Coke contract were too valuable to pass up. Over the course of the campaign, however, public concern about childhood obesity grew, helping to create a climate in which the board could no longer ignore advocates' concerns without the threat of litigation.

Strategies

In an analysis of 12 campaigns designed to change corporate practice (Freudenberg et al.,2009), my colleagues and I identified the following 11 strategies that these campaigns used to achieve their objectives: community organization and capacity building, media advocacy, policy advocacy, litigation, research and information gathering, letter writing, coalition building, counter marketing, public protest, community mobilization, and working directly with corporations. Most campaigns used multiple strategies with a mean of 4.3 strategies per campaign. Recently, several organizations have launched internet campaigns to change corporate practices, a low-cost strategy that national companies and retail chains seem to fear (Jones et al., 2006).

Some campaigns have chosen to start with educational strategies both as a way of first seeking to achieve their goals with the least intrusive methods and in order to win over supporters who might initially oppose more confrontational strategies. Other campaigning organizations limit their work to a single or a few strategies based on their strengths in, for example, litigation, community mobilization, or media advocacy. Several guidebooks help activists and policy advocates to select the strategy or strategies best matched to their goals and resources (Sen, 2003; Ritas, 2003; The Community Tool Box, 2009).

Intensity and Duration

For most public health interventions, evidence suggests that more is better, that is, more intensive contact with an intervention over an extended period of time yields better results. Public health campaigns vary in intensity, defined as the amount and quality of contact a campaign has with its participants, and duration, the time from the beginning to the end of the campaign, usually marked by victory or defeat. The Nestlé Boycott has lasted for decades while other encounters, such as the Ban *Trans* Fat lawsuit against Kraft Foods achieved their goals within a few weeks. To date, little empirical research has examined the impact of campaign intensity and duration on their success in modifying corporate practices.

Factors Associated with Success

In summary, based on a review of both academic and activist accounts (Nathanson, 1999; Freudenberg et al., 2009; John & Thompson, 2003; Sen, 2003; Brown et al., 2004), it appears that campaigns that use multiple methods, frame issues so as to mobilize support across constituencies, define specific and limited objectives, seize policy "windows of opportunity" (Kingdon, 1984), and are able to work across sectors and levels that are more successful than campaigns without these characteristics. These preliminary findings warrant further research.

Case History 3 The Treatment Action Campaign: Campaigning for the Rights of People with HIV/AIDS

The Treatment Action Campaign (TAC) was launched on International Human Rights Day in 1998 to "campaign for greater access to treatment for all South Africans, by raising public awareness and understanding about issues surrounding the availability, affordability, and use of HIV treatments" (Friedman & Mottiar, 2004). When a close friend of one of TAC's founders, Zachi Amat, died because he couldn't afford the antiretroviral medicines that would have saved his life, Ahmat, himself a veteran of the antiapartheid struggle and infected with HIV, pledged he would stage a drug strike, refusing to take antiretrovirals until they were available for all South Africans. "The only reason we don't have this medication in South Africa," he said, "is because we are poor, not because it doesn't exist"(Powers, 2003).

TAC realized South Africa could never afford the antiretrovirals until the Western pharmaceutical companies lowered their prices – or dropped the patent. So TAC decided to begin its campaign by focusing on newborn babies infected with HIV because their mothers were not given a dose of the antiretroviral drug AZT, manufactured by Glaxo, an international pharmaceutical company. By joining with the South African government, labor, and religious organizations, TAC hoped to shame Glaxo into lowering its price. A few years earlier South Africa had passed legislation that allowed the country to bypass patents and provide more affordable generic drugs. In 1998, however, 39 drug companies filed suit in South Africa's High Court to overturn the rule and the Clinton Administration lobbied aggressively to prevent South Africa from making its own generic antiretrovirals (Powers, 2003).

TAC then formed an alliance with four other global health organizations, Doctors without Borders, ACT UP, Health Gap, and the Consumer Project on Technology to reverse the U.S. position. By staging demonstrations at campaign stops for U.S. Presidential candidate Al Gore, eventually the activists persuaded the U.S. to drop its opposition to generic drugs. After several months of continued protests in South Africa, in 2000 Glaxo agreed to halve the price of AZT in South Africa (Powers, 2003), and soon other companies also lowered prices. Unfortunately, however, it took TAC and its allies another seven years to make antiretrovirals widely available in South Africa, not because of the practices of the drug industry but because of the opposition to antiretrovirals by then South African President Thembo Mbeki. By 2008, about 470,000 South Africans with HIV were estimated to be receiving antiretroviral therapy and another 524,000 were still in need of treatment (Treatment Action Campaign, 2008). TAC continues to campaign for changes in government and pharmaceutical industry practices that will make treatment more accessible. Throughout its history, its goal has been to create the moral unity that can serve as a catalyst for individual and collective action.

Campaigns and Social Movements

Campaigns are the building blocks but also the manifestations of social movements. While not every campaign is part of a social movement, those that are can ride the wave of activism that movements generate, often landing further up the beach of policy change than those campaigns without such momentum. In this section, we consider first some of the social movements that have supported campaigns to change corporate health practices, then analyze whether the cumulative efforts to change corporate health practices have the potential to become a social movement in their own right.

Social Movements and Campaigns to Change Corporate Practices

Social movements are groupings of people who organize over time to redress grievances and promote social justice. Charles Tilly (2004), a leading theorist of social movements, has identified three main elements that define movements: campaigns, which he describes as sustained, organized public efforts to make collective claims on authorities; a repertoire of both conventional and contentious strategies and tactics; and ongoing public representations of their positions, commitments, strength, and moral purpose. Table 16.1 lists linkages between some recent social movements and related public health campaigns to change corporate practices. It shows that many such campaigns have their roots in the social movements of the last several decades.

Movements have much to offer campaigns. First, they create "frames" that help to define the ways that participants, targets and observers think about the contested issues. For example, the environmental movement created the frame that people have the right to breathe air that will not sicken them, a more powerful and compelling frame than the tobacco industry's claim that individuals had the right to smoke. The concept of a right to breathable air helped tobacco control activists to overcome tobacco industry opposition to public smoking bans (Menashe & Siegel, 1998; Brandt, 2007).

TABLE 16.1. Linkages between Social Movements and Campaigns to Change Corporate Health Practices.

Movement for	Common aims of Movement and Public Health Campaigns	Examples of Campaigns	Selected References
Civil rights	End harmful corporate practices that target Blacks or Latinos	Stop Uptown cigarettes; ban tobacco and alcohol billboards in Black areas	Robinson & Sutton, 1994; Hackbarth et al. 2001; Brulle & Pellow, 2006.
Consumer protection	Stop corporate marketing and design practices that harm consumers	Nader campaigns for safer car designs, Action for Children's Television campaigns to restrict unhealthy food ads to children	Mayer, 1989; Khann et al., 2000

TABLE 16.1. Continued

Movement for	Common aims of Movement and Public Health Campaigns	Examples of Campaigns	Selected References
Corporate reform	Modify corporate structures and behaviors that undermine democracy or externalize costs to public	Shareholder resolutions in tobacco and Nestlé boycott	Graves et al., 2001; Guay & Doh, 2004.
Environmental justice	End practices that damage environment or are unsustainable	Campaigns to close polluting factories in low income areas or to force auto companies to produce less polluting vehicles	Bullard, 1993; Brulle & Pellow, 2006
Global justice	Stop corporate practices or policies that harm economy or well-being of lower income nations	Global treaties, campaigns, and alliances that restrict tobacco or pharmaceutical industries from selling unsafe products in developing world markets	People's Health Assembly, 2002; Blum, 2007
Health care for all	Prevent profit from dictating quality of or access to health care	Prescription Drug Project that seeks ban on pharmaceutical industry gifts to doctors; campaigns to lower price of essential drugs	Jasso-Aguilar et al., 2004; Waitzkin et al., 2005.
Occupational safety and health	End corporate practices that harm health or safety of workers	Campaigns to end exposures to toxic substances in workplace	Levenstein et al., 1984; Lipschutz, 2004.
Nuclear power safety	Require nuclear industry to follow safety standards	Campaigns to shut nuclear facilities or require stricter safety standards	Ackland, 2002; Walsh, 1988.
Women's rights	Withdraw or keep from market products that harm women's health	Campaigns against Dalkon shield, hormonal replacement therapy or mandatory HPV vaccination in absence of safety evidence	Hippert, 2002; Krieger et al., 2005.

Second, movements help to mobilize the human, organizational, cultural, intellectual, and financial resources that campaigns need to win (Edwards & McCarthy, 2004). The Treatment Action Campaign's success in forcing Glaxo to lower the price of antiretroviral drugs in South Africa played out in the context of global movements for human and health rights, North–South equality, action to contain AIDS, and against apartheid. The organizations and individuals that eventually supported the TAC goals were pulled into the conflict by these deeper currents as well as the specific tactics of the campaign.

Third, social movements can provide the setting in which campaigns can find allies in other sectors and at other levels that help them achieve victories. For example, the civil rights movement provided the context for the Coalition against Uptown Cigarettes to reach out to Black church groups, civil rights organizations and health professional organizations within Philadelphia. Similarly, the environmental movement provided the framework and common ground that joined several strata: local activists demonstrating to convince auto retailers to demand that car makers produce less polluting vehicles, statewide efforts to pass tougher emissions control standards in California and elsewhere, and national campaigns for federal legislation on auto fuel efficiency. Movements thus provide the glue that can bring together disparate campaign activities across sectors and levels.

Finally, social movements have the capacity to sustain the individuals and organizations working for change that discrete public health campaigns may lack. When Lois Gibbs, a leader of the campaign to cleanup toxic contamination in Love Canal, moved away from the area, an emerging national environmental justice movement was able to recapture her leadership potential in a new organization. For TAC and Zachi Ahmat, the antiapartheid struggle provided the moral foundation and tactical repertoire that guided their actions. With their moral and political visions and articulated grievances, movements can supply the energy and nurture the passion and commitment that are often needed to win significant victories.

To be fair, movements can also exact a toll on public health campaigns. With their broader goals, more clearly defined ideologies and sometimes more confrontational tactics, movements may deter some individual or organizations from participating in public health campaigns that are closely linked with a particular movement. Many movement strategies depend on polarization of supporters and opponents in order to escalate power struggles. Some public health campaigners may be uncomfortable with such strategies and some campaigns may be able to achieve their goals with less disruptive activities.

From Public Health Campaigns to a Social Movement

If social movements offer advantages that can extend, accelerate, and amplify the successes of discrete public health campaigns, it is logical to ask whether there can be an anticorporate public health movement. Wiist (2006) urges public health advocacy movements to make linkages with the anticorporate movement and Nathanson (1999) has argued that social movements can act as catalysts for public health policy change. Here we consider whether existing mobilizations that seek to change health-damaging corporate practices have the potential to be a movement in their own right.

A variety of scholars have defined the essential characteristics of social movements (Snow et al., 2004; Tilly, 2004) to include: multiple campaigns at local, regional, national and/or global levels that seek to achieve some common goals; articulated grievances; individuals and organizations recognized as national leaders; a developed political agenda; and a national presence in media and other public settings.

Table 16.2 assesses the extent to which public health campaigns to change corporate practices in six selected business sectors meet the criteria for social movements.. This review shows that many of these domains of activity meet some of the prerequisites for movement status—in each sector there are some common goals that can unify distinct campaigns, national and global organization that support and link campaigns, and some ongoing if sporadic media coverage. However, to date there have been few public health organizations or leaders who bridge these sectors of activity. Unlike the consumer movement of the later mid-20th century or the environmental movement of the 1970s and 1980s, current mobilizations to modify health-damaging corporate practices do not yet have a consistent voice in Washington, the media, or the mainstream political parties. For the most part, public health activists have not articulated a comprehensive critique of corporate structures nor advanced an alternative political agenda, although a few individuals and organizations have suggested what might serve as frameworks for such a platform, as summarized in Table 16.3.

Is there already a public health movement that could add corporate change to its agenda? Some observers have described such a movement but they usually describe late 19th century or early 20th century mobilizations (Szreter, 2002) or, more recently, efforts that are primarily aimed at forcing government to improve health-related living conditions rather than those seeking to change corporate practices that influence health (Milewa & DeLeeuw, 1996). In addition, the activities of the "new public health movement" are often "confined within the state rather then the expression of a social movement against the

TABLE 16.2. Characteristics of Campaigns to Change Corporate Practices in Various Sectors.

Industry Sector	Examples of Local, Regional, National or Global Campaigns	National Agenda	Selected National & Global Organizations	National Presence in Media
Alcohol	Municipal and state campaigns to increase alcohol tax; local campaigns to change zoning laws; demands to withdraw ads or products aimed at youth or minorities	Reduce availability of alcohol, especially to youth; restrict advertising; make industry more responsible for adverse effects of alcohol	Marin Institute; Center on Alcohol Marketing and Youth; Mothers Against Drunk Driving; Global Alcohol Policy Alliance	Sporadic
Automobile	National and state campaigns to improve vehicle fuel efficiency and safety; campaigns against SUVs	Make motor vehicles safer and less polluting; support mass transit and other forms of sustainable transportation; enforce vehicle safety and environmental standards vigorously	Apollo Alliance; Center for Auto Safety, Union of Concerned Scientists, Sierra Club; Natural Resources Defense Council; Center for Environmental Health	Sporadic
Firearms	Municipal, state, and national lawsuits against gun industry for failure to monitor retail sales; campaigns to improve gun safety standards; bans on assault rifles	Keep guns away from criminals, mentally ill, and other risk groups; Mandate safety standards for firearms; monitor retail sales more closely; enforce existing laws vigorously	Brady Center to prevent Gun Violence; Million Mom March; Coalition to Stop Gun Violence; States United to prevent Gun Violence; International Action Network on Small Arms; Control Arms Campaign	Sporadic, especially after episodes of gun violence

Sector	Campaigns	Goals	Organizations	Frequency
Food and beverages	Campaigns to end soda company "pouring rights" contracts, to ban junk food from schools, to restrict television advertising to children, to require calorie labeling, to withdraw unhealthy products from market or to tax unhealthy food	Make healthy food more available, affordable and accessible; reduce promotion and accessibility of unhealthy food; restrict deceptive health claims	National Action Against Obesity, Rudd Center for Food Policy and Obesity, Public Health Advocacy Institute, Strategic Alliance, Campaign for a Commercial-Free Childhood; Center for Science in the Public Interest; Corporate Accountability International; International Obesity Task Force	Consistent in last few years
Pharmaceutical	Campaigns to lower prices of needed drugs, to set and enforce more effective pre-market testing and safety standards, to lower windfall profits, to restrict direct-to-consumer advertising and physician gifts	Make life saving drugs more available and affordable to individuals and countries that need them; restrict deceptive or misleading advertising; focus drug development on most serious public health threats; require drug companies to complete safety and efficacy tests before marketing a drug	Prescription Project, No Free Lunch, Health Research Group, PharmedOut, Doctors without Borders, Health Action International	Sporadic, especially after news on drug risks
Tobacco	Campaigns to ban public smoking, restrict market-ing to youth, raise taxes on tobacco, require tobacco industry to pay damages	Make tobacco less available and more expensive; end marketing to young people, close loopholes on sales and taxes, require industry to pay costs of tobacco-related illnesses	**Action on Smoking and Health, American Legacy Foundation, Campaign for Tobacco-Free Kids,** Network for Accountability of Tobacco Transnationals, Corporate Accountability International	Consistent

TABLE 16.3. Elements of a Common Agenda for Public Health Campaigns to Change Corporate Practices.

Principles or Policy Goals

Corporation 2020 Corporate Design Goals
1. The purpose of the corporation is to harness private interests to serve the public interest.
2. Corporations shall accrue fair returns for shareholders, but not at the expense of the legitimate interests of other stakeholders.
3. Corporations shall operate sustainably, meeting the needs of the present generation without compromising the ability of future generations to meet their needs.
4. Corporations shall distribute their wealth equitably among those who contribute to wealth creation.
5. Corporations shall be governed in a manner that is participatory, transparent, ethical, and accountable.
6. Corporations shall not infringe on the right of natural persons to govern themselves, nor infringe on other universal human rights.

Source: http://www.summit2020.org/CorporateDesign.pdf

Goals for Strategic Corporate Initiative of Corporate Ethics International
1. Separate corporations and the state
2. Change international trade rules
3. Elevate community rights
4. Protect the commons
5. Transform corporate purpose
6. Tame giant corporations
7. Redirect capital

Source: Corporate Ethics International, 2007.

Policy Agenda to Reduce Harm from Corporate Practices
1. Provide consumers with a right-to-know the health consequences of legal products and companies with a duty-to-disclose such information.
2. Protect children and other vulnerable populations against targeted marketing that promotes unhealthy behavior.
3. Level the political playing field. Meaningful campaign finance reform, higher ethical standards for elected officials, more stringent oversight of lobbying, and stronger voter rights will make it easier for public health advocates to gain electoral, legislative or legal support for health promoting policies and to encourage healthier corporate practices.
4. Increase sanctions for deliberate distortions of science designed to protect corporate interests.

Source: Freudenberg & Galea, 2008.

Corporate Accountability International Standards of Political Conduct for Corporations
1. Lobbying: Corporations must fully and publicly disclose all lobbying activities around the world, including through trade associations and public relations campaigns.
2. Political Contributions: Corporations must end financial contributions to political candidates, parties and referenda worldwide.
3. Political Access: Corporations must not trade favors with or buy access to local, national or international public officials.

TABLE 16.3. Continued

4. Safeguards: Corporations must follow the precautionary principle and must not interfere in the development or implementation of global, national or local policies affecting human rights, health or the environment. Corporations must also require their subsidiaries and suppliers to abide by such policies.

5. Independent Oversight: Corporations must respect the independent authority of and refrain from "partnering" with institutions that set standards affecting their business.

6. International Institutions and Agreements: Corporations must accept policies that protect people, human rights and the environment and must not use trade agreements or governing institutions (such as the World Trade Organization) to preempt such policies or use them for private gain.

7. Local Control: Corporations must honor local control over natural and financial resources.

Source: http://www.stopcorporateabuse.org/files/pdfs/Corporate%20Accountability%20 International%20Standards%20of%20Political%20Conduct%20for%20Corporations.pdf

How to Curb Corporate Power—Subordinating Corporations to People
Ralph Nader
1. Crack down on corporate crime
2. Rein in imperial CEOs
3. Shore up the civil justice system
4. Regulate in the public interest
5. Trust-busting in the new century: start with the media
6. Get corporations out of our elections
7. Reclaim the constitution

Source: Nader, 2005.

state" (Stevenson & Burke, 1992), calling into question whether these activities meet the usual definition of a movement.

Moreover, it appears that today's anticorporate movement – an amalgam of the global justice, human rights, labor, and other movements (Crossley, 2002) – has developed closer links with the environmental and human rights movements than with the public health community, perhaps because the former already have a more activist orientation. Possible exceptions to this generalization are the global work around tobacco control and AIDS care, where the anticorporate movement and public health campaigners work more closely together.

In summary, campaigns to change health-damaging corporate practices meet some but not all of the defining characteristics of a social movement. Rather than affix a binary label (movement vs. nonmovement) to this phenomenon, it may be more helpful to consider these activities on a continuum from episodic and fragmented campaigns on one end to a coherent social movement with a defined agenda at the other.

In his analysis of the global anticorporate struggle, Crossley (2002), borrowing from Bourdieu (1993), suggests the term "protest field," rather than movement, to better depict the heterogeneity and diversity that these mobilizations represent. Others have called the global justice mobilizations a "movement of movements," again emphasizing the disparate, sometimes conflicting elements (Cox & Nilsen, 2007). In this sense, the campaigns described in this chapter may be considered "a movement of campaigns" with the potential to become a more cohesive and integrated social movement at some future point. In the final section, I examine some of the ways that public health activists, researchers, and professionals and their organizations can contribute to public health campaigns and movements that seek to modify corporate practices that harm health.

Roles for Public Health, Advocates, and Researchers

A growing body of evidence described in other chapters in this volume and elsewhere (Nestle, 2002; Freudenberg & Galea, 2007; Brandt, 2007; Jahiel, 2008) demonstrates that corporate practices have become major social influences on patterns of health and disease. As modifiable determinants of health, these practices offer promising arenas for intervention for primary prevention. In this chapter, I have described how public health campaigns can serve as vehicles for modifying corporate practices that harm health. How then can the public health community contribute most effectively to the success of these campaigns?

Scientific Contributions

Public health researchers can contribute to more effective and successful campaigns to change health-damaging corporate practices in two important ways. First, they can help to create a body of evidence that demonstrates the specific pathways by which corporate decisions on marketing, product design, retail distribution, and pricing influence health. Using methods and concepts from epidemiology, sociology, economics, law, and other disciplines, researchers can illuminate the mechanisms by which corporate practices influence health; estimate the risks attributable to various industries, products, and practices; and thus create an evidence base to guide policy makers and advocates in selecting priorities and targets for action.

Several universities have already established centers that provide information and support to public health campaigns that seek to change corporate practices. These include the Rudd Center for Food Policy and Obesity at Yale University; the Harvard Injury Control Research Center, which studies, among other things, the role of the gun industry in violence; the Center on Alcohol Marketing and Youth at Georgetown University; the Public Health Advocacy Institute at Northeastern University; the Center for Tobacco Control Research and Education at University of California, San Francisco; Corporations and Health Watch at City University of New York and others.

Increasing evidence shows that the growing corporate sponsorship of research on the health effects of tobacco, food, pharmaceuticals, and other products leads to biased science that distorts policy (Krimsky, 2003; Baba et al., 2005; Lesser et al., 2007; Sismondo, 2008). This trend makes it particularly important that independent researchers not be beholden to corporate sponsors produce evidence that can counteract these biases.

Second, public health researchers can study public health campaigns as an object of interest, seeking to identify more precisely the factors associated with more and less successful campaigns. A growing number of researchers are now comparing activism across sectors and strategies (Nathanson, 1999; Parmet & Daynard, 2000; Bohme et al., 2005; Freudenberg et al., 2009; Yach et al., 2005; West, 2007). Among the questions that warrant further scrutiny are:

- What role can public health campaigns that seek to end racial/ethnic targeting of unhealthy products play in reducing socioeconomic and racial/ethnic disparities in health?
- How can developed world activists avoid pushing undesirable products and practices to the developing world, where protections are lower and adverse impact potentially higher?
- What are the comparative benefits and costs of campaigns that cooperate with corporations versus those that use adversarial strategies?

By providing the evidence that activists, public health professional, and public officials can use to guide their involvement in public heath campaigns and their selection of targets, strategies, and partners, researchers can contribute to more effective practice.

Educational Contributions

Public health workers can also contribute to the public and professional education that supports public health campaigns. With their credibility, communications skills, and connections to various media channels, public health workers can help to organize community educational forums, frame campaign messages (Dorfman et al., 2005b), testify on behalf of campaigns, and develop community leaders (Hennessey et al., 2005), all tasks that fit within the competencies and job description of many health professionals.

Within academic public health programs, faculty can help students to develop the competencies to analyze the corporate role in health and disease; plan, support, and evaluate public health campaigns; create partnerships with advocacy organizations; and advocate for policies that reduce harmful corporate practices (Freudenberg, 2005; Jahiel, 2008; Wiist, 2006). Universities can also convene researchers, advocates, policy makers, and, as appropriate business leaders, to meet, exchange information, and consider policy options.

Political Contributions

Ultimately, policy decisions about corporate practices are based on politics and power as well as science and evidence. Some public health researchers and professionals prefer to stop at the line that divides science from politics while others argue that this line is in the mind of the beholder. In addition, say these more activist-oriented researchers, the public health ethic requires them to follow their evidence to the point where it has an impact on population health, even if that brings them into the political arena.

In practice, by carrying out the previously described research and educational tasks, public health professionals make political contributions: enhanced credibility in policy circles; access to the media; and the scientific, intellectual, and human resources that universities can provide. By analyzing what they have to offer and what a particular health campaign needs at a particular time, public health professionals can decide how best to support these campaigns.

In closing, public health campaigns have the potential to modify corporate practices that in the past few decades have become a significant social determinant of health. Public health professionals can play key roles in such campaigns by documenting the impact of corporate practices on population health; providing advocates with evidence to make their case; educating policy makers, advocate, and citizens; joining and helping to organize coalitions; and evaluating the impact of changes in harmful practices. In sum, by making these campaigns an object of study and by contributing to their success, public health researchers, professionals, and advocates can better fulfill their role of promoting health and preventing disease.

REFERENCES

Ackland L. *Making a Real Killing: Rocky Flats and the Nuclear West* (Rev. ed.). Albuquerque, NM: University of New Mexico Press; 2002.

Baba A, Cook DM, McGarity TO, Bero LA. Legislating "sound science": the role of the tobacco industry. *Am J Public Health.* 2005;95(Suppl. 1):S20–S27.

Baby Milk Action. *Briefing Paper: History of the Campaign*. Retrieved January 15, 2009. Available at: http://www.babymilkaction.org/pages/history.html. No publication date listed.

Blum JD. Distributive justice and global health: a call for a global corporate tax. *Med Law*. 2007;26(2):203–212.

Bohme SR, Zorabedian J, Egilman DS. Maximizing profit and endangering health: corporate strategies to avoid litigation and regulation. *Int J Occup Environ Health*. 2005;11(4):338–348.

Borra S, Kris-Etherton PM, Dausch JG, Yin-Piazza S. An update of trans-fat reduction in the American diet. *J Am Diet Assoc*. 2007;107(12):2048–2050.

Bourdieu P. *"Some Properties of Fields," in Sociology in Question*. London: Sage; 1993.

Brandt AM. *The Cigarette Century: The Rise, Fall and Deadly Persistence of the Product That Defined America*. New York: Basic Books; 2007.

Brown P, Mayer B, Zavestoski S, Luebke T, Mandelbaum J, McCormick S. Clearing the air and breathing freely: the health politics of air pollution and asthma. *Int J Health Serv*. 2004;34(1):39–63.

Brulle RJ, Pellow DN. Environmental justice: human health and environmental inequalities. *Annu Rev Public Health*. 2006;27:103–124.

Bullard RD. (ed.). *Confronting Environmental Racism: Voices from the Grassroots*. Boston: South End Press; 1993.

Burros M. A suit seeks to bar Oreos as a health risk. *The New York Times*. p. F5; May 14;2003.

Center for Science in the Public Interest. *Anyone's Guess: The Need for Nutrition Labeling at Fast-Food and Other Chain Restaurants*. Retrieved January 15, 2009, Available at: http://www.cspinet.org/restaurantreport. Published 2003.

Center for Science in the Public Interest. Trans Fat On the Way Out. Available at: http://www.cspinet.org/transfat/index.html. Published 2008. Accessed September 12, 2009.

Clinton WJ. Speech given at: alliance for a Healthier Generation Schools Forum; August 7, 2008; Little Rock AR. Available at: http://www.clintonfoundation.org/news/news-media/speech-alliance-for-a-healthier-generation-healthy-schools-forum. Published 2008. Accessed January 15, 2009.

The Community Tool Box. *Changing Policies* (Chapter 25). Available at: http://ctb.ku.edu/en/tablecontents/chapter_1025.htm. Published 2009. Accessed January 15, 2009.

Cox L, Nilsen AG. Social movements research and the 'Movement of Movements': studying resistance to neoliberal globalisation. *Sociology Compass*. 2007;1/2:424–442.

Cray C. Corporate campaigns: are we asking enough? *Rachel's Democracy & Health News*. 2007;94:1–6.

Crossley N. Global anti-corporate struggle: a preliminary analysis. *Br J Sociol*. 2002;53(4):667–691.

Dorfman L, Wallack L, Woodruff K. More than a message: framing public health advocacy to change corporate practices. *Health Educ Behav*. 2005a;32(3):320–336.

Dorfman L, Wilbur P, Lingas EA, Woodruff K, Wallack L. *Accelerating Policy on Nutrition: Lessons from Tobacco, Alcohol, Firearms, and Traffic Safety*. Berkeley, CA: Berkeley Media Studies Group. Available at: http://www.bmsg.org/pdfs/BMSG_AccelerationReport.pdf. Published 2005b. Accessed January 15, 2009.

Edwards B, McCarthy JD. Resources and social movement mobilization. In Snow DA, Soule S, Kriesi H (eds.). *The Blackwell Companion to Social Movements* (pp. 116–152). Ames, IA: Blackwell; 2004.

Ervin K. July 3; Stop selling junk food in schools, group says. *The Seattle Times*, p. B1; 2002.

Food and Drug Administration (FDA), HHS. Food labeling: trans fatty acids in nutrition labeling, nutrient content claims, and health claims. Final rule. *Fed Regist*. 2003;68(133):41433–41506.

Freudenberg N. Public health advocacy to change corporate practices: implications for health education practice and research. *Health Educ Behav*. 2005;32(3):298–319.

Freudenberg N, Bradley SP, Serrano M. Public health campaigns to change industry practices that damage health: an analysis of 12 case studies. *Health Educ Behav*. 2009;36(2):230–249.

Freudenberg N, Galea, S. The impact of corporate practices on health: implications for health policy. *J Public Health Policy*. 2008;29(1):86–104.

Friedman S, Mottiar, S. A moral to the tale: the Treatment Action Campaign and the Politics of HIV/AIDS. Durban, South Africa: centre for Civil Society and the School of Development Studies, University of KwaZulu-Natal. Available at: http://www.ukzn.ac.za/ccs/files/Friedman%20Mottier%20TAC%20Research%20Report%20Short.pdf. Published 2004. Accessed January 15, 2009.

Garofoli J. February 12; $7 million for suit on trans fats, McDonald's to pay heart association. *San Francisco Chronicle*, p. A1; 2005.

Graves SB, Waddock S, Rehbein, K. Fad and fashion in shareholder activism: the landscape of shareholder resolutions. *Business and Society Review*. 2001;106(4):293–314.

Grier S, Bryant CA. Social marketing in public health. *Annu Rev Public Health*. 2005;26:319–339.

Guay T, Doh JP, Sinclair G. Non-governmental organizations, shareholder activism, and socially responsible investments: ethical, strategic, and governance implications. *J Bus Ethics*. 2004;52:125–139.

Hackbarth DP, Schnopp-Wyatt D, Katz D, Williams J, Silvestri B, Pfleger M. Collaborative research and action to control the geographic placement of outdoor advertising of alcohol and tobacco products in Chicago. *Public Health Rep*. 2001;116(6):558–567.

Hennessey Lavery S, Smith ML, Esparza AA, Hrushow A, Moore M, Reed DF. The community action model: a community-driven model designed to address disparities in health. *Am J Public Health*. 2005;95(4):611–616.

Hippert C. Multinational corporations, the politics of the world economy, and their effects on women's health in the developing world: a review. *Health Care Women Int*. 2002;23(8):861–869.

Jacobson MF. Statement on Partially Hydrogenated Oils and Trans Fat. May 18,2004. http://www.cspinet.org/new/pdf/michael_jacobson_trans_statement.pdf. Published 2004. Accessed September 12, 2009.

Jahiel RI. Corporation-induced diseases, upstream epidemiologic surveillance, and urban health. *J Urban Health*. 2008;85(4):517–531.

Jasso-Aguilar R, Waitzkin H, Landwehr A. Multinational corporations and health care in the United States and Latin America: strategies, actions, and effects. *J Health Soc Behav*. 2004;45(Suppl.):136–157.

John S, Thomson S. *New Activism and the Corporate Response*. New York: Palgrave; 2003.

Jones P, Comfort D, Hillier D. Anti-corporate retailer campaigns on the internet. *Int l Retail Distribution Management*. 2006;34(12):882–891.

Khann SR, Vajpeyi R, Assunta M. Consumer Protection and Tobacco—NGO Strategies for Combating Tobacco Proliferation in Developing Countries of Asia. Paper Presented at: the World Health Organization International Conference on Global Tobacco Control Law, January 7–9, 2000; New Delhi India. Available at: https://www.who.int/tobacco/media/en/KHANNA2000X.pdf. Published 2000. Accessed January 15, 2009.

Kingdon JW. *Agendas, Alternatives, and Public Policies*. Ann Arbor, MI: University of Michigan; 1984.

Krieger N, Löwy I, Aronowitz R, et al. Hormone replacement therapy, cancer, controversies, and women's health: historical, epidemiological, biological, clinical, and advocacy perspectives. *J Epidemiol Community Health*. 2005;59(9):740–748.

Krimsky S. *Science in the Private Interest: Has the Lure of Profits Corrupted Biomedical Research*. Lanham, MD: Rowman-Littlefield Publishing Co.; 2003.

Kristal AR, Goldenhar L, Muldoon J, Morton RF. Evaluation of a supermarket intervention to increase consumption of fruits and vegetables. *Am J Health Promot*. 1997;11(6):422–425.

Lesser LI, Ebbeling CB, Goozner M, Wypij D, Ludwig DS. Relationship between funding source and conclusion among nutrition-related scientific articles. *PLoS Med*. 2007;4(1):e5.

Levenstein C, Boden LI, Wegman DH. COSH: a grass-roots public health movement. *Am J Public Health*. 1984;74(9):964–965.

Lipschutz RD. Sweating it out: NGO campaigns and trade union empowerment. *Dev Pract*. 2004;14(1&2):197–209.

Lofland J. *Social Movement Organizations: Guide to Research on Insurgent Realities*. New York: Aldine de Gruyter; 1996.

Manheim JB. Corporate Campaigns Labor's Tactic of the "Death of A Thousand Cuts." *Capital Research Center Labor Watch, January*. 2002;1–7.

Mayer R. *The Consumer Movement: Guardians of the Marketplace*. Woodbridge, CT: Twayne; 1989.

Menashe CL, Siegel M. The power of a frame: an analysis of newspaper coverage of tobacco issues—United States, 1985–1996. *J Health Commun*. 1998;3(4):307–325.

Milewa T, de Leeuw E. Reason and protest in the new urban public health movement: an observation on the sociological analysis of political discourse in the 'healthy city'. *Br J Sociol.* 1996;47(4):657–670.

Minkler M, Wallerstein N. (eds.). *Community-Based Participatory Research for Health From Process to Outcomes.* San Francisco, CA, Jossey-Bass; 2008.

Minkler M, Breckwich Vásquez V, Chang C, Miller J. *Promoting Healthy Public Policy through Community-Based Participatory Research: Ten Case Studies.* Oakland, CA: PolicyLink; 2008.

Nader R. October 10; How to curb corporate power. *The Nation.* 2005;20–24.

Nathanson CA. Social movements as catalysts for policy change: the case of smoking and guns. *J Health Polit Policy Law.* 1999;24(3):421–488.

Navarro M. August 8; Tobacco companies find Harlem wary. *The New York Times.* Available at: http://query.nytimes.com/gst/fullpage.html?res=9C0CE3DD143D F93BA3575BC0A966958260&sec=&spon=&pagewanted=all#. Published 1990. Accessed January 15, 2009.

Nestle M. *Food Politics: How the Food Industry Influences Nutrition and Health.* Berkeley, CA: University of California Press; 2002.

Noar SM. A 10-year retrospective of research in health mass media campaigns: where do we go from here? *J Health Commun.* 2006;11(1):21–42.

Oliver TR. The politics of public health policy. *Annu Rev Public Health.* 2006;27:195–233.

Parmet WE, Daynard RA. The new public health litigation. *Annu Rev Public Health.* 2000;21:437–454.

People's Health Assembly. People's charter for health. *J Public Health Policy.* 2002;23(4):387–398.

Pertschuk M. *Smoke in Their Eyes: Lessons in Movement Leadership from the Tobacco Wars.* Nashville, TN: Vanderbilt University Press; 2001.

Powers S. May 19; The AIDS Rebel: letter from South Africa. *The New Yorker.* 2003;54.

Randolph W, Viswanath K. Lessons learned from public health mass media campaigns: marketing health in a crowded media world. *Annu Rev Public Health.* 2004;25:419–437.

Ritas C. *Speaking Truth, Creating Power: A Guide to Policy Work for Community-Based Participatory Research Practitioners.* Community-Campus Partnerships for Health. Available at: http://depts.washington.edu/ccph/pdf_files/ritas.pdf. Published 2003. Accessed January 15, 2009.

Robinson RG, Sutton CD. The coalition against Uptown cigarettes. In Wright PA, Jernigan D (eds.), *Making News, Changing Policy: Case Studies of Media Advocacy on Alcohol and Tobacco Issues* (pp. 89–108). Rockville, MD: Center for Substance Abuse Prevention; 1994.

Rothman DJ, Chimonas S. New developments in managing physician-industry relationships. *J Am Med Assoc.* 2008;300(9):1067–1069.

Schroeder SA. Tobacco control in the wake of the 1998 Master Settlement Agreement. *N Eng J Med.* 2004;350:293–301.

Sen R. *Stir It Up: Lessons in Community Organizing and Advocacy*. San Francisco: Jossey-Bass; 2003.

Severson K. July 2, 2003; Kraft promises to take healthier approach to food. *San Francisco Chronicle*, p. A1; 2003.

Sierra Club. June 2; Press Release: Sierra Club announces three-year campaign to pressure automakers to improve fuel economy. Available at: http://www.commondreams.org/news2002/0612–08.htm. Published 2002. Accessed January 15, 2009.

Sierra Club. July 11; *Ford's Mercury Mariner Hybrid: A Better Way to Build an SUV*. Available at: http://www.sierraclub.org/mercurymariner/. Published 2005. Accessed August 15, 2005.

Simon M. *Appetite for Profit: How the Food Industry Undermines Our Health and How to Fight Back*. New York: Nation Books; 2006.

Sismondo S. How pharmaceutical industry funding affects trial outcomes: causal structures and responses. *Soc Sci Med*. 2008;66(9):1909–1914.

Snow DA, Soule S, Kriesi H. (eds.). *The Blackwell Companion to Social Movements*. Ames, IA: Blackwell; 2004.

Stevenson HM, Burke M. Bureaucratic logic in new social movement clothing: the limits of health promotion research. *Can J Public Health*. 1992;83(Suppl. 1):S47–S53.

Sustainable Development Commission. *Green, Healthy and Fair: A Review of Government's Role in Supporting Sustainable Supermarket Food*. London, England. Available at: http://www.sd-commission.org.uk/publications/downloads/GreenHealthyAndFair.pdf. Published 2008. Accessed January 15, 2009.

Szreter S. Rethinking McKeown: the relationship between public health and social change. *Am J Public Health*. 2002;92(5):722–725.

Tilly C. *Social Movements, 1768–2004*. Boulder, CO: Paradigm Publishers; 2004.

Treatment Action Campaign. Summary of HIV Statistics for South Africa. Available at: http://www.tac.org.za/community/keystatistics. Published 2008. Accessed January 15, 2009.

Waitzkin H, Jasso-Aguilar R, Landwehr A, Mountain C. Global trade, public health, and health services: stakeholders' constructions of the key issues. *Soc Sci Med*. 2005;61(5):893–906.

Wallack L. The California Violence Prevention Initiative: advancing policy to ban Saturday night specials. *Health Educ Behav*. 1999;26(6):841–858.

Wallack L, Winett L, Nettekoven L. The Million Mom March: engaging the public on gun policy. *J Public Health Policy*. 2004;24(3–4):355–379.

Walsh EJ. *Democracy in the Shadows: Citizen Mobilization in the Wake of the Accident at Three Mile Island*. Westport, CT: Greenwood Press; 1988.

West R. What lessons can be learned from tobacco control for combating the growing prevalence of obesity? *Obes Rev*. 2007;8(Suppl. 1):145–150.

Wiist WH. Public health and the anticorporate movement: rationale and recommendations. *Am J Public Health*. 2006;96:1370–1375.

Yach D, McKee M, Lopez AD, Novotny T. Improving diet and physical activity: 12 lessons from controlling tobacco smoking. *BMJ*. 2005;330(7496):898–900.

17

Public Health Infrastructure: Toward a Blueprint for Change

René I. Jahiel

This chapter proposes an adaptation of the public health infrastructure (PHI) of the United States to deal more effectively with health hazards to consumers, workers, and community residents induced by corporations in their quest for profits. It is predicated on significant support from the federal government and from public opinion. After a brief discussion of the PHI and the reasons for modifying it, the chapter deals with proposed changes in the scope of PHI, its knowledge and information component, education of the workforce in the schools of public health, new roles for the workforce, and changes in the organizational component, and, finally with a discussion of feasibility.

The PHI helps the nation to: (1) monitor health status; (2) diagnose and investigate health problems and hazards; (3) inform, educate and empower people on health issues; (4) mobilize communities to solve health problems; (5) develop policies and plans to support individual and community health; (6) enforce laws and regulations to protect health and safety; (7) assure provision of health care; (8) Assure a competent health workforce; (9) evaluate public health services; and (10) conduct research to solve health problems (Institute of Medicine, 2002).

The PHI includes the public health's knowledge and information workforce, and organizational systems (Baker, 2005). It has been criticized for weaknesses in dealing with chronic diseases attributed to fragmented and precarious funding; uneven and antiquated legal foundation; inadequate workforce; inconsistent application of information technology; and organizational deficits (Baker, 2005), and defects in number, training, and credentialing of the workforce (Gebbie & Turnock, 2006; Tilson & Berkowitz, 2006).

There may be more fundamental reasons. One of them, which is at the core of this chapter, is that modern public health approaches to prevention are focused on personal risk factors and behavior change and not on broader social causes (Pearce, 1996). The growth of social epidemiology has done little to change that approach because it has dealt with social issues as risk factors for the individual (Putnam & Galea, 2008). The slow progress in prevention of diseases caused by tobacco, alcohol, or unhealthy foods that are the main real causes of mortality (Mokdad, 2004), and the marked increase in prevalence of obesity (Sturm, 2003) and diabetes (Seidel, 2000) are evidence that this approach is not working.

Research over the past two decades reviewed in other chapters of this volume show that public health efforts at prevention of chronic diseases are opposed by large social forces and that the driving engine of these social forces are corporations (Spitzer, 2005; Wiist, 2006). Following earlier studies (Markowitz & Rosner, 2003), a body of knowledge in the field of public health studies of corporations has been brought together since 2005 (Freudenberg, 2005; Bohme et al., 2005; Michaels & Monforton, 2005; Spitzer, 2005; Wiist, 2006; Jahiel & Babor, 2007; Galea & Freudenberg, 2007; Jahiel, 2008). An extensive list of corporate strategies to influence health policy and health has been drawn (Wiist, this volume). Conceptually, the field is ready to extend the scope and content of PHI so that the public health community may better engage corporations to protect the public's health. This is not a development that can be achieved with addition of one or two corporation related components to PHI because corporations permeate each of the ten essential public health programs cited at the beginning of this chapter. The needed changes in PHI involve its scope; its information, workforce and organizational components; and the development of new disciplinary approaches, job slots, and educational programs. I will present a blueprint for these changes before assessing their feasibility.

Changes in the Scope of PHI

In order to address corporate issues, PHI must reach to the five levels of the induction of health hazards by corporation shown in Table 17.1, each of which has its own environment, actors, and forces. The initiation level is where corporate decision making to launch or modify products or processes occurs.

TABLE 17.1. Sites of Public Health Action on the Corporate Infrastructure.

Level	Environment	Object of surveillance and intervention
1	Initiation	Corporate headquarters' strategies and actions about new or modified products
2	Intermediate	Actions of conduits of corporate strategies –marketeers and distributors –lawyers and public relations –lobbyists –advertisers –scientists
3	Exposure	Actions of retailers –inducements in the environment –behavior of persons at risk
4	Post-Embodiment	Corporate responsibility for harm
5	Clinical	Corporate health services

The intermediate level is where corporate conduits carry out these decisions to protect and promote the corporations' products or processes. The exposure level is where consumers, workers, or community residents are exposed to the disease agents present in corporation products or processes. The postembodiment level is where these agents interact with the body in a manner that may produce disease. The clinical level involves another set of corporations, those that provide health services and goods for treatment or rehabilitation.

Knowledge and Information Component of the PHI

Wiist (2006) has analyzed the significance of corporations for public health. The PHI must deal with two issues that it has not been concerned with in the past. First, the only function of corporations is profit and growth. Second, corporations are part of a complex social system at the core of the economic activity of the nation, a fact that has two consequences: (1) a considerable body of knowledge must be mastered to understand the various relationships of corporations to the social system; and (2) the central position of corporations in the social system, along with their large size and wealth, certain legal protections, and positive feedbacks with governments, gives them considerable power for the defense of their economic interests.

Information is needed at the five levels shown in Table 17.1. At the initiation level, information about new products and production or marketing processes planned by the corporation is needed to conduct investigation of their health hazards before they have reached the public; and information about corporate efforts to influence governmental policies in matters such as regulation of permissible disease burden of these products or processes is needed to guide public health advocacy. At the intermediate level, information about corporate activities undertaken by the conduits for marketing, advertising, scientific disinformation, public relations, legal actions, and lobbying is needed for public health interventions targeting each of these activities. At the exposure level, information on strategies used to promote exposure of the public to corporation products or processes is needed to support intervention in the proximal environment of the public (such as price and taxation of products, control of physical access to products, or control of work environment). At the postembodiment level, information about the effects of the corporate products on the health of the public and the expenses incurred thereof by the State is needed to help respectively in class action suits and state attorney general law suits.

Education in the Schools of Public Health

The call made by Wiist (2006) to educate public health workers about the dangers to the public's health posed by corporations has been followed by discussions of the content of such education at meetings of the Industrial Diseases Study Group by Jahiel in Boston in 2006 and Freudenberg in Washington in 2007, and by a commentary at the Corporations and Health web site (Freudenberg, 2008), and the introduction of material on corporations in graduate public health courses by Jahiel at the University of Connecticut Health Center in Fall 2008 and Wiist at the University of Chile in January 2009, and the planning of such courses by Freudenberg and Markowitz at the City University of New York in Fall 2009, by Malone at University of California San Francisco in 2010 (personal communications from the teachers). Interest on education about corporations has focused on the schools of public health, because of their leading current position in public health, although eventually it should extend to all the educational institutions whose training is relevant to public health, particularly since their students are much more numerous than those in schools of public health and are usually in more direct contacts with members of the public. Thus, the following deals with only one of several educational components of PHI.

SPECIAL COURSE ON CORPORATIONS AND HEALTH. A special course on corporations and health would include the context of corporations in the contemporary social structure, their history, their growth in number and in size, their mergers, and their transnational impact; general knowledge of the nature of the corporate entity; measures of its activities and trends thereof; its relationships to domestic and international markets and trade, to public entities, and to laws and regulation of its activities and their implementation; and of various anticorporate movements (Wiist, 2006).

CORE CURRICULUM. The core curriculum taken by all public health students consists of five subjects: biostatistics; epidemiology; environmental science; social and behavioral sciences; and health policy and management. The reader is referred to a detailed listing of topics by Freudenberg (2008). In this section, I have highlighted certain general objectives.

Statistics. Health statistics are usually given as prevalence of diagnoses and their associated mortality. Students should also learn mortality and morbidity statistics based on the "true causes of death", such as tobacco, alcohol, obesity, unhealthy food (Mokdad et al, 2004), and, along the same lines true occupational and environmental causes of death due to specific agents in these environments. Furthermore, statistics on corporations that produce and promote such agents should be taught, including corporate profits, stock prices, bonuses and salaries of executives, ratio of executive to worker salaries, tax rates, amount spent on marketing, advertising and lobbying, and amount and type of political contributions (Wiist, 2006).

The course in statistics is the optimal place to teach the precautionary principle of public health (PPPH). Students are often taught to make judgments according to stringent criteria. However, the course in statistics educates them in notions of probability. The PPPH means that action should be taken even at lower levels of probability, depending upon the damage that would result from taking no action (Goldstein, 2001; Kriebel & Tickner, 2001; Martuzzi & Bertollini, 2004). The PPPH is particularly relevant for corporation-induced diseases, because corporations have repeatedly attempted to throw doubt on the weight of the scientific evidence by calls for more stringent criteria and additional studies that would delay intervention (Michaels & Monforton, 2005).

Epidemiology. Teaching of causal criteria to assess the role of an agent in causation of a disease (Rothman & Greenland, 1998) should be complemented by discussions of causal chains that lead from corporate decision making to actual embodiment of people with the agents present in corporate products. This should also include exposure of students to contemporary research to elucidate these causal chains and develop epidemiologic surveillance of corporations (Jahiel, 2008), and to assess the relative risk that is attributed to the individual and to the corporation.

Environmental Science Teaching should include comparison of toxicity thresholds of corporate products in the occupational or community environment enacted by different organizations or in different countries (Egilman & Bohme, 2005); issues of corporate justice as illustrated in studies of the hog industry (Wing, 1998; Okun, 1999; Wing et al., 2008), issues of duration of pollution of the environment (Litt et al., 2002), and issues of corporate social responsibility for sustainable environments (Mathur et al., 2005).

Social and behavioral sciences. The students should be informed of current research on models of corporate production of disease that present the corporation as a vector that carries a toxic agent (Sweanor, 1999; Le Gresley, 1999; Guardino & Daynard, 2007), as part of a vertically organized social system of production, marketing, retail distribution, and pricing, each of which may be harmful to health (Freudenberg & Galea, 2007), or as part of an integrated social network that may include government, consumer organizations, and various other firms (Freudenberg, 2005; Jahiel, 2008). Education should include an analysis of the methods corporations are using to promote their products or escape regulation (Wiist, this volume) Students should also be instructed on the roles of corporations in our society and on various modifications of or alternatives to the corporate structure and their expected feasibility in different political situations.

Health policy and management. The students should be informed about the various federal and state/local laws and regulations that deal with harmful corporate products or processes and with assessments of their relative efficacy and effectiveness (Babor et al., 2003). Information the courts' positions on corporate and public health objectives would include information on the canons of judicial decision making used by the courts (Daynard, 2002). Students should be taught about the anticorporate movement (Wiist, 2006) and successful local movements (Freudenberg et al., 2007), and about planning, coalition formation, and framing of information (Siegel & Doner, 2004). The management component of the course should educate students on the management tools used by corporations to promote their products, and on the management of public health advocacy and other interventions to protect the public.

ELECTIVE CURRICULUM, RESEARCH, AND INTERNSHIPS. In addition to core curriculum courses, corporation relevant material should be included in various electives. In Fall 2008, I gave a course on Chronic Disease Control to students in a graduate public health program with half of the material on corporations (two-thirds of that on industrial corporations as sources of agents of chronic diseases and one third on health services corporations); the course was well received: twice as many students registered for it as compared to previous years; and comments at the end of the course were favorable. Copies of the syllabus are available upon request.

Wiist (personal communication) gave a course on Economic Globalization and Health in January 2009 at the University of Chile where three out of seven topics were on corporations, with reference to their effects on health and health policy; it included sections on the history, purpose, and operations of for-profit corporations and on strategies for reforming corporations.

Freudenberg (2008) lists a number of subjects as electives relevant to corporations and health: "globalization and health; tobacco, alcohol and food industries; interdisciplinary perspectives on roles of government and corporations in health; public health strategies to modify corporate practices; and history of corporations and public health." He also suggested that students develop research projects on corporation and health and complete internships in research or advocacy organizations dealing with a corporate product such as tobacco.

The instruction of the public health workforce in existing and emerging knowledge about corporations and public health is essential to provide them with a framework that changes their conception of public health by demonstrating the pervasive influence of corporations on all phases of the health system, and to make them better allies of community advocates or state government officials who are engaged in legal or administrative actions to protect the public from corporation-induced harm or to recuperate State expenditures caused by such harm. However, it does not provide them with specific tools to help change the system in favor of the public's health. The following sections sketch five types of tools, some of which were once prominent in public health practice, but have atrophied and must be extensively reconstructed, while others are relatively new to public health. Each contributes to new formulation of a workforce specialty.

Design of and Education for New Public Health Workforce Specialties

LABORATORY. Public health laboratories, once the mainstay of public health, have markedly decreased numbers, staffing, and programs. As an indicator of this change, the laboratory section, once one of the largest in American Public Health Association (APHA), it is now reduced in status to a special program interest group or SPIG, because the number of its members is less than that required for a section. Yet, most state public health departments still have laboratories with an active organization the Association of Public Health Laboratories (APHL), and there are several laboratory facilities in federal institutions both of which may serve as nuclei to reconstruct a strong public health laboratory system. I give an example of what might have been accomplished with a laboratory that provides an independent assessment of corporate products, in the instance of addiction to nicotine in cigarettes. David Kessler describes the extensive cat and mouse game that he had to conduct for several years to obtain evidence of the addictive power of nicotine despite denials of by tobacco executives. Using information from whistle blowers, field investigations of domestic production, investigation of markets abroad, uncovering of a suppressed publication of experimental work demonstrating addictive properties, and painstaking reconstruction of the processes used by tobacco companies to prepare cigarettes with more addictive power, over a period of several years of work by dozens of workers from his agency, he built a case that forced tobacco company executives to admit that nicotine is addictive and that they enhanced the nicotine availability in cigarettes (Kessler, 2003). That information might have been obtained in a shorter time if the following requirements had been met: (1) the tobacco companies would have given an independent agency the information needed to replicate the preparation of cigarettes with tobacco and enhanced tobacco; (2) that agency would have a laboratory to (a) investigate the addictive properties of these preparations in laboratory animals; and (b) do human experimentation to investigate the addictive properties of cigarettes and cigarettes prepared with enhanced tobacco.

In general, I propose to establish laboratories in agencies that are independent from corporate funding, either in the federal government or as a self-standing agency. Such agencies would carry out laboratory studies on new or newly modified products submitted by corporations with all the information needed. An administrative mechanism would be developed to protect the confidentiality of that information. A similar mechanism has existed for years at the U.S. patent office. The laboratory would perform studies of (a) acute and chronic toxicity in animals; (b) acute and short-term chronic toxicity in human subjects; (c) in lieu of long-term (i.e., years or decade) chronic toxicity in human subjects, studies with indicators of such long-term processes, such as transformation of human cells in culture, tests for nucleic acid adducts in human chromosomes, or other approaches; while these indicators do not provide stringent evidence of chronic hazards, they provide enough probability of such to trigger the precautionary principle of public health.

Education for a concentration on the public health laboratory may initially require schools of public health to make cooperative educational undertaking with Science Departments of Graduate Schools, with Programs for laboratory education in technical colleges. Eventually, the schools of public health would have to establish their own departments of public health laboratory instruction.

EPIDEMIOLOGIC SURVEILLANCE. Epidemiologic surveillance is well developed at the Center for Disease Control and Prevention (CDC) and state laboratories, but it is usually limited to surveillance in the postembodiment environment and to some extent in the exposure environments of Table 17.1. A framework for epidemiologic surveillance in the four relevant environments has been presented (Jahiel, 2008). Epidemiologic surveillance of the initiation environment would be carried out with information on the corporation that would communicate to the government on its plans for new of modified products, or that would be derived from trade sources of information. It would be supplemented by appropriate laboratory studies as described in the preceding section. Epidemiologic surveillance of the intermediate environment involves surveillance of the conduits used by corporations to modify the environment of exposure. This includes surveillance of distributors to learn about the markets targeted by the companies; advertisements to learn about the framing used to promote use of the products; the scientific reports issued by the corporations to learn about the doubt that may be communicated to the public about scientific information on health hazards of the products; and the lobbying activities of the companies to learn about the companies' attempts to influence health policy. Education for a concentration in epidemiological surveillance would be conducted in the schools' epidemiology departments.

PUBLIC HEALTH ENGINEERING. Public health engineering to prevent water, food, and air transmission of disease was once a major branch of public health. The new public health engineers would deal with corporation-induced diseases and they have to know (1) the characteristics of the corporations, products, and manufacturing processes including their production costs as well as biological properties, and of those of alternative products that might be substituted with less toxic effects and (2) the marketing of the products and related features of corporations' interests and the potential assets and limitations in marketing alternative products.

For instance, formaldehyde vapors are a frequent contaminant of plastic products, and they have been tightly regulated in some countries such as Denmark (Mathur et al., 2005). The public health engineer would work with the surveillance specialists to study the markets for the product, and with the public health laboratory researchers to assess the role of formaldehyde in production and develop alternative formulations that result in a less toxic product without formaldehyde. Having done this, the public health engineers would assess these alternatives from the viewpoints of cost of preparation and quality, the barriers to change that may be present in marketing of the alternative, and they would develop ways to overcome these barriers. Depending upon the manner it is presented and the reaction of the company, this approach might lead to a confrontation between the company and public health, or to a mutually satisfactory relationship that would pave the way for the adoption of the less toxic material by the company.

The public health engineering concentration would develop a curriculum together with schools of engineering based on aspects of engineering appropriate to the prevention and management of corporation-induced diseases. A solid foundation would be given in physics, chemistry and chemical engineering, and economics, as well as in general aspects of system design and systems analysis. A special course would be given on the biochemistry, manufacturing, and marketing of food products, and on systemic aspects of substitution of less harmful products. Another special course would be given on design of transportation systems including automobiles, buses, trains to assess the harm associated with current transportation, and systems analysis of changes to less harmful transportation patterns. Another course would concern the pharmaceutical industry; it would deal with the efficacy, cost-effectiveness and cost-benefits of alternative medications, and other forms of treatment that do not employ medications. Another course would cover the alcoholic beverage industry, including the manufacturing and marketing of alcoholic beverages, and analysis of the harmful and beneficial aspects of these beverages; and social system analysis of alcoholic beverages. Each of these courses would also provide analysis and information on the economics of manufacturing, research, marketing and advertising by the industrial companies, and the distribution of gains to shareholders, other owners, executives, the state through taxation, and research and development. The general aim of these courses would be to provide knowledge that could be utilized to provide less harmful alternatives at lower costs to society.

Public health engineering departments would be involved in the integration of responses to different products. Public health engineers could be located in state public health departments to work on problems posed by large companies in the area, or with central research institutes especially organized for that purpose, or with agencies of the federal government.

POLICY DEVELOPMENT. The concentration on policy development would include an intensive course on corporations, such as the one proposed by Wiist (2006). Further training would include economics of industrial corporations;

communications about corporation products; corporation politics at the federal and local levels; advocacy, coalition formation, and action planning.

The course on economics would include (a) elements of accounting to be able to analyze the corporations' balance sheets; (b) intake–output analyses to analyze the flow of capital and resources through the system depicted in Table 17.1 that extends from the corporation to its retailers; (c) measures of social benefits/social harm ratio of corporate products; (d) cost analyses of the corporation's return to the state including the taxes received by the state on the one hand and the cost to the state's Medicaid and other divisions of services and goods paid by the state for the care of people harmed by the corporation's products; (e) transnational economic studies of corporate activities, including the cost of labor abroad, the cost of harm to environment, tariffs, and economic agreements; and (f) analysis of corporation profits and of executive pay scale and bonuses.

The course on communications would include (a) a study of the system of overt and covert communications between the corporations and their various associates and conduits (b) analysis of the framing of messages by corporations, including not only advertising, but also messages to policy makers, to the media, to scientific groups, and to law courts.

The course on corporation policies would include empirical studies of corporations in the food, tobacco, alcohol, care, and pharmaceutical sectors (as discussed in earlier chapters of this book) and syntheses to show the features common to corporations in these different sectors and to develop countervailing policy approaches.

SPECIALTY IN ADVOCACY STRATEGIES. The functions of this specialist would be to corral all the information that is available for the other specialists and develop strategies to offset the health hazards posed by the corporations at all the levels of Table 17.1. This specialist would have received training in coalition formation and action planning would include approaches that have been validated in public health marketing (Siegel & Doner, 2004) and case studies of community actions (Freudenberg, 2008).

Organizational Component

The federal government would provide the main initial site for the reorganization of this component, for three reasons. First, it comprises most of the agencies that have the basic knowledge and trained workers that could be modified to include the new knowledge, objectives, and trained workforce without having to recreate or markedly change an organizational component. Second, the reorganization under consideration could not take place unless it was backed by a federal government that is strongly on the side of the people to protect it from the toxic burden of the corporations' products. It appears that we are now in a period of change in the federal government's attitude toward corporations that might lead to significant opposition to the excesses of corporate profits. Third, an effort conducted by one or a few states is likely not to be followed for many years by other states, thus creating an inequality among states. However, grassroots organizations, including community coalitions organized on health issues, professional people and organizations, advocacy groups, and local public health agencies are an essential part of the PHI's organizational component because: (1) they have a better understanding of the local problems to be solved and barriers to the solutions; (2) their enthusiasm and commitment may be an important and needed support to the PHI; and (3) it is to such grassroots that the federal component of PHI is accountable.

Therefore, the following blueprint involves both federal and grassroot levels.

The main federal agencies that would be redesigned to carry out the reorganization of the PHI would be the CDC, its National Institute of Occupational Safety and Health (NIOSH) and National Institute of Health Statistics (NIHS) components, the National institutes of Health (NIH), the National Science Foundation (NSF), the Environmental Protection Agency (EPA), and the Food and Drug Administration (FDA). The subsequent development of job slots for the new public health workers would be organized in the Departments of Health and Human Services, Labor, and the Interior.

LABORATORY COMPONENT. The basic knowledge to design the laboratory system would be developed jointly by the NIH and the CDC. The laboratories would be attached to the federal public health agencies, the state departments of health, or the local school of public health. Its financing would be separate from that of other departments of the institutions to assure stability. Performance of the system would be evaluated by a special committee of the Institute of Medicine (IOM).

SURVEILLANCE COMPONENT. The surveillance component would be developed by the CDC with considerable input from the NSF or NSF sponsored commissions for the development of surveillance of the corporate decision-making process (initiation level). The Congressional Research Office and appropriate Executive branch departments might also provide input regarding the laws and regulations that govern the conduits in the intermediate environment. The CDC would have to add expertise in social and business sciences to its expertise in surveillance. The NIOSH and EPA would be involved in this program with regard to occupational and general environments.

PUBLIC HEALTH ENGINEERS. The public health engineering component would be developed in think tanks and universities with strong communication connections with the federal agencies. The reason for this choice is that the universities would have ready access to colleagues in schools of engineering and other schools trained in environmental engineering and in systems engineering; and to colleagues in schools of business that have training in marketing and other aspects of the public health engineering program. The development of research and subsequent curriculum development programs would be supported by grants from the federal government, with peer review by committees drawn from public health, engineering, and business, and representation of corporations and of anticorporate movement advocates. It would be important to make sure that corporate funding of university research, partnership, or facilities does not influence the committees. The schools and think tanks will participate in communication with the appropriate departments of the CDC, EPA, and NIH to coordinate diffusion of information about the program. It would be evaluated by a joint committee of the IOM and National Institute of Engineering.

POLICY DEVELOPMENT COMPONENT. The development of the public policy component will take place primarily in schools of public health with the help of federal grant programs to support hiring of new faculty members with the appropriate expertise in political science and political economics, and some ethnographers. This part of the program will also include a large input from community organizations, anticorporate advocates, and other representatives of the people, with representation as great as that of the academics. In order to keep the focus on public health, integration of the universities' programs should take place under the aegis of the Department of Health and Human Services, in collaboration with the Association of Schools of Public Health.

STRATEGY COMPONENT. This component has a specific function to help support various alternative approaches: confrontation between corporation and government or community, and cooperative endeavor between corporation and government or community. It would include experts in community organization, political science and community and government representatives, and it would work in association with the other four components. Its initial work would be performed in schools of public health or community organizations. Coordination among different sites would be performed by bottom-up commissions with representatives from the local work groups.

THE DEVELOPMENT OF JOB SLOTS Even before the guidelines and standards for the various activities described above are completed, the Department of Labor, working closely with the Departments of Health and Human Services and the Bureau of the Census, will develop plans to determine the size of the labor force needed in general and in various sites; to assess the availability of trained and trainable workers for these jobs; to develop cost-effectiveness and cost-benefits estimates of the inclusion of the various workers in federal and local public health agencies; and to make recommendations for federal grants for training and for grants to states and localities, tax or other incentives for the public and private jobs slots respectively.

Feasibility and Scenarios

The proposed program would prepare the public health infrastructure to defend the public's health against harm produced by corporations. But, is it feasible? The public health infrastructure would have to compete with the corporate infrastructure. Can the public health infrastructure and its allies develop enough countervailing power to match the corporations? The three factors that might support such countervailing power are a public convinced of the program's importance; a government that actively supports it; and a public health workforce mobilized to realize the program. Until recently, it was very unlikely that these three requirements could be met. However, the recent events in banking and Wall Street have made people much less confident in the judgment and good intentions of corporations and more aware of the harm they can inflicted to the nation. In this context, the public might be much more receptive to the concept that it is corporations, and not people's health behavior, that is the main culprit in the chronic disease epidemic, and it might be ready to do something about it. The stance of the new federal executive and legislative branches of government toward the corporate establishment is still uncertain. The public health community has yet to take a clear stand against corporation-induced harm to health; however, a well conducted information and motivation campaign might help to mobilize it for the program. Thus, the proposed program is not impossible a priori, and, therefore, it is appropriate to develop a strategy to implement it, so that the public health community is ready when the time comes for action.

Action may come as confrontation, where the government takes steps to limit corporate actions that result in harm, and as evolution, where the nature of the corporate entity is changed to give health concerns priority over financial ones. The two approaches are not mutually exclusive.

Several scenarios may be considered. The first is a predominantly court action oriented scenario. The history of past successes such as those against tobacco and asbestos, shows that the public health community may set the stage, for instance with surgeon general's reports, but that effective action came from class action suits or suits by the States that made the continued production of harmful products so onerous that the companies would become bankrupt, as Manville in the instance of asbestos (Delaney, 1998), or limit some of their activities, as the tobacco companies after the suit by the States' attorneys generals. A public health infrastructure reorganized as proposed in this chapter could help local or national coalitions in several ways: First, it would provide them with the services of a workforce with expertise on corporations; and its components would help in gathering evidence and developing strategies.

An alternative scenario is conceivable if the executive and legislative branches of the federal government lead the initiative to limit corporate harm. Such initiative may occur if corporation-induced chronic diseases increase to the point that the public demand action from the government, or, if it is included as part of a more general governmental action to limit corporation-induced harm to the economy, the middle and lower classes, and the health of the nation. In such eventualities, the federal government would take the initiative by reorganizing the federal public health agencies, possibly along the lines suggested in this chapter; by providing grants to schools of public health for curriculum and specialty developments such as the ones presented in this chapter; and by helping to create job slots for graduates of such programs through grants to the States and tax relief to private organizations. Funding from these programs might come from general revenue, from taxes on products that carry a disease burden, from a special levy on corporate entities that make such products.

An third scenario might develop if corporations that make products or with significant disease burden find themselves under such attacks that they welcome help from public health workforce, in order to survive. This scenario could have two versions: in one version, components of the corporations would be taken over by the government, in a situation analogous to current governmental intervention with financial corporation; in the other, corporations would support the financing of the services of the public health workforce; in this instance, co-optation by the financial interests of the corporations should be guarded against with adequate governmental regulation.

Finally, another scenario involves a sea change in the attitude of the nation toward money making, reversing the lionization of greed since 1980. This would be a general cultural change, rather than a political one. Such changes are difficult to predict. When they occur, they may diffuse rapidly through society. Again, two versions of this scenario are possible. In one version, the corporate structure would remain, but its culture would change to put less emphasis on the bottom line and more on health effects; however, such changes would be limited because of the very structural factors in corporations that promote the quest for profit. In the other version, the very concept of corporation would come under attack and alternative structures would be developed. Changes such as the ones suggested under the various scenarios develop at certain times in history with great rapidity. Forces that push toward one scenario or another may already be at work in the nation. It is important that the public health community does not find itself bypassed by the events, and that it is ready when the time comes with a blueprint for a reorganized public health infrastructure.

Conclusions

The proposed changes in the PHI would have seemed unrealistic only a few years ago, but that assessment must be reconsidered in view of changing attitudes toward corporations. The central element of the proposed program is the public health engineering component through which public health will directly engage corporations in addressing the health hazards of their products. It will be supported by four other elements (laboratory, corporate surveillance, policy, and strategy) and by general education of the public health workforce about corporations and health. The implementation of the program may lead to confrontations between government or community and corporations, or it may lead to cooperative endeavors, depending upon the pressures on corporations that exist at the time and the changes in the nature of corporations that might develop as a result. It is important that public health is not left behind when such time occurs and that it starts preparing now.

REFERENCES

Babor TF, Caetano R, Casswell S, et al. *Alcohol: No Ordinary Commodity*. New York: Oxford University Press; 2003.
Baker EL Jr, Potter MA, Jones DL, et al. The public health infrastructure and our nation's health. *Annu Rev Public Health*. 2005;26:303–318.
Bohme SE, Zorbedian G, Egilman DS. Maximizing profit and endangering health: corporate strategies to avoid litigation and regulation. *Int J Occup Environ Health*. 2005;11:338–348.

Daynard R. Regulating tobacco: the need for a public health judicial decision making canon. *J Law Med Ethics.* 2002;30:281–289.

Delaney KJ. *Strategic Bankruptcy:How Corporations and Creditors Use Chapter 11 to Their Advantage.* (Chapter 3: The Manville corporation: solving asbestos liability through bankruptcy). Berkeley: University of California Press; 1998.

Egilman DS, Bohme SE. Over a barrel: corporate corruption of science and its effect on workers and the environment. *Int J Occup Environ Health.* 2005;11(4):331–337.

Freudenberg N. Public health advocacy to change corporate practices: implications for health education practice and research. *Health Educ Behav.* 2005;32(3):298–319.

Freudenberg N. Commentary: teaching about corporations and health: bringing corporate practices into public health classrooms. Available at: http://www.corporationsandhealth.org/teaching_corp_and_health.php. Published 2008.

Freudenberg N, Bradley SPO, Serrano M. Public health campaigns to change industry practices that damage health: an analysis of 12 case studies. *Health Educ Behav.* 2007;36(2):230–249 (Epub ahead of print 2007).

Freudenberg N, Galea S. Corporate practices. In Galea S (ed.), *Macrosocial Determinants of Population Health.* New York: Springer; 2007.

Gebbie KM, Turnock BJ. The public health work force 2006: new challenges. *Health Aff.* 2006;25(4):923–933.

Goldstein BD. The precautionary principle also applies to public health actions. *Am J Pub Health.* 2001;91(9):1358–1361.

Guardino SD, Daynard R. Tobacco industry lawyers as disease vectors. *Tob Control.* 2007;16:224–228.

Institute of Medicine. *The Future of Public Health in the 21st Century.* Washington, DC: National Academy Press; 2002.

Jahiel RI. Corporation induced diseases, upstream epidemiologic surveillance, and urban health. *J Urban Health.* 2008;85(4):517–531.

Jahiel RI, Babor TF. Industrial epidemics, public health advocacy, and the alcohol industry: lessons from other fields. *Addiction.* 2007;102:1335–1339.

Kessler D. *A Question of Intent. A Great American Battle with a Deadly Industry.* New York: Public Affairs (Perseus books); 2003.

Kriebel D, Tickner J. Reenergizing public health through precaution. *Am J Pub Health.* 2001;91(9):13512–1355.

Le Gresley EA. 'Vector analysis' of the tobacco epidemic. Bulletin von Medicus Mundi Schweiz. Available at: http://www.medicusmundi.ch/mms/services/bulletin/bulletin199901/kap01/03legresley.html. Published 1999;(1):72.

Litt JS, Tran NL, Burke TA. Examining urban brownfields through the public health 'macroscope'. *Environ Health Perspect.* 2002;110(suppl. 2):183–193.

Markowitz G, Rosner D. *Denial and Deceit. The Deadly Politics of Industrial Pollution.* Berkeley: University of California Press; 2003.

Martuzzi M, Bertollini R. The precautionary principle: science and human health protection. *Int J Occup Environ Health.* 2004;17(1):43–46.

Mathur SK, Hackner CS, Aday LA. Sustainable environment. In: Aday LA (ed.),
    Reinventing Public Health: Policies and Practices for a Healthy Nation (pp. 65–105).
    San Francisco: Jossey Bass, 2005.

Michaels D, Monforton C. Manufacturing uncertainty: contested science and the
    protection of the public's health and of the environment. *Am J Pub Health.*
    2005;95(S1):S38–S48.

Mokdad AH, Marks JS, Stroup DF, Gerberding JL. Actual causes of death in the
    United States, 2000. *JAMA.* 2004;291:1238–1245.

Okun M. Human health issues associated with the hog industry. 32 pp. available at
    University of North Carolina-Chapel Hill Environmental Resource Program,
    Chapel Hill, NC; 1999.

Pearce N. Traditional epidemiology, modern epidemiology, and public health.
    Am J Pub Health. 1996;86:678–688.

Putnam S, Galea S. Epidemiology and the macrosocial determinants of health.
    J Public Health Policy. 2008;29:275–289.

Rothman KJ, Greenland S. *Modern Epidemiology,* 2nd ed. (pp. 6–28). Philadelphia,
    PA: Lippincott-Raven; 1998.

Seidel JC. Obesity, insulin resistance, and diabetes: a worldwide epidemic. *Br J Nutr.*
    2000;83(Suppl.1):55–58.

Siegel M, Doner L. *Marketing Public Health: Strategies to Promote Social Change.*
    Sudbury, MA: Jones & Bartlett; 2004.

Spitzer S. A systemic approach to occupational and environmental health.
    Int J Occup Environ Health. 2005;11:444–455.

Sturm R. Increase in clinically severe obesity in the United States 1986–2000.
    Arch Int Med. 2003;163:2146–2148.

Sweanor D. Why tobacco companies proceed as they do. Presented at INGCAT
    Meeting. Geneva, Switzerland. Available at: http://www.islamset.com/
    healthnews/smoking/INGCAT/David_Sweanor. html. Published 1999. Accessed
    May 15–16, 1999.

Tilson H, Markowitz B. The public health enterpriseÙ: Examining out twenty-first-
    century policy challenges. *Health Affairs.* 2006;25(4):900–910.

Wiist WH. Public health and the anticorporate movement: rationale and
    recommendations. *Am J Pub Health.* 2006;96(8):1370–1375.

Wing S. Whose epidemiology, whose health? *Int J Qual Health Care.*
    1998;28(2):241–152.

Wing S, Horton RA, Muhammad N, et al. Integrating epidemiology, education, and
    organizing for environmental justice: community health effects of industrial hog
    operations. *Am J Pub Health.* 2008;98(8):1390–1397.

18

Indigenous Peoples' Movements

Raymundo D. Rovillos

Social movements are generally defined as "the collective efforts by socially and politically subordinate people to challenge the conditions and assumptions of their lives... (These are) persistent, patterned, and widely distributed collective challenges to the status quo."[1] Usually differentiated from political parties, corporate interest groups or guerrilla movements, social movements "generally seek to reshape state policy rather than hold state power."[2]

The indigenous peoples' movements discussed in this book suggest that indigenous movements differ from other social movements in their goals, political orientation and forms of mobilization and political action. Their most distinctive characteristic is the centrality of ethnic identity as a mobilizing factor. The indigenous peoples' call for "putting history before us, and not behind us" is an explicit appeal to collective experience and memory as the basis of collective identity, consciousness and action. Thus history is revisited, ritual and other forms of identity markers are used as symbols, and cultural practices are politicized.

Identity as a mobilizing category is not devoid of any materiality. Indeed, "ethnicity cannot be politicized unless an underlying core of

Reprinted with permission from Victoria Tauli-Corpuz & Joji Cariño (Eds) (2004). *RECLAIMING BALANCE: Indigenous Peoples, Conflict Resolution & Sustainable Development.* Copyright © TEBTEBBA FOUNDATION, 2004 memories, experience, or meaning moves people to collective action."[3] Most of the indigenous authors in this book narrate their common histories of displacement from their ancestral lands, domains or territories. For indigenous peoples, land is inextricably linked with their identity. "Land is life" because it sustains the economic and cultural activities of indigenous peoples. Land is thus the space and source of cultural reproduction: territory is identity.

Indigenous movements are fairly recent phenomena. During the first half of the 20th century, indigenous peoples in Latin America, Asia and Africa participated in revolutions and political movements but their participation was based on their class (as peasants) rather than on their ethnic identity. For example, Juan León explains that for a long time since the 1960s, the Maya peoples joined other marginalized sectors of Guatemalan society in an armed struggle. "Even so, prior to the onset of the peace negotiations, the major objectives of the revolutionary movement did not include proposals from the indigenous peoples themselves." It was in the late 1980s, during the peace process, when the Maya activists themselves presented their common agenda both to the government of Guatemala and to the Unidad Revolucionaria Nacional Guatelmateca (URNG).

In other instances, ethnic concerns are subsumed within the context of religious movements. In Mindanao, Philippines, the armed movement led by the Moro National Liberation Front (MNLF) and the Moro Islamic Liberation Front (MNLF) has articulated their struggle for self-determination largely within the framework of religion, Islam. As Rolando Esteban remarks in his paper, "Islam has increasingly homogenized Moro culture as it became the basis of identity formation ... Islam has not only provided an ideology for the Moros but also provided a basis for the goal of an Islamic State."

Movements that are inspired by religion may also pose some dangers to indigenous peoples. Religious intolerance of difference can cause their marginalization. In Bangladesh, indigenous leaders see the rise of Islamic fundamentalism as a threat to their survival as a people. Islamic fundamentalism is intolerant of "other" cultures and seeks to homogenize them into "one world of Islam." This is especially difficult for the indigenous peoples of the Chittagong Hill Tracts (CHT) in Bangladesh since the majority of them are also Buddhists. Since the 1960s to the present, the CHT has been a scene of continuing violence (Roy).

Some indigenous leaders believe that indigenous movements should not be separated from broader social movements. Joan Carling of the Cordillera

Peoples Alliance in the Philippines sums up their lessons from decades of organizing and mobilizing work thus: "The major lesson learned from this political exercise is that genuine regional autonomy cannot be achieved if the national government is not truly democratic and independent." Carling believes that the clamor of indigenous movements for self-determination can only materialize under a nationalist and democratic regime.

However, as can be observed in many papers in this book, there has also been some tension between the ideology of nationalism and identity politics (Bom, Roy, Leon). A scholar has remarked that the problem with nationalism is that it remains captive to categories such as "progress," "reason," and "modernity," elements that are still alien to many indigenous peoples. He adds: "Obsessively concerned with the West and other forms of local elitism, nationalism fails to speak for its own people; on the contrary, it suppresses the politics of subalternity."[4]

Several cases cited in the papers illustrate this point. For example, nation-states' modernization programs have been designed within the framework of export-oriented industrialization. These growth-driven development projects, such as transnational corporate mining in India (Rebbapragada) and Indonesia (Chalid Muhamad), eco-tourism in Panama (Martínez), and hydroelectric projects in the Philippines (Carling), have displaced indigenous peoples from their lands, thereby causing or worsening poverty in these communities.

Nationalist movements, either of the Liberal Democratic or Marxist orientation, often fail to fully understand indigenous peoples' symbolic challenges to the status quo that offer alternative interpretations of individual and collective experience.[5] Juan León notes that one of the factors that led to the demise of the COPMAGUA, the national coalition of Mayas, was the yielding by its leaders to the political decisions of the URNG. In the process, COPMAGUA lost its autonomy and its strategic vision that planning must be based on the interests of the Mayan people themselves.

The left-wing political parties in Guatemala also failed to address cultural concerns and were often detached from representatives from their communities. Guerrilla movements usually could not provide land or justice, and frequently violated community cultural norms. Because of these, indigenous peoples sought alternative modes of social movement mobilization.

Another trend in contemporary indigenous movements is that they seek to break stereotypical representations of their identities as "marginalized," "poor" and "powerless." This shift in political orientation from the periphery to the center was largely a result of indigenous peoples' recognition of their inherent source of power—their knowledge, spirituality, and values of collectivity and community solidarity. Even non-indigenous peoples (mainstream society) are now going back to indigenous knowledge(s), values and practices as a viable alternative to the world's social and environmental crises.

To better understand indigenous peoples' efforts in changing their lives and the world, it is important to use a paradigm that recognizes the role of social actors and the concept of "human agency." Norman Long defines agency in the following manner:

> The notion of agency attributes to the individual actors the capacity to process a social experience and to devise ways of coping with life, even under the most extreme forms of coercion. Within the limits of information, uncertainty and other constraints that exist, social actors are "knowledgeable" and "capable."[6]

Within this framework, indigenous peoples become active "subjects" of social movements rather than passive objects. As actors, they are not treated as individuals that can be "aroused, organized and mobilized" for revolutionary and other political aims. Rather, indigenous peoples use their human agency to influence events, interpret and "socially construct" their social relations and their environments, and create their discourses in the light of these relationships. Thus, there can be multiple discourses and realities (as opposed to universal and particular discourses). This is because the construction of identities and the exercise of agency are influenced by different spatial (place) and temporal (time) contexts.

Indigenous peoples have expressed their voices and "human agencies" through their collective actions (movements) in a variety of ways. In turn, these movements use multifaceted and multilayered strategies to cope with their different conditions. What follows is a rendering of some of these strategies (as culled from the papers presented in this book).

Sanjay Bosu Mullick writes that indigenous peoples have gradually evolved a strategy of accommodation, in response to the challenges imposed by alien forces. Mullick posits:

> Over the ages, indigenous peoples have developed and practiced a social mechanism in which they accommodate and mold foreign social, political and economic elements compatible with their basic values and aspirations into their own social system, and reject totally

those that are incompatible. This has saved them time and again from compromising with or surrendering to opposing forces and in keeping their identity intact.

An example of the strategy of accommodation or localization that Mullick cites is the Indian indigenous peoples' conversion to Christianity during the British colonial period. He maintains that the indigenous peoples somehow made the church work in their favor as they succeeded in getting back a major portion of their lost land. In addition, the converts are now "engaged in local-izing the church by bringing in their traditional cultural ethos and practices."

A similar pattern of accommodation and localization can be seen in Latin America. Pilar Valencia informs us that in Colombia indigenous peoples have strengthened their claims over their resources by appropriating colonial prop-erty regimes, such as the *reguardos*. Introduced during the colonial times, the *reguardo* is a collective property under land deed. It was initially an instrument of domination by the Spanish crown. But over the course of more than a cen-tury, it has gradually become a tool for the defense of indigenous territorial rights.

These examples suggest that through time, indigenous peoples have selectively adopted various property regimes (primordial, colonial or modern) in their attempts to strengthen their claims over their territories. Above all, the strategy of accommodation and localization is a reflection of native agency.

Another strategy that indigenous peoples' movements have used is the revaluation of their indigenous institutions. Ariel Araujo writes that in 1983 in Argentina, "the indigenous peoples embarked upon a new process in which they reevaluated their traditional political institutions. This gave those institu-tions new momentum, and also led to the founding of political organizations to defend indigenous rights." Under a democratic system, institutions were created within the framework of provincial governments to which indigenous peoples elect their representatives. These institutions, generally known as the "Institutes of the Aborigines," are in charge of coordinating all the sectors of the State in the respective areas for purposes of implementing health, educa-tion, development, and housing programs as well as planning in indigenous territories.

A similar tact of creating local institutions of empowerment has been pur-sued by the Kuna peoples of Panama. Flaviano Martínez notes:

> The local assemblies and general assembly have provided the Kuna people with organizational self-empowerment. Thanks to these structures, they were able to confront external pressures from the

State and/or from domestic and foreign private sectors seeking to embark on large-scale economic projects in our communities.

Besides revaluating and strengthening their traditional institutions, indigenous peoples have also created "new" institutions of self-empowerment. These local, national and international indigenous peoples' organizations have become their instruments for policy advocacy and campaigns. In Nepal the Kirat Yakthung Chumlung (KYC) is working towards the restoration of the *Kipat* system, a traditional resource ownership and management system that was abolished by the state. In Kelian, Indonesia, communities affected by the large-scale mining of Rio Tinto have organized the Lembaga Kesejateraan Masharikat Tambang dan Lingkuran (LKMTL). Indigenous peoples in this country have actively participated in the formation of a national alliance of mining "struggle groups"—Mines, Minerals and People (MM&P). Multisectoral organizing with indigenous peoples as key players was also the approach followed by the Cordillera Peoples Alliance in the Cordillera, Philippines.

Legal rights protection is another strategy that indigenous movements have employed. In Australia the Aboriginal Legal Service System was created and developed by the National Aboriginal and Torres Strait Islander Legal Services Secretariat (NAILSS). Authors Bellear, Bond and Leslie assess this mechanism as largely and generally effective and efficient in bringing conflict situations involving indigenous peoples "along a path which emphasizes non-violent legal and political strategic action across all levels of the executive, legislative and judicial arms of government." The experience of NAILSS also shows that indigenous intellectuals have "learned the rules of the game" created by government and corporations. As a result, indigenous peoples now know "how to beat them at their own game."

In other instances, indigenous peoples have taken the path of armed movements as the ultimate means to prevent and reverse their marginalized status. In Mexico the indigenous peoples have waged a non-Marxist social movement, the Ejercito Zapatista de Liberacion Nacional (EZLN) or Zapatista movement. This movement takes up the discourse of human rights, democracy and autonomy as points of distinction from the old agrarian struggles.[7] In Burma indigenous peoples have formed their own political parties, the Karen National Association (KNA) and the Chin National Front (CNF). Liton Bom reports that these political parties have actively engaged in political struggle, employing different forms of protest—armed, legal, or both in the pursuit of their objectives.

During the last decade, indigenous movements have been internationalized, due in part to the push made by indigenous peoples themselves.

Indigenous peoples sought international support and protection because they lacked political access at home. This was exemplified by the Cordillera peoples' struggle against the World Bank's Chico Dam project in the Central Cordillera region during the Marcos dictatorship (see Carling).

The internationalization of indigenous movements was also a result of international campaigns and processes. For example, the UN Decade of Indigenous Peoples has brought to center stage the debate and further discourse on indigenous peoples in all the bodies and agencies of the UN system. The Decade has undoubtedly mobilized several local/village level organizations to participate in these international processes, where indigenous peoples were able to voice out their local issues and concerns in the global arena.

International processes/instruments, such as the UN Draft Declaration on the Rights of Indigenous Peoples, have encouraged indigenous peoples to examine and reexamine their past, revitalize their indigenous institutions, assert their claims over their land and resources and their right to self-determination (read, for instance, Bom, Carling, Limbu). The convergence of local demands and international norms/standards has resulted in a new form of political syncretism that is local but not parochial.[8]

Indigenous peoples' movements have undoubtedly impacted on the local, national and global society. These have attracted public attention and opened spaces for discourse on indigenous issues in civil society, guerrilla movements and dominant institutions, and nation-states. These institutions are now forced to deal (in various levels of sincerity) with the issues and concerns of indigenous peoples. How much of these issues and demands are recognized and addressed depends largely on the strength of the indigenous movements themselves, as history and recent experiences have taught them.

NOTES

1 Darnovsky, Epstein, and Flacks, (1995) cited in Brysk (2000), 33.
2 Ibid.
3 Esman, quoted by Brysk (2000).
4 Radhakrishan (1992), 88.
5 Kay B. Warren, *Indigenous Movements and Their Critics: Pan-Maya Activism in Guatemala* (Princeton: Princeton University Press, 1999), 5.
6 Norman Long, *Battlefields of Knowledge: The Interlocking of Theory and Practice in Social Research and Development* (London and New York: Routledge, 1992), 23.
7 Harvey, cited in Brysk, (2000).
8 Alison Brysk, *From Tribal Village to Global Village: Indian Rights and International Relations in Latin America* (California: Stanford University, 2000).

REFERENCES

Brysk, Alison. From Tribal Village to Global Village: Indian Rights and International Relations in Latin America. California: Stanford University, 2000.

Long, Norman and Long, A., eds. "From Paradigm Lost to Paradigm Regained?" Battlefields of Knowledge: The Interlocking of Theory and Practice in Social Research and Development. London and New York: Routledge, 1992.

Warren, Kay B. Indigenous Movements and Their Critics: Pan-Maya Activism in Guatemala. Princeton: Princeton University Press, 1998.

19

The New Politics of Consumption: Promoting Sustainability in the American Market Place

Maurie J. Cohen, Aaron Comrov, and Brian Hoffner

Introduction

More than a decade has passed since the Rio Earth Summit out sustainable development on the international policy agenda. Individuals and organizations with an interest in the concept have used this milestone to measure the progress that has been achieved formulating and implementing plans broadly consistent with the aims of sustainability (see, for example, Lafferty & Meadowcroft, 2000; OECD, 2002). Viewing the situation solely from the vantage point of the affluent countries, it is apparent that several nations have embraced the challenges of sustainable development—foremost among them the Netherlands, Norway, and Sweden—while others have evinced much greater caution.

By virtually all accounts, the United States is an anomaly in terms of how its national government has sought to reconcile conventional policy objectives with the goals of sustainable

This article reprinted with permission from *Sustainability: Science, Practice, & Policy* 2005;1(1):58–76.

development. The Clinton administration launched the President's Council on Sustainable Development (PCSD) in 1993 and its staff prepared a handful of laudable reports (see, for example, PCSD, 1999). However, these initiatives achieved little public visibility and, in terms of their political influence, have had no enduring effect. When George W. Bush assumed office in 2001, his decision to disband the PCSD occurred with hardly any notice. In a recent comprehensive review of the uptake of sustainable development as a policy concept in the United States, Gary Bryner (2000) explains that:

> [F]ew political leaders have been willing to take on the broader questions of American values of economic growth, consumption, technology, land use, transportation, and individual freedom. Most Americans seem determined to view economic growth as limitless, constrained only by unwise policy or business choices. They resist strongly the idea that limits should be placed on material consumption, and exhibit tremendous faith in technological solutions to whatever problems confront them. Their strong commitment to private property rights places major limits on political decisions which seek to promote environmental ends but which involve limitations on established patterns of property usage.

In their comparative assessment of sustainable development in several affluent countries, Lafferty and Meadowcroft (2000) caustically conclude that, "sustainable development had had virtually *no* impact on the operations of the US federal government. It is not just that the term itself has failed to catch on, but also that core values associated with the idea—particularly the global equity dimension—have failed to gain even formal political acceptance" (italics in original).

There is no reason to dispute these claims and, if anything, the status of sustainable development in the United States has eroded further since these authors prepared their evaluations. The Bush administration has embraced a domestic agenda that seeks to systematically dismantle many of the country's cornerstone pieces of environmental legislation (Cohen, 2004; see also Pope and Rauber, 2004; Alterman and Green, 2004). On the international front, hard-edged diplomacy and military intervention have supplanted humanitarian assistance and political empowerment as the preferred policy options.

Yet there are indications that the status of sustainable development in the United States is not as dire as this appraisal suggests. While it is true that the concept currently is all but nonexistent at the level of the national government, there are signs that individual states are moving, albeit with noticeable hesitation and little unison, toward fragile acceptance of some of the core tenets of sustainability. Several states, for instance, have launched their own climate change mitigation programs and others are beginning to grapple with the difficulties of discouraging suburban sprawl (Pew Center on Global Climate Change, 2002). Consistent with these efforts, a consortium of ten northeastern states has begun to negotiate the guidelines for a regional market to trade greenhouse gas emissions credits (Johnson, 2003a). For students of American environmental policymaking, this pattern of state progressiveness in the face of federal intransigence is not surprising. The historical record shows that, from air pollution regulation to managing toxic chemicals, the states have trailblazed virtually every new environmental policy idea implemented in the United States. It has only been after the states have demonstrated effectiveness, and an unwieldy system of differing state-based standards has come into view, that the government has taken action (see, for example, Andrews, 1999). With this experience in mind, the lack of enthusiasm for sustainable development at the national level becomes more understandable.

The intent here is not to contend that the system of American federalism is stealthily powering a sustainability revolution. Rather the claim is that policy innovation in large, diverse nations such as the United States is often not as readily discernible as it might be in smaller, more homogenous countries. Moreover, the constitutionally designed weakness of the national government in the United States heavily constrains opportunities for dynamic transformation. As a result, protest and local organization have been the engines of political change throughout American history. For these reasons, the study of sustainable development in spheres some distance removed from Washington, DC, may yield more encouraging results.

Lafferty and Meadowcroft (2000) usefully disaggregate the admittedly vague and elusive notion of sustainable development into five themes: the integration of economy and environment, the development of strategic plans and monitoring programs, the design of opportunities for participation and stakeholder involvement, the internationalization of environmental policy, and the movement toward sustainable production and consumption. Because of the challenge the reformulation of production and consumption practices poses to the core values of liberal democracy, these scholars characterize it as the most ambitious component of the sustainable development agenda. This distinction helps to frame further the bold aims of the following discussion, namely that there exists in the United States not only underappreciated resolve for sustainable development, but that some of the most notable activities are occurring within the most demanding thematic sphere.[1]

To give credence to this contention that a new politics of consumption is currently taking hold in the United States, this study casts a wide net. The following discussion organizes a diverse array of developments into three broad categories: social and political protest campaigns, lifestyle reinventions, and public policy initiatives.

First, it is axiomatic to observe that the United States has been at the forefront of the recent wave of globalization (see, for example, Green and Griffith, 2002; Bhagwati, 2002). Some commentators, such as Fabbrini (2002), contend that political resistance to globalization is most voluble in Europe and elsewhere, and is often tantamount to anti-Americanism. Lost in these discussions of international campaigns to confront American economic and cultural dominance is the fact that similar configurations have coalesced in the United States itself—indeed, the first major anti-globalization confrontation occurred in Seattle. While American activists, like their counterparts in other countries, have focused their attacks on international financial institutions, it is noteworthy that salient symbols of consumer culture (e.g. The Gap, Nike, and Starbucks) have also been prominent targets. This particular facet of the anti-globalization movement in the United States promotes sustainable consumption through three separate (though interdependent) forms of social and political protest: anti-consumerist, anti-television, and anti-advertising.

Second, other elements of this new politics of consumption embody a less impassioned approach and do not display the same kind of zealous and animated fervor. Predicated more on the reinvention of individual lifestyles than on overt social and political agitation, this set of initiatives to encourage sustainable consumption comprises several different strands. The following discussion focuses specifically on voluntary simplicity, ethical consumption, and slow food.

Finally, sub-national units of government in the United States have begun to implement a number of policy initiatives that have the implicit aim of promoting sustainable consumption. To be certain, government officials have not aggressively employed a language of sustainability to advance these programs. However, the correspondence between efforts to develop local greenhouse gas reduction schemes, to rebuild local economies, and to discourage the accumulation of consumer debt dovetail very closely with the aims of sustainable consumption.

Protest Politics and Sustainable Consumption

Consumption has been a pervasive element of social organization in the United States and, over the course of the last two centuries, this lifestyle form has inspired numerous political responses, ranging from the home economics movement of the nineteenth century to recent campaigns to foster consumer rights (Mayer, 1989; Furlough & Strikwerda, 1999). In some respects, the social agitation of the 1960s was fueled by a rebellion against mainstream consumer ideology. More recent protest politics have had a similar edge, as adherents have sought to expose what they construe as the falseness and the lack of authenticity inherent in mass consumerism. The following section focuses on three expressions of this anxiety: anti-consumerists protests, anti-television activism, and anti-advertising campaigns.

Anti-Consumerism

Among some youthful and vocal adherents, the disparagement of mass consumerism as a set of social practices, as well as attacks against some of its most emblematic symbols, has become a visible form of protest politics in the United States during the past decade. Activists have yet to construct many of the institutional features of a social movement, and instead rely on boisterous pranks designed to malign dominant expressions of contemporary consumer culture. Proponents are often disillusioned not only with material icons, but also evince a more general disenchantment with contemporary society (Zavestoski, 2002). While this disaffection derives from numerous sources, for analytic purposes it is instructive to group them into three broad categories—social, economic, and environmental.

First, anti-consumerist activists in the United States contend that consumption, or more specifically over-consumption, is harmful to both the individual and the wider society (DeGraaf et al., 2002; Schor, 1998). This cast of mind asserts that personal attachment to inanimate objects is psychologically stultifying and that consumers should more appropriately invest in education and other projects to foster societal improvement. Moreover, they maintain that rampant egoistic acquisition diminishes community solidarity and encourages artificial competition to accumulate. Proponents of this view fundamentally disagree with neo-classical economic principles, and assert in contrast that an undue emphasis on material acquisition constrains socioeconomic mobility and lowers the societal standards of living. In addition to these ills, activists stress that consumption drains away valuable time and money, ruins physical and mental health, threatens religious faith, and undermines civic institutions. The largest beneficiaries of consumption, this critique asserts, are its ubiquitous advocates. Anti-consumerism is also highly critical of the mainstream media for their defenselessness before powerful advertisers.

Second, American anti-consumerism activists assert that lifestyles founded on mass consumption oblige people to assemble a large arsenal of inexpensive products, many of which are produced under exploitive conditions (Bender & Greenwald, 2003; Broad, 2002). The relentless drive for cheaper goods leads to the loss of local employment and to the migration of production to offshore locations. Moreover, this form of uncritical consumerism erodes spiritual and cultural diversity. A retreat from a goods-oriented lifestyle will obstruct the march toward international homogenization and reduce the economic pressure on developing countries to abandon venerable traditions.

Finally, contemporary American anti-consumerism alleges that to create a sustainable and healthy world for future generations it is necessary to strive for the diffusion of more modest consumption practices (Myers & Kent, 2004; Princen et al, 2002).[2] One of the major drivers of this sensibility is a concern that the export of prevalent American lifestyles contributes to numerous ecological problems. Activists are especially mindful about dematerializing their consumption practices as a means of reducing their reliance on natural resources, disposable commodities, chlorine-based products, agricultural chemicals, virgin wood, meat, dairy products, processed foods, non-durable appliances, and consumables attributable to exploitive labor practices. A key precept of this philosophy is the encouragement of relatively modest lifestyles on a global level, as this will lead to a more environmentally sustainable economy and will resolve social ills stemming from an inequitable distribution of wealth.

These three currents of anti-consumerism presently flow like meandering rivulets of a stream. Despite their different emphases, activists view their goals as entirely practicable, because unchecked materialism is, by this view, a constructed social phenomenon rather than an indomitable feature of the human condition. By disabling the powerful engines driving prevailing consumption desires, people can assert themselves and steer away from the destructive and manipulative forces.

The tenor of anti-consumerism in the United States is at once low-key and loud. It is quiet in the sense that it does not have an organized mass following to communicate its message on a consistent basis. Activists are also relatively unobtrusive because they do not customarily advocate audacious acts of vigilantism and violent confrontation. Part of the reason for its current status is that anti-consumerism aside from its sometimes creative tactics, has yet to articulate an incremental program for achieving its political objectives. Anti-consumerism is also simultaneously loud in the sense that its recommendations and social commentary are markedly radical. Some adherents have also begun to promote strategies that are more aggressive and, in some cases, have used violence against property as a means of political expression.[3]

Anti-consumerism in the United States is not presently endowed with many of the organizational features commonplace among more established social movements. Few national organizations have taken up the mantle of this campaign as their primary mission, and existing environmental, social justice, and consumer organizations have been, at best, reluctant partners. Nonetheless, one prominent group working on this front is the Adbusters Media Foundation (AMF), a small, plucky group that has made strides to problematize consumerism and to give concrete form to an emergent social movement (Rumbo, 2002; Bordwell, 2002).

Based in Vancouver, AMF was founded by Danish-born activist Kalle Lasn in 1989. The organization currently publishes a quarterly magazine, entitled *Adbusters*, that reaches approximately 85,000 readers and has the appearance of an elite design magazine.[4] The publication's content is highly premised on irony and parody and is savagely critical of mainstream advertising, consumer products, and consumerism as a lifestyle. In place of paid advertisements, *Adbusters* publishes its own satirical versions of real print promotions, with the intent of using humor to expose the negative social, psychological, and environmental impacts of the products they depict. The magazine's funding comes from subscriptions, philanthropic contributions, and revenue derived producing promotional segments for Greenpeace.

Adbusters refers to its specific style of political expression as "culture jamming," a term coined in 1985 by a San Francisco-based music group called Negativland (Lasn, 1999). More specifically, the approach involves a kind of cultural jujitsu that seeks to turn the language of advertising and promotion against itself. Culture jammers also use civil disobedience and other provocative means to reclaim certain "strategic spaces" that have been appropriated for commercial purposes.[5] The specific spaces to which culture-jamming techniques are applied can be physical places, such as parks, promenades, and highways, as well as more subtly psychological and cultural spheres. The so-called "un-commercials" that appear in *Adbusters* are creative caricatures of familiar advertisements and, as such, are paradigmatic examples of culture jamming. This mode of resistance has begun to transcend the clever lampooning of cultural symbols to include vandalizing billboards and defacing other promotional media.[6]

In addition to publication of its magazine, AMF occasionally organizes boycotts, store sit-ins, mass sign-ins, and local demonstrations to challenge mainstream lifestyles and to raise public consciousness. AMF's largest event, and the activity through which the organization is most widely known, is its annual Buy Nothing Day (BND). BND is held in November of each year and is scheduled for the Friday following the American holiday of Thanksgiving, generally regarded as one of the most vigorous shopping days on the calendar. Promoted as "a third millennium holiday—a celebration of simplicity and frugality," BND has become an international event, and the number of countries participating in it grows each year. An emphasis on leading more modest lifestyles is central to AMF's mission, and the group maintains that less commercialism is essential for peace and global sustainability.

AMF exemplifies the contradictory temperament of anti-consumerism. The organization is, on one hand, quiet and cerebral and, on the other hand, loud and confrontational. Supporters advocate non-violence, yet endorse the goal of undermining existing centers of power and forging new ways to think about prevailing norms. AMF's protest methods may be generally peaceful, but its stated objective is irrefutably radical.

Anti-Television Activism

After a slow start caused by the onset of World War II, television in the United States diffused at a rapid rate (von Schilling, 2003; Barnouw, 1990). By 1950, 3.1 million households were watching, and just five years later this number had grown to 32 million. Today, 99% of American households have at least one television, and more than 50% of children in the United States have a set in their bedroom. The viewing equipment has been subject to a regular stream of technological improvements—color, cable, video compatible, DVD compatible, pay-to-view, high definition, and so forth. Television watchers can now even subscribe to services that allow one to delete commercials and to record one program while viewing another. An enthusiastic audience has eagerly embraced these upgrades and made substantial investments to acquire them.

Advertising has been a continual presence on American television since the earliest days of the medium, and the magnitude of commercial promotionalism that occurs today is remarkable by any measure. Thirty percent of network news programming is devoted to commercials, and the average American views 20,000 broadcast advertisements each year. Despite consistent corporate claims that these images do not increase consumption, marketing managers spent $40 billion in 1999 to develop and air their product inducements (Samuel, 2001).

A common social critique in recent decades has been to disparage television for its stultifying effects on viewers who spend long hours in front of the screen (see, for example, Mander, 1978). However, more recent appraisals adopt the opposite perspective. In fact, contemporary American critics of the technology insist that rather than contributing to passivity, television is notable for its motivational potential. It is an indisputable marketing precept that the comely images featured on television stimulate previously non-existent consumption urges. The role of advertising experts is not to promote this obvious fact, but to formulate the most appealing images and to convince viewers that material goods can satisfy their ethereal needs.

According to anti-television activists in the United States, this continual ramping up of consumption is not trivial. Excessive television viewing exacerbates environmental dilemmas by drawing ever-larger volumes of raw materials into production. The medium is also alleged to be responsible for an assortment of social problems. For example, even a family that watches an ordinary amount of television exposes itself to a heavy dose of advertising. Parents often find themselves having to work long hours to generate the income necessary to purchase the kaleidoscopic menu of goods that their children demand. These circumstances detract from parents' ability to foster meaningful social relationships and, to assuage the situation, the family watches more television and consumes more goods (Molnar, 1996; Fox, 1996; Boyles, 1998).

It was in the context of this emerging appraisal that a group of activists established TV-Free America (TVFA) in 1994. Prior to the launch of this organization, misgivings about television tended to find expression as part of larger initiatives focused, for example, on banning advertisements for alcohol, on ensuring programming with adequate educational value, or on prohibiting violent and sexually explicit broadcast content. TVFA endorsed a more basic agenda, namely one that encouraged viewers to disconnect the set.

Over the past decade, TVFA has evolved into the TV Turnoff Network (TVTON), and has continued to advance the perspective that excessive television viewing is highly problematic. With financial support from donations and the sale of products, TVTON serves as the educational arm for a more diffuse array of anti-television activism. For instance, the organization distributes fact sheets and coordinates special events to encourage alternative family- and community-based activities to replace long hours of television viewing. TVTON, as stated on the organization's website (http://www.tvfa.org) , seeks to "shift the debate from concerns about television's content toward an understanding that breaking free of TV is a fun, liberating, and enriching experience." In other words, TVTON is not concerned with censorship battles or changing the content of specific programming. Instead, the organization is engaging with what it sees as the core of the problem—the need to reduce the number of hours people spend in front of their televisions. Consistent with this objective, TVTON coordinates two annual public projects—a long-standing initiative known as TV Turnoff Week and a newer scheme called More Reading, Less TV.

TV Turnoff Week (TVTW) challenges adults, teenagers, and children to forsake television for one week each year. It is important to recognize that the guiding purpose of TVTW is not to create incentives for participants to demonstrate their ability to achieve this objective in the narrow sense, but rather to create space in which they can learn first-hand how satisfying life can be without (or at least with less) television. Volunteer coordinators distribute TVTW facilitation kits to community groups, schools, and religious organizations that include "screen free" activities, pledge cards, and instructional materials for arranging alternative activities. TVTW has expanded its reach every year since its establishment in 1995. According to its sponsors, 90% of the respondents to its annual survey report that they now watch less TV than they did prior to participating in TVTW, and two-thirds of the sample say that the changes they have made in their viewing habits may be permanent.

Anti-television activists contend that excessive television viewing is one of the leading reasons for poor school performance among young children. In response, TVTON has developed its More Reading, Less TC (MRLTV) campaign to confront head-on the link between television and literacy. MRLTV is a four-week campaign sponsored by the Educational Foundation of America that is relayed directly to students in their classrooms. Youngsters are encouraged figuratively and literally to "Bury the Television with Books." In practice this means that for every book a student reads he or she receives a colorful strip of paper to affix to the classroom television. The intent is that, by the end of the month-long initiative, the class will have accumulated enough strips to obscure the television in its entirety. According to its promoters, MRLTV serves as an especially good incentive for children who rarely pick up books, and TVTON reports that "poor readers" are more than twice as likely to seek out a book after participating in the program.

In addition to these two initiative, TVTON actively campaigns for the elimination of *Channel One*, the in-school television network that is mandatory viewing in most classrooms across the country. The organization disapproves of *Channel One* because advertisements are spliced into the regular programming and students have a difficult time distinguishing the educational content from the promotional inducements. TVTON also contends that *Channel One* is entirely inappropriate in an educational setting. Schools, for the most part, are the only relatively advertisement-free places in the United States, and administrators and teachers who allow this medium into the classrooms compromise the integrity of their profession.

The advocacy agenda promoted by TVTON includes several professional medical associations and is grounded in a large body of social scientific research documenting the personal and social problems associated with excessive television viewing. The following discussion organizes this array of adverse impacts into four categories: youth problems, societal effects, negative outcomes for families and communities, and individual consequences.

First, children in the United States between two and seventeen years of age watch, on average, twenty hours of television each week—the majority of which is spent without a parent or adult present. Research suggests the existence of a causal link between the number of hours school-age children view television and academic performance (see, for example, Clarke & Kurtz-Costed, 1997). Based on this evidence, the American Academy of Pediatrics has called for reductions in the amount of television that children watch (Lowry et al., 2002; Hu et al., 2003). Aside from attentiveness in school, it is apparent that children who spend a great deal of time in front of the television do not develop active lifestyles, and this has ramifications later in life (Crespo et al., 2001).

Second, anti-television activists are not blind to the positive social contributions that television in certain circumstances can make. For instance, the technology can break down the isolation of distance, deliver news and entertainment, and unify a large and diverse nation. However, they assert that television is responsible for bringing in its wake a host of intractable social problems. The situation is exacerbated in the United States because political culture discourages the kinds of public intervention—often in the form of restrictive regulation—that has been used in other countries. For instance, aside from broadcasters' fears about transgressing viewers' sensibilities, there are few constraints on violence on television. By the time the average American adolescent reaches the age of eighteen, he or she will have seen in excess of 200,000 violent acts and 16,000 murders on television. This phenomenon is not limited to programming ostensibly designed for entertainment. Between 1993 and 1996 there was a 20% downturn in the nation's homicide rate, but a seven-fold increase in homicide coverage on network news. The American Medical Association (AMA) reports that many youngsters cannot clearly distinguish between real life and fantasy because they are conditioned by television violence from a very early age. In response, the AMA has begun to assert that public policymakers should treat violence on television in the same way as they promote seatbelts and bicycle helmets.[7]

Third, anti-television activists contend that evidence links excessive viewing with a variety of negative outcomes for families and communities. They argue that the ubiquity of television has undermined interpersonal relationships because the technology offers the opportunity for virtual relationships with fictional characters, and these interactions then become substitutes for displaced family and communal contacts (Schor, 1998). Though it is hard to determine the extent to which the observation might be tainted by nostalgic yearnings, proponents of reduced television viewing point out that in earlier eras dinnertime was an opportunity for busy families to catch up with one another. What is somewhat more reliable is social survey data indicating that today 40% of families watch television while eating their evening meal.

Fourth, heavy television viewing appears to be taking a heavy toll on viewers' physical health, and medical studies have correlated certain ailments with precursor conditions, especially obesity. Anti-television activists highlight one recent study finding that, as television viewing increases, exercise drops off and consumption of snack foods grows. These circumstances contribute to weight gain and an affinity for passive recreation. Individuals who watch television for more than three hours per day are twice as likely to be obese as those who viewed it for less than one hour per day (Coon et al., 1998).

Finally, anti-television activists have begun to problematize television in much wider social and political terms. Some groups assert that the technology has a perverse effect because the major networks receive de facto subsidies in excess of $70 billion from political candidates who use public finds and contributions to purchase campaign commercials. This arrangement creates a system in which only electoral contestants who can afford to pay for television airtime have any chance of success. As such, television has become one of the driving forces sustaining the political status quo.[8]

Anti-Advertising Campaigns

As noted above, advertising is an omnipresent and unavoidable fact in the United States, especially as communicated by television. However, television is surely not the only medium for marketing goods and services, and producers seek to reach consumers through a multitude of other channels, including radio, billboard, telephone, postal mail, electronic mail, and so forth. To penetrate the thicket of competing messages, advertisers have developed increasingly invasive approaches. Ironically, many consumers have come to accept advertising as a value-natural—and in some cases wholly agreeable—feature of contemporary life. In some communication forms, it is virtually impossible to distinguish the actual content from the sales promotions. Nevertheless, a growing number of anti-advertising campaigns has begun to make some novel (and seemingly conservative) assertions, namely that advertising infringes on personal freedom, contributes to mental and physical harm, and impairs economic growth. The emergence of this discourse has generated some raucous forms of resistance and given birth to a loose alliance of organizations variously dedicated to stricter regulation (and in some cases outright abolition) of advertising.

Although it is unlikely that this confederation of anti-advertising organizations constitutes a social movement in the strict sociological sense, what is more interesting for current purposes is the high degree of issue differentiation that exists within this sphere. For instance, advocates have launched initiatives to oppose the use of commercialization of public education, to resist the use of paid promotions to sell tobacco, to work against the erection and continued use of billboards, and to stop the communication of advertisements by telephone, postal mail, and electronic mail.

Commercial Alert (CA), an advocacy organization founded by Ralph Nader in 1998, is the undisputed leader of the American anti-advertising movement. CA's stated mission is "to keep the commercial culture within its proper sphere, and to prevent it from exploiting children and subverting the higher values of family, community, environmental integrity and democracy" (http://www.commercialalert.org). The organization's activities focus on lobbying for legislation to regulate advertising and on preventing the proliferation of commercial content in public venues. For example, CA urged the top fifty advertising agencies in the country to boycott CNN's *Student News* after the program dropped its commitment to be commercial-free. Other initiatives have sought to encourage the prohibition of advertising on public transport vehicles, to persuade publishers from printing sales pitches for junk food in children's books, to pressure major league baseball teams to remove badges with product insignias from players' uniforms, and to discourage companies from patronizing *Channel One*, the controversial in-school television network.

A specific point of criticism against advertising that appears to have struck a chord in the American public mind over the past decade concerns the effects of commercial promotion on children. While it was not framed specifically as an anti-advertising campaign, efforts to discourage the tobacco company RJ Reynolds' from running its so-called Joe Camel advertisements dampened the effectiveness of a marketing tool deliberately aimed at children (DiFranza, 1991).

Aside from CA, there is a diverse network of smaller and less visible organizations working along similar lines.[9] Three groups are emblematic of the activity in this sphere. First, Stop Commercial Exploitation of Children (www.commercialexploitation.com) is specifically concerned with the harmful effects of advertising on youngsters. Second, Dads and Daughters (www.dadsanddaughters.org) is an incipient group committed to fostering meaningful relationships between fathers and their female children, an agenda that seeks to dampen the deleterious effects of advertising on young women. Finally, the Center for Commercial-Free Public Education (CCFPE) works to resist the encroachment of advertising in schools. Established in Oakland in 1993 to campaign against *Channel One*, the organization is one of many grassroots groups that have coalesced to oppose the news service.[10] Because CCFPE is larger and more established than most of its counterparts, it supports other local activists with information and training. The group coordinates initiatives to raise student consciousness about advertising in contemporary life, to encourage schools to become commercial-free, and to support parents who challenge the invasion of corporate promotions in schools.[11]

Tobacco companies have been a specific target of anti-advertising campaigners in the United States. The battle over tobacco advertising has been raging for as long as public health advocates have recognised that cigarettes were hazardous. The Badvertising Institute (BI) is one organization that has been at the forefront of the effort to ban the advertising of tobacco products, and it played a major role in the demise of the aforementioned Joe Camel. BI models itself as an educational group, but it also pursues an active advocacy agenda. One of its notable activities is the production of mock renditions of actual tobacco advertisements. BI also prepares educational materials for schools, organizes exhibits, and presents slideshows and workshops to advance the case against tobacco advertising.[12]

Other anti-advertising campaigns have sought to expose the tendency of some companies to make unsubstantiated claims. As consumers have expressed a preference for corporations with reputable social and environmental records, it has become common for advertisers to appropriate these themes for promotional purposes. Perhaps not surprisingly, the firms responsible for many familiar brands have sought to embellish their accomplishments, practices that activists have termed "bluewashing" and "greenwashing." The former refers to a company's tendency to exaggerate its commitment to social responsibility, and the latter denotes unjustified amplification of its environmental performance. One organization that has taken up the challenge of exposing instances of bluewashing and greenwashing is the ethical watchdog CorpWatch.

Anti-advertising activists in the United States have also taken their efforts to the nation's highways. Since the 1950's, efforts to impose prohibitions on outdoor advertising have been part of wider efforts to encourage highway beautification. Early federal legislation banning the erection of billboards in specific areas took effect in 1965, and several states—notably Vermont, Hawaii, Maine, and Alaska—adopted more exacting measures. Proponents of these laws, including Lady Bird Johnson, the wife of the former president, generally framed their concerns not in antagonistic terms denouncing advertising, but as appeals to an aesthetic sensibility. The organization Scenic America has been at the forefront on this issue since its inception and continues to provide resources to numerous state and local groups, such as Citizens for a Scenic Florida, Citizens for a Scenic Spokane, and Citizens for a Scenic North Nevada, that work to ban outdoor advertising in specific jurisdictions. More recently, these groups have spearheaded campaigns against telecommunications towers and other facilities deemed to disfigure the landscape.

Most encounters with advertising are situational experiences into which consumers insert themselves. Exposure to billboards, television commercials, and magazine inserts arguably occurs when individuals take purposeful action that brings them within reach of these commercial appeals. Consumers who are interested in practicing an especially vigilant form of avoidance behavior can actively avoid (or at least lessen) their encounters with these promotional inducements. For this reason, various forms of unprompted advertising, some of them quite ingenious, have come to be widely despised. Telemarketing calls, junk mail, and so-called unsolicited commercial e-mails (UCM) circumvent conventional defenses and become major sources of irritation. Public intolerance of these unduly intrusive modes of advertising is growing and, according to some observers, is prompting the biggest consumer backlash in decades. This response has assumed many different expressions and led to the formation of a host of organizations.

First, telemarketing involves the use of targeted voice- and fax-based telephone calls. These promotional practices have always had a dark side and over the years have attracted no shortage of unscrupulous operators. Nevertheless, during the past decade, more efficient dialing and messaging technologies have reduced the cost of reaching large numbers of households and the field has grown severalfold. Telemarketing firms are even setting up large-scale operations in India and other English-speaking countries, where they take advantage of low international calling rates to the United States to canvass on behalf of American companies. To defend themselves, would-be recipients of telemarketing solicitations can purchase and install an impressive number of gadgets that offer the promise of deterring telephone solicitors. Most of the numerous organizations working to thwart telemarketing adopt a similar approach that consists of offering consumers information on how to insulate themselves and enforce their legal rights. The groups also issue blanket advice discouraging the purchase of goods and services from telemarketers.

Anti-telemarketing organizations are also typically equipped to offer information regarding the Telephone Consumer Protection Act of 1991 (TCPA). TCPA prohibits unsolicited faxes and pre-recorded telephone sales calls, as well as providing states with the authority to create "do-not-call" lists.[13] Once an individual places herself on such a list, it becomes illegal to direct most telemarketing calls to her. Virtually all the anti-telemarketing groups support TCPA, but advocate for more restrictive legislation to impede the heavy flow of activity that continues to occur.

Second, unsolicited mailings, or junk mail, are a ubiquitous feature of life in the United States. Public tolerance for the seemingly relentless flow of postal promotions is higher than it is for telemarketing, perhaps because it is easier to discard an unopened envelope than it is to hang up on a polite telephone caller. While there are a few organizations that address this problem, none does so as vigorously as the Center for a New American Dream (CNAD), a new, somewhat anomalous upstart group. CNAD has created an entire campaign around the issue of eliminating junk mail. This organization does not view these mailings in terms of customary anti-advertising themes, but as a particularly egregious and offensive form of environmental disregard.

Finally, so-called unsolicited commercial e-mail, more commonly known as "spam," has become a common feature of mass computer use in recent years. Spam is not only a nuisance to most recipients, but it creates congestion on the Internet and overtaxes computing resources. The only thing that has grown faster than the volume of spam is the public reaction against it. While computer experts endorse the use of specially designed anti-spam software, it appears that the purveyors of these solicitations are able to stay a step ahead on the technological curve. In the absences of a credible technological fix, anti-spam activists have launched numerous organizations and websites to stem the rising tide of these electronic promotions. One group, the Coalition Against Unsolicited Commercial E-mail (CAUCE), is an example of organized resistance to spam. Aside from maintaining a website to which spam victims can turn for guidance, CAUCE lobbies for stringent legislation barring the distribution of unsolicited e-mail.

Lifestyle Reinventions and Sustainable Consumption

Vocal protest represents only one facet of the contemporary effort to forge a new politics of consumption in the United States. While culture jammers, anti-consumerism activists, and anti-advertising campaigners have formulated strident modes with which to express their anxieties about contemporary consumption-laden lifestyles, other sympathizers have chosen a more inward-looking approach focused on transforming personal values and practices. Termed lifestyle reinventions, this branch of the nascent sustainable consumption movement comprises voluntary simplifiers, ethical consumers, and slow food aficionados.

Voluntary Simplicity

Voluntary simplicity has been a preoccupation of both ancient prophets and modern social critics (Shi, 1985). Although contemporary adherents are likely to be familiar with popular proponents, such as Henry David Thoreau and Mahatma Gandhi, it is Duane Elgin's (1981) book that serves today as the inspirational bible. It is therefore appropriate to turn to this treatise for an operational definition.

> To live more voluntarily is to live more deliberately, intentionally, and purposefully—in short, it is to live more consciously. We cannot be deliberate when we are distracted from life. We cannot be intentional when we are not paying attention. We cannot be purposeful when we are not being present. Therefore, to act in a voluntary manner is to be aware of ourselves as we move through life. This requires that we not only pay attention to the actions we take in the outer world, but also that we pay attention to ourselves acting—our inner world. To the extent that we do not notice both inner and outer aspects of our passage through life, then our capacity for voluntary, deliberate, and purposeful action is commensurately diminished.

In other words, the decision to adopt a life of voluntary simplicity is a personal matter. Everyone is capable of determining where life is fraught with unnecessary complication. All have the capacity to recognize the clutter and pretense that weigh upon them and make the passage through this world more cumbersome and awkward. To live more simply is to become unburdened—to live more lightly, cleanly, and aerodynamically. It is to establish a more direct, humble, and unencumbered relationship with all aspects of life: the things that are consumed, the work that is done, the relationships that are maintained, and the connections that are created with nature and the cosmos. Simplicity of living means meeting life face-to-face. Voluntary simplicity, by extension, is about confronting life without unnecessary disruption and turmoil. It is about taking life as it is—straight and unadulterated.

Voluntary simplicity is not a lifestyle of deprivation, and this is often a critical point of misinterpretation by individuals who are unfamiliar with its aims. It is about discovering what is sufficient in life—based upon thoughtful analysis of one's values. Apropos for Elgin is Simone de Beauvoir's contention, "If all life does is maintain itself, then living is only not dying." If people look to non-material satisfactions, thus simplifying their lives, then they can establish a more meaningful existence and truly experience life. Voluntary simplicity is, then, about forging modest material needs to allow opportunities for people to surpass themselves and to find more satisfying, meaningful existences.

Early research on the extent to which people were actively pursuing voluntary simplicity in the United States suggested this mode of living had considerable appeal across a range of geographic regions (see, for example, Elgin & Mitchell, 1977; Leonard-Barton, 1981). There were indications that voluntary simplicity was distinct from other forms of lifestyle politics, popular during the 1970s, that stressed agrarian values and self-sufficiency. These studies also pointed to the fact that the vast majority of voluntary simplifiers were well-educated and had grown up under relatively affluent circumstances. In keeping with Ronald Inglehart's (1990) notion of post-materialism, they had conditioned cravings for material goods.

More recently Amitai Etzioni (1998) has conceptualized three forms of voluntary simplicity—downshifters, strong simplifiers, and holistic simplifiers. First, downshifters, according to this typology, are the most moderate, least intense simplifiers. These individuals tend to be financially secure, but for one reason or another choose to forego certain consumer items. Etzioni describes this group as being comprised of people who "dress down" to work, or drive unfashionable cars. There is no doubt a certain renegade status is associated with this lifestyle, and the irony is that while it may appear superficially simple, it is actually costly and engenders its own sort of commodification.

Second, strong simplifiers are people who have actively rejected high-paying jobs and lavish living in favor of less remunerative compensation and much more modest lifestyles. A widely read and cited New York Times report from the mid-1990s described this group as comprised of individuals who choose to buy and earn less, in exchange for more free time and less stress. This form of lifestyle politics involves a "quiet personal revolt against the dominant culture of getting and spending" (Goldberg, 1995).

Finally, Etzioni distinguishes a separate group of strong simplifiers that is comprised of individuals who embrace an ardent conception of "simple living," one that entails active abandonment of affluent lifestyles. However, this class of voluntary simplicity lacks the back-to-the-land ethos of the earlier era. With the explicit goal of leading simpler, less cosmopolitan lifestyles, strong simplifiers reside in various geographic locales, including older suburbs, gentrifying urban neighborhoods, smaller rural towns, and farmsteads. According to Etzioni, this group has a coherently articulate philosophy grounded in transcendentalism and is explicity anti-consumerist.

Several recent studies have sought to expound upon Etzioni's analytic framework and to shed further light on the motivations behind a purported shift toward voluntary simplicity. A particularly notable investigation, by

Margaret Craig-Lees & Constance Hill (2002), suggests that efforts to concep-
tualize voluntary simplicity solely in terms of behaviors deemed antagonistic
to material possessions might be overly narrow. These authors content that,
although all three of the themes associated with materialists concern physical
possessions, only one of the themes characterizing simplifiers has to do with
material goods. Voluntary simplifiers may reduce their material consumption,
but a life of poverty is not required and it is not necessary to sever all emotional
ties to goods. Craig-Lees & Hill take issue with how we conventionally understand materialism. We typically think of materialists as people who derive their
happiness and satisfaction from physical possessions. However, this study
questions whether it is indeed the case that materialists use possessions to
create significance, while non-materialists generate significance out of experiences. Craig-Lees & Hill found that voluntary simplifiers demonstrated greater
attachment to their homes than non-voluntary simplifiers did. In a finding
that departs from the conventional view, non-voluntary simplifiers were found
to be more likely to view their homes in non-emotive terms as smart investments and good buys. In this sense, the voluntary simplifiers, because of their
seemingly deep connection they developed with their possessions, appeared
more materialistic than their non-simplifying counterparts.

In a more recent essay, Elgin (2003) contributes to this discussion on how
to typologize voluntary simplicity, and generates a still more variegated schema
that distinguishes among choiceful simplicity, commercial simplicity, compassionate simplicity, ecological simplicity, elegant simplicity, frugal simplic-
ity, natural simplicity, political simplicity, soulful simplicity, and uncluttered
simplicity, by no means meant to be mutually exclusive. Elgin emphasizes
the artful tapestry in which individuals blend and combine elements of each
expression of simple living. Attached to each of these ten modes of voluntary
simplicity is a specific description, but for current purposes they can be aggregated into three main expressions: ecological awareness, frugal consumption,
and personal growth.

First, voluntary simplicity, at least in its contemporary form, has strong
intellectual roots in the environmental movement. In fact, Elgin issued his
landmark book soon after publication of the infamous *Limits to Growth*, prepared under the aegis of the Club of Rome. However, the patchy evidence that
does exist on the motivations behind the adoption of voluntary simplicity suggests that the connection between ecological awareness and voluntary simplicity is actually quite weak (see, for example, Maniantes, 2002). For instance, in
Craig-Lees & Hill's sample, only 10% of self-designated voluntary simplifiers
were members of environmental organizations, and only 25% identified the
environment as a primary reason for their lifestyle choice.

Second, some voluntary simplifiers are motivated by a personal commitment to frugality (Dacyczyn, 1998). This form of simple living seeks to resurrect the skills of thriftiness and to give them a new, more artful connotation. Mass consumerism and the quest for continual economic growth has denigrated the knowledge required to live without much regard for the value of money. Joe Dominguez & Vicki Robin's bestselling book *Your Money or Your Life* has been a particularly popular approach for reinvigorating enthusiasm for frugality. This volume provides readers with a nine-step program for achieving financial independence and establishing a sound relationship with money.

Finally, voluntary simplicity appears to be attracting attention because of a subtler and intangible promise for personal growth. In this sense, adherents seek to take on board certain lifestyle practices because they seem "right" and are suffused with greater authenticity. This quest for self-improvement also contains an element of spiritual enlightenment.

These three facets of voluntary simplicity have, over the past decade, generated a vast array of mass-market magazines, narrow-niche publications, product catalogs, websites, and other resources—a veritable industry of its own. These circumstances suggest that it is reasonable to raise the question whether this mode of sustainable consumption has, in the United States, passed the threshold of a social movement.[14] The very nature of voluntary simplicity makes it difficult to formulate a concise answer, mainly because there is a contradiction between the downscaling of lifestyles and the formation of a large-scale social movement with specific political intent (Maniates, 2002). Voluntary simplifiers embrace specific lifestyle choices, but the emphasis is on introspection and personal change rather than on creating a more ambitious political program. Another notable feature of voluntary simplicity in its current forms is the absence of vilification. In other words, social movements normally manifest a need to draw boundaries around their campaigns, and simplifiers are not seeking, at least presently, to articulate a social critique that assigns responsibility for the purported problems of consumerism.

Ethical Consumption

Adherents of ethical consumption maintain that consumers, by exercising care when making ordinary purchases, can recast the current system of social and political relations. More specifically, by steering clear of products manufactured under conditions that exploit vulnerable laborers or unduly degrade the environment, material consumption can become an engine for human and ecological betterment. The United Nations Platform for Action Committee (UNPAC) has developed a comprehensive guide to ethical consumption that includes recommendations to support local businesses, to assess the environ-mental costs of consumer purchases, to purchase second-hand goods, and to consider the transportation of products.

Although ethical consumption tends to enjoy greater public visibility in Europe, the Council on Economic Priorities (CEP) has spearheaded the move-ment in the United States (CEP, 1994). The CEP is a public interest research group funded by memberships, philanthropic grants, and donations. The or-ganization edits a keystone publication in the field of ethical consumption, entitled *Shopping for a Better World*, and encourages consumers to use their purchasing power as a vote—in as a way of conveying their preferences to oth-erwise inaccessible corporations. The group advocates that

> "Your choice of what car, washing machine, computer, or even
> breakfast cereal to buy may make more difference than you think,
> especially if you let companies know that social and environmental
> records affect your choices. Companies wield tremendous power,
> but individuals can influence corporate practices and can actually
> help change the world. It's simple, positive activism of casting your
> *economic vote* conscientiously." (CEP, 1994)

CEP's consumer guide rates several hundred companies on the basis of environmental performance, charitable donations, community outreach programs, women's and minority advancement, support for family-oriented employment policies, workplace issues, and information disclosure policies. The CEP Honor Roll recognizes firms that score especially well on these cri-teria, while the so-called X-rated list is reserved for the poorest performers. Consumers can use these assessments to guide their purchase decisions on virtually any product.

Social Accountability International (SIA), an affiliate of CEP, serves as the accreditation agency for these evaluations. Launched during the early 1990s in response to the weak and incompatible guidelines that individual firms were developing, SAI's mission is to create standards for workplace codes of con-duct and labor conditions worldwide. The group's first standard was Social Accountability 8000 (SA 8000), which provides a uniform measure for assess-ing workplace conditions and for independently gauging the compliance of specific industrial facilities. SA 8000 seeks to define objectively the relative quality of the workplace, and then to translate this information to consumers so that they can respond accordingly.

Co-op America, an NGO established in 1982 with a current membership of 50,000 individuals and 2,000 businesses, seeks to educate and empower peo-ple and organizations to use the economic system to promote positive change.

Within the constellation of American advocacy organizations, Co-op America is unique in that it does not campaign for equity and justice using conventional political or legal strategies; rather staff members strive to reorient economic relationships by promoting more conscientious consumer expenditures. The approach consists of two interlocking elements: Co-op America, on one hand, helps consumers identify companies that are committed to socially and environmentally acceptable practices and, on the other hand, assists companies to operate under these stricter standards. The organization coordinates several initiatives, including a green business program, a consumer education program, a corporate responsibility program, and a sustainable living program.

Global Exchange is a California-based human rights organization committed to environmental, political, and social justice. The group's campaigns promote democratic ideals and political empowerment both in the United States and abroad, and seek to highlight the connections between corrupt political systems and human rights abuses. In recent years, countries in which Global Exchange has been active include Brazil, Cuba, Colombia, and Mexico. Though its operational strategies vary across countries, the organization does not aim simply to press employers to pay better wages. Rather, Global Exchange seeks to improve human rights by educating people about oppressive political and social organizations.

Closely connected to the campaign for ethical consumption is the effort to support so-called fair trade as an alternative means of exchange (Rice, 2001; Browne et al., 2000). This strategy seeks to sidestep complex issues embedded in the political economy of globalization by directly linking ethical consumers with socially and environmentally conscientious growers and manufacturers. The intent is to simplify distribution to ensure that a larger portion of the sales price accrues to indigenous farmers and small-scale producers. By selling fair trade products at premium prices, sponsors offset higher transaction costs. TransFair USA, the leading fair trade organization in the country, works closely with the Fair Trade Federation (FTF). FTF is a network of retailers, wholesalers, and producers that have agreed to comply with a code of conduct calling for schemes that offer employees opportunities for advancement, provide equal employment opportunities, and engage in environmentally sustainable practices.

For the past decade, coffee has had an especially prominent position on the fair trade agenda. Coffee is the second largest commodity import in the United States (after oil) and Americans annually consume 20 percent of the world's total production. At the same time, the tendency for coffee plantations to promote unsafe and unhealthy working conditions has been a long-standing point of discussion (Tucker, 2000). To ameliorate some of the problems associated with coffee production, fair trade proponents have sought to educate consumers about the benefits of purchasing their beans from cooperatives, of avoiding higher yield varieties that require greater sun intensity (to discourage deforestation and biodiversity loss), and of supporting growers that pay workers equitable wages.

Increasingly, consumers are demanding fair trade coffee, and major purveyors such as Starbucks have been encountering pressure from their customers to offer a fair trade alternative. At present, fair trade coffee comprises only 1% of the global market with the majority of sales taking place through specialized fair trade retailers—many of them operating via the Internet. However, after considerable pressure from stakeholders, food industry giants such as Kraft and Proctor and Gamble have recently announced plans to launch fair trade coffee brands.

A related area of activism has sought to highlight the migration of garment manufacturing to low-wage havens in the developing world. Laborers working under substandard conditions throughout Asia and Latin America sew most of the clothing worn today by relatively affluent people in economically advanced countries. Developing countries often find themselves in the unfortunate position of bidding against one another to convince large corporations and their subcontractors to set up these facilities (Ross, 1997: see also Gonzalez, 2003).

In 1997, municipal officials in North Olmstead (Ohio) realized that nearly all of the garments their city purchased—from athletic equipment to police uniforms—came from overseas sweatshops. This recognition encouraged the city to pass the first law in the United States banning a government from purchasing products manufactured under sweatshop conditions. This initiative led to the notion of "sweat-free cities" and induced a number of major municipalities (including San Francisco, Cleveland, Philadelphia, and New York) to pass similar legislation.

The movement to protest the globalization of clothing manufacturing has moved from the chambers of municipal governments to college and university campuses. Indeed, the opposition to sweatshop labor has spurred one of the largest and most vocal forms of student activism in recent years. Directed by the group United Students Against Sweatshops, this wave of protest politics started when students began to examine their institutions ties to companies such as Nike and Reebok. The organization currently campaigns against "campus sweat" and has assembled a network of over 200 colleges and universities.

Action on many campuses has involved the elimination of sweatshop clothing adorned with the insignias of some of the most esteemed colleges and universities in the United States. To counter these protests, the Collegiate Licensing Company, a consortium of major educational institutions that negotiates with the distributors of these products, published a code of conduct and encouraged participating firms to endorse it. Because student activists viewed this assurance as insufficient—it did not contain a clause requiring full public disclosure, a provision demanding a living wage, or a statement concerning women's rights—this defensive action only intensified campus demonstrations.

The effort to resist the importation of apparel manufactured under substandard conditions has also given rise to a more general campaign. Leading this struggle has been the group Sweatshop Watch, an eclectic coalition of trade unions, civil rights groups, and immigrant rights organizations committed to eliminating sweatshop production. Sweatshop Watch focuses on both the domestic (especially California) and international dimensions of this form of exploitation.

The Slow Food Movement

Originally launched in 1989 by Carlo Petrini in response to the establishment of the first McDonald's restaurant in Rome, the slow food movement has assumed international significance and now maintains offices in Italy, Switzerland, Germany, and the United States (Kummer, 2002; Petrini, 2001). The major aims of the movement are to celebrate the joy of wholesome and nutritious food and to protect the gastronomic traditions of the: world's cultures in the face of the interlocking forces of modernization, standardization, and globalization. International membership in the slow food movement's 600 chapters, or *convivia*, has reached 70,000 food aficionados in 45 countries.

Slow food adherents argue for the importance of preserving the pleasures and qualities of everyday life from the relentless pursuit of speed and purported convenience by slowing down, and by celebrating traditional lifestyles. Though the movement does adopt some of the rhetoric of anti-globalization activists, particularly in terms of the threats posed by industrially produced food, the slow food movement does not embrace the rancorous political edge common among supporters of the wider campaign (Miele & Murdoch, 2002: Jones et al., 2003). In addition to apprehension about globalization foodies (in slow food parlance) express concern over what they interpret to be a ceaseless barrage of food regulations from national and multinational authorities. Instituted to promote food safety, many of these provisions have jeopardized the traditional food preparation methods favored by specialty businesses and

local food artisans.[15] The slow-food movement has not been passive in the face
of these regulatory directives, and the European wing of the international organization recently opened an office in Brussels to lobby against these measures. The effectiveness of slow food adherents has proved formidable, and
foodies delivered a petition to the European Commission with half-a-million
signatures demanding exemptions to many of the hygiene rules. In response
to these efforts, Italy received special dispensations for thousands of its small
food producers (Stille, 2001).

In addition to its commitment to the preservation of local culture, slow
food also embraces a certain environmental sensibility. Adherents support
"sustainability and biodiversity of the earth's bounty" as well as the consumption of seasonal and local foods (Nabhan, 2002). This particular brand of ecological consciousness shares many similarities with the sentiments expressed
by hunting and birding enthusiasts. Just as wildlife proponents are motivated
to protect valued habitats, the slow food's ecological commitments are tied to
the production of healthy and wholesome food.[16]

While much of the slow food movement's organizational resources remain
in Europe, it has had some notable success developing a base in the United
States. At present, more than 7.000 members subscribe to 70 American convivia and produce a national publication aptly named *The Snail*. The guiding
values of Slow Food USA are sustainability, cultural diversity, pleasure and
quality in everyday life, inclusiveness, and authenticity and integrity. One of
the major programs sponsored by the American arm of the movement is "Ark
USA" (part of the worldwide "Ark of Taste"). Ark USA seeks to identify, Protect,
and promote indigenous foods deemed to be in danger of "extinction." Slow
Food USA has established a committee that maintains a data bank to collect
information on cultivars, breeds, products, and producers, as well as restaurants and shops that sell Ark products. In the eyes of some observers, this project provides the slow food movement with a greater semblance of legitimacy
than it would otherwise have if it were simply dedicated to the pleasures of
indulging in traditional foods.[17]

The worldwide success of slow food, and its call for simpler lifestyles, has
inspired more ambitious activities in recent years and led to the establishment
of a new organizational infrastructure. Towns and cities around the world
are pledging to promote urban planning agendas geared toward improving
the quality of life by reducing the frenetic pace of social activity. Launched in
Italy in 2000, "Slow Cities" is an international organization that seeks to build
upon the successes of the slow food movement. If the intent of slow food is to
preserve the integrity and traditions of deliberate culinary pleasures, then the
slow cities offshoot is its geographic equivalent.

Designation as a slow city entails permitting more neighborhood restaurants, combating traffic and noise pollution, facilitating bicycling, planting trees, and maintaining parks and urban squares. These requirements translate into more practical measures: banning car alarms, television antennas, and neon signs. Slow cities are also encouraged to enlarge pedestrian areas and to move automobile parking lots to the edges of city centers. While these initiatives are only likely to be practicable for smaller cities, this does not mean that larger municipalities are discouraged from pursuing slow city status. To date, only four Italian cities (Orvieto, Greve, Bra, and Positano) have secured formal recognition as slow cities and a further forty jurisdictions in Italy are being considered for certification.[18] There are no American municipalities presently up for nomination to become slow cities, though given the similar commitments of slow cities and new urbanism it is likely only a matter of time before a worthy candidate steps forward.

Public Policy and Sustainable Consumption

As noted earlier, sustainable development has not been a central issue for governmental planning in the United States, and the adverse impacts of consumption have been even further removed from mainstream public policy agendas. Despite his loose endorsement of sustainability, President Clinton did little to advance the issue, and the current Bush administration has pursued an avowedly anti-environmental political program. Nonetheless, if one adopts a broad-minded view of sustainable consumption, there are indeed a number of officially sanctioned initiatives taking place in the United States that are fully consistent with the aims of this policy program.

Local Greenhouse Gas Reduction Schemes

While anthropogenic climate change has become, over the past two decades, a central international environmental policy issue, the American federal government continues to postpone substantive actions to reduce the country's greenhouse gas emissions. The lack of national action in this area has left a void that a handful of environmentally progressive states are now stepping forward to fill. Several states have created their own greenhouse gas reduction schemes and, among the northeastern states, a promising effort is afoot to create a regional market for trading emission credits (Johnson, 2003a).[19] The following section reviews the individual climate change policies of three of these states—New Jersey, New Hampshire, and Massachusetts.[20]

First, the New Jersey Department of Environmental Protection (NJDEP) issued in 1998 an administrative order calling for a statewide greenhouse gas reduction of 3.5% by 2005.[21] To support this objective, two years later NJDEP released the New Jersey Sustainability Green House Gas (GHG) Action Plan that advances strategies to achieve reductions in several specific areas, including energy conservation, transportation, innovative technologies, pollution prevention, waste management and recycling, and open space and natural resources protection. To measure progress, the plan establishes indicators predicated upon the total volume of GHG emissions (based on data developed by the Energy Information Agency), commuting by public transport, and annual mean surface air temperature.

Second, New Hampshire governor Jeanne Shaheen signed the Clean Power Act (CPA) into law in 2002. This legislation represented a milestone for state-level climate change policymaking, as it was the first instance in which a state required power plants to implement a four-pollutant emission reduction program. The CPA calls upon electric utilities operating in New Hampshire to cut their releases of sulfur dioxide, nitrogen oxides, mercury, and carbon dioxide by implementing new pollution control technologies or by participating in emission trading schemes. Because of the state's susceptibility to transboundary air pollution from other states, the CPA makes it more expensive for electric utilities to purchase emission credits from facilities outside of the region.[22]

Finally, Massachusetts, through implementation of its voluntary environmental stewardship program, represents a different state-based approach to sustainability and greenhouse gas reduction. This program requires participating businesses to commit to improve, over a three-year period, at least four aspects of their environmental performance. Intended for companies that already have environmental management systems in place and are in full compliance with all environmental regulations, this initiative seeks to secure improvements in energy conservation, water use, toxics, air emissions, discharges to water, solid and hazardous waste management, and product performance.

On a complementary front, the International Council for Local Environmental Initiatives (ICLEI) assists municipal and county governments in the United States and elsewhere in organizing their own proactive anti-climate change policies. ICLEI, a new institutional entity that operates under United Nations auspices, serves, in its own words, as the "international environmental agency for local governments" (International Council). Through the provision of policy guidance, training, and technical assistance, the organization presently serves more than 350 sub-national governmental units that are committed to building a global movement of localities committed to sustainable development.

ICLEI has developed its Cities for Climate Protection Campaign (CCP) to support local governments in formulating and implementing policies to achieve measurable local greenhouse gas reductions, to improve air quality, and to enhance urban livability and sustainability. Two cities in the United States that exemplify the ICLEI's mission are Burlington, Vermont and Austin, Texas.

Both residents and visitors frequently characterize Burlington as a politically liberal community with a palpable new-age ethos, though this description captures only a portion of what invariably is a much more complex political economy. Throughout the 1980s and 1990s, the municipal government championed environmental and social projects that established a nascent culture of sustainabilty.[23] In partnership with ICLEI, Burlington has begun to formulate an alternative community model, one rooted in the ideals of sustainability and good urban governance. Much of the city's sustainability planning has occurred within the context of its so-called Legacy Project, a multi-stakeholder initiative that aims to embrace residents from all communities and economic sectors and to initiate a dialogue for giving direction to local development over the next thirty years. The program calls upon people to articulate this vision of the future in accordance with five major themes: economy, neighborhoods, governance, youth and life skills, and environment. The challenge for municipal leaders has been to reconcile Burlington's seemingly inevitable growth with its commitment to sustainability. The city's pioneering experience with sustainability planning has brought forth two especially notable outcomes. The Burlington Eco-Info Project provides residents with easy access to data on local air, water, land, and energy trends, and the Education for Sustainability Program trains schoolteachers to incorporate sustainability issues into their curricula.

Many observers admire Austin, the capital of Texas and home to the state university's main campus, for its relatively progressive municipal politics.[24] The city's CCP campaign seeks to shift 5% of local electricity production to renewable sources. To meet this objective, Austin's municipally owned utility has implemented a variable pricing scheme to induce residents to favor nonpolluting forms of electricity. In this manner, Austin expects renewable energy to account for approximately one half of its expected increase in electricity demand . By generating 340 million kw/year from renewable sources primarily wind—this Texas city will reduce its annual carbon dioxide emissions by approximately 255,000 tons.

Relocalization Schemes

In the United States over the past decade, there has been an outpouring of public policy initiatives to bolster local economic autonomy. Campaigns to

encourage consumers to buy indigenously produced goods, to support community-based agriculture, and to legitimize local currency programs have proliferated.[25] This wave of relocalization is, to a large extent, a defensive reaction
to the forces of globalization that are disembedding economic activities from
their situated contexts. Efforts to promote relocalization can be quite diverse,
but they all share the objective of enhancing the sustainability of community
enterprises and rekindling direct relationships between producers and consumers. This section reviews three broad categories of this phenomenon: local
promotion schemes, novel modes of agricultural production and consumption, and local currency programs.

First, the mantra to "buy American," especially during periods of nationalist fervor or economic retrenchment, is familiar to consumers across the
United States. Over the past two decades, states and cities have refashioned
this strategy to promote the relocalization of economic activity by encouraging
consumers to favor locally produced goods and services. Examples of these
so-called "buy local" campaigns can be found in virtually all parts of the country and take a variety of different forms. For instance, the Savannah, Georgia
Chamber of Commerce organizes a drive to support local businesses through
public education and the distribution of "buy local" emblems.[26] A business
promotion group in western North Carolina utilizes a logo to promote local
commerce with the slogan, "Buy Local—Western North Carolina is Worth
It."[27] An organization in Pittsburgh, Pennsylvania, encourages consumers to
purchase compact discs from local musicians.[28]

Agricultural commodities—especially fruits and vegetables—have been
especially popular targets for policy initiatives to relocalize consumption. The
sophistication of buy local schemes has improved markedly over the years, and
appeals to geographic familiarity today are likely to rely on integrated promotional strategies developed by professional marketing specialists.[29] While all
states use this approach to varying degrees, New Jersey, New York, California,
and Massachusetts have demonstrated the most consistent commitment.

First, New Jersey claims to be the first state in the country to launch a
local campaign to promote its homegrown agricultural products. State agricultural officials began marketing local produce under the slogan "Jersey Fresh"
in 1983. The campaign has utilized radio, television, and billboards, as well
as colorful signage in supermarkets, to encourage consumers to purchase
local agriculture. The state's department of agriculture also provides grants to
marketing associations that would like to sell their products in more distant
locales. For instance, organizations designed to promote specific crops use the
Jersey Fresh moniker to advertise to consumers in Virginia and Montreal.[30] In
this way, the campaign has evolved into a regional marketing tool to increase

state exports, undermining claims that this program is ultimately about fostering local sustainability.

Second, New York has devised a similar approach to market its agricultural products. The state's department of agriculture uses the slogan "Pride of New York" to persuade consumers to buy locally grown produce. The New York campaign relics largely on conventional advertising and in-store displays to showcase the state's agricultural products. In addition to this statewide program, New York's distinct regions have initiated their own promotional efforts to relocalize consumption at an even more proximate level of geographic scale {Hilchey, 2000; see also Moskin, 2004).

Third, agriculture officials in California have developed a coordinated program for marketing the state's prodigious output of fruits and vegetables to local consumers. This promotional effort is part of the state' s familiar and long-standing export-oriented campaigns to encourage the consumption of locally grown raisins and peaches. More recent initiatives to relocalize consumption at the sub-state level in Placer and Sonoma Counties are typical of programs launched elsewhere in California. Placer County utilizes the conventional portfolio of marketing strategies, including print and radio advertising, public education, and supermarket displays, to enhance public awareness of local agriculture. Sonoma County, in part because of its reliance on wine production, has begun to formulate appeals that stress not only that local products are "Sonoma Grown," but that they are: "Sonoma Made" as well.[31]

Finally, Massachusetts appears to have the most sophisticated campaign to promote the relocalization of agricultural production and consumption. The state's success is largely attributable to the creation of an array of public-private partnerships, and to savvy marketing. Agriculture officials in Massachusetts have set up a separate division called "Massgrown" that provides financial and logistical resources to support state agricultural products, and that licenses its slogan: "MASS grown... and fresher!" The state also actively supports farmers' markets, "agritourism," and pick-your-own farms.[32] Despite its relatively small size, Massachusetts has also promoted the development of several sub-state level promotional initiatives. Especially notable is Community Involved in Sustaining Agriculture (CISA), an organization dedicated to encouraging the consumption of agricultural produce from the western part of the state. ClSA actively draws attention to how the programs it facilitates can offset the damaging affects of globalization, and its campaign slogan, "Be a Local Hero-Buy Locally Grown." has attracted national attention.

While the proliferation of buy local campaigns has been widespread, policymakers in the United States have actually been employing a much broader portfolio of strategies to promote the relocalization of food production and consumption. Three notable innovations include community-supported agriculture (CSA), direct marketing of agricultural produce, and community gardening.

CSAs are a latent outgrowth of profound demographic shifts in the United States. The process of rural-urban migration that has reshaped the national landscape over more than 100 years was accompanied (and in many instances motivated by) sweeping technological advances in agricultural efficiency and automated product processing (Hinrichs, 2000). As the size of farmholdings increased and people were displaced from local agricultural economics, they sought new opportunities in the expanding cities. At present, less than 2% of the American population is directly engaged in farming. The disappearance of the American family farm has become a popular focal point for critiques highlighting the dark side of capitalism and globalization.

It is from this nexus that CSAs have grown, and there are today an estimated 1,000 of these agricultural enterprises operating across the country.[33] A CSA consists of a community of consumers who enter into a seasonal "subscription" agreement with a local farm. In return for a preseason payment (normally a few hundred dollars), the farm owner supplies his subscribers with fresh agricultural products on a weekly basis. Farmers and subscribers satisfy one another's respective needs. On one hand, farmers obtain access to a flexible form of financing and a direct distribution channel for their produce. On the other hand, subscribers receive a personal connection to the food they are consuming and the knowledge that it comes from a local source. The relationship is also founded on the fact that most CSAs are committed to sustainable farming practices, and that subscribers often contribute their own labor during the growing season. Hence, a system has evolved in which both farmers and subscribers can insulate themselves from industrialized modes of agriculture and get a foothold for relocalizing themselves against the forces of mass consumerism and globalization.[34]

Another form of alternative production and consumption of agricultural produce is the concept of "direct marketing," which entails the distribution of fruits and vegetables without reliance on corporate mechanisms. While CSAs fall within this rubric, another common example is the growing popularity of farmers' markets (Grey, 2000). Farmers' markets are as old as agriculture itself. but their numbers began to wane in the United States following World War II with the advent of the modern supermarket. By 1960 there were fewer than 100 farmers' markets nationwide. During the past two decades, there has been renewed interest in this mode of engaging producers and consumers and today there are an estimated 2,400 farmers' markets operating around the country. The resurgence of this mode of direct marketing is in part attributable to a backlash against mainstream agriculture. The success of farmers' markets resides in their ability to exploit the anonymity of the industrial food system with its tendency to produce goods that must conform to standardized guidelines regarding size, color, taste, and so forth.

A final, if understated, example of the innovative production and consumption of agricultural produce is provided by community gardening (see, for example, von Hassell, 2002). There are more than 10,000 community gardens in the United States, many of them located in the country's most economically depressed neighborhoods. The transitory and uncertain disposition of the land parcels used to operate community gardening schemes often means that it is difficult for devotees to gain secure title to their plots. However, policymakers in some cities—New York City has one of the largest and most successful community garden programs in the country—have devised strategies to ensure long-term tenancy.

Proponents of community gardening often frame the practice as an opportunity for low-income urban residents to reconnect to the local environment and to gain a degree of political empowerment—while at the same time growing their own wholesome food. Viewed from a slightly different perspective, it becomes apparent that community gardening is also an instance of the relocalization of agriculture and the promotion of sustainable consumption.

While local promotion schemes and innovations in agriculture both clearly demonstrate a trend in the United States toward new consumption practices, the most conscious and dedicated efforts to create systems of proximate exchange are local currency initiatives. Long before national governments began issuing their own legal tender, and before monetary policy became a central function of centralized authorities, local currency was the norm. The modernization of national economics, however, has meant the demise of community-based scrip (Helleiner, 2002). More recently, a number of cities in the United States have seen the emergence of local currency schemes (or local exchange trading systems) designed to strengthen the local economy by stemming the outflow of money to distant locations and facilitating meaningful relationships between buyers and sellers.

The precise organizational characteristics of different systems vary, but the essential features are that the scheme is self-regulating and allows users to manage the money supply within a set of specified boundaries (normally a single municipality). Specially designated script serves as the means of exchange and participants negotiate the value they will attach to particular exchange transactions (organizers generally peg the value of a currency unit, and its exchange rate with conventional currency, according to the average hourly wage in the community).

Local currency systems began to develop a following in the early 1980s with the introduction of the first modern scheme on Vancouver Island, British Columbia. At present, there are an estimated sixty communities in the United States with some form of local currency, with especially vibrant systems operating in Ithaca, New York and Madison, Wisconsin (Shuman, 1998). What many of these cities share is a recognition that globalization is a doubled-edged sword and that local currency systems can ameliorate some of the dislocation and instability that frequently comes in its wake.

Consumer Credit

The use of consumer credit to drive the cycle of production and consumption in the United States is a relatively new phenomenon. The country's move away from a cash economy to a credit economy has enabled consumers to embrace the instantaneous gratification that comes from being able to purchase goods without the need to save first for extended periods. An outcome of the widespread availability of credit cards, coupled with the endless enticements of mass consumerism, has contributed to an array of social problems associated with the accumulation of large personal debt loads and financial insolvency (Warren & Warren-Tyagi, 2003: Calder, 1999). The easy availability of consumer credit, often carrying exorbitant interest rates, contributed to a wave of consumer activism during the late 1960s, and this political agitation gave rise to the first generation of modern consumer protection legislation. The most notable public policy initiative to curb unscrupulous purveyors of credit was the Consumer Credit Protection Act (CCPA) of 1968. In particular, the CCPA's so-called truth-in-lending provisions require lenders to state in clear language the terms and conditions of their offers.

Despite this groundbreaking legislation, the past thirty years have seen a massive accumulation of consumer debt in the United States. By 1999, per capita consumer debt had exceeded $30.000, nearly 50% more than it had been ten years earlier. Overall, American consumers are now in debt to the tune of $2 trillion, with approximately one-third of this amount payable on high-interest credit cards. The typical American household carried forward each month $7,500 in unpaid credit card debt, a two-fold increase in just ten years. 13% of families in the United States have outstanding balances that exceed 40% of their household income, a situation that means 90% of each monthly payment is solely dedicated to paying interest. The inevitable outcome of this situation is an ever-mounting number of personal bankruptcies—more than 1.3 million in 1999 alone.

As vendors have saturated the credit card market, they have aggressively sought to cultivate new markets, especially among university students. These companies regularly organize carnival-type promotional events, complete with loud music, games, and gifts. Accordingly, 32% of undergraduate students had four or more credit cards in 2000, and the average overall credit card balance was more than $2,700. Nearly 10% of these students owed more than $7,000 on their credit cards.[35]

In response to this dilemma, many universities now offer bankruptcy counseling to their students, and at all levels of education new courses in financial literacy have become part of the curriculum. There has even been new legislation to restrict campus access for credit card vendors and to tighten lending terms (USGAO, 2001). For instance, the College Student Credit Card Protection Act (CSCCPA) of 1999 imposes a number of new standards, including a restriction on issuing large-limit accounts to student, a prohibition on increasing credit limits without a parental co-signer, and a disallowance of open-ended consumer credit plans for full-time students with no annual income.

Conclusion

Though it is possible to point to various efforts to catalyze a new public dialogue about consumerism in American society, the question remains whether this inchoate activity has the potential to coalesce into a coherent social movement. It is probably too early to offer any firm assessments, but the mélange of initiatives described above does seem to denote a certain level of public discomfort in the United States—at least among some social segments—with contemporary mass consumption. Of noteworthy interest is that this unease does not stem primarily from concern about accumulating ecological harm, and environmental themes are at best peripheral considerations for Americans skeptical of consumerist lifestyles. In this sense, the oppositional political agenda developing around consumption in the United States is—at least for the moment—less about "sustainable" consumption than it is about "critical" consumption.

Public opinion polling has regularly demonstrated the prevalence of environmental values in the United States, but these sensibilities tend to be relatively shallow and superficial. For instance, environmental politics rarely plays a major role in determining the outcome of American elections, and few voters in the country cast their ballots according to candidates' environmental records.[36] For this reason, there is a certain futility in propounding a political program to address the growing social problematization of consumption in the United States with appeals to how environmental gains will derive from more purposive lifestyles. While the clumsiness that accompanies environmentalists' efforts to talk about consumption is evidence of some profound difficulties, scrappy organizations such as the Center for the New American Dream appear to have learned this lesson. To the extent that critical consumption matures as a domestic political discourse, it will almost invariably be driven by relatively prosaic concerns about, for instance, working hours, leisure time, and family life, An array of less tangible misgivings about the insidious affects of commercialism and the lack of authenticity engendered by consumerist lifestyles may also prove important.

All of this suggests that efforts to reconfigure consumption practices in the affluent countries will proceed along different trajectories, and will be conditioned in specific places by political culture and institutional constraints. It is difficult to imagine an American political administration, regardless of party affiliation, embracing a meaningful program to move the country toward alternative modes of consumption, The economic risks are simply too high and the political payoffs too elusive. Progress in the United States to realign consumption practices will come from a combination of social activism and targeted resistance, but first it will be necessary for the various strands of the nascent critical consumption movement to forge a common identity and to launch a new politics of consumption.

NOTES

1 It is also important not to underestimate the monumental obstacles to sustainable development in the United States. For instance, income among Americans is more unevenly distributed than it has been in half a century and the country has the greatest income inequality among economically advanced nations. Moreover, while European nations have made considerable strides modernizing their environmental policymaking institutions during the past decade, the United Slates remains strongly committed to an increasingly ineffectual administrative model.

2 Anti-consumerism activists are actually reticent about employing the term "sustainable consumption" because of suspicions about the international organizations that are responsible for its popularization.

3 For instance, individuals associated with the Earth Liberation Front (ELF) have destroyed new suburban homes under construction and, perhaps most famously, burned down a $12 million ski lodge in Colorado (Brown, 2003).

4 Although *Adbusters* is based in Canada, American consumers constitute its primary focal point and most of the magazine's subscribers are based in the United States (Lindsay. 2002).

5 The group Project Billboard employs similar strategies to communicate anti-war and other messages of political protest. The organization was recently involved in a dispute with Clear Channel Communications over a provocative billboard that would be visible to participants at the Republican National Convention in New York City (Preston. 2004).

6 At this point, culture jamming begins to meld with other more familiar forms of political protest associated with certain radical environmental organizations in the United States.

7 See the letter endorsed by the American Medical Association and other allied organizations in support of TV-Turnoff Week, available at http://www.tvturnoff. org/healthgroups%20pr%2002.htm.

8 In a related vein, critics denounce television for reducing political awareness because the medium encourages viewers to focus their attention on fictional characters rather than real events. TVFA contends that 59% of Americans can name all of the Three Stooges, while only 17% can identify three justices on the Supreme Court.

9 An especially prominent focus for activists seeking to limit advertising to children has been to block the penetration of promotional inducements in schools. In recent years, as school districts have struggled with the rising costs of education, a growing number of them have turned to advertising as a supplemental source of revenue. At many schools, it is customary for corporate marketing messages to appear on book covers, hallways, athletic facilities, and buses. Especially prominent are soda manufacturers that have negotiated exclusive "pouring" contracts to sell their products in vending machines and at school events. Sponsored educational materials are also regularly mailed free of charge to teachers and principals for use in the classroom.

10 While CCFPE and many of the groups that are part of its alliance promote secular values, evangelical Christian organizations have also targeted *Channel One*. Obligation and the Eagle Forum are two groups that oppose the advertising, as well as the programming, on *Channel One* on religious grounds. These organizations coordinate boycotts of *Channel One's* parent company and offer parents a "tool kit" for removing the news service from their children's schools. As a mark of its political sophistication, this activist network has reached beyond its traditional base to recruit into their fold many national education associations.

11 A measure of the high level of concern that exists regarding the effects of advertising on children is that this campaign is not confined to groups of intrepid grassroots activists. For instance, the American Academy of Pediatrics took a stand on the issue in 1995 that called for more vigorous regulation of advertising aimed at children.

12 Many other anti-smoking groups, such as the American Lung Association and the Coalition for Women Against Smoking, oppose tobacco advertisements, but they do not make it the main focus of their campaigns.

13 There now exists a federal do-not-call list designed to limit intrusive telemarketing appeals (Richtel, 2003).

14 Consistent with the approach taken by this analysis is the tendency among self-described voluntary simplifiers to reject the contention that they are carriers of a broader political agenda. Adherents of simpler lifestyles are likely to equate social movements with superficial changes in "style of life" (as opposed to more penetrating changes in "way of life"). The extended comments of one of Elgin's respondents are illuminating: "This is a country of media hype, and [simple living] is good copy. The media is likely to pick up on it...and create a movement. I hope they won't. The changes we're talking about are fundamental and take a lot of time... If it is made into a movement, it could bum itself out. I hope it spreads slowly. This way the changes will be more pervasive, Voluntary Simplicity is the kind of thing that people need to discover for themselves."

15 For example, the European Union's food and sanitary regulations stipulate that the traditional curing of Tuscan pig lard be done in stainless steel containers, instead of marble vats. Advocates of the traditional process argue that the marble vats are essential to creating the right flavor and texture for the lard. Another rule prohibits baking pizzas in traditional wood-burning ovens that contain carcinogenic ash (Smith, 2000).

16 One commentator has called Slow Food the "gastronomic version of Greenpeace: a defiant determination to preserve unprocessed, time-intensive food from being wiped off the culinary map" (Osborne. 2001).

17 The number of endangered foods listed in the Ark of Taste program numbers ninety worldwide, with nine of them indigenous to the United Stales: Dry Monterey Jack Cheese, Green Mountain Potatoes, Blenheim Apricots, Creole Cream Cheese, Heritage Turkeys, New Mexican Native Chiles, Delaware Bay Oysters, Heritage Clone Zinfandel, and naturally grown wild rice.

18 Full accreditation is currently pending for forty cities, including Canale, Loreto, Penne, Todi, and Trevi (Kennedy, 2001).

19 The Conference of New England Governors and Eastern Canadian Premiers in 2000 also adopted a coordinated climate change plan that includes regional targets, state and provincial commitments to implement their own greenhouse gas reduction schemes, and statements of intent to develop specially tailored educational outreach programs.

20 In addition to the northeastern stales, California has also been a leader in the development of a state-level greenhouse gas reduction program.

21 The target is calculated in CO_2 equivalent units and requires the state to reduce its greenhouse gas emissions by approximately 20 million CO_2 equivalent tons (NJDEP, 1999). Current projections indicate that the state will likely not achieve its reduction target, largely because of increases in emissions from transport vehicles.

22 The CPA calls for annual emission reductions of 75% for sulfur dioxide and 70% for nitrogen oxides by the end of 2006 and a reduction of carbon dioxide 1990 levels by 2010.

23 See the website at http://www3.iclei.org/localstrategies/sumrnary/burlington2.html.

24 See the website at http://www3.icIei.org/iclei/casedetail.cfm?pid=40.

25 During the aftermath of the attacks against the World Trade Center and the Pentagon, these appeals have assumed a certain nationalistic significance. Promotional inducements now regularly beseech consumers to purchase domestic (and indeed local) goods and services as a patriotic gesture (Shenon, 2001; Rather, 200l). A similar phenomenon occurred immediately following the capture of Saddam Hussein in Iraq (Morgan. 2003).

26 See the website http://www.buylocalsavannah.com.

27 See the website http://www.mtnmicro.org/pages/about_us/subsidiaries html.

28 See the website http://www.mtnmicro.org/pages/about_us/subsidiaries.html.

29 A cursory review of these initiatives suggests that geographically defined regions within particular states have developed more proficient programs for promoting their agricultural products.

30 See the website http://www.state.nj.us/agriculture/markets/jerseyfresh.htm.

31 See the websites http://www,sonoma-county.org/agcomm/pdf/2001_Crop_Report.pdf and http://www placergrown.com.

32 See the website http://www.state.ma.us/dfa/massgrown/index.htm.

33 As described by Cone & Myhre (2000), the CSA concept actually developed in Japan and Europe prior to coming to the United States. The first CSA in the country was established in western Massachusetts in 1985.

34 So-called buying clubs, which are gaining in popularity in some cities, represent a variation of the essential CSA concept (Johnson, 2003b).

35 Nellie Mae, a quasi-government agency that issues education loans, conducts an annual survey of credit card usage among students. See the website http://www.nelliemae.com/library/research_8.html.

36 The bizarre outcome that characterized the presidential election in 2000 is more an exception than the rule. George W, Bush 's victory was, at least in part, attributable to the Green Party's ability in diverting several thousand votes from Vice-President Al Gore in Florida. Had Gore been able to secure even a few hundred of these ballots, he would have prevailed in Florida and the protracted controversy surrounding the election's outcome would have been averted.

REFERENCES

Alterman, E. & Green, M. 2004. *The Book on Bush: How George W. Bush (Mis)Leads America*, New York: Viking.

Andrews, R. 1999. *Managing the Environment, Managing Ourselves. A History of American Environmental Policy*, New Haven: Yale University Press.

Barnouw, E. 1990. *Tube of Plenty: The Evolution of American Television*, 2nd ed., New York: Oxford University Press.

Bender, D. & R. Greenwald (Eds.). 2003. *Sweatshop USA: The American Sweatshop in Historical and Global Perspective*, New York: Routledge.

Bhagwati, J. 2002. "Coping with antiglobalization: A trilogy of discontents," *Foreign Affairs* 81(1):2–7.

Bordwell, M. 2002. "Jamming culture: Adbusters' hip media campaign against consumerism," pp. 237–253 in T. Princen, M. Maniates, & K. Conca (Eds.), *Confronting Consumption*, Cambridge. MA: MIT Press.

Boyles, D. 1998. *American Education and Corporations: The Free Market Goes to School*, New York: Garland.

Broad, R. (Ed.). 2002. *Global Backlash: Citizen Initiatives for a Just World Economy*, Lanham, MD: Rowman and Littlefield.

Brown, P. 2003. "Enabling and disabling, ecoterrorists," *The New York Times*, November 16 (section 4): 14.

Browne, A., P. Harris, A. Hofny-Collins, N. Pasieczmk, & R. Wallace. 2000. "Organic production and ethical trade: definition, practice, and links," *Food Policy* 25(1):69–89.

Bryner, G. 2000. "The United States: sorry—not our problem," pp. 373–302 in W. Lafferty & J. Meadowcroft (Eds.), *Implementing Sustainable Development: Strategies and Initiatives in High Consumption Societies*, New York: Oxford University Press.

Calder, L. 1999. *Financing the American Dream: A Cultural History of Consumer Credit*, Princeton: Princeton University Press.

CEP, Council on Economic Priorities. 1994. *Shopping for a Better World: The Quick and Easy Guide to All Your Socially Responsible Shopping*, San Francisco: Sierra Club Books.

Clarke, A. & Kurtz-Costes, B. 1997. "Television viewing, educational quality of the home environment, and school readiness," *Journal of Educational Research* 90(5):279–285.

Cohen, M. 2004. "George W. Bush and the Environmental Protection Agency: A midterm appraisal," *Society and Natural Resources* 17(1):69–88.

Cone, C. & Myhre, A. 2000. "Community-supported agriculture: A sustainable alternative to industrial agriculture?" *Human Organization* 59(2):187–197.

Coon, K., Goldberg, J., Rogers, B., & Tucker, K. 2001. "Relationships between use of television during meals and children's food consumption patterns," *Pediatrics* 107(1):167.

Craig-Lees, M. & Hill, C. 2002. "Understanding voluntary simplifiers," *Psychology and Marketing* 19(2):187–210.

Crespo, C., Smit, E., Troiano, R., Bartlett, S., Macera, C., & Andersen, R. 2001. "Television Watching, Energy Intake, and Obesity in US Children: Results from the Third National Health and Nutrition Examination Study, 1988–1994," *Archives of Pediatrics and Adolescent Medicine* 155:360–365.

Dacyczyn, A. 1998. *The Complete Tightwad Gazette: Promoting Thrift as a Viable Alternative Lifestyle*, New York: Villard Books.

DeGraaf, J., D. Wann, T. Naylor, D. Horsey, & S. Simon. 2002. *Affluenza: The All-Consuming Epidemic*, San Francisco: Berrett-Koehler.

DeVaney, A. (Ed.). 1994. *Watching Channel One: The Convergence of Students, Technology, and Private Business*, Albany: State University of New York Press.

DiFranza, J., Richards, J., Paulman, P., Wolfgillespie, N., Fletcher, C., Jaffe, R., & Murray, D. 1991. "RJR Nabisco's cartoon camel promotes camel cigarettes to children," *Journal of the American Medical Association* 266(22):3149–3153.

Elgin, D. 1981. *Voluntary Simplicity: Toward a Way of Life that is Outwardly Simple, Inwardly Rich,* New York: William Morrow.

Elgin, D. 2003. "The garden of simplicity." http://www.simpleliving.net/ webofsimplicity/the_garden_of_simplicity.asp.

Elgin, D. & Mitchell, A. 1977. "Voluntary simplicity: lifestyle of the future," *Ekistics* 45:207–212.

Etzioni, A. 1998. "Voluntary Simplicity: Characterization, Select Psychological Implications, and Societal Consequences," *Journal of Economic Psychology* 19(5):619–643.

Fabbrini, S. 2002. "The domestic sources of European Anti-Americanism," *Government and Opposition* 37(1):3–14.

Fox, R. 1996. *Harvesting Minds: How TV Commercials Control Kids,* Westport, CT: Praeger.

Furlough, E. & C. Strikwerda (Eds.). 1999. *Consumers Against Capitalism? Consumer Cooperation in Europe, North America, and Japan, 1840–1990,* Lanham, MD: Rowman and Littlefield.

Goldberg, C. 1995. "Choosing the joys of a simplified life," *The New York Times,* Sept. 21: C1.

Gonzalez, D. 2003. "Latin sweatshops pressed by US campus power," *The New York Times,* April 4: A1.

Green, D. & Griffith, M. 2002. "Globalization and its discontents," *International Affairs* 78(1):49–68.

Grey, M. 2000. "The industrial food system and its alternatives in the United States: An introduction," *Human Organization* 59(2):143–150.

Helleiner, E. 2002. "Think globally, transact locally: the local currency movement and green political economy" pp. 255–273 in T. Princen, M. Maniates, & K. Conca (Eds.), *Confronting Consumption,* Cambridge, MA: MIT Press.

Hilchey, D. 2000. "BUY-LOCAL marketing programs taking root in New York," *Smart Marketing,* July.

Hinrichs, C. 2000. "Embeddedness and local food systems: notes on two types of direct agricultural market," *Journal of Rural Studies* 16(3):295–303.

Hu, F., Li, T., Colditz, G., Willett, W., & Manson, J. 2003. "Television watching and other sedentary behaviors in relation to risk of obesity and type 2 diabetes mellitus in women." *Journal of the American Medical Association* 289(14):1785–1791.

ICLEI, International Council for Local Environmental Initiatives. 2005. http://www. iclei.org. January 19, 2005.

Inglehart, R. 1990. *Culture Shift in Advanced Industrial Society,* Princeton, NJ: Princeton University Press.

Johnson, K. 2003a. "Ten states to discuss curbs on power-plant emissions," *The New York Times,* July 25:B5.

Johnson, K. 2003b. "In concrete city, fruit of the land," *The New York Times*, October 27:B1.

Jones, P., Shears, P., Hillier, D., Comfort, D., & Lowell, J. 2003. "A return to traditional values? A case study of slow food," *British Food Journal* 105(4–5):297–304.

Kennedy, F. 2001. "Why life is sweeter in the slow lane." *The Independent (London)*, July 3: 7.

Kummer, C. 2002 *The Pleasures of Slow Food: Celebrating Authentic Traditions, Flavors, and Recipes*, New York: Chronicle Books.

Lafferty, W. & J. Meadowcroft (Eds.). 2000 . *Implementing Sustainable Development: Strategies and Initiatives in High Consumption Societies*, New York: Oxford University Press.

Lasn, K. 1999. *Culture Jamming: The Uncooling of America*, New York: William Morrow.

Leonard-Barton, D. 1981. "Voluntary simplicity lifestyles and energy conservation," *Journal of Consumer Research* 8(3):243–252.

Lindsay, G. 2002. "Ad busted in times square," *Folio: The Magazine for Magazine Management* 21(4):13.

Lowry, R., Wechsler, H., Galuska, D., Fulton, J., & Kann, L. 2002. "Television viewing and its association with overweight, sedentary lifestyle, and insufficient consumption of fruits and vegetables among US high school students," *Journal of School Health* 72(10):413–421.

Mander, J. 1978. *Four Arguments for the Elimination of Television*, New York: William Morrow.

Maniates, M. 2002. "In search of consumptive resistance: The voluntary simplicity movement," p. 199–235 in T. Princen, M. Maniates, & K. Conca (Eds.), *Confronting Consumption*, Cambridge, MA: MIT Press.

Mayer, R. 1989. *The Consumer Movement: Guardians of the Marketplace*, Boston: Twayne Publishers.

Miele, M. & Murdoch, J. 2002. "'The: practical aesthetics of traditional cuisines: Slow food in Tuscany," *Sociologica Ruralis* 42(4):312–328.

Molnar, A. 1996. *Giving Kids the Business: The Commercialization of America's Schools*, Boulder: Westview Press.

Morgan, M. 2003. "Indices forge ahead after Iraq breakthrough," *Financial Times*, December 16: 46.

Moskin, J. 2004. "Eat your vegetables: Easier said than done," *The New York Times*, July 21: C1.

Myers, N. & Kent, J. 2004. *The New Consumers: The Influence of Affluence on the Environment*, Washington, DC: Island Press.

Nabhan, G. 2002. *Coming Home to Eat: The Pleasures and Politics of Local Foods*, New York :W. W. Norton.

NJDEP, New Jersey Department of Environmental Protection. 1999. *New Jersey Sustainability Action Plan*, Trenton: NJDEP.

OECD, Organization for Economic Cooperation and Development. 2002. *Governance for Sustainable Development: Five OECD Case Studies,* Paris: OECD.

Osborne, L. 2001. "The year in ideas: A to Z: Slow food," *The New York Times Magazine,* December 9: 100.

PCSD, President's Council on Sustainable Development. 1999. *Towards a Sustainable America: Advancing Prosperity, Opportunity, and a Healthy Environment for the 21st Century,* Washington, DC: Government Printing Office.

Petrini, C. 2001. *Slow Food: Collected Thoughts on Taste, Tradition, and the Honest Pleasures of Food,* White River Junction, VT: Chelsea Green.

Pew Center on Global Climate Change. 2002. *Climate Change Activities in the United States,* Philadelphia: Pew Charitable Trust.

Pope, C. & Rauber, P. 2004. *Strategic Ignorance: Why the Bush Administration is Recklessly Destroying a Century of Environmental Progress,* San Francisco: Sierra Club Books.

Preston, J. 2004. "Antiwar group settles dispute with company on times square ad," *The New York Times,* July 16: B2.

Princen, T., M. Maniates, & K. Conca (Eds.). 2002. *Confronting Consumption,* Cambridge: MIT Press.

Rather, J. 2001. "Shop till you drop survives, but economists remain wary," *The New York Times,* September 30 (Sect. 14 (LI)):8.

Rice, R. 2001. "Noble goals and challenging terrain: Organic and fair trade coffee movements in the global marketplace," *Journal of Agricultural and Environmental Ethics* 14(1):39–66.

Richtel, M. 2003. "After delays, US prepares to enforce do-not-call list," *The New York Times,* October 11: C2.

Ross, A. (Ed.). 1997. *No Sweat: Fashion, Free Trade, and Rights of Garment Workers,* New York: Verso.

Rumbo, R. 2002. "Consumer resistance in a world of advertising clutter: The case of *Adbusters,*" *Psychology and Marketing* 19(2):127–148.

Samuel, L. 2001. *Brought to You By: Postwar Television and the American Dream,* Austin: University of Texas Press.

Schor, J. 1998. *The Overspent American; Upscaling, Downshifting, and the New Consumer,* New York: Basic Books.

Shenon, P. 2001. "Washington makes a patriotic pitch," *The New York Times,* November 4 (Sect. 5): 3.

Shi, D. 1985. *The Simple Life: Plain Living and High Thinking in American Culture,* New York: Oxford University Press.

Shuman, M. 1998. *Going Local: Creating Self-Reliant Communities in the Global Age,* New York: Free Press.

Smith, J. 2000. "EU rules leave a bad taste in Italians' mouths: Regulations often conflict with culinary traditions," *The Washington Post,* August 7: A1.

Stille, A. 2001. "Slow food," *The Nation,* August 20.

Tucker, R. 2000. *Insatiable Appetite: The United States and the Ecological Degradation of the Tropical World*, Berkeley: University of California Press.

USGAO, United States General Accounting Office. 2001. *Consumer Finance: College Students and Credit Cards*, Washington, DC: Government Printing Office.

von Hassell, M. 2002. *The Struggle for Eden: Community Gardens in New York City*, Westport, CT: Bergin and Garvey.

von Schilling, J. 2003. *The Magic Window: American Television, 1939–1953*, New York: Haworth Press.

Warren, E. & Warren-Tyagi, A. 2003. *The Two-Income Trap: Why Middle-Class Mothers and Fathers are Going Broke*, New York: Basic Books.

Zavestoski, S. 2002. "The social-psychological bases of anticonsumption attitudes," *Psychology and Marketing* 19(2):149–165.

20

Spiritual Activism and Liberation Spirituality: Pathways To Collective Liberation

Claudia Horwitz and Jesse Maceo Vega-Frey

There is a new culture of activism taking form in the world—a new paradigm for how we work, how we define success, how we integrate the fullness of who we are and what we know into the struggle for justice. Activists are being asked to examine our current historical moment with real intimacy, with fresh eyes, fire, and compassion. Many of the once-groundbreaking methods we know and use have now begun to rot. Many of our tactics are now more than simply ineffective—they are dangerous.

For agents of change, and all those who we work with, the detriment is twofold. We are killing ourselves and we are not winning. A life of constant conflict and isolation from the mainstream can be exhausting and demoralizing. Many of our work habits are unhealthy and unsustainable over the long haul. The structures of power have become largely resistant to our tactics. Given the intensity of our current historical circumstance it would be easy for us to rely on what we know, to fall back upon our conditioning and our historical tendencies, in our efforts to create change under pressure. Many lessons of the past carry wisdom; others are products and proponents of dysfunctional systems and ways of being in the world. A new paradigm requires a complex

Reprinted by permission of the authors. Originally published May 2006. http://www. stonecirdes.org/thoughts/writing/liberation.html relationship with history; we must remember and learn from the past, but we cannot romanticize it.

Neither do we presume that the answer lies only in the new, the innovative, and the experimental. We carry the hearts and minds of the ancient ones of many traditions, across time and continents, while also connecting to the resources that surround us. Our intention is to survive and flourish in the landscape that we find ourselves living in. A new philosophy and practice of social change is emerging, one that grows out of an ethic of sustainability, spirituality, and a broader understanding of freedom. We are weaving old threads together in new forms and new ways of being.

Spiritual Activism and Liberation Spirituality

At its best, this new paradigm, which some of us are calling "spiritual activism" or "liberation spirituality" is revolutionary. It provides us with deepened competencies and tools to go forward in this tangle of conditions history has prepared for us and to assume the roles we're being asked to play. While the field growing up around this new paradigm is varied and vast, we are beginning to see each other and understand what we share:

- a deep commitment to spiritual life and practice;
- a framework of applied liberation;
- an orientation towards movement-building; and
- a desire for fundamental change in the world based on equity and justice.

We are moving toward a *doing* that grows more deliberately out of *being*; an understanding that freedom from *external* systems of oppression is dynamically related to liberation from our *internal* mechanisms of suffering. It provides us with a way to release the construct of "us versus them" and live into the web of relationship that links all. Instead of being limited by the reactions of fight or flight, we encounter a path that finds fullness in presence. The humility of not-knowing allows truth to appear where fear once trapped us. We recognize the pervasive beauty of paradox, the dynamic tension between two simultaneous truths that seem contradictory. We enlarge our capacity to hold contradictions and to be informed by them. And our movements for change are transformed as a result.

Swimming in the Dominant Culture

The culture of activism in the United States is like a fish swimming in murky waters. It lives and breathes in the dominant culture and it is greatly impacted by its nature. Even as we are attempting to change this culture, we easily overlook how it has impacted us and how we recreate it. As we begin to understand and reckon with these attributes, we start to unravel their influence. Like anything, the more we invite and allow ourselves to notice and name what is, the more space, opportunity, and permission conditions have to change.

All too often we are limited in our capacity to connect deeply with ourselves, with each other, and with reality because of deep instability in our being. We are knocked around by the tumult of our daily lives, battered by the constant barrage of bad news, of over-work and despair. We work more hours than our bodies and psyches can stand. We may deceive ourselves about the very nature of possibility and the openings for change, get stuck in postures of despair and cynicism or find ourselves caught up in a rigid relationship to time, task, and relationship. More is more, more is better. Long-term vision is sacrificed for immediate and inadequate gains. Opportunities for collaboration become mired in competition. Our anxiety around scarcity and the sense of a world on the verge of collapse disables us and disconnects us from our own internal sources of wisdom, vision, and spaciousness. None of these tendencies are inherently wrong but they are limiting if not balanced with a more holistic and revolutionary approach.

From Suffering to Liberation

Because the ups and downs can be unbearable, many of us learn to intuitively disconnect from our bodies, our environments, our emotional worlds, and other people around us. We feel incapable of functioning in a world of deep intimacy and so we protect ourselves with the armor of anger, denial, self-neglect, and abuse—all in an effort to shield us from the depression, disenchantment, and discouragement we fear would overwhelm us if we gave it space. Our strategies often emanate from this place of suffering, forged of anguish and a polarized understanding of the forces at work in the world. It's vital that we learn how to see our own suffering, to have some ongoing relationship with the internal pain that has immeasurable impact on the people around us, the work we do, and our own happiness. If we're not healthy, we can't think as clearly. If we're only working out of anger, we reproduce the energy and momentum of destruction. If our visions for the world tend toward the fantastical or the apocalyptic, they cannot act as good guides for action.

We can look around the globe today and see how individual suffering comes to life in collective forms and how society is a manifestation and projection of our own internal turmoil. Individual hatreds lead to violence of all forms—state-sanctioned oppression, war, domestic and sexual abuse. Greed leads to unjust economic system, distrust of others, the construction of individuals as mere factors of production, non-livable wages, exploitation of natural resources, and the insatiable desire to consume regardless of cost. Delusion in the news, media, and advertisements promote a sense of individualism and isolation, over-consumption and hubris on an individual and national level. We're familiar with these forms of collective suffering because they are much of the motivating forces behind our quest for justice.

And yet we know it doesn't have to be this way. We know human beings have access to a wellspring of wisdom, good will, and compassion. So, how do we begin to change our selves, our organizations and institutions, our society, our world? What are the tactics that lend themselves to the kind of transformation we are seeking in the world?

We desire freedom. We desire a way of being that expresses the best of what we have to offer as human beings—our truth, our joy, our complex intelligence, our kindness. For some, freedom comes when we experience ourselves and the world around us as sacred, when we have a consistent awareness of the divine and our embodiment of it. For some, freedom is paying attention to what is and accepting it, even as we also want space to dream about what could be, without censorship. Freedom thrives in individual wholeness and in strong, flexible relationships with others. We want to see deeply and we want to be seen. We want to remember, over and over again, how our destinies are woven together. We want a spirituality that holds the liberation of all people at the center and an activism that is not void of soul.

A liberated society and person is one that can hold the truth of different ways, perspectives, and mind states at once, where there is a complete acceptance of *the way things are* that also holds a prophetic vision of *how things could be*. We want collective liberation and we get there through spiritual practice, liberatory forms, a liberatory relationship to form, skillful group process, and embracing difference and unity.

Collective Liberation Through Spiritual Practice

Spiritual practice builds a reservoir of spaciousness and equanimity that can provide us with access to our deepest capacities in the midst of great turmoil and difficulty, tension, and conflict. The key is in the ability to deeply and compassionately connect with our experience in any moment without clinging or rejecting, allowing for *what is* to arise and be engaged with wisdom without friction or resistance. Real, meaningful change can only happen in these places of compassionate and powerful acceptance of our own capacities and our personal and societal limitations. When we clearly open to *what is* we gain the ground to imagine what might be possible. And in the places where we cannot be as breezy as we want to be we try to develop compassion for ourselves and each other, gentleness with our learning edges that allows us the space to grow where we can. We can create communities of practice, where ancient and traditional wisdom and practices are made relevant and current; they are shared in community. We can bring a depth of practice and learning to our spiritual path, and a strengthening of our own emotional container. Attaining some level of mastery in our own tradition or practice accelerates our learning and enhances our ability to experience and receive the wisdom and gifts from other traditions.

Collective Liberation Through Liberatory Forms

How do we embody ways of being and create ways of working that make real freedom possible? We do it by creating forms that lean toward freedom. We live in a world of form. Institutions, buildings, bodies, ideas—all are the forms which we use to negotiate and navigate through our interrelated lives. There are certain forms—institutions and practices—that function to quash, limit, or undermine our freedom. Some of the more obvious, all manifestations of collective suffering, include prisons, slavery, and totalitarian regimes. Some forms tend to promote liberation:

- collective struggle in the form of grassroots movements, unions, and locally-based organizing
- farms, food cooperatives, and community supported agriculture models
- religious and spiritual communities that call forth ecstatic expression, nurture contemplative refuge and build strong community
- justice-centered retreat centers that offer an oasis for incubation
- creative protests that convey urgent messages in unexpected forms
- experiential and direct education that values students as experts of their own experience
- artistic venues that capture reality in compelling and unchartered ways
- forms of communication that leave us feeling animated and inspired rather than drained and beat up
- local merchants founded in an ethic of fair economics and community interest
- communal and intentional living experiments

Collective Liberation Through a Liberatory Relationship to Form

New, innovative forms that aim for justice and lean toward freedom do not guarantee true liberation. We know the depths of suffering and oppression that can be found within our so-called revolutionary institutions- from unions to collectives to communist systems of government. This is because *form itself is not freedom*. Our willingness and ability to develop a revolutionary relationship to forms, to institutions, to ideas, to practices, is equally important to our success as the forms themselves.

There are numerous examples of physical, mental, and spiritual liberation occurring within the confines of oppressive forms such as prisons or slavery. Nelson Mandela, Malcom X, Aung San Suu Kyi, and Victor Frankel all had profound experiences of awakening while in the confines of prison walls. True freedom is realized when we develop the internal capacity to not be the victim or captive of any form, of any experience, of any condition. This means deeper understandings of who we are and what is needed in a given moment are based on realities beyond the conceptual, the intellectual, the known. This depth comes through contemplative practice, through worship, through communion with the divine, through ceremony. When we act out of *faith* (not necessarily in a divine being or external force) and align fiercely with *what is* we gain power, strength, and presence that enables our actions to be driven by wisdom and compassion rather than craving, aversion, and delusion.

Collective Liberation Through Skillful Group Process

We can practice liberation in our group forms, appreciating the energetic and intellectual dimensions of a group field when real skillfulness is present. We recognize liberation in a group; we see it, we hear it, or we feel it. We can sense when a group is operating with a high degree of wellbeing in their culture. Sometimes it is most visible in models of leadership and decision-making which operate with honesty, respect, and cultural relevancy. Privilege, power, and rank are acknowledged and engaged. Issues below the surface of daily life are consistently brought to light. When groups are operating with a certain level of internal and external freedom, change is not shunned, but welcomed. Relationships are resilient; people feel supported and challenged in good balance. There is value placed on imagination and intuition, on creativity and story, both a mode of individual expression and a way of accessing the collective psyche.

Much has been written about skillful group process. In brief, it entails deep listening, moving from a place of faith, the ability to hold space for dissent, understanding the roles and needs of both individuals and the group as a whole, and taking decisive action when appropriate. Skillful group facilitators recognize there is a dance between structure and flexibility, between knowing and not knowing, between cutting each other some slack and prodding each other to be more rigorous. The organizing principles of collective liberation encourage authenticity and disagreement. We embrace conflict as a powerful tool for learning and growth. We see times of challenge and struggle as an opportunity to go deeper.

Collective Liberation Through Embracing Difference and Unity

One of the fatal flaws of both spiritual and progressive movements is the inability to powerfully embrace both difference and unity. When unity becomes a habit, conformity results, and we don't have enough creativity to thrive. When differences dominate, we don't have enough unity to accomplish anything significant. Too easily, we view difference with suspicion and fear, a factionalism disintegrates rather than strengthens. We lose space for varied expressions of our humanity. Or, we get caught in the trap of wanting everyone to agree to one strategy for collective movement. The work of politics disallows dissent or distinction in favor of expediency and the "party line" or it results in rebellion, marginalization, and fragmentation. In the spiritual world, an insistence on "the oneness of all life" or submissive faith in God can prevent a healthy attending to meaningful conflict, the realities of oppression, and the internal and external methods of domination and control.

We can create ways of being and acting that are strong enough for both difference and unity. Our ability to work powerfully across multiple lines of difference is dependent upon our ability to connect intimately with our selves, our vision, and each other. We believe that the fundamental purpose of connecting around a common experience of humanity, of living and breathing in our oneness, is to be able to healthily engage, explore, and celebrate our very real differences as people. And that engaging in collective and individual spiritual practice is a method that uniquely allows for the skillful development of both of these capacities. We are learning to be inclusive in a way that doesn't disable us, more willing to see that we can be allied without being the same. Unity that is complete connectedness is called "*love.*" But love is more than the expression of deep emotion or the pull to intimacy. It is a love that can become intimate with grief, stand firmly in the fire of conflict, and witness horror without recoiling. It is the kind of love that keeps our senses open and does not shrink from truth. It is relentlessly inclusive.

Moving Forward...

Spiritual activism and liberation spirituality are ways of being and acting that encourage an intimacy that retains discernment. With ease and with care, we can find ways to link the powerful urges for freedom inside ourselves with the collective urge for freedom that humanity has known since the beginning of time. We can commit to ongoing analysis of and consciousness around our dominant culture, its forces of oppression and how these affect our work. We can develop a nuanced understanding of what it means to live and work across multiple lines of difference. And we can create the conditions that allow us to move from suffering to collective liberation.

Appendix

This list of organizations and their web site URLs is intended to be illustrative, not complete or comprehensive.

Organizations Whose Primary Focus is Reform of the Corporation

Centre for Research on Multinational Corporations
http://somo.nl/

Corporate Accountability International
http://www.stopcorporateabuse.org/

Corporate Crime Reporter
http://www.corporatecrimereporter.com/

Corporate Ethics International
http://corpethics.org/

Corporate Watch (UK)
http://www.corporatewatch.org/

Corporate Watch: Holding Corporations Accountable
http://www.corpwatch.org/

Corporations and Health Watch
http://www.corporationsandhealth.org/index.php

European Coalition for Corporate Justice
http://www.corporatejustice.org/

Multinational Monitor
http://multinationalmonitor.org/

Our World Is Not For Sale
http://www.ourworldisnotforsale.org/

Program on Corporations, Law & Democracy
http://www.poclad.org/

Reclaim Democracy: Restoring Citizen Authority Over Corporations
http://www.reclaimdemocracy.org/

The Center for Corporate Policy
http://www.corporatepolicy.org/index.htm

Organizations that Include Corporate Reform in Their Activities

Center for Human Rights and Environment: Corporate Accountability and Human Rights
http://www.cedha.org.ar/en/initiatives/corporate_social_liability/

Center for Media and Democracy: PRWATCH
http://www.prwatch.org/

Center for Science in the Public Interest
http://www.cspinet.org/

Interfaith Center on Corporate Responsibility
http://www.iccr.org/

International Forum on Globalization
http://www.ifg.org/

Good Jobs First Corporate Subsidy Watch
http://www.goodjobsfirst.org/corporate_subsidy/overview.cfm

Polaris Institute
http://www.polarisinstitute.org/corporations

Public Citizen's Corporate Crime Center
http://www.citizen.org/_corpcrime/

The Alliance for Democracy: Corporate Globalization/Positive Alternatives
http://www.thealliancefordemocracy.org/html/eng/1133-AA.shtml

The Global Policy Forum: Transnational Corporations
http://www.globalpolicy.org/socecon/tncs/indxmain.htm

Source Watch Portal: Global Corporations
http://www.sourcewatch.org/index.php?title=Portal:Global_Corporations

War on Want: Corporations and Conflict
http://www.waronwant.org/campaigns/corporations-and-conflict

Organizations that Focus on Democracy

Alliance for Lobbying Transparency (UK)
http://www.lobbyingtransparency.org/

Center for Civil Society
http://www.ccsindia.org/ccsindia/index.asp

Center for Digital Democracy
http://www.democraticmedia.org/about_cdd

Citizen Works: Tools for Democracy
http://www.citizenworks.org/

Community Environmental Legal Defense Fund Democracy School
http://celdf.org/DemocracySchool/tabid/60/Default.aspx

Free Press: Reform Media. Transform Democracy
http://www.freepress.net/

Highlander Research and Education Center
http://www.highlandercenter.org/

Network Institute for Global Democratization
http://www.nigd.org/nan/nan-doc-store/10–2006/wsf-2009-dilemmas-of-
decision-making-on-the-periodicity-of-the-forums

Open Secrets: Center for Responsive Politics
http://www.opensecrets.org/

Platform
http://platformlondon.org/

The Forum on Privatization and the Public Domain
http://www.forumonpublicdomain.ca/about

Citizenship and Activists Organizations

Attac: The World is not For Sale
http://www.attac.org/

Citizens Trade Campaign
http://www.citizenstrade.org/index.php

Focus on the Global South
http://focusweb.org/

International Council on Human Rights
http://www.ichrp.org/

Interfaith Working Group in Trade and Investment
http://www.tradejusticeusa.org/

La Via Campesina: International Peasant Movement
http://viacampesina.org/main_en/index.php

Maquiladora Health and Safety Support Network
http://mhssn.igc.org/

People's Health Movement
http://www.phmovement.org/cms/

People's Global Action
http://www.nadir.org/nadir/initiativ/agp/en/index.html

Third World Network
http://www.twnside.org.sg/

Women's International League for Peace and Freedom
http://www.wilpf.org/

World Social Forum
http://www.forumsocialmundial.org.br/index.php?cd_language=2&id_menu=

Indigenous People's Health and Rights

Center for World Indigenous Studies
http://cwis.org/

Cultural Survival
http://www.culturalsurvival.org/home

Indigenous Environmental Network
http://www.ienearth.org/

Indigenous Peoples Biodiversity Information Network
http://www.ibin.org/

Indigenous People's Council on Biocolonialism
http://www.ipcb.org/publications/other_art/globalization.html

Indigenous Peoples Survival Foundation
http://www.indigenouspeople.org/

Indigenous Peoples Task Force
http://www.indigenouspeoplestf.org/

International Indian Treaty Council
http://www.treatycouncil.org/home.htm

International Work Group for Indigenous Affairs
http://www.iwgia.org/sw617.asp

Tebtebba: Working for the Recognition and Protection of Indigenous People's
Rights
http://www.tebtebba.org/

Underrepresented Nations and Peoples Organization
http://www.unpo.org/

United Nations Permanent Forum on Indigenous Issues
http://www.un.org/esa/socdev/unpfii/

About the Contributors

Emily Ardolino, A.B.
Emily Ardolino received a Bachelors of Arts degree from Brown University in Anthropology with a focus on public health. She currently works as a researcher in occupational health and corporate ethics at Never Again Consulting.

Katherine A. Campbell, J.D., M.P.H.
Katherine Campbell is a Staff Attorney with the Center for Science in the Public Interest in Washington, D.C. www.cspinet.org.

Maurie J. Cohen, Ph.D.
Maurie Cohen is Associate Professor in the Graduate Program in Environmental Policy Studies at the New Jersey Institute of Technology, University Heights, Newark, New Jersey.

Aaron Comrov
Aaron Comrov was a student at the New Jersey Institute of Technology, University Heights, Newark, New Jersey at the time when this article, reprinted here, was initially published.

Charlie Cray, B.A.
Charlie Cray is with the Center for Corporate Policy in Washington, D.C. He is the author of numerous reports about corporate reform and coauthor of the book, *The People's Business: Controlling Corporations and Restoring Democracy.*

David Egilman, M.D., M.P.H.

David Egilman is Clinical Associate Professor in the Department of Community Health at Brown University. He teaches, and precepts residents in the Family Medicine Department. He has published on issues of health and safety, including the corporate corruption of science in the asbestos, beryllium, pharmaceutical, and other industries, and served as an expert witness at the request of injured patients and corporate defendants in tort and other litigation. He founded Global Health through Education Training and Service (GHETS) a nonprofit that provides grants and technical assistance to primary care-oriented medical and nursing schools in Africa, Asia, and Latin America.

Diane Farsetta, Ph.D.

Diane is the Senior Researcher at the Center for Media & Democracy (CMD) in Madison, Wisconsin. Diane coauthored CMD's three reports on sponsored public relations videos in newscasts, which led to the Federal Communications Commission's first-ever investigation of the matter. She has contributed chapters to the two-volume academic review "Battleground: The Media" and the Project Censored books "Censored 2007" and "Censored 2008." In addition to CMD, Diane's reporting has been published by The Progressive and the Bulletin of the Atomic Scientists magazines and numerous web sites. She has a background is in radio reporting and scientific research.

Nicholas Freudenberg, Dr.P.H.

Nicholas Freudenberg is Distinguished Professor of Public Health and Director of the Doctor of Public Health Program at Hunter College and the Graduate Center, City University of New York. He is also founder and director of Corporations and Health Watch www.corporationsandhealth.org, a resource for researchers, activists, and public health professionals seeking to reduce health damaging corporate practices.

Brian Hoffner

Brian Hoffner was a student at the New Jersey Institute of Technology, University Heights, Newark, New Jersey at the time when this article, reprinted here, was initially published.

Stephen Gardner, J.D.

Steve is Director of Litigation for the Washington, D.C.-based Center for Science in the Public Interest, www.cspinet.org. He served as Counsel to the National Consumer Law Center, Assistant Dean of Clinical Education and

Visiting Assistant Professor of Law at Southern Methodist University School of Law, Assistant Attorney General for the State of Texas, Assistant Attorney General for the State of New York, Students Attorney at the University of Texas, and a staff attorney at the Legal Aid Society of Central Texas. He authored or coauthored The Practice of Consumer Law, Unfair and Deceptive Acts and Practices, and Consumer Class Actions.

Claudia Horwitz

Claudia Horwitz is Director of Stone Circles in Mabane, North Carolina, an organization that supports activists in deepening their capacity for social transformation through fellowships, workshops, and trainings in connecting the inner realm of spirit with the outer realm of social change work. www.stonecircles.org/.

René I. Jahiel, M.D., Ph.D.

René Jahiel, M.D., Ph.D. (microbiology). Formerly research professor of medicine at New York University. Created NYC Pre-Natal Diagnostic Lab in 1970s. Cowriter, Dellums bill for a National Health System in 1970s–80s. Chair, Committee on Health Services Research at American Public Health Association (APHA) 1979–1986. Founding member and past chair of APHA Disability Forum. Research in homelessness, disability, and social epidemiology 1990s–present. Currently President of Ecole Libre des Hautes Etudes (ELDHE), a not-for-profit international think tank in public health, and chair of its study group on industrial diseases; adjunct teaching faculty at the University of Connecticut Graduate Program in Public Health.

Jane Lethbridge, M.A., M.Sc.

Jane Lethbridge is Principal Lecturer/MPA Programme Leader in the Business School and a researcher at the Public Services International Research Unit (PSIRU), University of Greenwich, London, United Kingdom. Her main research interests are the global commercialization of health and social care, European social dialogue, trade union responses to neoliberal policies, and involving public sector workers in improving public services. She has worked with Public Services International (PSI) and the European Federation of Public Services (EPSU) since 2001.

Ruth E. Malone, R.N., Ph.D., FAAN

Ruth Malone is Professor of nursing and health policy and Vice Chair, Department of Social & Behavioral Sciences, School of Nursing, University of California, San Francisco. She received the American Legacy Foundation's Sybil Jacobs Award for tobacco industry documents research, and she has been a Fulbright Distinguished Scholar. She served as a tobacco industry documents consultant to the Centers for Disease Control, the U.S. Department of Justice in its fraud and racketeering civil case against the tobacco industry, and a WHO expert panel member on the tobacco industry. She is editor of the BMJ international journal *Tobacco Control*.

Mari Margil, M.P.P.

Mari Margil is the Associate Director for the Community Environmental Legal Defense Fund, Portland, Oregon. She is involved with campaign and organizational strategy, outreach, media, and leads the organization's fundraising efforts. In 2008, she traveled to Ecuador where she assisted the country's Constitutional Assembly on the rewriting of their Constitution. Prior to joining the Legal Defense Fund, Mari was the Director of Corporate Transformation for Corporate Ethics International, conducting corporate accountability campaigns targeting multinational "big box" retailers. She received her Master's degree in Public Policy and Urban Planning from Harvard University's John F. Kennedy School of Government.

Thomas E. Mertes, M.A., ABD

Tom Mertes is the administrator of Center for Social Theory and Comparative History at UCLA and teaches US history courses for UCLA Extension. He is the editor of, and a contributor to, *A Movement of Movements: Is Another World Really Possible?* which grew out of his work as an editor for the *New Left Review*.

Judith A. Pojda, Ph.D.

Judith Pojda holds a Ph.D. in Nutrition and Communications from Cornell University and a B.S. in Food Science. She has worked on hunger issues overseas through agencies such as the United Nations, Catholic Relief Services and the U.S. Peace Corps. As a recipient of an undergraduate travel scholarship in 1986, Judith researched global food distribution policies. She believes that there must be a strong public nutrition component to the discipline of public health, and that the examination of nutritional consequences of corporate agribusiness influences is key to alleviating hunger. She has coordinated the Agribusiness Accountability Initiative since 2006.

Leon S. Robertson, Ph.D.

Leon S. Robertson is retired. During 1978–1998 he occupied various positions in the Institution for Social and Policy Studies and the Department of

Epidemiology and Public Health at Yale University. He previously served on the faculties of Harvard University Medical School and Wake Forest University. He was also Senior Behavioral Scientist in the Insurance Institute for Highway Safety. Dr. Robertson is coauthor of six books and the sole author of six, as well as 148 articles in the scientific literature http://nanlee.net/cv/Page_ix.html. His latest book is *Injury Epidemiology*, 3rd Edition, 2007 published by Oxford University Press.

Jesse Maceo Vega-Frey
Jesse Maceo Vega-Frey leads programs at Stone Circles, a cross-cultural, multiracial community in Mabane, North Carolina for social justice and a sustainable and sacred relationship with the natural world. www.stonecircles.org/.

Raymundo D. Rovillos, Ph.D.
Raymundo Rovillos is Dean of the College of Social Science and Assistant Professor of History at the University of Philippines, Baguio.

Lainie Rutkow, J.D., M.P.H.
Lainie Rutkow is a doctoral candidate in the Department of Health Policy and Management at the Johns Hopkins University Bloomberg School of Public Health in Baltimore, Maryland.

Stephen P. Teret, J.D., MPH
Stephen Teret is a Professor in the Department of Health Policy and Management, and the Director of the Center for Law and the Public's Health at the Johns Hopkins Bloomberg School of Public Health in Baltimore, Maryland.

Shelley K. White, M.P.H., O.T.R.
Shelley White is a doctoral candidate in the Sociology Department at Boston College in Chestnut Hill, Massachusetts, and holds a Masters degree in International Public Health. She recently served as Policy Analyst at the University of Southern Maine and consultant with the Maine Department of Health and Human Services on HIV/AIDS policy and programming. She has also consulted with the international nonprofit organization, Free the Children, on international development and organizational policy. Shelley studies and has published on such topics as global HIV/AIDS and public health, globalization and political economy, human rights, development, and social change.

William H. Wiist, D.H.Sc., M.P.H., M.S.

William H. Wiist is a Professor in the Department of Health Sciences at Northern Arizona University, the Special Assistant to the Executive Dean of the College of Health and Human Services, and is a Senior Scientist in the Interdisciplinary Health Policy Institute. He is an officer of the Trade & Health Forum, and a representative of the Public Health Education and Health Promotion Section to the Governing Council of the American Public Health Association. He has been an administrator in a public health department and directed not-for-profit and for-profit health organizations.

Donald W. Zeigler, Ph.D.

Donald W. Zeigler is Director, Long Range Health Care Trends, American Medical Association, Chicago, IL. Donald was the lead author of the 2005 World Medical Association "Statement on Reducing the Global Impact of Alcohol on Health and Society" and published "International Trade Agreements Challenge Tobacco and Alcohol Control Policies" (Drug and Alcohol Review, 2006) and "The Alcohol Industry and Trade Agreements: A Preliminary Assessment" (Addiction, 2009, Suppl. 1). He serves on the Governing Council and the Trade and Health Forum of the American Public Association and the Advisory Board of the Center for Policy Analysis on Trade and Health.

Index

Note: Page numbers followed by *f, t,* and *n* indicates figures, tables, and notes respectively.

public health community
  educational contributions, 443–44
  political contributions, 444
  scientific contributions, 442–43
  and social movements, 433–42,
    434–35*t*
  strategies, 431
  success factors, 432
  target, 426–27
  Treatment Action Campaign, 429,
    430, 432–33, 436
Public health engineering, 459–60, 463
Public health infrastructure (PHI), 451
  benefits, 451
  communications, course on, 461
  economics, course on, 461
  epidemiologic surveillance, 459
  feasibility, 464
  knowledge and information
    component, 453–54
  organizational component, 461–62
    job slot development component,
     464
    laboratory component, 462
    policy development
     component, 463
    public health engineering
     component, 463
    strategy component, 463
    surveillance component, 462–63
  policy development, 460–61
  public health engineering, 459–60,
    463
  public health laboratories, 457–58, 462
  public health schools education, 45,
    454–57
    elective curriculum, 457
    environmental science, 456
    epidemiology, 455
    health policy and management, 456
    internships, 457
    research, 457
    social and behavioral sciences, 456

    special course on corporation and
     health, 45, 454–55
    statistics, 455
  scenarios, 465–66
  scope, changes in, 452–53
  specialty in advocacy strategies, 461
  weaknesses, 451–52
Public health laboratories, 457–58, 462
Public health professionals, 18, 30, 34,
  45, 46, 74, 89–90, 444. *See also*
  Advocacy/advocate(s)
  actions, 51
  in agribusiness sector, 281–82, 284,
    293
  antibiotic resistance, 285
Public health researchers, 45, 442–43
Public health workforce, 457–61, 464, 465
Public images, 17, 120–24
Publicly financing candidate elections,
  324
Publicly owned corporations, 100–101,
  313
Public-private partnerships, 385–86
Public relations (PR), 28–33, 116, 118–19
  adapting to changing media, 131–33
  and advertising, distinction between,
    119
  audio news releases (ANRs), 118
  corporate front groups, 33
  CSR, 32–33
  for public images, 120–24
  framing, 32
  funding health professions
    organizations, 30
  impact on public policy, 128–30
  issue management, 126
  junk science argument, 31
  news, 30–31
  partnering with NGOs, 121
  responding to criticism/threats,
    124–27
  spinning, 31–32
  spokespersons, 29